Cardiovascular Trials Review

Ninth Edition

Edited by:

Robert A. Kloner, MD, PhD
Yochai Birnbaum, MD

Studies compiled by:

Robert A. Kloner, MD, PhD
Yochai Birnbaum, MD

Robert A. Kloner, MD, PhD
Director of Research, Heart Institute
Good Samaritan Hospital
Professor of Medicine
Cardiovascular Division
University of Southern California
Los Angeles, CA

Yochai Birnbaum, MD
Medical Director
Cardiac Intensive Care Unit
Medical Director
The Heart Station
Professor of Medicine
Edward D. & Sally M. Futch
Professorship in Cardiology
Division of Cardiology
University of Texas Medical Branch
Galveston, TX

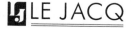

Dedicated to the memory of

Philip Kloner 1925–1997

Dedicated to the memory of

Malka and Hanoch Birnbaum

Contents

Table of Contents

Subjects

Section	Page

Trials Listing

1d. Acute Myocardial Infarction — Anticoagulation After Myocardial Infarction

1e. Acute Myocardial Infarction — Early vs Late Intervention After Acute Myocardial Infarction

1f. Acute Myocardial Infarction — Remodeling After Infarction

Contents

2. Acute Treatment of Stroke

3. Unstable Angina/Non-Q-Wave Infarction/Non-ST-Elevation Myocardial Infarction or Acute Coronary Syndrome

Page	Acronym/Title

Contents

5c. Interventional Cardiology — Medical Therapy, Including Antiplatelet Therapy, for Prevention of Complications and Restenosis with Angiography and Percutaneous Coronary Intervention

5d. Interventional Cardiology — Irradiation for Preventing Restenosis After Percutaneous Coronary Intervention

5e. Interventional Cardiology — Covered Stents and Drug-Eluting Stents

5f.   Interventional Cardiology — Other Therapy Including Transmyocardial Laser Revascularization

7. Congestive Heart Failure

Contents

8. Lipid-Lowering Studies

Page	Acronym/Title

9. Arrhythmia

Page	Acronym/Title

10.   Anticoagulation for Atrial Fibrillation

11.   Deep Vein Thrombosis/Pulmonary Embolism

14a. Preliminary Reports — Acute Myocardial Infarction

14b. Preliminary Reports — Unstable Angina/Non-Q-Wave Infarction/Non-ST-Elevated Myocardial Infarction or Acute Coronary Syndrome

14c. Preliminary Reports — Interventional Cardiology

14d. Preliminary Reports — Hypertension

Introduction

The purpose of *Cardiovascular Trials Review,* Ninth Edition, is to review those trials that have made a major impact on the practice of clinical cardiology within the last 5 years. We have included only studies that were published in English and concentrated mainly on publications that have appeared since 1999 and have studied either pharmacological or device therapy. The text is divided into major headings of diseases such as myocardial infarction and unstable angina. In general, we gave priority to prospective randomized trials with preference to multicenter studies. In this ninth edition, we have added more than 150 new entries and focused on trials from 2003–2004. We have included some smaller studies that describe the new drug-eluting stents and gene therapy.

The front section of the book reviews articles already in print. The preliminary reports section concentrates on studies that have been presented or discussed in abstract or other form at major cardiology meetings within the last year. Some of these studies are ongoing clinical trials. The Trials Listing sets forth studies by disease categories, which are in the Subjects section. The Trials Index at the back of the book alphabetically lists acronyms and the corresponding pages on which the trials can be found, followed by the names of trials without acronyms.

We continue to be amazed by the increasing number of new, large clinical trials in the literature. Since the early '90s there has been a virtual explosion of growth in the number of these trials. An article by Cheng (*Am Heart J.* 1999;137:726–765) listed more than 2250 cardiology trials with acronyms. It is common for some acronyms to be used for more than one study (example: PREVENT).

Unfortunately, we were not able to include all studies in this text. There are many excellent studies that may not appear in this book. However, a review of the trials included in this book should give readers a flavor of the types and designs of major clinical trials that have influenced the practice of clinical cardiology.

The drugs, indications for drugs, and drug dosages may or may not be approved for general use by the US Food and Drug Administration. Physicians should consult the package inserts and/or the *Physicians' Desk Reference* for drug indications, contraindications, side effects, and dosages as recommended.

Robert A. Kloner, MD, PhD   Los Angeles, July 2004
Yochai Birnbaum, MD

1. Acute Myocardial Infarction
a. Thrombolytic Therapy

ASSENT (Substudy)

Assessment of the Safety and Efficacy of a New Thrombolytic Agent

Title	Safety of the weight-adjusted dosing regimen of tenecteplase in the ASSENT Trial.
Authors	Angeja BG, Alexander JH, Chin R, et al.
Reference	Am J Cardiol 2001;88:1240-1245.
Disease	Acute myocardial infarction (MI).
Purpose	To determine the safety of single-bolus tenecteplase (TNK) vs tissue plasminogen activator (tPA) across a range of weight and dose categories.
Design	Randomized, double-blind, multicenter.
Patients	Acute MI with ST-segment elevation or left bundle branch block.
Follow-up	30 days.
Regimen	Patients randomized to TNK (plus placebo tPA bolus and infusion) or tPA (plus placebo TNK bolus). TNK and TNK bolus given according to weight-adjusted protocol. TNK given as 5 doses ranging from 30-50 mg adjusted by estimated weight. tPA given as 15 mg bolus, then 0.75 mg/kg infusion, up to 50 mg, over 30 minutes and 0.50 mg/kg, up to 35 mg, over 60 minutes. Dosing of both TNK and tPA based on weight estimated at admission—not requiring actual measurement.
Add'l Tx	Heparin (also weight adjusted), aspirin.

Results	Primary end point was 30-day all-cause mortality. Secondary end point was intracranial hemorrhage. Weight category and dose of TNK correlated for patients <60 kg weight, 30 mg of TNK (94%); 60-69 kg, 35 mg (92%); 70-79 kg, 40 mg (88%); 80-89 kg, 45 mg (87.6%); for ≥90 kg, 50 mg (93%). Rates of death with TNK vs tPA did not differ by any weight category: <60 kg weight (12.5% vs 11.5% with TNK and tPA, respectively); 60-69 kg (8.2% vs 9.0%); 70-79 kg (5.6% vs 5.5%), 80-89 kg (4.7% vs 5.4%) and ≥90 kg (4.9% vs 4.0%; all=NS). Rates of intracranial hemorrhage were also not different with TNK vs tPA: <60 kg (2.2% vs 2.3%); 60-69 kg (1% vs 1.3%); 70-79 kg (1.2% vs 1.1%), 80-89 kg (0.7% vs 0.5%), and ≥90 kg (0.5% vs 0.5%; all p=NS).
Concl.	Across range of estimated weights corresponding to each TNK dose, TNK was as effective and safe as tPA.

ASSENT-2

Assessment of the Safety and Efficacy of a New Thrombolytic-2

Title	Single bolus tenecteplase compared with front loaded alteplase in acute myocardial infarction: The ASSENT-2 double-blind randomized trial.
Authors	Assessment of the Safety and Efficacy of a New Thrombolytic (ASSENT-2) Investigators.
Reference	Lancet 1999;354:716-722.
Disease	Acute myocardial infarction.
Purpose	To assess whether body weight adjusted single bolus of tenecteplase would have comparable safety and efficacy as front loaded 90 minute infusion of alteplase in acute myocardial infarction.
Design	Randomized, placebo-controlled, double-blind, multicenter.
Patients	16,949 patients, ≥18 years old, with symptoms suggesting acute myocardial infarction started within 6 hours of randomization, ST elevation in ≥2 leads or left bundle branch block. Patients with blood pressure >180/110 mm Hg, use of glycoprotein IIb/IIIa inhibitors within the preceding 12 hours, contraindications to thrombolytic therapy, and current therapy with oral anticoagulants were excluded.
Follow-up	30 days.
Regimen	Randomization to tenecteplase (30-50 mg) + placebo alteplase or placebo tenecteplase + front loaded alteplase. Tenecteplase or placebo was administered as a single bolus over 5-10 seconds, alteplase or placebo was administered as a 15 mg bolus followed by 0.75 mg/kg infusion over 30 minutes and than 0.50 mg/kg infusion over 60 minutes.
Add'l Tx	All patients received oral aspirin 150-325 mg/d and IV heparin for 48-72 hours.

Results	8461 patients were assigned to receive tenecteplase and 8488 patients to receive alteplase. Covariate adjusted 30-day mortality rate was similar at 6.18% for tenecteplase vs 6.15% for alteplase (relative risk [RR] 1.004; 95% CI=0.914-1.104). Tenecteplase and alteplase were equally effective in all prespecified subgroups, except for a lower mortality in the tenecteplase assigned patients who were treated >4 hours after onset of symptoms (7.0% vs 9.2%; RR 0.766; 95% CI=0.617-0.952; p=0.018). Strokes occurred in 1.78% of the tenecteplase vs 1.66% of the alteplase assigned patients (p=0.555). Intracranial hemorrhages occurred in 0.93% vs 0.94%, respectively (p=1.00). Bleeding was noted in 26.4% in the tenecteplase group vs 28.9% in the alteplase group (p=0.0003). Major bleedings occurred in 4.66% vs 5.94%, respectively (p=0.0002).
Concl.	The tenecteplase and alteplase assigned patients had similar 30-day mortality. Tenecteplase was safe and was associated with less bleedings than alteplase. Tenecteplase is easy to administer (a single bolus dose) and effective for acute myocardial infarction.

ASSENT-3

Assessment of the Safety and Efficacy of a New Thrombolytic Regimen-3

Title	Efficacy and safety of tenecteplase in combination with enoxaparin, abciximab, or unfractionated heparin: the ASSENT-3 randomised trial in acute myocardial infarction.
Authors	The ASSENT-3 Investigators.
Reference	Lancet 2001;358:605-613.
Disease	Acute myocardial infarction.
Purpose	To compare the safety and efficacy of a combination of full-dose tenecteplase (TNK-tPA) + enoxaparin, full-dose tenecteplase + IV unfractionated heparin (UFH), and half-dose of tenecteplase + abciximab.
Design	Randomized, open-label, multicenter.
Patients	6095 patients, ≥18 years old, within 6 hours of onset of chest pain, ≥0.1 mV ST elevation in ≥2 limb leads or ≥0.2 mV in ≥2 precordial leads, or left bundle branch block. Patients with blood pressure >180/110 mm Hg, use of glycoprotein IIb/IIIa inhibitors in the preceding 7 days, any known history of stroke, transient ischemic attack, or dementia, current treatment with oral anticoagulants or heparin, known thrombocytopenia (<100,000 cells/μL), renal insufficiency, sustained cardiopulmonary resuscitation over 10 minutes in 2 weeks preceding enrollment, pregnancy, lactation, or contraindication to thrombolytic therapy were excluded.
Follow-up	30 days.

ASSENT-3

Assessment of the Safety and Efficacy of New Thrombolytic Regimens

Title	Outcome of urgent and elective percutaneous coronary interventions after pharmacologic reperfusion with tenecteplase combined with unfractionated heparin, enoxaparin, or abciximab.
Authors	Dubois CL, Belmans A, Granger CB, et al.
Reference	J Am Coll Cardiol 2003;42:1178-1185.
Disease	Acute myocardial infarction.
Purpose	To evaluate percutaneous coronary intervention in the ASSENT-3 trial, which evaluated co-therapy with abciximab, enoxaparin, or unfractionated heparin with tenecteplase in patients with acute myocardial infarction.
Design	Open-label, randomized trial in a prehospital setting.
Patients	Patients in the ASSENT-3 study who subsequently underwent an elective (n=1064) or urgent (n=716) percutaneous coronary intervention.
Follow-up	1 year.
Regimen	Tenecteplase combined with unfractionated heparin, enoxaparin, or abciximab followed by percutaneous coronary intervention (elective or urgent).

Results	No significant differences among the 3 treatment regimens in clinical end points (30-day mortality, in-hospital reinfarction, in-hospital refractory ischemia, 1-year mortality) were observed in patients who underwent elective PCI. There was a trend toward fewer in-hospital reinfarctions with abciximab and enoxaparin compared with unfractionated heparin (UFH) (0.5% and 0.6% vs 1.5%). The incidence of bleeding complications was similar in the 3 treatment arms. Fewer abciximab- and enoxaparin-treated patients needed urgent PCI compared with UFH-treated patients (9.1% vs 11.9% vs 14.3%; p<0.0001), but outcomes in these patients were generally less favorable (30-day mortality 8.2%, 5.4%, and 4.5%; 1 year mortality 11%, 8.5%, and 5.6%; in-hospital reinfarction 3.9%, 2.5%, and 2.7%; major bleeding complications 8.8%, 7%, and 3.4%, in the abciximab, enoxaparin, and UFH groups, respectively). The higher 1-year mortality and major bleeding rates with abciximab were significant in pair-wise comparisons (p=0.045 and p=0.012, respectively).
Concl.	With elective PCI, clinical outcomes were similar with the 3 antithrombotic co-therapies. Fewer patients needed urgent PCI with abciximab and enoxaparin treatment, but clinical outcomes were less favorable in this selected population, especially with abciximab.

ASSENT-3 (1-Year Mortality)

Assessment of the Safety of a New Thrombolytic-3

Title	Efficacy of tenecteplase in combination with enoxaparin, abciximab, or unfractionated heparin: one-year follow-up results of the Assessment of the Safety of a New Thrombolytic-3 (ASSENT-3) randomized trial in acute myocardial infarction.
Authors	Sinnaere PR, Alexander JH, Bogaerts K, et al.
Reference	Am Heart J 2004;147:993-998.
Disease	Acute myocardial infarction.
Purpose	In the ASSENT-3 study, it was observed that full-dose tenecteplase + enoxaparin or half-dose tenecteplase + abciximab decreased complications of acute myocardial infarction vs full-dose tenecteplase + unfractionated heparin. This study assesses the outcome of these fibrinolytic regimens on 1-year mortality.
Design	Randomized, multicenter.
Patients	5942 patients in whom 1 year vital status data were available as part of the ASSENT-3 trial.
Follow-up	1 year.
Regimen	As per the ASSENT-3 trial. Patients were randomized to full-dose tenecteplase + weight-adjusted unfractionated heparin (1976 completed 1-year follow-up) vs full-dose tenecteplase + enoxaparin (1993 completed 1-year follow-up) vs half-dose tenecteplase + reduced-dose unfractionated heparin + abciximab (1973 completed 1-year follow-up).
Add'l Tx	Aspirin.

Results   The primary outcome was 1-year mortality. 1-year mortality rates were 7.9% for the full-dose tenecteplase + unfractionated heparin group (UFH); 8.1% for the full-dose tenecteplase + enoxaparin group; and 9.3% for the half-dose tenecteplase + abciximab group (p=NS). Pair-wise comparisons failed to show a significant difference in mortality among the treatment regimens. Subgroups that were at increased risk at 1 year after acute MI were elderly or female patients; patients with low body weight, previous MI, anterior wall MI, and diabetes. Patients with diabetes had a higher risk of death when treated with abciximab vs when treated with UFH (p=0.027).

Concl.   Mortality at 1 year was similar among patients who were treated with full-dose tenecteplase + enoxaparin or half-dose tenecteplase + abciximab vs patients who received full-dose tenecteplase + weight-adjusted UFH.

ER-TIMI

Results of the Early Retavase-Thrombolysis in Myocardial Infarction (ER-TIMI) 19 Trial

Title	Evaluation of the time saved by prehospital initiation of reteplase for ST-elevation myocardial infarction.
Authors	Morrow DA, Antman EM, Sayah A, et al.
Reference	J Am Coll Cardiol 2002;40:71-77.
Disease	Acute myocardial infarction.
Purpose	To assess the feasibility of and the amount of time saved by prehospital administration of the fibrinolytic reteplase in patients who have an acute ST-elevation myocardial infarction (STEMI).
Design	Patients were ≥18 years old and eligible if they had ischemic discomfort lasting ≥30 minutes within the previous 12 hours and showed ST-segment elevation ≥0.1 mV in 2 or more contiguous limb leads or ≥0.2 mV in 2 or more contiguous precordial leads, or new left bundle branch block on a 12-lead ECG obtained in the field. Exclusion criteria included: cardiogenic shock or pulmonary edema requiring intubation, suspected aortic dissection, systolic blood pressure >180 mm Hg or diastolic BP >110 mm Hg at any time, known history of stroke, transient ischemic attack, intracranial neoplasm, arteriovenous malformation or aneurysm, active bleeding or history of bleeding diathesis, major surgery, trauma or internal bleeding within the previous 4 weeks, oral anticoagulation use in the past 3 days, suspected cocaine or amphetamine-induced MI, known or suspected pregnancy.

Patients	Patients were ≥18 years old and eligible if they had ischemic discomfort lasting ≥30 minutes within the previous 12 hours and showed ST-segment elevation ≥0.1 mV in 2 or more contiguous limb leads or ≥0.2 mV in 2 or more contiguous precordial leads, or new left bundle branch block on a 12-lead ECG obtained in the field. Exclusion criteria included: cardiogenic shock or pulmonary edema requiring intubation, suspected aortic dissection, systolic blood pressure >180 mm Hg or diastolic BP >110 mm Hg at any time, known history of stroke, transient ischemic attack, intracranial neoplasm, arteriovenous malformation or aneurysm, active bleeding or history of bleeding diathesis, major surgery, trauma or internal bleeding within the previous 4 weeks, oral anticoagulation use in the past 3 days, suspected cocaine or amphetamine-induced MI, known or suspected pregnancy.
Regimen	Initial evaluation and treatment followed the Advanced Cardiac Life Support recommendations for patients with suspected MI. A brief history, physical examination, and 12-lead ECG were taken by paramedical personnel and transmitted by telephone to a medical control physician who determined the patient's eligibility for study entry. Eligible patients were immediately treated with 325 mg aspirin (unless contraindicated) and 10 U of reteplase (rPA) given as an IV bolus over 2 minutes, with a second bolus of 10 U of rPA 30 minutes later. If time to the hospital was greater than 30 minutes, the second bolus of rPA was given in the ambulance. Unfractionated heparin was given (either in the field or hospital, depending on transport time) intravenously as a bolus of 60 U/kg (maximum 4000 U) and an initial infusion of 12 U/kg/h (maximum 800 U/h) upon enrollment. After arrival in the emergency department, patients were immediately evaluated by an emergency physician; if fibrinolysis was deemed unnecessary, patients then received medical therapy without a second bolus of rPA. If fibrinolysis was deemed necessary, patients could receive a second bolus of rPA or undergo immediate coronary angiography without the second bolus of rPA.
Add'l Tx	β-blockers, nitrates, calcium antagonists, and other medications were allowed and used at the discretion of the treating physician.

Results   The primary end point was the amount of time saved by administration of rPA in a prehospital setting vs in-hospital administration. The control was a population of patients with ST-elevation myocardial infarction (STEMI) who had been transported to the hospital and given a fibrinolytic in the hospital (without any pre-hospital administration) 6 to 12 months before the initiation of this study. 313 patients were evaluated in the prehospital group. The control population contained 630 patients. The median time from arrival of emergency medical service (EMS) to the first bolus of rPA (prehospital) was 31 minutes (25%-75% range: 24-37 minutes), whereas the time from EMS arrival to in-hospital administration of fibrinolytic (the control group) was 63 minutes (25%-75% range: 48-89 minutes), which produced a median time saved of 32 minutes ($p<0.0001$). At 30 minutes after EMS arrival, 49% in the prehospital group had received an initial bolus of rPA compared with 5% of control patients ($p<0.0001$). 1 hour after EMS arrival, 97% of prehospital group patients had received a bolus; less than half of the control group had received a bolus ($p<0.0001$). Patients in the prehospital group also achieved infarction resolution faster: when measured by percent ST resolution from baseline (STRES), the time until approximately 50% of the prehospital patients achieved full STRES was 30 minutes earlier than the corresponding time for the control group (120 vs 150 minutes). Compared with control, the total time from first medical contact to emergency department arrival was increased by 14 minutes in the prehospital group (42 vs 28 minutes).

Concl.   Pre-hospital administration of a fibrinolytic therapy to patients with ST-elevation MI is feasible and significantly reduces the time to reperfusion.

TIMI-4

Thrombolysis in Myocardial Infarction-4

Title	a. Comparison of front loaded recombinant tissue type plasminogen activator, anistreplase, and combination thrombolytic therapy for acute myocardial infarction: Results of the Thrombolysis in Myocardial Infarction-(TIMI) 4 trial. b. Rescue angioplasty in the thrombolysis in myocardial infarction-(TIMI) 4 trial.
Authors	a. Cannon CP, McCabe CH, Diver DJ, et al. b. Gibson CM, Cannon CP, Greene RM, et al.
Reference	a. J Am Coll Cardiol 1994;24:1602-1610. b. Am J Cardiol 1997;8:21-26.
Disease	a. Acute myocardial infarction.
Purpose	a. To compare 3 regimens of thrombolytic therapy: anistreplase (APSAC), front loaded recombinant tissue type plasminogen activator (rt-PA), or combination of the 2 agents. b. To determine the angiographic and clinical outcomes of patients with a patent coronary artery 90 minutes after thrombolysis compared to those that had an occluded infarct artery at this time treated with either rescue or no-rescue angioplasty.
Design	a. Randomized, double-blind, multicenter study.
Patients	a. 382 patients with acute myocardial infarction <80 years old <6 hours from onset of symptoms with chest pain >30 minutes and ST segment elevation ≥0.1 mV in ≥2 contiguous leads or with new left bundle branch block.
Follow-up	a. 90 minutes and 18-36 hour coronary angiography. Predischarge technetium-99m sestamibi scan. 6 week and 1 year follow-up.
Regimen	a. Front loaded rt-PA; APSAC (Eminase); or a combination of rt-PA and APSAC.
Add'l Tx	a. Heparin (5000 U bolus and infusion) and aspirin 325 mg/d. Intravenous and oral metoprolol.

Results	a. At 90 minutes, the incidence of TIMI grade 3 flow was 60.2%, 42.9%, and 44.8% of the rt-PA, APSAC, and combination-treated patients (rt-PA vs APSAC; p<0.01; rt-PA vs combination; p=0.02). The incidence of unsatisfactory outcome (death, severe heart failure, LVEF <40%, reinfarction, TIMI grade flow <2 at 90 minutes or 18-36 hours, reocclusion, major hemorrhage, or severe anaphylaxis) was 41.3%, 49%, and 53.6% for the rt-PA, APSAC, and combination therapy (rt-PA vs APSAC, p=0.19; rt-PA vs combination, p=0.06). 6 week mortality was 2.2%, 8.8%, and 7.2%, respectively (rt-PA vs APSAC, p=0.02; rt-PA vs combination, p=0.06).

b. The incidence of TIMI 3 flow was higher after successful rescue angioplasty (87%) than after successful thrombolysis (65%; p=0.002) and the number of frames needed to opacify standard landmarks was lower (that is flow was faster) with PTCA compared to thrombolysis. In-hospital adverse events occurred in 29% of successful rescue PTCA patients and 83% of failed rescue PTCAs (p=0.01). Among patients in whom rescue PTCA was performed (including successes and failures) 35% experienced an adverse event, which was the same as 35% incidence in patients not undergoing rescue PTCA. These values tended to be higher than 23% incidence of adverse events in patients with patent arteries following thrombolysis (p=0.07). |
| Concl. | a. Front loaded rt-PA is associated with higher rates of early reperfusion and trends toward better clinical outcome and survival than either APSAC or a combination of rt-PA and APSAC.

b. While restoration of flow at 90 minutes with rescue PTCA was superior to successful thrombolysis, the incidence of adverse events for strategy of rescue PTCA was not improved over no rescue PTCA. |

GUSTO-III (1 Year)

Global Utilization of Streptokinase and tPA for Occluded Coronary Arteries-III

Title	Survival outcome 1 year after reperfusion therapy with either alteplase or reteplase for acute myocardial infarction. Results from the global utilization of streptokinase and tPA for occluded coronary arteries (GUSTO) trial.
Authors	Topol EJ, Ohman EM, Armstrong PW et al.
Reference	Circulation 2000;102:1761-1765.
Disease	Acute myocardial infarction.
Purpose	Determine 1 year outcome of myocardial infarct treated with tPA (alteplase) vs rPA (reteplase) and to compare outcomes at 30 days and with previous GUSTO-1 trial.
Design	See GUSTO-III (1997) entry.
Patients	14,674 patients with acute MIs: 9885 reteplase and 4789 alteplase patients.
Follow-up	1 year.
Regimen	tPA 100 mg over 90 minutes; rPA 20 MU given as 2 boluses of 10 MU 30 minutes apart.
Add'l Tx	As per GUSTO-III.
Results	Mortality rate for tPA was 11.06%; for rPA it was 11.20% at 1 year (p=0.77). The absolute mortality difference of 0.14% was not statistically significant. There were no treatment differences in pre-specified groups: by age, infarct location, and time-to-treatment. Pattern of survival after 30 days showed a convergence between the 2 groups. For survivors at 30 days, the 1-year mortality rates were 4.07% in the tPA group vs 3.99% in rPA group (p=0.81). Mortality rate after 30 days in GUSTO-1 was 2.97%; while in this study it was 4.02% (p<0.001). This difference may have been related to higher risk patients (older, anterior MI, higher blood pressure, more females) in GUSTO-III vs GUSTO-I.

Concl.   rPA and tPA resulted in similar 1-year survival in patients with acute MIs. Higher long-term mortality rate in GUSTO-III vs GUSTO-I may have been secondary to higher risk patients in the more recent study.

GUSTO-V

Global Utilization of Strategies to Open Occluded Coronary Arteries-V

Title	Reperfusion therapy for acute myocardial infarction with fibrinolytic therapy or combination reduced fibrinolytic therapy and platelet glycoprotein IIb/IIIa inhibition: the GUSTO-V randomised trial.
Authors	The GUSTO-V Investigators.
Reference	Lancet 2001;357:1905-1914.
Disease	Acute myocardial infarction.
Purpose	To compare the effects of reteplase alone with a combination of a reduced dose of reteplase with abciximab in patients with ST elevation acute MI.
Design	Randomized, open-label, multicenter.
Patients	16,588 patients, ≥18 years old, within 6 hours of onset of symptoms of acute MI, ST segment elevation or new left bundle branch block. Patients with active bleeding, noncompressible vascular puncture site, blood pressure >180/110 mm Hg, oral anticoagulant therapy, stroke within the preceding 2 years, body weight >120 kg, or platelet count <100,000 cells/μL were excluded.
Follow-up	30 days.
Regimen	Randomization to reteplase 10 U × 2, 30 minutes apart (n=8260), or to abciximab 0.25 mg/kg bolus followed by 0.125 μg/kg/min for 12 hours + reteplase 5 U × 2, 30 minutes apart (n=8328).
Add'l Tx	All patients received aspirin 150 mg on enrollment and daily thereafter (75-325 mg/d). All patients received intravenous heparin with a target activated partial thromboplastin time 50-70 seconds. Coronary angiography and percutaneous coronary intervention or coronary artery bypass graft surgery were permitted. The use of nonstudy abciximab for patients in the reteplase alone group was permitted if PCI was performed within 24 hours of enrollment and recommended if performed >24 hours after enrollment.

Results   24-hour mortality was 2.3% in the reteplase group and 2.2% in the reteplase + abciximab group (RR 0.96; 95% CI=0.78-1.18), 7-day mortality was 4.5% and 4.3%, respectively (RR 0.97; 95% CI=0.83-1.12). 30-day mortality was 5.9% in the reteplase group vs 5.6% in the reteplase + abciximab group (RR 0.95; 95% CI=0.84-1.08; p=0.43). Nonfatal disabling stroke occurred in 0.3% of the patients in the reteplase group and in 0.2% of the patients in the combination group (OR 0.76; 95% CI=0.43-1.37; p=0.37). Intracranial hemorrhage occurred in 0.6% of the patients in each group. Among patients >75 years old, intracranial hemorrhage occurred in 1.1% of the patients in the reteplase group vs 2.1% in the combination group (OR 1.91; 95% CI=0.95-3.84; p=0.069), and among patients ≤75 years of age, intracranial hemorrhage occurred in 0.5% vs 0.4%, respectively (OR 0.76; 95% CI=0.46-1.24; p=0.27). Death or reinfarction occurred in 8.8% in the reteplase group vs 7.4% in the combination group (RR 0.83; 95% CI=0.74-0.93; p=0.0011). 8.6% of the patients in the reteplase group vs 5.6% in the combination group underwent PCI within 6 hours of therapy (RR 0.64; 95% CI=0.56-0.72; p<0.0001), and 0.1% of the patients in both groups underwent CABG within 6 hours of enrollment. 27.9% and 25.4%, respectively, underwent PCI within the first 7 days (RR 0.88; 95% CI=0.82-0.94; p<0.0001), and 3.7% and 3.0% of the patients, respectively, underwent CABG within 7 days after enrollment (RR 0.81; 95% CI=0.68-0.96; p=0.013). Reinfarction occurred in 3.5% of the patients in the reteplase group vs 2.3% in the combination group (p<0.0001). 20.6% of the patients in the reteplase group vs 16.2% of the patients in the combination group died, experienced reinfarction or underwent urgent revascularization within the first 7 days (RR 0.75; 95% CI=0.69-0.81; p<0.0001). Thrombocytopenia (<50,000 cells/ μL) occurred in 0.1% and 1.2% of the patients, respectively (p<0.0001). Severe bleeding occurred in 0.5% in the reteplase group vs 1.1% in the combination group (p<0.0001), moderate bleeding in 1.8% vs 3.5%, respectively (p<0.0001), and 4.0% vs 5.7% of the patients, respectively, had transfusion (p<0.0001).

Concl.   The combination of reduced dose of reteplase with 12-hour infusion of abciximab was not superior to standard reteplase regimen. The combination therapy was associated with a reduction in the secondary end points, including reinfarction. However, the combination therapy was also associated with an increased risk of nonintracranial bleeding complications and a trend towards an increased risk for intracranial hemorrhage among patients older than 75 years.

GUSTO V

Global Utilization of Strategies to Open Occluded Coronary Arteries V

Title	Mortality at 1 year with combination platelet glycoprotein IIb/IIIa inhibition and reduced-dose fibrinolytic therapy vs conventional fibrinolytic therapy for acute myocardial infarction. GUSTO V randomized trial.
Authors	Lincoff AM, Califf RM, Van de Werf F, et al.
Reference	JAMA 2002;288:2130-2135.
Disease	Acute myocardial infarction.
Purpose	To compare 1-year clinical outcome after treatment with standard dose of reteplase vs a combination of abciximab with lower dose of reteplase for ST-elevation acute myocardial infarction.
Design	Randomized, open-label, multicenter.
Patients	16,588 patients who had been enrolled in the GUSTO V trial (see above).
Follow-up	1 year.
Regimen	See GUSTO V, 30-day study.
Add'l Tx	See GUSTO V, 30-day study.
Results	Data on mortality was available for 16,453 patients (99.2%). All-cause mortality was 8.38% in the reteplase group and 8.38% in the combination therapy group (hazard ratio [HR] 1.00; 95% CI=0.90-1.11; p>0.99). 7-day reinfarction rate was 3.5% in the reteplase group and 2.3% in the combination group (p<0.001). Subgroup analysis showed that 1-year mortality with reteplase alone and with the combination treatment was comparable in men, women, and patients <75 yr old, patients >75 yr old, patients with and without diabetes, patients with anterior MI, and patients with non-anterior MI.
Concl.	Combination therapy with abciximab and a reduced dose of reteplase did not reduce 1-year mortality compared with standard dose reteplase alone in patients with ST-elevation acute MI.

SPEED

Strategies for Patency Enhancement in the Emergency Department. Global Use of Strategies to Open Occluded Arteries (GUSTO-IV Pilot)

Title	Trial of abciximab with and without low-dose reteplase for acute myocardial infarction.
Authors	SPEED Group.
Reference	Circulation 2000;101:2788-2794.
Disease	Acute myocardial infarction.
Purpose	To explore the effects of low-dose reteplase with standard dose abciximab, aspirin, and heparin in patients with acute MI and the effect on reperfusion, bleeding, and clinical outcome.
Design	Randomized, multicenter, angiographic study.
Patients	528 patients with acute MI.
Follow-up	30 days.
Regimen	Phase A: Patients randomized 4:1 to abciximab bolus with infusion alone (n=63) or with 5, 7.5, 10 U, 5 U + 2.5 U, or 5 U + 5 U of reteplase (total n=241). Phase B: Tested best phase A strategy (abciximab plus 5 U + 5 U reteplase) vs 10 U + 10 U of reteplase alone (n=109). The reteplase boluses were given 5 minutes following abciximab bolus. In those randomized to 2 boluses, the second reteplase bolus was given 30 minutes after the first. Bolus of abciximab was 0.25 mg/kg and infusion was 0.125 µg/kg/min for 12 hours.
Add'l Tx	Aspirin. Phase A: IV heparin 60 U/kg and additional weight-adjusted heparin bolus or infusion during angiography and intervention. Following the results of TIMI-14, the initial bolus of heparin in Phase B abciximab-reteplase 5 + 5 U group was reduced from 60 to 40 U/kg, patients in the reteplase-only group received 70 U/kg heparin bolus.

Results	Primary end point was TIMI grade 3 flow at 60-90 minutes. Results of Phase A: 62% of abciximab-reteplase 5 + 5 U group demonstrated TIMI 3 flow; 27% of abciximab-only patients demonstrated TIMI 3 flow (p=0.001). Results of Phase B: 54% of the abciximab-reteplase 5 + 5 U group had TIMI 3 flow vs 47% of the reteplase-only group (p=0.32). There was a nonsignificant trend for TIMI frame counts to be lower among split dose reteplase groups than single bolus groups. TIMI frame count was more often normal in patients receiving split reteplase (5 + 5 or 5 + 2.5 U at 36% and 38%, respectively) than in the abciximab only group (16%; p=0.02). Patients given abciximab-reteplase 5 + 5 U and standard dose heparin had a trend toward greater reperfusion (61%) vs patients given abciximab-reteplase 5 + 5 U and low-dose heparin (51%; p=NS). 11.4% of patients underwent transfusion by day 14 or discharge. Major bleeding was observed in 3.3% of abciximab-only groups and 9.2% of abciximab-reteplase groups. In Phase A, major bleeding occurred in 3.3% of patients on abciximab alone, 5.3% for abciximab + 5 U + 5 U; in Phase B major bleeding occurred in 9.8% abciximab-reteplase 5 + 5 U and 3.7% for reteplase alone. Major bleeding occurred in 6.3% of patients given abciximab-reteplase 5 U + 5 U on standard heparin and 10.5% on low-dose heparin (p=NS).
Concl.	Early, complete reperfusion was enhanced by adding reteplase to abciximab vs reteplase alone, in patients with acute MIs.

SPEED (GUSTO-IV Pilot)

Early Percutaneous Coronary Intervention Strategies for Patency Enhancement in the Emergency Department. Global Use of Strategies to Open Occluded Coronary Arteries IV

Title	Facilitation of early percutaneous coronary intervention after reteplase with or without abciximab in acute myocardial infarction. Results from the SPEED (GUSTO-IV Pilot) trial.
Authors	Herrmann HC, Moliterno DJ, Ohman EM, et al.
Reference	J Am Coll Cardiol 2000;36:1489-1496.
Disease	ST segment elevation acute MI.
Purpose	To determine the role of early percutaneous coronary intervention in a trial encouraging its use after thrombolysis and glycoprotein IIb/IIIa inhibition for acute MI.
Design	As per SPEED.
Patients	Patients with ST-segment elevation acute MI within 6 hours of chest pain onset who underwent PCI with planned initial angiography.
Follow-up	30 days.
Regimen	Drug regimens as per SPEED study. Comparisons between early PCI (n=323) and non-PCI patients (n=162).
Add'l Tx	As per SPEED study.

Results	Procedural success (defined as post-PCI residual stenosis ≤50% with TIMI grade 3 flow) occurred in 88% of patients in the early PCI group. 30-day composite incidence of death, reinfarction, or urgent revascularization rate in early PCI group was 5.6%. These included death (3.4%), reinfarction (1.2%), and urgent revascularization for severe ischemia (1.6%). 6.5% had major bleeding; 9.0% required blood transfusion. The 162 patients not undergoing early PCI had higher rates of reinfarction (4.9%), urgent revascularization (9.3%), composite of major outcomes (16.0%) and transfusions (16.0%) were higher. Overall clinical success (freedom from death, reinfarction, urgent revascularization, major bleeding, or transfusion at 30 days) was 85.4% for early PCI patients and 70.4% for patients not undergoing early PCI (p<0.001). Patients with TIMI flow grade 0 or 1 before PCI underwent early PCI more often. Patients who received abciximab plus reteplase (5 units + 5 units) had an 86% incidence of TIMI grade 3 flow at about 90 minutes.
Concl.	Early PCI in combination with abciximab and reduced-dose reteplase was safe and effective.

InTIME-II

Intravenous nPA for Treatment of Infarcting Myocardium Early-II

Title	Intravenous nPA for the treatment of infarcting myocardium early. InTIME-II, a double-blind comparison of single-bolus lanoteplase vs accelerated alteplase for the treatment of patients with acute myocardial infarction.
Authors	The InTIME-II Investigators.
Reference	Eur Heart J 2000;21:2005-2013.
Disease	Acute myocardial infarction.
Purpose	To compare the safety and efficacy of lanoteplase (nPA) and accelerated alteplase regimen in patients with acute myocardial infarction.
Design	Randomized, double-blind, multicenter.
Patients	15,078 patients, >18 years old (median age 61.1 years), who presented within 6 hours of onset of symptoms and ≥0.1 mV ST segment elevation in ≥2 adjacent limb leads, or ≥0.2 mV in ≥2 precordial leads. Patients with new or presumed new left bundle branch block were also included. Patients at an increased risk of bleeding, previous stroke or transient ischemic attack, blood pressure over 180/110 mm Hg, Killip Class 4 on admission, thrombocytopenia, and those who had received abciximab in the preceding 24 hours were excluded.
Follow-up	180 days.
Regimen	Randomization to nPA 120 KU/kg as a single bolus (n=10051) or front loaded alteplase (n=5027).
Add'l Tx	All patients received oral aspirin 150-325 mg or IV aspirin 150-500 mg before initiation of study medication. Oral aspirin 100-325 mg/d was administered during the study period. All patients received intravenous heparin (a bolus of 70 U/kg, followed by an infusion of 15 U/kg/h, with a target activated partial thromboplastin time of 50-70 s) for 24-48 hours.

Results	Confirmation of an acute myocardial infarction was made in 96% of the patients. The median time from onset of symptoms to therapy was 2.83 and 2.9 hours in the lanoteplase and alteplase groups, respectively, with 25% of the patients treated within 2 hours, 50% between 2 and 4 hours, and 22% between 4 and 6 hours of symptoms. 24-hour mortality rate was 2.4% in the lanoteplase and 2.5% in the alteplase group. 30-day mortality was 6.75% and 6.61%, respectively (RR 1.02). At 6 months, the Kaplan-Meier estimates of death were 8.7% for lanoteplase and 8.9% for alteplase, and at 1 year, 10.0% and 10.3%, respectively. 30-day stroke rate was 1.87% in the lanoteplase and 1.53% in the alteplase group (p=0.135). Hemorrhagic strokes occurred often in the lanoteplase group (1.12% vs. 0.64%; p=0.004). The combined end point of death or disabling stroke at 30 days occurred in 7.2% and 7.0%, respectively (p=NS). Major nonintracranial bleeding occurred in 0.5% and 0.6% of the lanoteplase and alteplase groups, respectively, and moderate bleeding in 2.4% and 2.4%, respectively. However, minor bleedings occurred more often in the lanoteplase group (19.7% vs. 14.8%; p<0.0001). There was no difference in the incidence of reinfarction (5.0% and 5.5%) or revascularization (25.8% and 26.9%) at 30 days between the lanoteplase and alteplase groups.
Concl.	Mortality was comparable between the single-bolus weight-adjusted lanoteplase and accelerated alteplase regimen groups. Lanoteplase was associated with slightly higher risk of intracranial bleeding and minor hemorrhages. The simplified single bolus regimen should shorten the time interval between admission to treatment and be especially convenient for prehospital or emergency department administration.

1. Acute Myocardial Infarction — a. Thrombolytic Therapy

TUCC

***Randomized Trial Confirming the Efficacy of Reduced Dose
Recombinant Tissue Plasminogen Activator in a Chinese
Myocardial Infarction Population and Demonstrating
Superiority to Usual Dose Urokinase***

Title	A randomized trial confirming the efficacy of reduced dose recombinant tissue plasminogen activator in a Chinese myocardial infarction population and demonstrating superiority to usual dose urokinase: the TUCC trial.
Authors	Ross AM, Gao R, Coyne KS, et al.
Reference	Am Heart J 2001;142:244-247.
Disease	Acute myocardial infarction.
Purpose	To compare the efficacy and safety of reduced-dose tissue plasminogen activator (tPA) with standard-dose urokinase in patients from the Republic of China with acute myocardial infarction.
Design	Randomized, open-label.
Patients	342 patients, ≤70 years old, with ST elevation acute myocardial infarction within 12 hours of onset of symptoms. Patients with previous stroke, active bleeding, bleeding diathesis, recent trauma, blood pressure >170/110 mm Hg and unresponsive cardiogenic shock were excluded.
Follow-up	90-minute angiography. 30-day clinical follow-up.
Regimen	Randomization to tPA (bolus 8 mg, followed by 42 mg over 90 minutes) or urokinase (1.5 million units over 30 minutes).
Add'l Tx	All patients received aspirin >300 mg immediately and 50 mg/d thereafter. All patients received 5000 IU heparin bolus followed by infusion.

Results	The study was terminated prematurely by the Data and Safety Monitoring Board. 330 patients (96%) underwent angiography at 90 minutes. Mean body weight was 69 kg. TIMI flow grade 3 at 90 minutes was achieved by 48.2% in the tPA group vs 28.3% in the urokinase group (p=0.001). TIMI flow grade 2-3 was achieved by 79.3% vs 53.0%, respectively (p=0.001). LVEF at 90 minutes was 58.6%±11.4% in the tPA group vs 54.7%±12.7% in the urokinase group (p<0.01). 30-day mortality was 6% in the tPA and 3% in the urokinase group (p=0.28).
Concl.	A lower dose of tPA was more effective than a standard dose of urokinase in Chinese patients with acute myocardial infarction. It seems that even after considering body weight, in the Chinese population a dose that is significantly lower than the standard recommended dose of tPA was very effective. Further dose-response studies should be conducted to determine the appropriate doses in different ethnic groups to avoid overdosage.

INTEGRITI

Integrilin and Tenecteplase in Acute Myocardial Infarction Substudy

Title	Improved speed and stability of ST-segment recovery with reduced-dose tenecteplase and eptifibatide compared with full-dose tenecteplase for acute ST-segment elevation myocardial infarction.
Authors	Roe MT, Green CL, Giugliano RP, et al.
Reference	J Am Coll Cardiol 2004;43:549-556.
Disease	Acute myocardial infarction.
Purpose	To evaluate the impact of combination reperfusion therapy with reduced-dose tenecteplase + eptifibatide on continuous ST-segment recovery and angiographic results.
Design	INTEGRITI: randomized trial. Substudy: continuous ST-segment monitoring.
Patients	140 patients enrolled in the INTEGRITI trial.
Follow-up	24-hour monitoring.
Regimen	Dose-combination regimen of half-dose tenecteplase (0.27 µg/kg) + high-dose eptifibatide (2 boluses of 180 µg/kg separated by 10 min, 2 µg/kg/min infusion) or full-dose tenecteplase (0.53 µg/kg).
Results	On 24-hour continuous 12-lead ST-segment monitoring, the combination regimen was associated with a faster median time to stable ST-segment recovery (55 vs 98 minutes; p=0.06), improved stable ST-segment recovery by 2 hours (89.6% vs 67.7%; p=0.02), and less recurrent ischemia (34% vs 57.1%; p=0.05) compared with full-dose tenecteplase. There was an NS trend toward greater ST-segment recovery at 30 minutes (57.7% vs 40.6%) and 60 minutes (82.7% vs 65.6%; p=0.08) with this combination regimen. These findings correlated with trends towards improved angiographic results at 60 minutes including improved TIMI flow grades, frame counts, and myocardial perfusion grades.

Concl.   Combination therapy with reduced-dose tenecteplase and high-dose eptifibatide may be a promising reperfusion regimen for acute ST-segment elevation MI. These findings call into question the relationship between biomarkers of reperfusion success and clinical outcomes. Larger studies and studies of patients with larger infarcts are needed to determine whether enhanced speed and stability of ST-segment recovery and improved angiographic flow patterns seen with the combination regimen will translate into improved clinical outcomes.

1. Acute Myocardial Infarction

b. Primary Percutaneous Transluminal Coronary Angioplasty vs Primary Stenting vs Thrombolytic Therapy

1. Acute Myocardial Infarction — b. Primary PTCA vs. Primary Stenting vs. Thrombolytic Therapy

35

1. Acute Myocardial Infarction — b. Primary PTCA vs. Primary Stenting vs. Thrombolytic Therapy

Title	TIMI frame count immediately after primary coronary angioplasty as a predictor of functional recovery in patients with TIMI 3 reperfused acute myocardial infarction.
Authors	Hamada S, Nishiue T, Nakamura S, et al.
Reference	J Am Coll Cardiol 2001;38:666-671.
Disease	Acute myocardial infarction (AMI).
Purpose	To determine whether corrected Thrombolysis in Myocardial Infarction (cTIMI) correlates to improved functional and clinical outcome following percutaneous transluminal coronary angioplasty in patients with acute MI.
Design	Observational study.
Patients	104 patients admitted with first acute MI who underwent PTCA during the first 12 hours of onset of MI.
Follow-up	1-month echocardiographic follow-up.
Regimen	Aspirin, 3000 U IV heparin, primary PTCA.

Results	Angiogram used corrected TIMI frame count technique of Gibson et al. (Circulation 1996;93:879-888) in which number of cineangiographic frames are counted from initial contrast opacification of proximal coronary artery to opacification of distal arterial landmark, corrected for length of the left anterior descending artery. Values greater or equal to 23 in this study were characterized as slow TIMI flow. 45 patients exhibited TIMI 3 slow flow (cTIMI frame count ≥23) and 59 had TIMI 3 fast flow (cTIMI frame count <23). Baselines characteristics and admission echocardiographic wall motion score index was similar between these 2 groups. The TIMI 3 fast group exhibited improvement in echocardiographic wall motion score index (1.33±0.52) compared to the TIMI 3 slow group (0.60±0.34; $p<0.001$). TIMI 3 slow group had a higher rate of pericardial effusion and intractable heart failure (27% and 36%) compared to the TIMI 3 fast group (10% and 17%; $p<0.005$ slow vs fast). The cTIMI frame count correlated with change in echocardiographic wall motion score index ($r=0.60$; $p<0.001$) after adjusting for a number of confounding variables.
Concl.	Lower cTIMI frame count of the infarct related artery correlated with better LV functional recovery and better clinical outcome following PTCA for acute MI.

Long-Term Benefit of Primary Angioplasty as Compared with Thrombolytic Therapy for Acute Myocardial Infarction

Title	Long-term benefit of primary angioplasty as compared with thrombolytic therapy for acute myocardial infarction.
Authors	Zijlstra F, Hoorntje JCA, DeBoer M-J, et al.
Reference	N Engl J Med 1999;341:1413-1419.
Disease	Acute myocardial infarction.
Purpose	To compare the long-term efficacy of primary angioplasty vs thrombolytic therapy for acute myocardial infarction.
Design	Prospective, randomized, multicenter.
Patients	395 patients with acute myocardial infarction. 194 were assigned to primary angioplasty; 201 to streptokinase.
Follow-up	5±2 years.
Regimen	Primary coronary angioplasty or streptokinase (1.5 million units IV over 1 hour).
Add'l Tx	All patients received aspirin and heparin.

Results	The infarct related coronary artery was patent in 90% of the angioplasty group vs the streptokinase group (65%; p<0.001). Prior to discharge 26% of the streptokinase group vs 14% of the angioplasty group had LV ejection fraction <40% (p=0.006). Over ≈5 years, 24% of the streptokinase group died vs 13% of the angioplasty patients (RR 0.54; 95% CI=0.36-0.87). 22% of the streptokinase patients and 6% of the angioplasty patients experienced nonfatal reinfarction (RR 0.27; 95% CI=0.15-0.52). The incidence of death due to cardiac causes correlated with a lower LV ejection fraction. Reinfarctions were more common in the streptokinase group both within the first 30 days of enrollment and after 30 days of enrollment. The combined outcomes of death and nonfatal reinfarction were lower in the angioplasty compared to the streptokinase group during the first 30 days (RR 0.13; 95% CI=0.05-0.37 and after 30 days of ran-domizations (RR 0.62; 95% CI=0.43-0.91). There were fewer readmissions for ischemia in the angioplasty group compared to the streptokinase group.
Concl.	Primary coronary angioplasty for acute myocardial infarction was associated with lower incidence of death and nonfatal reinfarction compared to streptokinase, over 5 years of study.

Stenting vs Balloon Angioplasty for Acute Myocardial Infarction

Title	Long-term outcome and cost-effectiveness of stenting vs balloon angioplasty for acute myocardial infarction.
Authors	Suryapranata H, Ottervanger JP, Nibbering E, et al.
Reference	Heart 2001;85:667-671.
Disease	Acute myocardial infarction.
Purpose	To assess the long-term clinical outcome and cost-effectiveness of stenting vs balloon angioplasty in patients with acute MI.
Patients	227 patients with acute MI, within 6 hours from onset of symptoms and coronary anatomy suitable for stenting.
Follow-up	Clinical follow-up for 24 months. Repeated coronary angiography at 6 months. Radionuclide ventriculography at predischarge and at 6 months.
Regimen	Randomization to balloon angioplasty (n=115) or Palmaz-Schatz stenting (n=112).
Add'l Tx	Thrombolytic therapy, glycoprotein IIb/IIIa inhibitors, and intravascular ultrasound were not used.

Results	2 patients, assigned to stenting, underwent balloon angioplasty alone and 15 patients (13%) of the balloon angioplasty group, crossed over to stenting. The combined end point of death and reinfarction at 24 months occurred in 4% of the patients in the stent group and in 11% of the patients in the balloon group (p=0.04). 2-year mortality was 3% in each group (p=1.00), and reinfarction occurred in 1% in the stent group vs 9% in the balloon group (p=0.01). 13% in the stent group vs 34% in the balloon group underwent target vessel revascularization (p=0.0003). Cumulative cardiac event-free survival at 2 years was 84% and 62%, respectively (p=0.0002). The average in-hospital total cost was 21,484 Dutch guilders in the stent group and 18,625 in the balloon group (p=0.0001). However, the total follow-up costs were 9939 vs 14,308 Dutch guilders, respectively (p=0.028), and therefore, the average total cost per patient was comparable between the stent (31,423 Dutch guilders) and the balloon (32,933 Dutch guilders) groups (p=0.83). 197 patients (87%) underwent follow-up angiography. Minimal lumen diameter was 2.56±0.63 mm and 2.17±0.48 mm after PCI in the stent and balloon group, respectively (p<0.0001). At 6 months, minimal lumen diameter was 2.04±0.63 mm and 1.64±0.83 mm, respectively (p=0.0002). The percent of diameter stenosis immediately after PCI was 18.0%±6.5% in the stent group and 29.1%±9.2% in the balloon group (p<0.0001), and at follow-up 33.4%±18.8% and 47.3%±23.6%, respectively (p<0.0001). Angiographic restenosis occurred less often in the stent group (11.9% vs 34.4%, respectively [p=0.0002]). LVEF increased significantly in both groups.
Concl.	In patients with acute MI, primary stenting resulted in better long-term clinical outcome and 6-month angiographic results than primary balloon angioplasty without increased costs.

***Randomized Comparison of Direct Stenting with
Conventional Stent Implantation in Selected Patients with
Acute Myocardial Infarction***

Title	A randomized comparison of direct stenting with conventional stent implantation in selected patients with acute myocardial infarction.
Authors	Loubeyre C, Morice M-C, Lefevre T, et al.
Reference	J Am Coll Cardiol 2002;39:15-21.
Disease	Acute myocardial infarction.
Purpose	To determine whether direct stenting was associated with better outcome compared to primary angioplasty with stenting for acute myocardial infarction.
Design	Randomized, single-center trial.
Patients	206 patients with acute myocardial infarction.
Follow-up	In-hospital study.
Regimen	102 patients had direct stenting of the infarct-related vessel; 104 patients had pre-dilatation with percutaneous transluminal coronary angioplasty (PTCA) prior to stenting (conventional stenting).
Add'l Tx	Aspirin, heparin. Glycoprotein (GP) IIb/IIIa inhibitors were optional; use of intracoronary verapamil or adenosine could be used in cases of slow or no-reflow; ticlopidine for one 1 month.

Results	End points were final TIMI frame count, a composite angiographic end point including angiographic events as distal embolization, slow-flow, or no-reflow, ECG evidence of microvascular reperfusion injury, persistent ST segment elevation, and a composite clinical end point of in-hospital mortality and reinfarction. Direct stent implantation failed in 8 patients. In these patients pre-dilatation was necessary for stenting. Cumulative angiographic end point of slow-flow, no reflow, distal embolization occurred in 28 patients in the PTCA-followed by stenting group vs 12 in the direct stent group (p=0.01). Final TIMI 3 grade was 95.1% in the direct stent group vs 93.3% in the PTCA-followed by stent group (p=NS). There was no significant difference in the corrected TIMI frame count at 31.5 ± 17 in the direct stent group vs 35.2 ± 20 in the PTCA followed by stent group (p=NS). Resolution of ST-segment elevation was improved after direct stenting. There were 38% of patients who had no ST-segment resolution after PTCA stenting vs 20% with direct stenting (p=0.01). Clinical outcomes did not differ between groups. Death and/or recurrent MI occurred in 6 patients after PTCA stenting vs 2 after direct stenting (p=0.28).
Concl.	Direct stenting can be safe and effective in selected acute MI patients. Direct stenting may reduce microvascular injury with less no- and slow-reflow and better resolution of ST-segment elevation.

Randomized Comparison of Primary Angioplasty and Thrombolytic Therapy

Title	Reperfusion therapy in elderly patients with acute myocardial infarction.
Authors	de Boer M-J, Ottervanger J-P, van't Hof AWJ, et al.
Reference	J Am Coll Cardiol 2002;39:1723-1728.
Disease	Acute myocardial infarction (AMI).
Purpose	To determine outcome of primary coronary angioplasty vs thrombolytic therapy in patients older than 75 years of age with AMI.
Design	Prospective, randomized.
Patients	87 patients 76 years or older with AMI and no contraindications to thrombolytic therapy.
Follow-up	30 days; 1 year; 2 years.
Regimen	Patients were randomized to primary angioplasty (n=46) or streptokinase (1.5 million U IV over 1 hour; n=41).
Add'l Tx	Aspirin, nitroglycerin, heparin. If patients received stent, ticlopidine.

Results	Primary end point was death, reinfarction, and stroke at 30 days. Secondary end point included this composite at 1 year. The 30-day primary end point occurred in 4 (9%) of patients randomized to primary coronary angioplasty vs 12 (29%) who received streptokinase (p=0.01; RR 4.3; 95% CI=1.2-20.0). At 30 days 7% in the angioplasty group died vs 22% in the thrombolytic group (p=0.04). This benefit was maintained at 1 year where the composite was reached in 6 (13%) primary angioplasty patients vs 18 (44%) thrombolytic patients (p=0.001; RR 5.2; 95% CI=1.7-18.1) At 1 year, 11% of the angioplasty group and 29% in the thrombolytic group had died (p=0.03). Procedural success rate for angioplasty was 90%. 51% of patients treated with angioplasty received a stent. At 24 months the composite end point of death, reinfarction, and stroke was 9 (20%) in the angioplasty and 18 (44%) in the thrombolytic group (p=0.003; RR 3.1; 95% CI=1.4-7.0). At 24 months there were 7 deaths in the angioplasty group (15%) vs 13 (32%) in the streptokinase group (p=0.04). Enzymatic infarct size by lactic dehydrogenase and ejection fraction did not differ between groups.
Concl.	Primary coronary angioplasty had a significant benefit on clinical outcomes over IV streptokinase in patients with AMI over the age of 75 years.

Air PAMI

Air Primary Angioplasty in Myocardial Infarction Study

Title	A randomized trial of transfer for primary angioplasty vs on-site thrombolysis in patients with high-risk myocardial infarction. The Air PAMI study.
Authors	Grines CL, Westerhausen DR, Grines LL, et al.
Reference	J Am Coll Cardiol 2002;39:1713-1719.
Disease	Acute myocardial infarction (AMI).
Purpose	To determine the best reperfusion strategy for patients with high-risk AMI in centers without percutaneous transluminal coronary angioplasty (PTCA) capability—either on-site thrombolysis vs transfer for primary PTCA.
Design	Randomized, multicenter.
Patients	138 patients with high-risk AMI (age >70 years, anterior MI, Killip class II/III, heart rate >100 bpm, systolic blood pressure <100 mm Hg), eligible for thrombolysis.
Follow-up	30 days.
Regimen	Patients were randomized to either emergent transfer for primary PTCA (n=71) or on-site thrombolysis (n=67). PTCA included stenting for residual lesions >30%. Thrombolysis included the drug considered standard of care at the admitting hospital.
Add'l Tx	Oxygen, nitroglycerin, oral aspirin, or β-blockers; heparin.

Results	Primary end point was major adverse cardiac events (MACE) defined as the combined occurrence of death, nonfatal reinfarction, or disabling stroke at 30 days. At 30 days, MACE occurred in 8.4% of the transfer group vs 13.6% of the thrombolytic group (p=0.331). This 38% reduction did not achieve statistical significance due to inability to recruit necessary sample size. Time from hospital arrival to treatment was delayed in the transfer group (155 minutes vs 51 minutes; p<0.0001) due to initiation of transfer (43 minutes) and transport time (26 minutes). The mean distance of transfer was 32±36 miles. Air transfer (helicopter) was used for longer distances (57 miles) vs ground transfer (26 miles). 79% of patients were transferred by ambulance; 21% by helicopter. No patient died or required CPR during transfer. Of the transfer patients 87% achieved normal TIMI 3 flow with primary PTCA. Those patients randomized to transfer had a shorter hospital stay (6.1±4.3 vs 7.5±4.3 days (p=0.015) and less clinical ischemia (12.7%) than the reperfusion group (31.8%; p=0.007).
Concl.	There was a nonsignificant trend toward improved outcomes in high-risk AMI patients transferred to an interventional center for primary PTCA vs on-site thrombolysis. Additional study will be required.

1. Acute Myocardial Infarction — b. Primary PTCA vs. Primary Stenting vs. Thrombolytic Therapy

Stent-PAMI

Stent-Primary Angioplasty in Myocardial Infarction

Title	Coronary angioplasty with or without stent implantation for acute myocardial infarction.
Authors	Grines CL, Cox DA, Stone GW, et al.
Reference	N Engl J Med 1999;341:1949-1956.
Disease	Acute myocardial infarction.
Purpose	To compare outcomes in patients with acute myocardial infarction undergoing primary angioplasty to angioplasty with implantation of a heparin-coated Palmaz-Schatz stent.
Design	Randomized, multicenter.
Patients	900 patients with acute myocardial infarction undergoing emergency catheterization and angioplasty.
Follow-up	6-6.5 months.
Regimen	Patients with vessels appropriate for stenting were randomized to angioplasty alone (n=448) or angioplasty with stenting (n=452).
Add'l Tx	Aspirin, ticlopidine, heparin and, if no contraindications, β-blockers.

1. Acute Myocardial Infarction — b. Primary PTCA vs. Primary Stenting vs. Thrombolytic Therapy

49

Results	Based on angiograms performed immediately after the procedure, stenting was associated with a larger mean minimal luminal diameter (2.56±0.44 mm) compared to angioplasty alone (2.12±0.45 mm; p<0.001). There was a trend toward slightly lower incidence of TIMI 3 grade flow in stented (89.4%) vs angioplasty alone group (92.7%) but this was not statistically significant (p=0.10). The combined primary end point at 6 months of death, reinfarction, disabling stroke, or target vessel revascularization because of ischemia occurred in fewer patients that received stents (12.6%) compared to the angioplasty alone group (20.1%; p<0.01). At 6 months mortality rates were 4.2% in the stent groups and 2.7% in the angioplasty group (p=0.27). Decrease in composite end point was secondary to decreased need for target vessel revascularization. The incidence of angina at 6 months was lower in the stent group (11.3%) compared to the angioplasty alone group (16.9%; p=0.02). Late angiograms at 6.5 months showed that patients who received stents had a larger minimal diameter, less residual stenosis, and a lower rate of restenosis (20.3% vs 33.5%; p<0.001).
Concl.	Implantation of a stent for acute myocardial infarction "has clinical benefits beyond those of primary coronary angioplasty alone."

CAPTIM

Comparison of Angioplasty and Prehospital Thrombolysis in Acute Myocardial Infarction

Title	Primary angioplasty vs prehospital fibrinolysis in acute myocardial infarction: a randomised study.
Authors	Bonnefoy E, Lapostolle F, Leizorovicz A, et al.
Reference	Lancet 2002;360:825-829.
Disease	Acute myocardial infarction.
Purpose	To compare outcome of prehospital thrombolysis with primary angioplasty in patients with ST elevation acute myocardial infarction.
Design	Randomized, open-label, multicenter.
Patients	840 patients within 6 hours of onset of symptoms and ≥0.2 mV ST elevation in ≥2 contiguous leads or LBBB. Patients with contraindications to thrombolytic therapy or increased risk of bleeding, severe renal or hepatic disease, aortofemoral bypass, or any condition that could prevent femoral artery access were excluded. Patients in cardiogenic shock, with a history of CABG, current oral anticoagulant therapy, and those in whom the duration of transfer to the hospital was expected to be >1 hour were not included.
Follow-up	30 days.
Regimen	Patients were randomized to prehospital thrombolysis (alteplase 15 mg as a bolus followed by 0.75 mg/kg over 30 minutes and then, 0.50 mg/kg over 60 minutes) with a transfer to a hospital with an interventional facility (n=419) or to direct transfer for primary angioplasty (n=421).
Add'l Tx	All patients received aspirin 250-500 mg and intravenous heparin 5000 U. Intravenous heparin infusion was continued for ≥48 hr. Patients who underwent stenting received thienopyridine for 1 month.

Results	The median time from onset of symptoms to treatment was 130 minutes in the thrombolysis group and 190 minutes in the PTCA group. 400/419 patients assigned thrombolysis (95.5%) received the therapy, 1.2% underwent primary angioplasty, and 3.3% did not receive reperfusion therapy. 26.0% of the patients assigned thrombolysis underwent rescue PTCA immediately after thrombolysis. 405/421 patients assigned PTCA (96.2%) underwent angiography and 364 (86.5%) underwent angioplasty. 303 patients in the primary angioplasty group received stents and 97 patients received GP IIb/IIIa inhibitors. 85.4% of the patients in the thrombolysis group vs only 14.3% in the PTCA group underwent non-study angiography within 30 days. 14.3% of the patients in the PTCA group vs 70.4% in the thrombolysis group underwent nonscheduled PCI within the first 30 days. 30-day mortality was 3.8% in the thrombolysis group and 4.8% in the PTCA group (risk difference -0.93; 95% CI=-3.67 to 0.81; p=0.61). Reinfarction occurred in 3.7% in the thrombolysis group vs 1.7% in the PTCA group (risk difference 1.99; 95% CI=-0.27 to 4.24; p=0.13). 1.0% of the patients in the thrombolysis group vs 0 in the PTCA group had a disabling stroke (p=0.12). The composite end point of death, reinfarction, and disabling stroke occurred in 8.2% in the thrombolysis group vs 6.2% in the PTCA group (risk difference 1.96; 95% CI=-1.53 to 5.46; p=0.29). Recurrent ischemia was noted in 7.2% and 4.0% of the patients, respectively (p=0.09). Severe bleeding occurred in 0.5% of the patients in the thrombolysis group vs 2.0% in the PTCA group (p=0.06), and cardiogenic shock from randomization to hospital discharge in 2.5% vs 4.9%, respectively (p=0.09).
Concl.	A strategy of primary angioplasty was not better than prehospital thrombolysis (with transfer to a hospital with an interventional facility) in patients within 6 hours of onset of acute MI.

1. Acute Myocardial Infarction — b. Primary PTCA vs. Primary Stenting vs. Thrombolytic Therapy

CCP

Cooperative Cardiovascular Project

Title	Primary coronary angioplasty vs thrombolysis for the management of acute myocardial infarction in elderly patients.
Authors	Berger AK, Schulman KA, Gersh BJ, et al.
Reference	JAMA 1999;282:341-348.
Disease	Acute myocardial infarction.
Purpose	To compare the efficacy of primary PTCA and thrombolysis in elderly patients with acute myocardial infarction.
Design	Observational.
Patients	80,356 patients, ≥65 years old with acute myocardial infarction, ≤12 hours of onset of symptoms and without contraindications to thrombolytic therapy. Patients with cardiogenic shock were excluded.
Follow-up	1 year.
Regimen	Primary PTCA or thrombolytic therapy.

1. Acute Myocardial Infarction — b. Primary PTCA vs. Primary Stenting vs. Thrombolytic Therapy

53

Results	28,955 patients presented within 6 hours of onset of symptoms and with ST segment elevation or LBBB. Among those, only 44.7% received reperfusion therapy within 6 hours of hospitalization. 18,645 patients (23.2%) received thrombolytic therapy and 2038 patients (2.5%) underwent primary PTCA within 6 hours after hospital arrival. The remaining 59,673 patients (74.2%) did not receive reperfusion therapy within the first 6 hours after hospital arrival, and 54,989 patients (68.4%) did not receive reperfusion therapy at all. Mean time to treatment after admission was 68.3±54.4 minutes in the thrombolysis group vs 142.6±68. 1 minute in the primary PTCA group (p<0.001). 30-day mortality was 8.7% in the primary PTCA group vs 11.9% in the thrombolysis group (p=0.001). 1-year mortality was 14.4% vs 17.6%, respectively (p=0.001). After adjusting for baseline cardiac risk factors the hazard ratio of death at 30 days was 0.74 (95% CI=0.63-0.88), and at 1 year it was 0.83 (95% CI=0.73-0.94). Patients undergoing primary PTCA had less cerebral hemorrhages (0.2% vs 1.4%; p=0.001), stroke (2.1% vs 3.0%; p=0.03), post infarction angina (24.0% vs 29.6%; p=0.001) and reinfarction (4.0% vs 5.3%; p=0.009) than the patients receiving thrombolytic therapy. However, among patients who presented within 6 hours of onset of symptoms and were eligible for thrombolytic therapy, 30-day mortality was insignificantly smaller with primary PTCA (10.1% vs 12.0%; p=0.06). Eventually, 39.2% of the patients receiving thrombolytic therapy underwent coronary angioplasty, 12.4% underwent PTCA and 6.3% CABG. After stratification of the patients by age, gender, hypertension, prior heart failure and the location of myocardial infarction, the benefit of primary PTCA persisted. The benefit of primary PTCA was still apparent when patients were stratified by hospital's volume of acute myocardial infarction patients (<150 per year vs ≥150 per year) and the presence of on-site catheterization laboratory.
Concl.	In patients, ≥65 years old, with acute myocardial infarction, primary PTCA was associated with a modest decrease in 30-day and 1-year mortality. In the subgroup analysis of patients eligible for thrombolytic therapy, the benefit of primary PTCA was not statistically significant.

C-PORT

The Atlantic Cardiovascular Patient Outcomes Research Team

Title	Thrombolytic therapy vs primary percutaneous coronary intervention for myocardial infarction in patients presenting to hospitals without on-site cardiac surgery. A randomized controlled trial.
Authors	Aversano T, Aversano LT, Passamani E, et al.
Reference	JAMA 2002;287:1943-1951.
Disease	Acute myocardial infarction (MI).
Purpose	To determine whether treating acute MI with percutaneous coronary intervention (PCI) is better than thrombolytic therapy in hospitals that lack on-site cardiac surgical programs.
Design	Randomized, controlled trial, multicenter.
Patients	451 patients eligible for thrombolytic therapy, with acute MI with ST-segment elevation.
Follow-up	6 months.
Regimen	Following development of a formal primary PCI program at the 11 community hospitals without a cardiac surgical program, patients were randomized to primary PCI (n=225) or tissue plasminogen activator treatment (15 mg followed by an infusion of 0.75 mg/kg for 30 minutes and then 0.5 mg/kg for 60 minutes; n=226).

Results	Primary outcome was a 6-month composite of death, recurrent MI and stroke. Median hospital length was also determined. PCI was successful in 96% of patients in whom it was attempted. 63% had stents and 76% had glycoprotein IIb/IIIa receptor antagonists. The incidence of the composite end point was 10.7% in the primary PCI group vs 17.7% in the thrombolytic group (p=0.03) at 6 weeks and was 12.4% vs 19.9% (p=0.03) at 6 months. At 6 months, death occurred in 6.2% of primary PCI patients vs 7.1% for thrombolytic patients (p=NS); recurrent MI occurred in 5.3% of primary PCI patients vs 10.6% of thrombolytic patients (p=0.04) and stroke occurred in 2.2% of primary PCI patients vs 4.0% of thrombolytic patients (p=0.28). The primary PCI group had a shorter median length of stay (4.5 days) vs the thrombolytic group (6.0 days; p=0.02). 2 thrombolytic patients required emergency CABG following elective PCI at a tertiary center. No patient in the primary PCI group was sent for emergency CABG to a tertiary center.
Concl.	Primary PCI for acute MI at hospitals without on-site cardiac surgical programs was associated with better 6-month outcomes than thrombolytic therapy.

PACT

Plasminogen Activator Angioplasty Compatibility Trial

Title	A randomized trial comparing primary angioplasty with a strategy of short acting thrombolysis and immediate planned rescue angioplasty in acute myocardial infarction: The PACT trial.
Authors	Ross AM, Coyne KS, Reiner JS, et al.
Reference	J Am Coll Cardiol 1999;34:1954-1962.
Disease	Acute myocardial infarction.
Purpose	To determine the efficacy and safety of a short acting and reduced dose fibrinolytic regimen rt-PA coupled with PTCA as the primary recanalization modality.
Design	Randomized, double-blind, placebo-controlled, multicenter.
Patients	606 patients with acute myocardial infarction.
Follow-up	1 year.
Regimen	IV bolus of rt-PA (50 mg) given over 3 minutes or an IV placebo bolus and then angiography. If infarct artery was TIMI grade 0, 1, 2, immediate angioplasty; if it was TIMI grade 3, a second bolus of assigned study drug could be given.
Add'l Tx	Heparin, aspirin.

Results	The primary end points were patency at the time of initial angiography, technical results of the PTCA, complication rates, LV function (LV angiogram), and time to restored patency after angioplasty. The patency rates (TIMI flow grade 2 or 3) at the time of arrival in the catheterization laboratory were 34% with placebo vs 61% with rt-PA (p=0.001). Both rescue and primary PTCA restored TIMI 3 levels of flow in closed arteries at 77% and 79%, respectively. Stenting was done in 26% of patients in each group. The LV ejection fraction (EF) obtained at the first angiogram (following angioplasty if angioplasty was done) was 57.7±14.1% in the placebo group and 59.4±13.8% in the rt-PA group (p=NS). Follow-up LV function assessed on repeat or convalescent angiogram (at day 5-7) revealed an LVEF of 58.4±12.5% in the placebo group and 58.2±13.0% in the rt-PA group (p=NS). Patients arriving in the catheterization laboratory with TIMI flow grade 3 had convalescent LVEF of 62.4% vs those with later mechanical restoration (primary or planned rescue PTCA) of 57.9% (p=0.004). Lowest convalescent LVEF was seen in patients who never achieved TIMI flow grade 3 (EF=54.7%). No difference in adverse events occurred between placebo vs rt-PA patients, including the incidence of major hemorrhage (13.5 vs 12.9%, respectively).
Concl.	A tailored thrombolytic regimen with subsequent PTCA, if needed, leads to better early recanalization prior to arrival to the catheterization lab that facilitates better LV function and no adverse events.

PRAGUE

*Primary Angioplasty in Patients Transferred from General
Community Hospitals to Specialized PTCA Units with or
Without Emergency Thrombolysis*

Title	Multicenter randomized trial comparing transport to primary angioplasty vs immediate thrombolysis vs combined strategy for patients with acute myocardial infarction presenting to a community hospital without a catheterization laboratory.
Authors	Widimsky P, Groch L, Zelizko M, et al.
Reference	Eur Heart J 2000;21:823-831.
Disease	Acute myocardial infarction.
Purpose	To compare 3 reperfusion strategies for patients with acute myocardial infarction presenting initially to hospitals without catheterization facility: 1) IV streptokinase; 2) transport to primary angioplasty; or 3) thrombolysis with streptokinase during transfer to immediate coronary angioplasty.
Design	Randomized, open-label, multicenter.
Patients	300 patients with acute myocardial infarction and ST elevation or bundle branch block who presented to 17 participating hospitals without catheterization facility within 6 hours of onset of symptoms.
Follow-up	30 days.
Regimen	Randomization to: 1) IV streptokinase (n=99); 2) thrombolytic therapy during transportation for immediate angioplasty (n=100); or 3) immediate transportation for primary angioplasty without thrombolytic therapy (n=101).
Add'l Tx	Angioplasty was performed in all patients with TIMI flow 0-2 in the infarct related artery. In case of TIMI flow 3, angioplasty was performed at the discretion of the operator. Stents were implanted whenever anatomically suitable or when suboptimal results were achieved by balloon angioplasty.

Results	2 patients from the thrombolytic therapy + PTCA had ventricular fibrillation during transportation. No complications occurred during transportation in the PTCA without thrombolysis group. Median time from admission to reperfusion was 106 minutes and 96 minutes in the groups transferred for PTCA with and without thrombolysis, respectively. TIMI flow before angioplasty was 2 and 3 in 17% and 30% of the patients transferred with thrombolytic therapy and 15% and 12%, respectively, of the patients transferred without thrombolysis. PTCA was performed acutely in 82 and 91 of the patients transferred with and without thrombolysis. After PTCA, 91% and 92% of the patients transferred with and without thrombolysis had TIMI flow 3 and 5% and 3%, respectively, TIMI flow 2. 30-day mortality was 14% in the thrombolysis without PTCA, 12% in the PTCA + thrombolysis, and 7% in the PTCA without thrombolysis. Reinfarction occurred in 10%, 7%, and 1% (p<0.03), respectively, whereas stroke occurred in 1%, 3%, and 0 of the patients, respectively. The combined end point of death/reinfarction/stroke at 30 days occurred in 23%, 15%, and 8%, respectively (p<0.02).
Concl.	Transferring patients with acute myocardial infarction from community hospitals to a tertiary center for primary angioplasty is feasible and safe. Compared with the strategy of thrombolytic therapy, transfer for primary angioplasty was associated with less reinfarction and the combined end point of death/reinfarction/stroke at 30 days. The combined strategy of thrombolysis + PTCA was not associated with better outcome than thrombolytic therapy alone.

PRAGUE-2

Primary Angioplasty in Patients Transported From General Community Hospitals to Specialized PTCA Units with or Without Emergency Thrombolysis-2

Title	Long distance transport for primary angioplasty vs immediate thrombolysis in acute myocardial infarction. Final results of the randomized national multicenter trial—PRAGUE-2.
Authors	Widimsky P, Budesinsky T, Vorac D, et al.
Reference	Eur Heart J 2003;24:94-104.
Disease	Acute myocardial infarction.
Purpose	To compare intravenous streptokinase infusion vs immediate transport for primary PCI in patients with ST-elevation acute myocardial infarction who are admitted to hospitals without PCI facilities.
Design	Randomized, open-label, multicenter.
Patients	850 patients with ST-elevation acute myocardial infarction, within 12 hours of onset of symptoms, distance from the admitting hospital to the PCI center <120 km, and feasibility for transportation within 30 minutes after randomization. Patients with contraindications to thrombolytic therapy and those without femoral pulsations were excluded.
Follow-up	30 days.
Regimen	Randomization to streptokinase (1.5 million units over 45 minutes) or transport for PCI.
Add'l Tx	All patients received aspirin 500 mg IV, fraxiparin 0.8 mL subcutaneously for 3 days and clopidogrel 75 mg/d for 1 month.

1. Acute Myocardial Infarction — b. Primary PTCA vs. Primary Stenting vs. Thrombolytic Therapy

61

Results	The study was terminated prematurely by the ethical committee because the mortality was 2.5-fold higher in the thrombolysis group than in the PCI group among patients treated >3 hours of the onset of symptoms. The distance between the primary hospitals and the PCI centers was 5-120 km. The transport time for PCI was 48±20 minutes. 425 patients (99%) randomized to PCI were transported. 4 patients were not transported because of hemodynamic deterioration. During transportation there were 2 deaths and 3 ventricular fibrillations that were successfully defibrillated. (Complications during transport occurred in 1.2% of the patients). PCI was performed in 89% of all patients assigned PCI. The success rate was 88%. Stents were implanted in 63% of all PCIs. The 30-day mortality was 10% in the streptokinase group and 6.8% in the PCI group (p=0.12). Among the 299 patients randomized >3 hours after onset of symptoms (average of 5 hours and 6 minutes), mortality was 15.3% in the streptokinase group and 6.0% in the PCI group (p<0.002). Among the 551 patients randomized within 3 hours of onset of symptoms (average of 1 hour and 41 minutes) mortality was 7.4% and 7.3%, respectively (p=NS). Death, reinfarction or stroke occurred in 15.2% of the patients in the streptokinase group vs 8.4% in the PCI group (p<0.003). Reinfarction occurred in 3.1% and 1.4% of the patients, respectively (p=NS), and stroke in 2.1% and 0.2%, respectively (p<0.03). Left ventricular ejection fration by echocardiogram at 30 days was 51%±9% in the streptokinase group and 50%±8% in the PCI group (p=NS).
Concl.	Long-distance transportation of patients with acute MI from community hospitals to tertiary PCI centers is safe and feasible. PCI resulted in significantly lower mortality in patients presented >3 hours after onset of symptoms. For patients presenting within the first 3 hours of onset of symptoms streptokinase infusion and transport for PCI were comparable.

SHOCK

Should We Emergently Revascularize Occluded Coronaries for Cardiogenic Shock?

Title	a. Early revascularization in acute myocardial infarction complicated by cardiogenic shock. b. 1-year survival following early revascularization for cardiogenic shock.
Authors	a. Hochman JS, Sleeper LA, Webb JG, et al. b. Hochman JS, Sleeper LA, White HD, et al.
Reference	a. N Engl J Med 1999;341:625-634. b. JAMA 2001;285:190-192.
Disease	Acute myocardial infarction complicated by cardiogenic shock.
Purpose	To evaluate the effect of early revascularization in patients with acute myocardial infarction complicated by shock.
Design	Randomized, multicenter.
Patients	302 patients with acute myocardial infarction and cardiogenic shock (confirmed by both clinical and hemodynamic criteria). Mean age was 66 years; 32% were women; 55% were transferred from other hospitals.
Follow-up	6 months.
Regimen	Patients were randomized to emergency revascularization (n=152) or intensive medical therapy and thrombolysis (n=150). Angioplasty or coronary bypass surgery had to be performed as soon as possible within 6 hours of randomization. 150 patients were randomized to medical stabilization—intensive medical therapy and thrombolytic therapy. Intra-aortic balloon counterpulsation was recommended in both groups.
Add'l Tx	As needed.

Results	a. The primary end point was death from all causes at 30 days and the secondary end point was survival at 6 months. Time from onset of myocardial infarction to shock was 5.6 hours (median value). Among patients randomized to early revascularization, 64% received angioplasty and 36% surgery. At 30 days, 46.7% of the revascularization group died and 56.0% of the medical-treatment group died (p=0.11). At 6 months, mortality was significantly lower among patients who received early revascularization (50.3%) vs those that received medical treatment (63.1%; p=0.027). Success rate for early revascularization of the culprit-vessel was 77% for the group assigned to early revascularization. Successful angioplasty in the group assigned to early revascularization was associated with a lower 30-day mortality (38%) vs those that had an unsuccessful angioplasty (79%; p=0.003). Acute renal failure occurred in 13% assigned to revascularization and 24% to those assigned to medical therapy (p=0.03).
	b. 1-year survival was 33.6% for the medical-treatment group vs 46.7% for the early revascularization group (13.2% absolute difference in survival; 95% CI=2.2%-24.1%; p<0.03; RR 0.72; 95% CI=0.54-0.95). Only age (<75 vs ≥75 years) interacted significantly with the treatment strategy (p<0.03). The benefit of early revascularization was apparent only for patients <75 years old (51.6% survival in the early revascularization group vs 33.3% in the initial medical therapy group. Among patients ≥75 years old, survival was 20.8% vs 34.4% for the early revascularization and medical therapy groups, respectively. There was no interaction between the treatment effect and gender, randomization 6 hours or less after onset of symptoms, anterior acute myocardial infarction, prior myocardial infarction, diabetes mellitus, hypertension, transfer to referral center, and contraindications to thrombolytic therapy. Among the 1-year survivors (n=90), 83% were in New York Heart Association class I or II.
Concl.	a. In patients with acute myocardial infarction and cardiogenic shock, emergency revascularization did not significantly decrease overall mortality at 30 days but did reduce overall mortality at 6 months. "Early revascularization should be strongly considered for patients with acute myocardial infarction complicated by cardiogenic shock."
	b. Early revascularization significantly reduced 1-year mortality, especially in those younger than 75 years.

STAT

Stenting vs Thrombolysis in Acute Myocardial Trial

Title	Stenting vs thrombolysis in acute myocardial infarction trial (STAT).
Authors	Le May MR, Labiraz M, Davies RF, et al.
Reference	J Am Coll Cardiol 2001;37:985-991.
Disease	Acute ST elevation MI.
Purpose	To compare primary stenting with accelerated tissue plasminogen activator (t-PA) in patients with acute ST elevation MI.
Design	Randomized, single-center.
Patients	123 patients with acute ST elevation MI.
Follow-up	6 months.
Regimen	Percutaneous transluminal coronary angioplasty predilation and then stenting (n=62) of the infarct related artery vs accelerated tPA and heparin (n=61).
Add'l Tx	In stent patients: abciximab at discretion of investigator, heparin, aspirin, ticlopidine.
Results	Primary end point was composite of death, reinfarction, stroke, or repeat target vessel revascularization for ischemia at 6 months. Primary end point occurred in 24.2% of stent vs 55.7% of tPA patients (p<0.001). 3 patients in stent group and 2 in tPA group died (p=NS). Reinfarction occurred in 6.5% of the stent and 16.4% of tPA patients (p=0.096). Stroke occurred in 1.6% of the stent group and 4.9% of the tPA group (p=NS). Target vessel revascularization for ischemia occurred in 14.5% of stent patients and 49.4% of tPA patients (p<0.001). Also, recurrent unstable angina occurred in 9.7% of the stent group vs 26.2% of the tPA group (p=0.019). Patients receiving stents had an initial hospitalization length-of-stay of 4 days vs 7 days in the tPA group. (p<0.001).
Concl.	Primary stenting for acute MI reduced the composite end point of death, reinfarction, stroke, or repeat target vessel revascularization for ischemia compared to accelerated tPA.

STENTIM-2

Stenting in Acute Myocardial Infarction-2

Title	A comparison of systematic stenting and conventional balloon angioplasty during primary percutaneous transluminal coronary angioplasty for acute myocardial infarction.
Authors	Maillard L, Hamon M, Khalife K, et al.
Reference	J Am Coll Cardiol 2000;35:1729-1736.
Disease	Acute myocardial infarction.
Purpose	To compare the outcome of patients with acute myocardial infarction treated with systematic stenting vs conventional balloon angioplasty with provisional stenting.
Design	Randomized, open-label, multicenter.
Patients	211 patients, >18 years old, within 12 hours of onset of ST elevation acute myocardial infarction. Patients who had received thrombolytic therapy or were in cardiogenic shock were not included. In addition, patients with a history of coronary artery bypass grafting, percutaneous coronary intervention within the preceding 6 months, contraindications to heparin, aspirin or ticlopidine, renal or hepatic disease, and body weight <40 kg or >100 kg were excluded. Angiographic inclusion criteria were vessel diameter <3.00 mm, TIMI flow grade <3 and diameter stenosis of the culprit lesion >70%. Patients with left main stenosis >50%, severe multivessel disease, massively calcified lesions, or bifurcation lesions involving a major side branch were excluded.
Follow-up	12 months clinical follow-up with a stress test and repeated angiography after 6 months.
Regimen	After coronary angiography and before crossing the lesion with a guide wire, patients were randomized to either routine stenting (Wiktor GX stent, Medtronic, Minneapolis, MN; n=101) or standard balloon angioplasty (percutaneous transluminal coronary angioplasty; n=110).

Add'l Tx	All patients received 500 mg aspirin IV and ≥5000 IU heparin. After sheath removal, all patients received low molecular weight heparin for >48 hours, aspirin 160-300 mg/d. Patients who underwent stenting received, in addition, ticlopidine 250 mg × 2/d for 1 month. ACE inhibitors and β-blockers were permitted.
Results	Angiographic success (TIMI flow grade 3 and residual diameter stenosis <50%) was documented in 86.0% of the patients in the stent group and 82.7% of the patients in the PTCA group (p=0.5). 3 patients (3%) in the stent group did not receive a stent and underwent PTCA alone. 40 patients (36.4%) in the PTCA group underwent stenting. Mean hospital stay was 10.4±8.9 days in the stent group and 10.0±5.5 days in the PTCA group (p=0.71). 1 patient in the stent group vs zero patients in the PTCA group died (p=0.48). Reinfarction occurred in 4.0% and 3.6% of the patients, respectively (p=1.0). Zero patients in both groups underwent CABG and 5.0% vs 5.4% in the stent and PTCA groups needed repeat revascularization (p=0.9). In-hospital event-free survival was 95.0% in the stent group and 94.5% in the PTCA group (p=0.87). The event-free survival at 6 months was 81.2% in the stent group and 72.7% in the PTCA group (p=0.14). 16.8% of the patients in the stent group vs 26.4% in the PTCA group underwent repeat revascularization (p=0.1), whereas 15.8% vs 26.4% underwent repeat PCI (p=0.06). The event-free survival at 1 year was 80.2% in the stent group and 71.8% in the PTCA group (p=0.16). At 1 year, 17.8% vs 28.2% of the patients, respectively, underwent repeat revascularization (p=0.1). The minimal lumen diameter after PCI was 2.38±0.39 mm in the stent group vs 2.11±0.49 mm in the PTCA group (p<0.001). Post-PCI residual stenosis was 19.4±8.1% in the stent group vs 28.5±10.8% in the PTCA group (p<0.001). 90% of the patients underwent repeat angiography at 6 months. Restenosis occurred in 25.3% of the patients in the stent group vs 39.6% in the PTCA group (p=0.0427). Reocclusion occurred in 7.2% vs 6.3%, respectively (p=0.79). The average diameter stenosis at 6 months was 42.5±21.7% in the stent group and 46.8±19.7% in the PTCA group (p=0.16). MLD at 6 months was 1.66±0.73 mm and 1.50±0.62 mm, respectively (p=0.10). LVEF at 6 months was comparable (56.3±10.5% vs 56.5±10%, respectively; p=0.92).

Concl.   In patients with acute MI undergoing primary PCI for acute reperfusion therapy, routine stenting using the Wiktor stent resulted in less restenosis and a trend toward less clinical events and repeat revascularization than a strategy of standard PTCA with provisional stenting.

STOPAMI

Stent vs Thrombolysis for Occluded Coronary Arteries in Patients with Acute Myocardial Infarction

Title	Coronary stenting plus platelet glycoprotein IIb/IIIa blockade compared with tissue plasminogen activator in acute myocardial infarction.
Authors	Schömig A, Kastrati A, Dirschinger J, et al.
Reference	N Engl J Med 2000;343:385-391.
Disease	Acute myocardial infarction.
Purpose	To determine whether the combination of coronary artery stenting plus blockade of platelet glycoprotein IIb/IIIa receptors salvage a greater amount of myocardium than fibrinolysis with accelerated infusion of alteplase, in patients with acute MI.
Design	Randomized.
Patients	140 patients with ST elevation acute myocardial infarcts who presented within 12 hours of symptoms.
Follow-up	6 months.
Regimen	Patients were randomized to thrombolysis vs stenting. Patients randomized to thrombolysis (n=69) bolus of 15 mg alteplase followed by 90-minute infusion 0.75 mg/kg (maximal dose 50 mg) over 30 minutes, followed by 0.5 mg/kg (maximal dose 35 mg) over 60 minutes. IV heparin for 48 hours. Patients randomized to stent (n=71) received 2500 U heparin intra-arterially and abciximab (0.25 mg/kg followed by infusion of 10 µg/min for 12 hours); ticlopidine 250 mg bid for 4 weeks and aspirin 100 mg bid indefinitely.

Results	Primary end point was degree of myocardial salvage that was determined by means of serial scintigraphic studies utilizing technetium (Tc) 99m sestamibi. Tc 99m sestamibi injected after randomization but before initiation of assigned therapy; single-photon-emission computed tomography performed within 6-8 hours after injection. Follow-up scintigraphic study done about 10 days later. Secondary end point was composite of the following clinical outcomes: death, reinfarction, stroke within 6 months of randomization. Patients that received stents plus abciximab had smaller final infarct sizes (median of 14.3% of the LV; 25th and 75th percentiles of 6.8% and 24.5%) vs patients that received thrombolysis (19.4%; 25th and 75th percentiles of 7.9% and 34.2%; p=0.02). A salvage index (% of the LV that was salvaged, divided by % that was comprised on initial perfusion defect) in the stent group was 0.57 vs 0.26 in the thrombolysis group (p<0.001). Incidence of death, reinfarction or stroke at 6 months was 8.5% in stent group vs 23.2% in thrombolysis group (p=0.02; RR 0.34; 95% CI=0.13-0.88).
Concl.	Coronary stenting plus abciximab resulted in more myocardial salvage and better clinical outcome than fibrinolytic therapy with the tissue plasminogen activator, alteplase.

1. Acute Myocardial Infarction — b. Primary PTCA vs. Primary Stenting vs. Thrombolytic Therapy

STOPAMI-3

Stent or PTCA for Occluded Coronary Arteries in Patients with Acute Myocardial Infarction Ineligible for Thrombolysis

Title	A randomized trial comparing myocardial salvage achieved by coronary stenting vs balloon angioplasty in patients with acute myocardial infarction considered ineligible for reperfusion therapy.
Authors	Kastrati A, Mehilli J, Nekolla S, et al.
Reference	J Am Coll Cardiol 2004;43:734-741.
Disease	Acute myocardial infarction.
Purpose	To assess myocardial salvage achieved by reperfusion with percutaneous coronary intervention and to compare stenting with percutaneous transluminal coronary angioplasty in patients with acute myocardial infarction ineligible for thrombolysis.
Design	Randomized, open-label study.
Patients	611 patients with acute myocardial infarction ineligible for thrombolysis (lack of ST-segment elevation on the electrocardiogram, presentation >12 hours after symptom onset, contraindications to thrombolysis).
Follow-up	6 months.
Regimen	Coronary artery stenting (n=305) or percutaneous transluminal coronary angioplasty (n=306).
Results	The main outcome of the study was the proportion of the initial myocardial perfusion defect assessed by single photon emission computed tomography that was salvaged by reperfusion. Both stenting and PTCA resulted in substantial myocardial salvage. Among patients who underwent stenting, the median size of the salvage index was 0.54 (25th and 75th percentiles: 0.29, 0.87) vs a median of 0.50 (0.26, 0.82) among patients who underwent PTCA. The 6-month mortality rate was not significantly different between the groups, 8.2% with stenting and 9.2% with PTCA. The combined incidence of death or recurrent MI was 10.5% in either group.
Concl.	Stenting and PTCA provide similar benefits in patients with MI ineligible for thrombolysis.

Title	A comparison of coronary angioplasty with fibrinolytic therapy in acute myocardial infarction.
Authors	Andersen HR, Nielsen TT, Rasmussen K, et al.
Reference	N Engl J Med 2003;349:733-742.
Disease	Acute myocardial infarction.
Purpose	To determine whether the benefit of primary angioplasty over fibrinolysis is maintained for patients with acute myocardial infarction who are transported from a community hospital to an invasive cardiology medical center.
Design	Randomized, multicenter.
Patients	1572 patients with acute myocardial infarction with ST-segment elevation. Patients had to be randomized within 12 hours.
Follow-up	30 days.
Regimen	Patients were randomized to treatment with primary angioplasty or accelerated IV alteplase (15 mg bolus and infusion of 0.75 mg/kg body weight over 30 minutes, followed by 0.5 mg/kg for 60 minutes). Patients randomized to thrombolysis also received aspirin, β-blockade, and unfractionated heparin. Patients randomized to angioplasty received aspirin, β-blockers, and unfractionated heparin, as well as glycoprotein IIb/IIIa inhibitors given at the discretion of the physician. Stenting of the culprit lesion was attempted in all patients. Ticlopidine or clopidogrel was given qd for 1 month after stenting. 1129 patients were enrolled at 24 referral hospitals without angioplasty facilities; 433 at 5 invasive treatment centers.

Results	Primary end point was the composite of death from any cause, clinical reinfarction, or disabling stroke at 30 days. Procedure-related reinfarction was not counted toward the primary end point. The primary end point was reached at 8.5% of patients in the angioplasty group vs 14.2% of those in the fibrinolytic group (p=0.002), and among patients randomized at referral hospitals. For patients enrolled in the invasive treatment centers, 6.7% of angioplasty patients achieved the primary end point vs 12.3% in the thrombolytic group (p=0.05). Better outcome in the angioplasty group was primarily related to a decrease in rate of reinfarction (1.6% vs 6.3% in the thrombolytic group; p<0.001). There was no significant difference in rate of death or stroke alone between the 2 therapies. Transfer from a referral to an invasive treatment center occurred within 2 hours in 96% of patients.
Concl.	Optimal clinical success of reperfusion is accomplished by primary PCI rather than on-site thrombolysis, even when invasive therapy requires transfer to an invasive treatment facility. However, the transfer should take 2 hours or less.

1. Acute Myocardial Infarction — b. Primary PTCA vs. Primary Stenting vs.
Thrombolytic Therapy

1. Acute Myocardial Infarction
c. Acute Anticoagulation/ Antiplatelet

Eptifibatide vs Placebo in Patients Receiving Thrombolytic Therapy

Title	Safety and efficacy of eptifibatide vs placebo in patients receiving thrombolytic therapy with streptokinase for acute myocardial infarction. A phase II dose escalation, randomized, double-blind study.
Authors	Ronner E, van Kesteren HA, Zijnen P, et al.
Reference	Eur Heart J 2000;21:1530-1536.
Disease	ST elevation acute myocardial infarction.
Purpose	To assess the efficacy and safety of a combination of full dose streptokinase with escalating doses of eptifibatide in achieving TIMI 3 flow in patients with ST elevation acute myocardial infarction.
Design	Randomized, placebo-controlled, double-blind, multicenter.
Patients	181 patients, ≥18 years old, with chest pain and ST elevation in ≥2 leads within 6 hours of onset of symptoms. Patients with previous cerebrovascular disease, previous coronary artery bypass graft surgery, current anticoagulant therapy and contraindications to thrombolytic therapy were excluded.
Follow-up	Coronary angiography at 90 minutes and 7 days. ST segment at baseline and at 3 hours.
Regimen	Randomization to placebo or eptifibatide in 3 different continuous infusion rates (0.75; 1.33; and 2.0 µg/kg/min). Placebo or eptifibatide (180 µg/kg) bolus was administered IV over 10 minutes. Infusion was continued for 72 hours.
Add'l Tx	All patients received a loading dose of aspirin 250-500 mg, continued with ≥80 mg/d, and 1.5 million IU of streptokinase over 60 minutes. Heparin was not administered.

Results	Study drug was discontinued because of bleeding or loss of hemoglobin in 9 patients receiving eptifibatide. In another 23 patients, study drug was discontinued prematurely due to various causes without differences among treatment groups. Study drug was discontinued in 15% in the placebo group and in 21%, 18%, and 20% in the 3 eptifibatide groups. Major bleeding occurred in none of the placebo group and in 7%, 18%, and 17% in the 3 eptifibatide groups (p<0.01). TIMI 3 flow was observed at 90 minutes in 31% in the placebo group and in 46%, 42%, and 45% in the 3 eptifibatide groups (p=0.07). TIMI 2-3 at 90 minutes was observed in 61% in the placebo vs 78%, 74%, and 83% in the 3 eptifibatide groups (p=0.02). Reocclusion was not noted in either the placebo or the 0.75 eptifibatide group, but occurred in 2 and 3 patients in the 1.33 and 2.0 eptifibatide groups. At day 7, TIMI 2-3 flow was noted in 89% in the placebo group vs 92%, 89%, and 87% in the 3 eptifibatide groups (p=0.99). Left ventricular ejection fraction was comparable among the 4 groups. There were no differences in the percentage of patients achieving complete (>70%) ST resolution at 3 hours (49% in the placebo group vs 41%, 38%, and 55%, in the 3 eptifibatide groups (p=NS). There were no differences in mortality, reinfarction and need for PCI among groups.
Concl.	A combination of aspirin, streptokinase and eptifibatide resulted in higher patency of the infarct-related artery and higher rates of complete reperfusion (TIMI 3) at 90 minutes, but not at day 7. This combination was associated with excess risk of bleeding.

1c

Enoxaparin vs Unfractionated Heparin After Thrombolytic Therapy for Acute Myocardial Infarction

Title	Randomized comparison of enoxaparin with unfractionated heparin following fibrinolytic therapy for acute myocardial infarction.
Authors	Baired SH, Menown IBA, McBride SJ, et al.
Reference	Eur Heart J 2002;23:627-632.
Disease	Acute myocardial infarction.
Purpose	To compare the safety and efficacy of unfractionated heparin and enoxaparin following thrombolytic therapy for acute myocardial infarction.
Design	Randomized, open-label.
Patients	300 patients who received thrombolytic therapy (streptokinase 1.5 million units over 60 minutes, anistreplase 30 U, or front-loaded alteplase 100 mg (for those previously treated with thrombolytic therapy) for ST elevation acute myocardial infarction. Patients with contraindications to thrombolytic therapy were excluded.
Follow-up	90 days.
Regimen	Randomized to unfractionated heparin (bolus 5000 U followed by 30,000 U/24 hours with a target activated partial thromboplastin time 2-2.5 times normal; n=151) or enoxaparin (IV bolus 40 mg followed by 40 mg every 8 hours; n=149) for 4 days.
Add'l Tx	Aspirin 75-300 mg/d. Patients at risk for left ventricular mural thrombus received intravenous unfractionated heparin 5000-10,000 U every 6 hours for an additional 3 days after the first 4 days of study treatment.

Results	The primary end point of death, nonfatal myocardial reinfarction or readmission for unstable angina at 90 days occurred in 36.4% of the patients in the unfractionated heparin group vs 25.5% of the patients in the enoxaparin group (OR 0.7; 95% CI=0.49-0.99; p=0.04). Cardiac mortality was 10.6% with unfractionated heparin and 6.0% with enoxaparin. Nonfatal myocardial reinfarction occurred in 19.9% vs 14.8% of the unfractionated heparin and enoxaparin groups, respectively, and readmission for unstable angina occurred in 6.0% vs 4.7%, respectively. Logistic regression analysis showed that left ventricular failure, hypertension, and the use of unfractionated heparin rather than enoxaparin were independently associated with recurrent events. Clinically significant hemorrhage, mandating at least temporary cessation of the study drug, was noted in 4% in the unfractionated heparin and in 3% in the enoxaparin group (p=NS). The overall costs for 4-day anticoagulant treatment were €77.67 for unfractionated heparin and €39.33 for enoxaparin.
Concl.	Compared with unfractionated heparin, 4-day treatment with enoxaparin after thrombolytic therapy for acute myocardial infarction resulted in a lower incidence of 90-day mortality, reinfarction and readmission for unstable angina.

Intracoronary vs Intravenous Abciximab in Acute Coronary Syndromes

Title	Reduction of major adverse cardiac events with intracoronary compared with intravenous bolus application of abciximab in patients with acute myocardial infarction or unstable angina undergoing coronary angiography.
Authors	Wöhrle J, Grebe O, Nusser T, et al.
Reference	Circulation. 2003;107:1840-1843.
Disease	Coronary artery disease, percutaneous intervention.
Purpose	To determine whether the administration of abciximab by the intracoronary route is associated with a decreased incidence of major adverse cardiac events compared to the usual intravenous route.
Design	Retrospective.
Patients	403 consecutive patients who had unstable angina or acute myocardial infarction.
Follow-up	30 days.
Regimen	Patients received a 20 mg bolus of abciximab either intravenously (n=109) or via an intracoronary route (n=294). Both groups then received 12 hours of intravenous infusion of 10 mg. All patients received 500 mg of aspirin and heparin adjusted to an activated clotting time of >280 seconds. Stent placement was left to the operator's discretion for use in case of dissection or if there was a residual lumen stenosis of >50%. Patients who had stents placed received 500 mg/d of ticlopidine or clopidogrel 75 mg/d for at least 4 weeks as well as aspirin 100 mg/d.

Results   A major adverse cardiac event (MACE) was defined as acute MI, need for urgent revascularization, or death. The 2 groups were similar in terms of risk profile, cardiac history, and clinical presentation. The rate of MACE was significantly lower ($p < 0.0008$) in the patients who received abciximab through the intracoronary route (10.2%, 30 incidents of MACE in 294 patients) vs the IV route (20.2%, 22 incidents of MACE in 109 patients). The significantly reduced rate of MACE was also seen in the subgroups of patients with stent placement (intracoronary vs IV, 10.7% vs 20.3%; $p < 0.05$), balloon angioplasty alone (8.8% vs 20.0%; $p = 0.07$), and patients without cardiogenic shock (2.8% vs 13.5%; $p < 0.0003$). Post-procedural reference diameter and acute gain were not significantly different between patients with and without a MACE. The components of MACE in the patients who received intracoronary vs IV abciximab were: urgent revascularization, 0.3% vs 4.6%, $p < 0.002$; recurrent MI, 0.3% vs 2.8%, $p < 0.04$; and death 9.5% vs 15.6%, $p < 0.09$. In patients who had TIMI 0/1 flow prior to the procedure, there was a significantly decreased risk of MACE with the intracoronary administration of abciximab (11.8%) compared to IV (27.5%). However, the incidence of MACE was not different if the TIMI flow before the procedure was TIMI 2/3 (intracoronary vs IV, 6.7% vs 7.7%).

Concl.   The intracoronary application of abciximab was associated with a lower risk of major adverse cardiac events in patients undergoing emergency coronary angioplasty for acute MI or unstable angina.

ADMIRAL

Abciximab Before Direct Angioplasty and Stenting in Myocardial Infarction Regarding Acute and Long-Term Follow-Up

Title	Platelet glycoprotein IIb/IIIa inhibition with coronary stenting for acute myocardial infarction.
Authors	Montalescot G, Barragan P, Wittenberg O, et al.
Reference	N Engl J Med 2001;344:1895-903.
Disease	Acute myocardial infarction.
Purpose	To compare the effects of early administration of abciximab before primary stenting vs stenting alone in patients with acute MI.
Design	Randomized, double-blind, placebo-controlled, multicenter.
Patients	300 patients, >18 years old, with ST segment elevation acute MI, within 12 hours of onset of symptoms. Patients with bleeding diathesis, administration of thrombolytic therapy for the current event, neoplasm, a limited life expectancy, childbearing potential, recent stroke or surgery, excessive hypertension despite therapy, oral anticoagulant therapy, and contraindications or hypersensitivity to aspirin, ticlopidine or heparin were excluded.
Follow-up	Repeat angiography at 24 hours and after 6 months.
Regimen	Randomization before arterial sheath insertion and coronary angiography to placebo or abciximab (0.25 mg/kg bolus followed by 0.125 µg/kg/min for 12 hours).
Add'l Tx	All patients received aspirin and IV heparin 70 U/kg. After percutaneous coronary intervention, patients received heparin infusion at an initial rate of 7 U/kg/h for 24 hours with target activated partial thromboplastin time 1.5-2.0 times the control value. All patients underwent coronary angiography and primary PTCA. If the infarct-related-artery was >2.5 mm, without extensive calcifications, a stent was placed. Ticlopidine 250 mg bid was administered for 30 days.

Results   PCI was attempted in 92% of the patients in the abciximab group and in 95% of the patients in the placebo group. 92% of the patients who underwent PCI received ≥1 stent and 32% received ≥2 stents. Before PCI, 16.8% of the patients in the abciximab group vs 5.4% in the placebo group had TIMI 3 flow grade (p=0.01), and 9.1% vs 5.4%, respectively, had TIMI 2 flow grade (p=0.34). Immediately after PCI, 95.1% of the patients in the abciximab group vs 86.7% of the patients in the placebo group had TIMI 3 flow grade (p=0.04), and 2.9% vs 4.5% had TIMI 2 flow grade (p=0.58). The rate of procedural success was 95.1% in the abciximab group vs 84.3% in the placebo group (p=0.01). 24 hours after PCI 95.9% in the abciximab vs 92.6% in the placebo group had TIMI 3 flow grade (p=0.33), and 0 vs 4.9% had TIMI 2 flow grade (p=0.02). 6 months after PCI 94.3% in the abciximab vs 82.8% in the placebo group had TIMI 3 flow grade (p=0.04), whereas 2.9% vs 5.2% had TIMI 2 flow grade (p=0.50), and 1.4% vs 10.3% had TIMI 0 flow grade (p=0.03). Reocclusions were detected in 2.9% of the abciximab group vs 12.1% of the placebo group (p=0.04). LVEF after 6 months was 61.1%±10.6% in the abciximab group vs 57.0%±11.1% in the placebo group (p=0.05). Death, reinfarction, or target vessel urgent revascularization at 30 days occurred in 6.0% of the patients in the abciximab group vs 14.6% in the placebo group (RR 0.41; 95% CI=0.18-0.93; p=0.01). 30-day mortality was 3.4% in the abciximab group vs 6.6% in the placebo group (RR 0.51; 95% CI=0.17-1.52; p=0.19). Urgent target vessel revascularization occurred in 1.3% and 6.6% of the patients, respectively (RR 0.20; 95% CI=0.04-0.94; p=0.02). 6-month mortality was 3.4% in the abciximab group vs 7.3% in the placebo group (RR 0.46; 95% CI=0.16-1.36; p=0.13). Death, reinfarction, or urgent target vessel revascularization at 6 months occurred in 7.4% vs 15.9%, respectively (RR 0.46; 95% CI=0.22-0.93; p=0.02). Death, reinfarction or any revascularization at 6 months occurred in 22.8% in the abciximab vs 33.8% in the placebo (RR 0.68; 95% CI=0.41-0.97; p=0.03). Major bleeding occurred in 0.7% in the abciximab and in zero of the placebo-treated patients (p=0.31). Minor bleeding occurred in 12.1% vs 3.3%, respectively (p=0.004). Groin hematoma was observed in 6.0% vs 0.7%, respectively (p=0.009).

Thrombocytopenia (<100,000 platelets/mm^3) was observed in 4.7% vs 1.3%, respectively (p=0.08), but severe thrombocytopenia (<50,000 platelets/mm^3) was observed in 1.3% of the patients in each group (p=1.00). The subgroup of patients who received their randomly assigned treatment with abciximab early, before hospitalization (ambulance or emergency department), had a greater benefit than those who received abciximab in the coronary care unit or catheterization laboratory. Patients with diabetes mellitus had a significant benefit from abciximab (6-month mortality 0 vs 16.7%; p=0.02).

Concl.	Early administration of abciximab before primary PCI for ST elevation acute MI improved coronary patency before and after stenting and at 6 months after PCI and was associated with better clinical outcome and preservation of left ventricular systolic function.

AMI-SK

Acute Myocardial Infarction Streptokinase

Title	Improved reperfusion and clinical outcome with enoxaparin as an adjunct to streptokinase thrombolysis in acute myocardial infarction.
Authors	Simoons ML, Krzeminska-Pakula M, Alonso A, et al.
Reference	Eur Heart J 2002;23:1282-1290.
Disease	Acute myocardial infarction.
Purpose	To evaluate the efficacy and safety of enoxaparin in patients with ST-elevation acute myocardial infarction treated with streptokinase.
Patients	496 patients, ≥18 years old, within 12 hours of onset of ST-elevation acute myocardial infarction. Patients with contraindications to streptokinase, cardiogenic shock, blood pressure >180/110 mm Hg, use of GP IIb/IIIa inhibitors, use of oral anticoagulants, current use of heparin or low molecular weight heparin, liver disease or renal insufficiency were excluded.
Follow-up	Coronary angiography at day 5-10. 30-day clinical follow-up.
Regimen	Randomization to enoxaparin (n=253) or placebo (n=243), started within 1 hour of streptokinase infusion. Enoxaparin was started as an IV bolus 30 mg and then subcutaneous 1 mg/kg every 12 hours for a minimum of 3 days and a maximum of 8 days (or until coronary angiography).
Add'l Tx	All patients received streptokinase 1.5 million U over 1 hour and aspirin 100-325 mg/d for ≥30 days. The use of GP IIb/IIIa inhibitors was prohibited, unless PCI was performed.

Results   491 patients received streptokinase. The median time from onset of symptoms to therapy was 3.3 hours in the enoxaparin group and 2.8 hours in the placebo group. The median duration of therapy was 5 days in both groups. The coronary angiography was considered evaluable for assessment of myocardial perfusion in 389 patients. TIMI grade 3 flow was 70.3% in the enoxaparin group and 57.8% in the placebo group (p=0.01). Corrected TIMI frame counts were better in the enoxaparin group (p=0.003). Coronary patency (TIMI flow grade 2 or 3) was better with enoxaparin (87.6% vs 71.7%; p<0.001). ST resolution at 90 minutes and 180 minutes was better in the enoxaparin group. Complete resolution of ST-segment elevation at 90 minutes was achieved by 15.7% of the patients in the enoxaparin group vs only 11.2% in the placebo group, partial ST resolution in 46.7% and 37.8%, respectively, and no ST resolution in 37.6% and 51.1% of the patients, respectively (p=0.012). At 180 minutes, complete ST-segment resolution was achieved by 36.3% in the enoxaparin group vs only 25.4% in the placebo group, partial ST resolution in 44.4% and 43.5%, respectively, and no ST resolution in 19.2% and 31.0%, respectively (p=0.014). 30-day mortality was 6.7% in the enoxaparin group and 7.0% in the placebo group (p=NS). Reinfarction occurred less often in the enoxaparin group (2.4% vs 7.4%; p=0.01). The combined end point of death, recurrent MI or angina was noted in 13.4% in the enoxaparin group and in 21.0% in the placebo group (p=0.03). 29.6% of the patients in the enoxaparin group vs 28.0% in the placebo group underwent revascularization (p=NS). Major bleeding occurred more often in the enoxaparin group (4.8% vs 2.5%; p=0.2). None of the patients in the enoxaparin vs 1.3% in the placebo had a stroke (p=0.1).

Concl.   Enoxaparin therapy for 5 days after streptokinase infusion for ST-elevation acute MI improved ST resolution at 90 minutes and 180 minutes, patency rates at day 5-10, and reduced the risk for adverse clinical events at 30 days.

ASSENT Plus

Assessment of the Safety and Efficacy of a New Thrombolytic Plus

Title	Low molecular weight heparin (dalteparin) compared to unfractionated heparin as an adjunct to rt-PA (alteplase) for improvement of coronary artery patency in acute myocardial infarction—the ASSENT Plus study.
Authors	Wallentin L, Bergstrand L, Dellborg M, et al.
Reference	Eur Heart J 2003;24:897-908.
Disease	Acute myocardial infarction.
Purpose	To evaluate the safety and efficacy of 4-7 days of dalteparin compared to 48 hours of unfractionated heparin, as an adjunct to alteplase in patients with ST-elevation acute myocardial infarction.
Design	Randomized, open-label with blinded evaluation of the primary end points, multicenter.
Patients	439 patients, ≥18 years old, with ST-elevation acute myocardial infarction, within 6 hours of onset of symptoms. Patients with hypertension, use of GP IIb/IIIa inhibitors within 24 hours, recent trauma or surgery, history of stroke or transient ischemic attack, dementia, current therapy with oral anticoagulants, renal insufficiency, and pregnancy were excluded.
Follow-up	Coronary angiography 96 hours to 7 days after initiation of therapy. Clinical follow-up for 30 days.
Regimen	Patients were randomized to unfractionated heparin (UFH), a bolus of 4000-5000 IU followed by an infusion of 800-1000 IU/h for 48 hours with a target aPTT of 50-75 sec) (n=213) or to dalteparin (a bolus of 30 anti-Xa IU/kg IV and thereafter, 120 anti-Xa IU/kg subcutaneous bid for 4-7 days) (n=221).
Add'l Tx	All patients received alteplase ≥100 mg over 90 minutes and aspirin 150-325 mg/d. The use of GP IIb/IIIa inhibitors was discouraged during the first 24 hours after randomization.

Results	202 patients in the dalteparin and 176 in the UFH group underwent coronary angiography at a median of 6 days after randomization. TIMI flow grade 3 was detected in 69.3% of the patients in the dalteparin group and in 62.5% in the UFH group (OR 1.11; 95% CI=0.96-1.28; p=0.163). TIMI flow grade 0-1 was detected in 13.4% and 24.4% of the patients, respectively (OR 0.55; 95% CI=0.35-0.85; p=0.006). Intraluminal thrombi were detected in 18.9% of the patients in the dalteparin group vs 27.3% in the UFH group (p=0.053). 7-day mortality was 2.3% in the dalteparin group and 3.8% in the UFH group. Recurrent MI within 7 days occurred in 1.4% and 5.4%, respectively (p=0.059). Death or MI within 7 days occurred in 3.6% and 8.1% of the patients, respectively (p=0.010). 30-day mortality was 4.1% in the dalteparin group vs 5.2% in the UFH group. After cessation of the dalteparin treatment there was an increased rate of recurrent infarction leading to a 30-day reinfarction rate of 6.5% in the dalteparin group and 7.0% in the UFH group. 30-day revascularization rate was 50.7% and 55.8%, respectively. There were no significant differences in major bleeding (3.7% vs 4.6%) or stroke (0.9% vs 0.5%) at 30 days between the groups.
Concl.	Among patients with ST-elevation acute MI who are treated with alteplase, adjunctive therapy with dalteparin for 4-7 days reduced the risk of early coronary events; however, after cessation of therapy there was an increase in reinfarction rate which might eliminate any long-term advantages.

CADILLAC

Controlled Abciximab and Device Investigation to Lower Late Angioplasty Complications

Title	Comparison of angioplasty with stenting, with or without abciximab, in acute myocardial infarction.
Authors	Stone GW, Grines CL, Cox DA, et al.
Reference	N Engl J Med 2002;346:957-966.
Disease	Acute myocardial infarction (AMI).
Purpose	To compare the effects of primary balloon angioplasty and stenting with or without abciximab in patients with AMI.
Design	Randomized, 2 × 2 factorial, open-label, multicenter.
Patients	2082 patients, >18 years old, with ≥30 minutes chest pain with <12 hours of onset of symptoms, and ST elevation in ≥2 contiguous leads or left bundle branch block, or other ECG patterns and high-grade coronary stenosis associated with regional wall motion abnormalities. Patients in cardiogenic shock, bleeding diathesis, allergy to abciximab, recent (<6 weeks) major surgery, gastrointestinal or genitourinary bleeding in the preceding 6 months, stroke in the preceding 2 years, hepatic dysfunction, renal impairment, thrombocytopenia, leukopenia, recent thrombolytic therapy, and severe noncardiac illness were excluded. After angiography, only patients with an occlusion of a native coronary artery with a lesion ≤64 mm in length and a reference diameter of 2.5-4.0 mm were included. Patients who needed surgery, multivessel angioplasty, or with anatomy unsuitable for stenting were not included. In addition, patients without a need for revascularization were not included.
Follow-up	12 months. 900 consecutive patients underwent follow-up angiography at 7 months.

Regimen	Patients were randomized in a 2×2 factorial design to PTCA alone (n=518), PTCA + abciximab (n=528), stenting alone (n=512), and stenting + abciximab (n=524). The stents used were MultiLink or MultiLink Duet (Guidant, Santa Clara, CA), 2.5-4.0 mm in diameter. Abciximab was given as a bolus of 0.25 mg/kg followed by 12 hours infusion at a rate of 0.125 μg/kg/min.
Add'l Tx	All patients received aspirin (oral 324 mg or IV 250 mg), ticlopidine 500 mg or clopidogrel 300 mg, heparin 5000 IU, and IV β-blocker (if not contraindicated) before coronary angiography. Crossover to stenting was permitted, if residual stenosis after percutaneous transluminal coronary angioplasty (PTCA) was >50% or if they had ≥type C dissection. Abciximab could be administered to the PTCA alone or stenting alone patients, if "no-reflow" or residual thrombus was noted. All patients received aspirin 325 mg/d, and ticlopidine or clopidogrel for 4 weeks.
Results	Of the 2681 patients enrolled, 2082 patients (77.7%) met the angiographic inclusion criteria and were randomized. 16% of the patients assigned PTCA crossed over to stenting. Less than 10% of the patients assigned stenting underwent PTCA alone. Minimal lumen diameter after PCI was significantly greater for the stenting groups (median 2.20, 2.15, 2.64, and 2.70 for the PTCA, PTCA + abciximab, stenting, and stenting + abciximab group, respectively [p<0.001]). Median residual stenosis after PCI was 25.2%, 25.2%, 11.7%, and 10.8%, respectively (p<0.001). The percentage of patients achieving TIMI grade flow 3 was comparable among the groups (94.7%, 96.1%, 94.5%, and 96.9%, respectively [p=0.16]). The composite end point of death, reinfarction, revascularization, or disabling stroke at 30 days occurred more often in the PTCA alone group (8.3%) than in the PTCA + abciximab (4.8%), stenting alone (5.7%), or stenting + abciximab (4.4%) group (p=0.02). There was no difference in 30-day mortality (p=0.31), reinfarction (p=0.97), or disabling stroke (p=0.79) among the groups. Revascularization for ischemic target vessel rates were lower with stenting than PTCA and with, than without, abciximab (5.6%, 3.4%, 3.2%, and 1.6%, respectively [p=0.004]). Subacute thrombosis occurred less often with abciximab (1.9%, 0.8%, 1.0%, and 0.0%, respectively [p=0.01]). There were no significant differences among the groups in the rate of severe, moderate, or intracranial hemorrhages. However, more patients

receiving (4.2%) than not receiving (1.9%) abciximab needed transfusions (p=0.002). Thrombocytopenia (<100,000 cells/mm^3) occurred more often with abciximab (1.4%, 4.0%, 2.6%, and 4.0%, respectively [p=0.02]). There were no significant differences among the groups in the rates of death (p=0.23), reinfarction (p=0.64), or disabling stroke (p=0.64) at 6 months. Revascularization of ischemic target vessel was noted in 15.7%, 13.8%, 8.3%, and 5.2%, respectively (p<0.001). The composite end point of death, reinfarction, revascularization, or disabling stroke at 6 months occurred less often in the stent groups (20.0%, 16.5%, 11.5%, and 10.2%, respectively [p<0.001]). Stenting alone was superior to PTCA alone (p<0.001), and stenting alone was not inferior to PTCA + abciximab (p<0.001). Among the 900 patients who were scheduled to undergo repeat angiography at 7 months, data was available for 636 patients. Restenosis occurred in 40.8% after PTCA and 22.2% after stenting (p<0.001). Reocclusion was noted in 11.3% and 5.7%, respectively (p=0.01). Abciximab therapy did not change the rates of restenosis or reocclusion. LVEF and regional wall motion in the infarct zone improved to a comparable extent in all 4 groups.

Concl.	Stent implantation (with or without abciximab therapy) was better than PTCA alone for reducing the rate of the composite end point of death, reinfarction, revascularization, or disabling stroke at 30 days and 6 months in patients undergoing primary PCI for acute myocardial infarction. The difference was mainly related to a reduction in the rates of revascularization of ischemic target vessel. Routine stenting resulted also in better angiographic results at 7 months. Abciximab reduced the rates of subacute thrombosis and recurrent ischemia leading to repeat revascularization of the target vessel. However, abciximab was not associated with better TIMI grade flow, and did not reduce the rates of restenosis and late cardiac events.

CADILLAC

Controlled Abciximab and Device Investigation to Lower Late Angioplasty Complications Trial

Title	Benefits and risks of abciximab use in primary angioplasty for acute myocardial infarction.
Authors	Tcheng JE, Kandzari DE, Grines CL, et al.
Reference	Circulation 2003;108:1316-1323.
Disease	Acute myocardial infarction.
Purpose	To assess early and late outcomes by abciximab assignment in patients randomized to primary stenting angioplasty and abciximab vs no abciximab.
Design	Open-label, 2 × 2 factorial design, randomized, multicenter.
Patients	2082 patients with acute myocardial infarction. Patients had to have clinical symptoms of myocardial infarction for <12 hours and either 1 mm ST-segment elevation or high-grade angiographic stenosis with associated regional wall motion abnormality.
Follow-up	30 days and 12 months.
Regimen	Patients were randomized to 1 of 4 reperfusion strategies: 1) percutaneous transluminal coronary angioplasty; 2) percutaneous transluminal coronary angioplasty + abciximab; 3) MultiLink stent implantation; 4) MultiLink stent implantation with abciximab. Abciximab given as 0.25 mg/kg IV bolus followed by 0.125 mg/kg/min infusion for 12 hours.
Add'l Tx	Aspirin, ticlopidine, heparin.

Results	At 30 days, the composite end point of death, MI, ischemia-driven targetvessel revascularization, or disabling stroke was reduced by abciximab therapy (4.6% vs 7.0%; relative risk [RR] 0.65; 95% CI=0.46-0.93; p=0.01). This was driven largely by a decrease in target vessel revascularization in the abciximab group (2.5%) vs control group (4.4%; RR 0.57; 95% CI=0.35-0.91; p=0.02). Abciximab also reduced subacute thrombosis. However at 12 months, the rates of the composite end point did not differ significantly between controls (18.4%) vs abciximab-treated patients (16.9%; RR 0.92; 95% CI=0.76-1.10; p=0.29). This reflected the fact that abciximab did not reduce restenosis and the need for target vessel revascularization. Also, at 1 year, abciximab was not associated with significant reductions in any of the individual components of the primary outcome. In an angiographic substudy done at 7 months (N=656), abciximab did not improve the rates of restenosis, infarct artery reocclusion, or degree of myocardial salvage.
Concl.	Abciximab given during primary PCI for acute MI improved 30-day cardiac eventfree survival, primarily by reducing the need for ischemiadriven target vessel revascularization. However, at 1 year, abciximab no longer affected the primary composite end point, primarily because it did not prevent restenosis or the need for target vessel revascularization at this time.

ENTIRE-TIMI-23

Enoxaparin and TNK-tPA with or Without GP IIIb/IIIa Inhibitor as Reperfusion Strategy in ST Evaluation MI— Thrombolysis in Myocardial Infarction-23

Title	Enoxaparin as adjunctive antithrombin therapy for ST elevation myocardial infarction. Results of the ENTIRE-Thrombolysis in Myocardial Infarction (TIMI) 23 Trial.
Authors	Antman EM, Louwerenburg HW, Baars HF, et al.
Reference	Circulation 2002;105:1642-1649.
Disease	ST elevation acute myocardial infarction.
Purpose	To evaluate low-molecular-weight heparin, enoxaparin, as adjunctive therapy in patients with ST elevation myocardial infarction using full-dose tenecteplase and combination therapy of half-dose tenecteplase + abciximab.
Design	Open-label, dose-ranging study, randomized, multicenter.
Patients	483 patients with ST elevation acute myocardial infarction presenting within 6 hours of symptoms.
Follow-up	30 days.
Regimen	All patients were given aspirin. They were then randomized to either full-dose tenecteplase (TNK) 0.53 mg/kg or combination therapy: abciximab (0.25 mg/kg bolus and then a 12-hour infusion at 0.125 µg/kg/min) and half-dose TNK (0.27 mg/kg); and randomized to either unfractionated heparin (60 U/kg bolus and infusion of 12 U/kg/h ≥36 hours) or to enoxaparin. Enoxaparin regimens included ones with and without an initial IV bolus of 30 mg, with dose ranging for the first 2 subcutaneous injections; followed by 1.0 mg/kg subcutaneously every 12 hours.

HERO-2

Hirulog and Early Reperfusion or Occlusion-2 Trial

Title	Thrombin-specific anticoagulation with bivalirudin vs heparin in patients receiving fibrinolytic therapy for acute myocardial infarction: the HERO-2 randomised trial.
Authors	The HERO-2 Trial Investigators.
Reference	Lancet 2001;358:1855-1863.
Disease	Acute myocardial infarction (AMI).
Purpose	To compare the effects of unfractionated heparin and bivalirudin, a thrombin-specific anticoagulant, on clinical outcomes of patients with AMI who are receiving streptokinase for fibrinolysis.
Design	Randomized, open-label, multicenter.
Patients	17,073 patients, median age 61.8 years (interquartile range 51.9-70.4), within 6 hours of onset of symptoms suggesting AMI, and ≥1 mm ST elevation in ≥2 adjacent ECG leads or presumably new left bundle branch block. Patients at high risk of bleeding, or who had previous stroke, transient ischemic attack within the last 6 months, current oral anticoagulant therapy, low-molecular-weight heparin therapy within the last 12 hours, blood pressure >180/110 mm Hg, and previous treatment with streptokinase were excluded.
Follow-up	30 days.
Regimen	Patients were randomized to bivalirudin (bolus 0.25 mg/kg, followed by an infusion of 0.5 mg/kg/h for 12 hours, and 0.25 mg/kg/h for the next 36 hours) or intravenous heparin (bolus 5000 units, followed by an infusion of 800-1000 units/h (adjusted to body weight) for 48 h. The infusion rate was titrated to maintain an activated partial thromboplastin time of 50-75 seconds.
Add'l Tx	All patients received aspirin 150-325 mg and streptokinase 1.5 million units over 30-60 minutes. Intravenous β-blockers were recommended.

Results   30-day mortality was 10.8% in the bivalirudin group vs 10.9% in the heparin group (OR 0.99; 95% CI=0.90-1.09; p=0.85). After adjusting for baseline risk factors, the mortality rates were 10.5% and 10.9%, respectively (p=0.46). Reinfarction within the first 96 hours occurred in 1.6% of the bivalirudin group vs 2.3% in the heparin group (OR 0.70; 95% CI=0.56-0.87; p=0.001). In-hospital reinfarction occurred in 2.8% and 3.6%, respectively (OR 0.78; 95% CI=0.66-0.93; p=0.005). Death or reinfarction occurred in 12.6% of the patients in the bivalirudin vs 13.6% in the heparin group (OR 0.92; 95% CI=0.83-1.01; p=0.07). Strokes occurred in 1.3% in the bivalirudin vs 1.0% in the heparin group (p=0.07). Intracranial hemorrhage occurred in 0.6% vs 0.4%, respectively (p=0.09). Severe noncerebral bleeding occurred in 0.7% in the bivalirudin group vs 0.5% in the heparin group (p=0.07). Mild bleeding occurred in 12.8% vs 9.0%, respectively (p<0.0001). Transfusions were administered to 1.4% of the patients in the bivalirudin group vs 1.1% in the heparin group (p=0.11).

Concl.   Bivalirudin infusion after streptokinase reduced the adjudicated reinfarction rate within 96 hours by 30%; however, it was not associated with reduction of mortality. Bivalirudin was associated with a small absolute increase risk of mild and moderate bleeding.

HIT-4

Hirudin for the Improvement of Thrombolysis-4

Title	Recombinant hirudin (lepirudin) for the improvement of thrombolysis with streptokinase in patients with acute myocardial infarction. Results of the HIT-4 Trial.
Authors	Neuhaus K-L, Molhoek GP, Zeymer U, et al.
Reference	J Am Coll Cardiol 1999;34:966-973.
Disease	Acute myocardial infarction.
Purpose	To compare hirudin vs heparin as adjunctive therapy to thrombolysis with streptokinase in patients with acute myocardial infarction.
Design	Randomized, double-blind, multicenter.
Patients	1205 patients with acute myocardial infarction presenting within 6 hours of chest pain. ST segment elevation had to be present on the ECG.
Follow-up	90-minute angiography in substudy; 30-day clinical outcomes, 1 year mortality.
Regimen	IV bolus of lepirudin (0.2 mg/kg body weight) or placebo given before streptokinase (1.5 million U IV over 60 minutes) followed by subcutaneous lepirudin (0.5 mg/kg) or unfractionated heparin 12,500 IU twice daily over 5-7 days beginning within 30 minutes of streptokinase. Dose adjustments by aPTT if needed.
Add'l Tx	Aspirin 300 mg loading dose and then 100-200 mg/d.

Results	Primary end point of early and complete patency of infarct artery at 90 minutes after start of drug in angiographic substudy. Secondary end points were composite and individual incidences of death, nonfatal stroke, nonfatal reinfarction, rescue PTCA, or refractory angina, within 30 days; individual incidences of strokes, resolution of ST elevation, and 1 year mortality. Angiographic substudy included 447 patients. Complete patency, defined as TIMI grade 3 flow, occurred in 40.7% (85/209) of lepirudin patients and 33.5% (70/209) of heparin treated patients (p=0.16). There was a nonsignificant trend toward higher TIMI 3 patency rates in lepirudin patients (43.2%) and heparin patients (36.8%) when treatment started within 180 minutes of symptoms vs when it occurred after more than 180 minutes (37.4% lepirudin and 27.6% heparin). Complete ST resolution tended to be higher with lepirudin (28%) than heparin (22%; p=0.05) at 90 minutes but this was not significantly different at 180 minutes (52% vs 48%; p=0.18). There was no difference in combined or individual clinical events between groups. Combined end point occurred in 22.7% of lepirudin and 24.3% of heparin groups (p=NS). 1-year mortality was 9.8% with lepirudin and 8.9% with heparin (p=NS). Total stroke occurred in 1.2% of lepirudin and 1.5% of heparin patients. Hemorrhagic stroke occurred in 0.2% of lepirudin and 0.3% of heparin patients. Major bleeding occurred in 3.3% and 3.5% of lepirudin and heparin groups, respectively.
Concl.	Lepirudin did not significantly improve restoration of blood flow of the infarct artery vessel by angiography but did improve ST segment resolution at 90 minutes.

INTRO AMI

Integrilin and Low-Dose Thrombolysis in Acute Myocardial Infarction Study

Title	Eptifibatide and low-dose tissue plasminogen activator in acute myocardial infarction. The Integrilin and Low-Dose Thrombolysis in Acute Myocardial Infarction (INTRO AMI) trial.
Authors	Brener SJ, Zeymer U, Adgey AAJ, et al.
Reference	J Am Coll Cardiol 2002;39:377-386.
Disease	Acute myocardial infarction.
Purpose	To determine whether the glycoprotein IIb/IIIa inhibitor eptifibatide and reduced-dose tissue plasminogen activator (t-PA) enhances infarct artery patency at 60 minutes vs full dose tPA.
Design	Open-label, dose-finding phase; formal randomization during confirmation phase; multicenter.
Patients	ST elevation acute myocardial infarction patients. Phase A, n=344 (dose finding); Phase B, n=305 (randomization phase).
Follow-up	Acute angiographic then 30-day clinical follow-up.
Regimen	Phase A: Single or double bolus (30 minutes apart) of 180, 180/90, or 180/180 µg/kg eptifibatide followed by an infusion of 1.33 or 2.0 µg/kg per minute plus 25 or 50 mg of tPA.Phase B: Randomized to: 1) Double bolus eptifibatide 180/90 (30 minutes apart) and 1.33 µg/kg per minute infusion with 50 mg tPA (group 1); 2) 180/90 (10 minutes apart) and 2.0 µg/kg per minute with 50 mg tPA (Group 2); or 3) full-dose, weight adjusted tPA (Group 3).
Add'l Tx	Aspirin, weight-adjusted heparin, angiography at 60 minutes and 90 minutes.

Results   Primary end point was incidence of TIMI flow grade 3 at 60
           minutes after tPA bolus. Secondary end point was incidence of
           TIMI flow grade 3 at 90 minutes. Phase A results: 180/90/1.33
           μg/kg per minute eptifibatide plus 50 mg tPA resulted in the
           best rate of TIMI flow grade 3 at 65% and 78% at 60 and 90
           minutes, respectively. Phase B results: TIMI flow grade 3 at 60
           minutes was achieved in 42%, 56%, and 40% of groups 1, 2,
           and 3, respectively ($p=0.04$, group 2 vs group 3). At 90 minutes
           TIMI flow grade 3 was 53%, 62%, 54% respectively, suggesting
           a persistent advantage of combination therapy (Group 2) over
           control (Group 3). Median corrected TIMI frame count was
           38, 33, and 50 for Groups 1, 2, and 3, respectively ($p=0.02$).
           Incidence of death, reinfarction, and revascularization at 30 days
           was similar among groups. Incidence of death was 4%, 5% and
           7%, respectively. Incidence of reinfarction was 8%, 2%, and
           3% respectively. Major bleeding occurred in 8%, 11%, and 6%
           respectively. Intracerebral hemorrhage occurred in 1%, 3%, and
           2% respectively ($p=NS$).

Concl.   Double-bolus eptifibatide (10 minutes apart) with a 48-hour
           infusion and half dose tPA (Group 2) improved quality and
           speed of reperfusion without adverse effects on safety.

ISAR-2

Intracoronary Stenting and Antithrombotic Regimen-2

Title	Effect of glycoprotein IIb/IIIa receptor blockade with abciximab on clinical and angiographic restenosis rate after the placement of coronary stents following acute myocardial infarction.
Authors	Neumann F-J, Kastrati A, Schmitt C, et al.
Reference	J Am Coll Cardiol 2000;35:915-921.
Disease	Coronary artery disease, acute myocardial infarction.
Purpose	To evaluate the effects of abciximab on restenosis after stent implantation following acute myocardial infarction.
Design	Prospective, randomized, single-blinded.
Patients	401 patients with ST segment elevation acute myocardial infarction undergoing coronary angiography and stent implantation within 48 hours after onset of symptoms.
Follow-up	Angiographic follow-up at 6 months, clinical follow-up for 12 months.
Regimen	Before stent placement patients were randomized to abciximab (n=201) (0.25 mg/kg bolus, followed by a 10 µg/min continuous infusion for 12 hours) + heparin (2500 U intra-arterially), or to heparin alone (n=200) (10,000 U intra-arterially), followed by 1000 U/hour for 12 hours after sheath removal.
Add'l Tx	Before angiography, all patients received 5000 U heparin and 500 mg aspirin intravenously. Different types of slotted tube stents were used. All patients received ticlopidine 250 mg bid for 4 weeks and aspirin 100 mg/d throughout the study.

Results   In 14 patients of the heparin alone group, the operators administered nonstudy abciximab. At 30 days any cardiac event (death, reinfarction, and target lesion revascularization) occurred in 5.0% of the abciximab group vs 10.5% of the heparin alone group (relative risk [RR] 0.47; 95% CI=0.25-0.88; p=0.038). Death occurred in 2.0% vs 4.5%, respectively (RR 0.44; 95% CI=0.17-1.18; p=0.16), and myocardial infarction occurred in 0.5% vs 1.5%, respectively (RR 0.33; 95% CI=0.01-4.09; p=0.62). 3% vs 5.0% of the patients in the abciximab and heparin treated patients underwent target lesion revascularization (p=0.30), whereas 3.5% vs 4.5% needed blood transfusion (p=0.79). At 1 year abciximab was associated with 5.7% absolute reduction in cardiac events (death, reinfarction, or target lesion revascularization; p=NS). Among the 397 patients with successful revascularization, 292 patients underwent repeated angiography at 6 months. There were no differences in minimal luminal diameter, % diameter stenosis, and restenosis rate between the 2 groups both immediately after stenting and at 6 months. Restenosis occurred in 31.1% of the abciximab group vs 30.6% of the heparin group. Late luminal loss was 1.26±0.85 mm with abciximab and 1.21±0.74 mm with heparin (p=0.61).

Concl.   Abciximab reduced the rates of death, reinfarction, and target lesion revascularization within the first 30 days following coronary stent insertion after acute myocardial infarction. However, abciximab did not reduce angiographic restenosis rates and was not associated with additional clinical benefits beyond the first 30 days.

MINT

Myocardial Infarction with Novastan and tPA

Title	A multicenter, randomized study of argatroban vs heparin as adjunct to tissue plasminogen activator (tPA) in acute myocardial infarction: MINT Study.
Authors	Jang I-K, Brown DFM, Giugliano RP, et al.
Reference	J Am Coll Cardiol 1999;33:1879-1885.
Disease	Acute myocardial infarction.
Purpose	To compare the small molecule, direct thrombin inhibitor, argatroban to heparin in patients with acute myocardial infarction who were reperfused with tPA.
Design	Randomized, multicenter, angiographic trial (tPA), single blind.
Patients	125 patients with acute myocardial infarction who presented within 6 hours.
Follow-up	90-minute angiography; 30 days.
Regimen	Front loaded tPA and aspirin. Patients then randomized to either low dose argatroban (100 μg/kg bolus plus infusion of 1.0 μg/kg/min), high dose argatroban (100 μg/kg bolus plus 3.0 μg/kg/min. infusion) or heparin as 70 U/kg bolus and 15 U/kg/h infusion up to 1500 U/h. Patients then underwent a 90 minute angiogram. In patients not requiring PTCA, infusion continued for 48-72 hours.
Add'l Tx	IV nitroglycerin prior to angiography; other meds as per physician.

Results	The primary end point was percentage of patients with TIMI grade 3 flow; secondary end point was corrected TIMI frame count at 90 minutes. TIMI grade 3 occurred in 56.8% of low dose argatroban (p=0.2 vs heparin), 58.7% of high dose argatroban patients, (p=0.13 vs heparin) and 42.1% of heparin patients. In those patients that presented after 3 hours, high dose argatroban resulted in more frequent TIMI 3 flow (57.1%) compared to heparin (20%; p=0.03). Corrected TIMI flow rates did not differ significantly among the 3 groups (30.4±3.4 in low dose argatroban, 28.0±2.4 in high dose argatroban, and 39.0±4.6 in the heparin group; p=0.19). Major bleeding occurred in 2.6% of low dose, 4.3% of high dose argatroban, and 10% of heparin patients (p=NS). At 30 days the composite end point of death, recurrent MI, cardiogenic shock, congestive heart failure, revascularization and recurrent ischemia was 32.0% with low dose, 25.5% of high dose, and 37.5% with heparin (p=NS).
Concl.	In patients with delayed presentation of MI, argatroban enhanced reperfusion with tPA vs heparin. There was a trend (although not significantly different) toward lower rates of major bleeding and other adverse events with argatroban vs heparin.

PENTALYSE

Pentasaccharide as an Adjunct to Fibrinolysis in ST Elevation Acute Myocardial Infarction

Title	A synthetic factor-Xa inhibitor (ORG31540/SR9017A) as an adjunct to fibrinolysis in acute myocardial infarction. The PENTALYSE study.
Authors	Coussement PK, Bassand J-P, Convens C, et al.
Reference	Eur Heart J 2001;22:1716-1724.
Disease	Acute myocardial infarction, thrombolysis.
Purpose	To evaluate the efficacy and safety of ORG31540/SR90107A, a synthetic pentasaccharide selective inhibitor of factor-Xa, as an adjunct to alteplase in patients with ST-segment elevation acute myocardial infarction.
Design	Randomized, open-label, dose ranging, multicenter.
Patients	333 patients, 21-75 years old, within 6 hours of onset of ST elevation acute myocardial infarction. Patients with contraindications to thrombolytic therapy, blood pressure >180/110 mm Hg, previous coronary artery bypass grafting (CABG), recent coronary stent insertion, and renal failure were excluded.
Follow-up	Patients underwent coronary angiography at 90 minutes and on day 5-7. Clinical follow-up for 30 days.
Regimen	Randomization to unfractionated heparin (a bolus of 5000 U followed by an infusion of 1000 U/h for 48-72 hours with target activated partial thromboplastin time 50-75 seconds) or pentasaccharide in 3 doses (low, 4-6 mg; medium, 6-10 mg; high, 10-12 mg). Doses were adjusted to body weight. The first dose of pentasaccharide was administered IV, and subsequent treatment continued SC for 5-7 days.
Add'l Tx	All patients received aspirin 150-325 mg/d and IV front loaded alteplase over 90 minutes. In cases that underwent rescue percutaneous coronary intervention (PCI) and glycoprotein IIb/IIIa inhibitor was given, the study drug was discontinued.

Results 326 patients received ≥1 dose of the study medication. At 90 minutes, 68% of the heparin group, and 65%, 69% and 60% of the low-, medium-, and high-dose pentasaccharide, respectively had TIMI 3 flow. On the follow-up angiogram, 75% of the patients treated with heparin vs 81%, 88%, and 89% of the patients in the low-, medium-, and high-dose pentasaccharide groups had TIMI 3 flow (p=0.1 pentasaccharide vs heparin). Among the 155 patients with TIMI 3 at 90 minutes and who did not undergo PCI, there was a trend toward less reocclusion with pentasaccharide (0.9% vs 7.0% with heparin; p=0.065). 30-day mortality was 2.5% in the pentasaccharide groups vs 1.2% in the heparin group. Reinfarction occurred in 3.8% vs 3.6%, respectively. 39% of the patients treated with pentasaccharide vs 51% of the patients in the heparin group underwent revascularization within 30 days (p=0.054). Intracranial hemorrhage or blood transfusion occurred in 7.1% of the patients in both the heparin and pentasaccharide groups.

Concl. Pentasaccharide was as safe and effective as unfractionated heparin in patients treated with alteplase for ST elevation acute myocardial infarction. 5-7 days of subcutaneous administration of pentasaccharide was associated with a trend toward less reocclusion and fewer revascularizations.

PRIME

Promotion of Reperfusion in Myocardial Infarction Evolution

Title	Multicenter, dose-ranging study of efegatran sulfate vs heparin with thrombolysis for acute myocardial infarction: The Promotion of Reperfusion In Myocardial Infarction Evolution (PRIME) trial.
Authors	The PRIME Investigators.
Reference	Am Heart J 2002;143:95-105.
Disease	Acute myocardial infarction.
Purpose	To compare the effects of efegatran, a direct thrombin inhibitor, and unfractionated heparin on the success of reperfusion with tissue plasminogen activator (tPA) in patients with acute myocardial infarction.
Design	Randomized, single-blind, dose-ranging, phase II, multicenter.
Patients	336 patients, 21-75 years old within 12 hours of onset of ischemic symptoms who had ≥0.1 mV ST elevation in ≥2 leads. Patients with contraindications to alteplase (tPA), heparin, or aspirin were excluded. Patients with internal bleeding in the preceding 3 months, child bearing potential, liver or renal impairment, history of central nervous system damage and other advanced illnesses, anemia or thrombocytopenia, allergic asthma, prolonged cardiopulmonary resuscitation, major trauma, blood pressure ≥180/110 mm Hg, cardiogenic shock, left bundle branch block or paced rhythm, use of warfarin, or administration of heparin within 6 hours before randomization were excluded. Patients who underwent thrombolytic therapy, angiography, or revascularization in the preceding 14 days were not included.
Follow-up	Coronary angiography at 90 minutes and day 5-7. 30 days clinical follow-up.

Regimen	Randomization in a 3:1 ratio to efegatran sulfate or unfractionated heparin (n=83) for 72-96 hours. Efegatran was administered in 5 different doses [1] bolus 0.05 mg/kg, infusion 0.3 mg/kg/h (n=15); 2) bolus 0.075 mg/kg, infusion 0.6 mg/kg/h (n=98); 3) bolus 0.1 mg/kg, infusion 0.8 mg/kg/h (n=23); 4) bolus 0.2 mg/kg, infusion 1.0 mg/kg/h (n=75); or 5) bolus 0.3 mg/kg, infusion 1.2 mg/kg/h (n=42)].
Add'l Tx	All patients received accelerated, weight-adjusted tPA. All patients received aspirin 325 mg/d.
Results	90-min TIMI grade flow 3 was achieved by 54% of the patients in the heparin group and by 27% in the low-dose efegatran (dose 1), 56% in the intermediate dose efegatran (dose 2 and 3), and 58% in the high dose efegatran (dose 4 and 5). 90-min TIMI grade flow 2-3 was achieved by 77% of the patients in the heparin group, by 78% in the intermediate-dose efegatran, and by 80% in the high-dose efegatran. The median (25th, 75th percentiles) of LVEF at 90 minutes was comparable in the heparin (56% [45, 61]) and intermediate (53% [46, 59]) and high (52% [45, 59]) doses of efegatran. Rescue angioplasty was performed in 25% of the patients in the heparin group and in 24% in the intermediate- and 24% in the high-dose efegatran groups. At day 5-7, TIMI grade flow 3 was detected in 86% of the patients in the heparin group vs 74% and 76% in the intermediate- and high-dose efegatran. Reocclusion occurred in 4.6% of the patients in the heparin group and in 12% and 10% in the intermediate- and high-dose efegatran groups, respectively (p=0.768). The primary end point of the study (TIMI grade flow <3) was achieved by 53.0% of the patients in the heparin group and in 53.8% of the efegatran treated patients (p=0.90). The rates of major bleeding and bleeding requiring transfusions were comparable among the groups. The combined end point of death, stroke, reinfarction, new heart failure, or refractory ischemia occurred in 23% of the patients in the heparin group and in 34% and 30% in the intermediate- and high-dose efegatran groups (p=0.231). Continuous ST monitoring showed that the median time to steady-state ST recovery was longer for the heparin group (154 minutes [54-302]) than for the efegatran groups (107 minutes [10-180]) (p=0.025). Late ST re-elevation occurred in 25% vs 11%, respectively (p=0.029).

Concl.   As an adjunctive to thrombolytic therapy with tPA, efegatran had
          no advantage over unfractionated heparin in achieving reperfu-
          sion and was even associated with a trend toward increased rates
          of clinical events, although it was associated with faster time to
          resolution of ST elevation and prevention of ST re-elevation.

TIGER-PA

Tirofiban Given in the Emergency Room Before Primary Angioplasty Pilot Trial

Title	Adjunctive platelet glycoprotein IIb/IIIa receptor inhibition with tirofiban before primary angioplasty improves angiographic outcomes.
Authors	Lee DP, Herity NA, Hiatt BL, et al.
Reference	Circulation 2003;107:1497-1501.
Disease	Acute myocardial infarction.
Purpose	To determine if early administration of tirofiban is safe and feasible before primary angioplasty, and whether there is benefit from such early administration in patients with acute myocardial infarction.
Design	Randomized, prospective, single-center.
Patients	100 patients. Patients were included if they had symptoms of acute MI with onset of chest pain in the prior 12 hours, were suitable candidates for percutaneous revascularization, and had ECG that showed ≥ 0.1 mV ST-segment elevation in 2 or more contiguous leads or new left bundle-branch block. Exclusion criteria were cardiogenic shock, use of intra-aortic balloon pump, and known bleeding tendency.
Follow-up	30 days.
Regimen	Patients were randomized to administration of tirofiban in the emergency room or before catheterization. The dose of tirofiban was 10 mg/kg over 3 minutes as a bolus, followed by 0.15 mg $\times$ kg^{-1} $\times$ min^{-1} for 24 hours. The early administration of tirofiban was accompanied with a bolus of heparin 70 U/kg followed by 5 U/kg/h, and late administration of tirofiban was accompanied by 100 U/kg bolus of heparin and then a maintenance dose of 10 U/kg/h. All other medications were given at the discretion of the treating physician. If the culprit lesion was $\leq 50\%$ as seen on angiography, revascularization was not performed. If a stent was placed, clopidogrel (300 mg orally, then 75 mg/d for at least 28 days) or ticlopidine (500 mg orally, then 250 mg bid for at least 28 days) was required.

Results   The angiographic end points were initial and final thrombolysis in MI (TIMI) grade flow, corrected TIMI frame count, and TIMI myocardial perfusion grade of the culprit vessel. There were no significant differences between the 2 groups in patient characteristics or presentation. The early treatment group received tirofiban for an average of 33 minutes (19-45 minutes) before percutaneous intervention. The percentage of patients with initial TIMI grade 3 flow before angioplasty was 32% in the early group and 10% in the late group, a significant difference (p=0.007). The corrected initial TIMI frame counts were significantly decreased in the early group (44±20 vs 66±23; p=0.005). TIMI grade 3 myocardial perfusion was observed in 32% in the early group and 6% in the late group (p<0.001). The final TIMI-grade flow, final corrected TIMI-frame count, and final TIMI myocardial perfusion grades were similar between the 2 groups. There were 5 minor bleeds in the early group and 3 in the late group (p=0.47), with 1 major bleed in each group. At 30 days, there were fewer adverse events (composite of death, recurrent MI, or rehospitalization) in the early group vs the late group (6% vs 10%; p=0.47). There were no significant differences in each of the individual outcomes.

Concl.   In this pilot study, tirofiban administration early in the emergency room to patients with acute MI was associated with improved initial angiographic outcomes, and was safe and feasible in patients undergoing primary angioplasty.

VITAL

Vasoflux International Trial for Acute Myocardial Infarction Lysis

Title	Randomized comparison of a novel anticoagulant, vasoflux, and heparin as adjunctive therapy to streptokinase for acute myocardial infarction: results of the VITAL study (Vasoflux International Trial for Acute Myocardial Infarction Lysis).
Authors	Peters RJG, Spickler W, Theroux P, et al.
Reference	Am Heart J 2001;142:237-243.
Disease	Acute myocardial infarction.
Purpose	To compare the angiographic results after thrombolysis with streptokinase with heparin or vasoflux, a derivative of low-molecular-weight heparin that inhibits activation of factor X by factor IXa and enhances fibrin-bound thrombin inactivation by heparin cofactor II.
Design	Randomized, phase II, dose-finding, single-blind, multicenter.
Patients	277 patients, >18 years old, with ST elevation acute myocardial infarction (or new left bundle branch block), who could be randomized within 6 hours of onset of symptoms. Patients with uncontrolled hypertension, hemodynamic instability, renal or liver disease, prior stroke, bleeding history, or diathesis were excluded.
Follow-up	60- and 90-minute angiography. Clinical follow-up for 30 days.
Regimen	Randomization to IV vasoflux (1, 4, 8, or 16 mg/kg bolus, followed by 1, 4, 8, or 16 mg/kg/h) (n=37, 52, 63, and 66, respectively) or IV unfractionated heparin (bolus 70 U/kg, followed by 14 U/kg/h) (n=59).
Add'l Tx	All patients received aspirin 150-350 mg/d, starting before study drug administration. All patients received streptokinase 1.5 million U over 45-60 minutes. The use of glycoprotein IIb/IIIa inhibitors and other anticoagulant agents was prohibited.

Results	15 patients did not undergo angiography at 90 minutes. TIMI 3 flow grade at 60 minutes was seen in 25% of the patients in the heparin group, and in 21%, 26%, 21% and 31% in the vasoflux 1, 4, 8, and 16 mg/kg groups, respectively. TIMI 3 flow grade at 90 minutes was seen in 41% of the patients in the heparin group and in 36%, 35%, 36%, and 42% in the vasoflux 1, 4, 8, and 16 mg/kg groups, respectively. The median corrected TIMI frame count at 90 minutes was comparable between the heparin (37) and the 1, 4, 8, and 16 mg/kg vasoflux groups (44, 38, 37, and 36, respectively). Major bleeding occurred more frequently in the vasoflux 16 mg/kg group (28%) than in the heparin group (8%) or vasoflux 1 mg/kg (9%), 4 mg/kg (10%), or 8 mg/kg (13%)(p=0.01 vs heparin). None of the patients had intracranial hemorrhage. Bleeding at instrumented sites occurred in 15% of the patients in the heparin group and in 11%, 14%, 23%, and 28% in the vasoflux 1, 4, 8, and 16 mg/kg, respectively. There were no statistically significant differences among the groups in 30-day mortality, recurrent myocardial infarction, or need for urgent revascularization.
Concl.	As an adjunctive therapy to aspirin and streptokinase, vasoflux was not better than unfractionated heparin in improving angiographic results and was associated with increased risk of bleeding at the higher doses. Targeting factor IXa and heparin cofactor II may not improve the results of thrombolysis with streptokinase.

Title	A randomized trial comparing primary infarct artery stenting with or without abciximab in acute myocardial infarction.
Authors	Antoniucci D, Rodriguez A, Hempel A, et al.
Reference	J Am Coll Cardiol 2003;42:1879-1885.
Disease	Acute myocardial infarction.
Purpose	To compare the outcome in patients with acute myocardial infarction treated with stenting alone vs stenting + abciximab.
Design	Randomized, multicenter.
Patients	400 patients with ST-segment elevation, acute myocardial infarction, admitted within 6 hours of symptoms.
Follow-up	6 months.
Regimen	Following coronary angiography, patients were randomized to stenting alone or stenting + abciximab. Stenting had to be attempted with carbo-film-coated tubular stent. Patients randomized to abciximab received a bolus of 0.25 mg/kg body weight followed by a 12-hour infusion of 0.125 µg/kg/min.
Add'l Tx	Aspirin, heparin, ticlopidine, or clopidogrel.

Results	Primary end point was composite of death from any cause, reinfarction, target vessel revascularization, and stroke within 1 month. Incidence of primary end point was lower in abciximab group (4.5%) vs stent-alone group (10.5%; p=0.023). Components of the primary end point tended to be lower in the abciximab group. Death at 30 days was 3.5% in stenting + abciximab group vs 4% in the stenting-alone group. Reinfarction at 30 days was 4.5% in stenting-alone group vs 0.5% in stenting + abciximab group (p=0.010). ST-segment reduction ≥50% at 30 minutes was 68% in the stenting-alone group vs 85% in the stenting + abciximab group (p<0.001). Infarct size assessed by 1 month technetium-99m sestamibi scintigraphy was smaller in the abciximab + stenting group (median=12.50) vs the stenting-alone group (median=16.6; p=0.067). There was no detectable scintigraphy defect in 18% of stenting + abciximab patients vs 8% of stenting-alone patients (p=0.032). At 6 months death had occurred in 4.5% of stenting + abciximab group vs 8.0% of stenting-alone group (p=0.148). Reinfarction at 6 months occurred in 1% of stenting + abciximab group vs 5.5% of the stenting-alone group (p=0.011). 6 month repeat target vessel revascularization and restenosis rates were similar in the stenting + abciximab vs stenting-alone group.
Concl.	Abciximab + infarct-related artery stenting should be considered routine therapy in patients with ST elevation acute MI.

ACE

Abciximab and Carbostent Evaluation Trial

Title	Abciximab-supported infarct artery stent implantation for acute myocardial infarction and long-term survival. A prospective, multicenter, randomized trial comparing infarct artery stenting plus abciximab with stenting alone.
Authors	Antoniucci D, Migliorini A, Parodi G, et al.
Reference	Circulation 2004;109:1704-1706.
Disease	Acute myocardial infarction.
Purpose	To determine the effect of abciximab on 1-year survival and other major adverse cardiac events of patients with acute myocardial infarction undergoing routine infarct artery stenting.
Design	Multicenter, unblinded, randomized, controlled trial.
Patients	400 patients with ST-segment elevation acute myocardial infarction.
Follow-up	1 year.
Regimen	Abciximab + stenting (n=200) or stenting alone (n=200).
Results	At 1 year, the survival rate was 95%±2% in the abciximab group and 88%±2% in the stent-only group, (p=0.017). Cardiovascular death occurred in 10.5% of stent-alone patients vs 5% of stent + abciximab patients (p=0.04). The reinfarction rate was 1% in the abciximab group and 6% in the stent-only group. There was no significant difference between the groups in rates of target-vessel revascularization (16.5% in the abciximab group vs 17.5% in the stent-only group).
Concl.	Adjunctive abciximab with infarct artery stenting for acute MI yielded improved 1-year survival and a lower reinfarction rate. This trial showed that abciximab may prevent target-vessel failure in the early phase by virtue of its antiplatelet effect and provide better myocardial reperfusion by virtue of its antithrombotic and anti-inflammatory effects.

BRAVE

Bavarian Reperfusion Alternatives Evaluation

Title	Early administration of reteplase plus abciximab vs abciximab alone in patients with acute myocardial infarction referred for percutaneous coronary intervention: a randomized controlled trial.
Authors	Kastrati A, Mehilli J, Schlotterbeck K, et al.
Reference	JAMA 2004;291:947-954.
Disease	Acute myocardial infarction.
Purpose	To assess whether early administration of reteplase + abciximab produces better results than abciximab alone in patients with acute myocardial infarction referred for percutaneous coronary intervention.
Design	Multicenter, open-label, randomized, controlled study.
Patients	253 patients with ST-segment elevation acute myocardial infarction presenting within 12 hours of onset of symptoms.
Follow-up	6 months.
Regimen	The combination of a half-dose of reteplase (two 5-U boluses 30 minutes apart) + a standard dose of abciximab (0.25 mg/kg bolus, 0.125 µg/kg/min infusion up to a maximum of 10 µg/min for 12 hours) (n=125) or standard-dose abciximab alone (n=128).
Add'l Tx	Patients referred for percutaneous coronary intervention.

Results   The main outcome measure was final infarct size by single pho-
           ton emission computed tomography with technetium-99m ses-
           tamibi, performed 5-10 days after randomization in 228 patients
           (90.1% of the sample). The median (interquartile range) of the
           final infarct size of the left ventricle was 13% (3%-28%) in the
           combination therapy group and 11.5% (3%-26.3%) in the
           abciximab-only group (p=0.81). The mean difference in final
           infarct size between the groups was 1.3% (95% CI=-3.1 to
           5.7). Within 6 months, a composite secondary end point event
           (death, recurrent MI, or stroke) occurred in 8 patients (6.4%)
           in the combination therapy group and 6 patients (4.7%) in the
           abciximab group (relative risk 1.4; 95% CI=0.5-3.9; log-rank
           p=0.56). Major bleeding complications occurred in 7 patients
           (5.6%) in the combination therapy group and in 2 (1.6%) in
           the abciximab group (p=0.16). 2 patients in each group died
           within 30 days of randomization, and 5 in each group died
           within 6 months.

Concl.   Early administration of reteplase + abciximab did not lead to
           a reduction in infarct size compared with abciximab alone in
           patients with acute MI referred for PCI. Further, clinical out-
           come was not improved by combination therapy. The larger
           ongoing FINESSE trial should yield more information on the
           outcome with the combination therapy.

On-TIME

Ongoing Tirofiban in Myocardial Infarction Evaluation

1c

Title	Facilitation of primary coronary angioplasty by early start of a glycoprotein 2b/3a inhibitor: results of the ongoing tirofiban in myocardial infarction evaluation (On-TIME) trial.
Authors	van't Hof AWJ, Ernst N, de Boer M-J, et al.
Reference	Eur Heart J 2004;25:837-846.
Disease	Acute myocardial infarction.
Purpose	To assess the effects of adding tirofiban to aspirin and IV heparin on the initial thrombolysis in myocardial infarction flow of the infarct-related artery in patients with ST elevation myocardial infarction transported for primary coronary intervention.
Design	Randomized, double-blind, placebo-controlled, multicenter.
Patients	507 patients, ≤80 years old, with ST elevation (>0.2 mV in precordial leads or >0.1 mV in limb leads) who could undergo primary angioplasty within 6 hours of onset of symptoms. Women <50 years old, patients who received thrombolytic therapy in the preceding 24 hours, patients treated with oral anticoagulants, those with contraindication to glycoprotein IIb/IIIa inhibitors, patients on hemodialysis, and patients with Killip class III or IV were excluded.
Follow-up	Angiography prior to primary angioplasty. 1-year clinical follow-up.
Regimen	Patients were randomized to tirofiban (10 µg/kg bolus followed by 0.15 µg/kg/min infusion) or placebo.
Add'l Tx	All patients received IV aspirin 250 mg and heparin 5000 IU before transportation. All patients underwent coronary angiography. Before angioplasty, all patients received a second bolus of the study drug (tirofiban for those who received placebo and placebo for those who received tirofiban initially) and then all patients received open-label tirofiban 0.15 µg/kg/min for 24 h. All patients received clopidogrel for 1 month and aspirin, β-blockers, statins, and angiotensin-converting enzyme inhibitors.

Results	A total of 251 patients were randomized to early tirofiban and 256 to tirofiban in the catheterization laboratory (late). Pretreatment time was 59 minutes longer (11-178 min) in the early vs the late group. A total of 14 patients (3%) did not have an acute MI. TIMI flow in the infarct-related artery could be assessed in 487 (99%) patients with confirmed MI. The initial TIMI flow grade was 3 in 19% of the patients in the early group compared to 15% in the late group (p=0.22). TIMI 2-3 flow was present in 43% of the early group vs 34% in the late group (p=0.04). Less patients in the early group had TIMI 0 flow (44% vs 59%). Intracoronary thrombus was found in 25% of the patients in the early group vs 32% in the late group (p=0.06). Thrombus or fresh occlusion was diagnosed in 60% vs 73% of the patients, respectively (p=0.002). A preangioplasty myocardial blush grade 2 or 3 was present in 30% of the patients in the early group vs only 22% in the late group (p=0.04). The postangioplasty TIMI flow was 3 in 90% of the patients in the early group and in 91% in the late group (p=0.74). There was no difference in myocardial blush grade or TIMI frame count postangioplasty between the groups (p=0.87 and p=0.76, respectively). 30-day mortality was 3.7% in the early group and 0.8% in the late group (p=0.03). Recurrent infarction occurred in 1.2% and 0.8% of the patients, respectively (p=0.65). Major bleeding occurred in 4.5% and 3.2% of the patients, respectively (p=0.47). 1-year mortality was 4.5% in the early group and 3.7% in the late group (p=0.66). After 1 year, death or reinfarction occurred in 7.0% of the patients in each group (p=0.99).
Concl.	Early initiation of tirofiban was not effective in improving initial TIMI 3 flow of the infarct-related artery. Although early tirofiban therapy was associated with better patency rate (TIMI 2-3 flow), a significantly lower intracoronary thrombus load and a better myocardial tissue perfusion before angioplasty, there was no difference between the groups in the postangioplasty angiographic results or clinical outcome. Routine initiation of tirofiban before primary angioplasty is not justified.

SASTRE

Reperfusion Regimens in ST-Elevation MI

Title	Comparison of reperfusion regimens with or without tirofiban in ST-elevation acute myocardial infarction.
Authors	Martinez-Rios MA, Rosas M, Gonzales H, et al.
Reference	Am J Cardiol 2004;93:280-287.
Disease	Acute myocardial infarction.
Purpose	To determine if a conjunctive strategy for reperfusion, using the glycoprotein IIb/IIIa inhibitor tirofiban + either reduced-dose alteplase or primary stenting percutaneous coronary intervention, improves thrombolysis in myocardial infarction flow and thrombolysis in myocardial infarction perfusion grade scores compared with the conventional strategies of either full-dose alteplase or primary stenting percutaneous coronary intervention alone.
Design	Multicenter, prospective, 2-parallel, phase II, open-label, randomized, angiographic trial.
Patients	144 patients with acute ST-elevation myocardial infarction presenting <6 hours of symptoms.
Follow-up	30 days.
Regimen	"Conjunctive" strategy of low-dose alteplase (50 mg) and tirofiban (0.4 µg/kg/min, 30-minute bolus, infusion of 0.1 µg/kg/min) or tirofiban + stenting; or "control" treatment with full-dose alteplase (100 mg) or stenting.
Add'l Tx	Aspirin, IV heparin, and additional medical therapy at the discretion of the physician.

Results	All patients underwent coronary angiography at 90 minutes. The primary end point was TIMI grade 3 flow at 90 minutes. Secondary end points were TIMI perfusion (TMP) rates, a composite end point at 30 days (death, reinfarction, refractory ischemia, stroke, CHF, revascularization, or pulmonary edema), and bleeding or hematologic variables. Rate of TIMI 3 flow at 90 minutes for alteplase alone patients was 42% vs 66% for those who received low-dose alteplase and tirofiban. Standard stenting yielded TIMI 3 flow in 81% vs 92% when tirofiban was used. Significantly higher rates of TMP grade 3 were observed when tirofiban was used as the adjunctive treatment with alteplase (66% vs 47%) and stenting (73% vs 55%). The composite clinical end point was more likely to be achieved in patients who received standard regimens compared with conjunctive regimens (hazard ratio 5.8; 95% CI=1.27-26.6; p=0.023). Better outcomes were achieved when a combination of TIMI 3 flow and TMP grade 3 was achieved, independent of the reperfusion regimen. The bleeding rates were 2.8% for standard and conjunctive regimens with tirofiban.
Concl.	Tirofiban as a conjunctive therapy for lytic and stenting regimens improves TIMI 3 flow rates as well as TMP 3 rates. These are associated with better clinical outcomes and no increase in the risk of major bleeding. The findings of this study support the hypothesis that platelets play an important role in the atherothrombotic process and in disturbances of microcirculation and tissue perfusion.

TETAMI

Tirofiban in Acute MI in Patients Ineligible for Reperfusion

Title	The safety and efficacy of subcutaneous enoxaparin vs intravenous unfractionated heparin and tirofiban vs placebo in the treatment of acute ST-segment elevation myocardial infarction patients ineligible for reperfusion (TETAMI): a randomized trial.
Authors	Cohen M, Gensini GF, Maritz F, et al.
Reference	J Am Coll Cardiol 2003;42:1348-1356.
Disease	Acute myocardial infarction.
Purpose	To determine whether enoxaparin is better than unfractionated heparin and whether tirofiban is better than placebo in patients with acute ST-segment elevation myocardial infarction who do not receive timely reperfusion.
Design	International, multicenter, randomized, double-blind, double-dummy, placebo-controlled, parallel-group study.
Patients	1224 patients with ST-segment elevation myocardial infarction ineligible for acute reperfusion.
Follow-up	30 days.
Regimen	Enoxaparin, enoxaparin + tirofiban, unfractionated heparin, or unfractionated heparin + tirofiban.
Add'l Tx	Aspirin.

Results	The primary efficacy end point was the 30-day combined incidence of death, reinfarction, or recurrent angina; the primary analysis was the comparison of the pooled enoxaparin and unfractionated heparin (UFH) groups. The incidence of the primary efficacy end point was not significantly different between the pooled enoxaparin and UFH groups: 15.7% vs 17.3% (OR 0.89; 95% CI=0.66-1.21). Similar results were observed for the tirofiban and placebo groups, 16.6% vs 16.4% (OR 1.02; 95% CI=0.75-1.38). The major hemorrhage rate was 1.5% for enoxaparin vs 1.3% for UFH (OR 1.16; 95% CI=0.44-3.02) and 1.8% for tirofiban vs 1% for placebo (OR 1.82; 95% CI=0.67-4.95). TIMI minor hemorrhage occurred in 4.2% of patients, with no significant difference between groups. Safety profiles were similar among the groups. The most common nonbleeding adverse event was heart failure (7%) followed by chest pain (5.4%) and hypotension (4.8%). A total of 14.7% of patients had a serious adverse event, with similar rates among groups.
Concl.	Enoxaparin did not significantly reduce the 30-day incidence of death, reinfarction, or recurrent angina compared with UFH in patients with ST-segment elevation MI who were ineligible for reperfusion. The safety and efficacy of enoxaparin are similar to those for UFH.

1. Acute Myocardial Infarction
d. Anticoagulation After Myocardial Infarction

Warfarin, Aspirin, or Both After Myocardial Infarction

Title	Warfarin, aspirin, or both after myocardial infarction.
Authors	Hurlen M, Abdelnoor M, Smith P, et al.
Reference	N Engl J Med 2002;347:969-974.
Disease	Myocardial infarction.
Purpose	To evaluate the efficacy and safety of warfarin, aspirin, or both after acute MI in preventing morbidity and mortality.
Design	Open, randomized, prospective, multicenter.
Patients	3630 patients, randomized to aspirin (n=1206), warfarin (n=1216), or aspirin + warfarin (n=1208). Eligible patients were <75 years, hospitalized for acute MI, as defined according to World Health Organization recommendations: history of typical chest pain; electrocardiographic changes consistent with MI; and a creatine kinase level >250 U/L, aspartate aminotransferase >50 U/L, or both, likely of cardiac origin. Patients were excluded if they had either an indication for or contraindication to any study drugs, malignant disease, or anticipated poor compliance.
Follow-up	Mean 4 years.
Regimen	Warfarin, with a target international normalized ratio (INR) of 2.8-4.2, or aspirin 160 mg/d, or aspirin 75 mg/d together with warfarin with a target INR of 2.0-2.5.

Results	The primary outcome was a composite of death, nonfatal reinfarction, or thromboembolic stroke. The secondary outcomes were each of the above analyzed separately. The primary outcome occurred in 20% of the aspirin group, 16.7% of the warfarin group (relative risk (RR) compared to aspirin 0.81; 95% CI=0.69-0.95; p=0.03) and 15.0% of the warfarin + aspirin group (RR compared to aspirin 0.71; 95% CI=0.60-0.83; p=0.001). The difference in primary outcome between the groups receiving warfarin was not statistically significant. The number of reinfarctions in the aspirin plus warfarin group was less than in the aspirin group (69/1208 vs 117/1206; RR 0.56; 95% CI=0.41-0.78; p<0.001). Reinfarction also occurred less frequently in the warfarin only group compared to the aspirin group (90/1216 vs 117/1206; RR 0.74; 95% CI=0.55-0.98; p=0.03). The incidence of thromboembolic stroke was similar in the warfarin groups (17/1208 in the combined group, 17/1216 in the warfarin-only group) and smaller than in the aspirin group (32/1206); RR 0.52 (95% CI=0.28-0.98), p=0.03 for combined group vs aspirin; RR 0.52 (95% CI=0.28-0.97), p=0.03 for warfarin only vs aspirin. There was no statistically significant difference in the incidence of death across the 3 groups. A total of 69 major bleeding episodes were recorded: 8 in the aspirin group, 33 in the warfarin group, and 28 in the combined group. The rate ratio of bleeding episodes between aspirin and warfarin was 0.25 (95% CI=0.10-0.60), which was significant.
Concl.	Warfarin, alone or in combination with aspirin, was more effective than aspirin alone in preventing nonfatal reinfarction and thromboembolic stroke, as well as reducing the incidence of the composite end point of reinfarction, stroke, and death. Usage of warfarin was associated with a slightly higher risk of bleeding.

APRICOT-2

Antithrombotics in the Prevention of Reocclusion in Coronary Thrombolysis Trial-2

Title	Aspirin plus coumarin versus aspirin alone in the prevention of reocclusion after fibrinolysis for acute myocardial infarction.
Authors	Brouwer MA, van den Bergh PJPC, Aengevaeren WRM, et al.
Reference	Circulation 2002;106:659-665.
Disease	Acute myocardial infarction.
Purpose	To determine whether aspirin and coumarin is superior to aspirin alone in preventing reocclusion in patients who have undergone fibrinolysis for ST elevation myocardial infarction.
Design	Randomized, open-label, multicenter.
Patients	308 were randomized: 135 to the aspirin plus coumarin group, 139 to the aspirin only group. Eligible patients had chest pain for ≥30 minutes and ≤6 hours and were unresponsive to nitrates. Patients were treated with fibrinolysis if ST elevation was ≥0.2 mV in ≥2 contiguous precordial leads or ≥0.1 mV in ≥2 limb leads. Exclusion criteria were age >75 years; a contraindication to antithrombotic therapy; patients with an infarct-related vessel that was a bypass graft; infarct-related stenosis that was previously dilated; patients with left main stem stenosis or unidentifiable culprit lesion.
Follow-up	3 months.

Regimen	Fibrinolytic agents were anistreplase (30 U in 5 minutes), strep-tokinase (1.5 million U in 30-60 minutes), reteplase (2 boluses of 10 U, 30 minutes apart), or accelerated recombinant tissue-type plasminogen activator. All patients received aspirin starting at 160 mg and then 80 mg qd. Unfractionated heparin was given intravenously for 48 hours as a bolus of 5000 U followed by an infusion of 24,000 U over 24 hours, with a target activated partial thromboplastin time twice the control. Coronary angiography was performed within 48 hours after study entry, and patients were eligible if they had TIMI grade 3 flow. Patients were then randomized: in 1 group, patients continued to use aspirin 80 mg daily, and heparin was discontinued at 48 hours; in the other group, coumarin was added to the 80 mg of aspirin, with heparin being continued until a target international normalized ratio between 2.0-3.0 was achieved, after which heparin was discontinued.
Results	The primary end point was reocclusion of the involved artery, defined as TIMI grade 2 flow or less, determined by angiography at 3-month follow-up. The secondary end point was event-free survival: an event was defined as all-cause death, reinfarction, or revascularization. Clinical and angiographic characteristics were similar between the 2 groups at baseline. Angiographic follow-up was available for 251 of the 274 enrolled patients (92%). Reocclusion occurred in 19 of 123 patients (15%) in the aspirin + coumarin group, and 36 of 128 (28%) in the aspirin-only group (relative risk [RR] 0.55; 95% CI=0.33-0.90; p<0.02). The difference was mostly accounted for by a reduced occurrence of TIMI grade 0-1 flow: 11/123 (9%) patients in the combined group vs 25/128 (20%) (RR 0.46; 95% CI=0.24-0.89; p<0.02). The secondary end point, event-free survival, occurred in 116/135 (86%) patients in the combined group vs 92/139 (66%) patients in the aspirin-only group (p<0.01). In the combined group, there were significantly fewer reinfarctions (3 vs 11; p<0.05) and revascularizations (17 vs 43; p<0.01), but little difference in deaths (1 vs 0). There were 7 bleeding complications as defined by the TIMI criteria in the combined group vs 4 in the aspirin alone group; this difference was not significant.
Concl.	The combination of aspirin and coumarin is superior to aspirin alone in preventing reocclusion and revascularization in patients with ST-elevation MI. The addition of coumarin was not associated with a significantly increased risk of bleeding.

ASPECT-2

Antithrombotics in the Secondary Prevention of Events in Coronary Thrombosis-2

Title	Aspirin and coumadin after acute coronary syndromes (the ASPECT-2 study): a randomised controlled trial.
Authors	van Es RF, Jonker JJ, Verheugt FW, et al.
Reference	Lancet 2002;360:109-113.
Disease	Coronary artery disease.
Purpose	To compare the efficacy of high-intensity coumadin, aspirin plus moderate-intensity coumadin, and aspirin alone in patients after an acute coronary event.
Design	Randomized, open-label, multicenter.
Patients	999 patients within 8 weeks of admission for an acute myocardial infarction or unstable angina. Patients with established indications for oral anticoagulant therapy or platelet inhibitors (after PCI) were excluded. In addition, patients with contraindications to the study drugs, planned revascularization, serious comorbidity, increased risk of bleeding, anemia, or platelet disorder, and history of stroke were not included.
Follow-up	Patients were followed for a median of 12 months (range 0-26 months).
Regimen	Randomization to aspirin (100 mg/d of pulverized carbasalate calcium) (n=336); coumadin with a target INR 3.0-4.0 (n=330); or to aspirin plus coumadin with a target INR of 2.0-2.5 (n=333).

Results   The study was terminated earlier than planned in 1999 because of slow patient recruitment. Mean INR in the high-intensity anticoagulation group was 3.2±1.1 and in the combination therapy group 2.4±0.9. Eighty percent of the patients received beta-blockers, 33% ACE-inhibitors, and 54% to 60% received statins. The primary end point (death, MI, or stroke) occurred less often in the high-intensity anticoagulation group (5%; hazard ratio [HR] vs aspirin 0.55; 95% CI=0.30-1.00; p=0.0479) or the combination therapy group (5%; HR 0.50; 95% CI=0.27-0.92; p=0.03) than in the aspirin alone group (9%). All-cause mortality was 4% in the aspirin alone group; 1% in the high-intensity anticoagulation group (HR vs aspirin 0.28%; 95% CI=0.09-0.82); and 3% in the combination group (HR 0.60; 95% CI=0.26-1.36). Myocardial infarction occurred in 4%, 4%, and 3% of the patients, respectively. 12% of the patients in the aspirin group, 10% in the high-intensity anticoagulation group, and 10% in the combination group underwent revascularization. There was no difference in the rate of stroke among groups (1%, 0, and 0.3%, respectively). Major bleeding occurred in 1%, 1%, and 2%, respectively. 1% of the patients in each group needed transfusion. Minor bleeding occurred in 5% of the patients in the aspirin group, 8% in the high-intensity anticoagulation group, and 15% in the combination group.

Concl.   High-intensity anticoagulation (Target INR 3.0-4.0) or medium-intensity anticoagulation (Target INR 2.0-2.5) and low-dose aspirin were more effective than low-dose aspirin alone (80 mg/d) in patient with recent MI or unstable angina that were treated conservatively without revascularization.

CARS (Substudy)

Coumadin Aspirin Reinfarction Study (Substudy)

Title	Initiation of hormone replacement therapy after acute myocardial infarction is associated with more cardiac events during follow-up.
Authors	Alexander KP, Newby LK, Hellkamp AS, et al.
Reference	J Am Coll Cardiol 2001;38:1-7.
Disease	Myocardial infarction (MI); coronary artery disease.
Purpose	To examine association between hormone replacement therapy (HRT) and risk of cardiovascular events in a secondary cohort of the CARS.
Design	Substudy analysis of CARS trial.
Patients	1857 postmenopausal women post-MI patients, who were prior/current hormone replacement users (therapy begun before enrollment) or were new users if they began HRT during the study; or never users.
Follow-up	≈24 months.
Regimen	As part of CARS trial, patients with recent MI (3-21 days) were randomized to aspirin vs warfarin. The use of HRT in this analysis was left up to the discretion of the patient and physician. It included estrogen only or estrogen/progestin.
Add'l Tx	Other usual care as per CARS.

Results	413 (22%) took hormone replacement at randomization or within the prior 2 years. 111 (6%) began hormones during study follow-up and were classified as new users, while 1333 women (72%) never took HRT. The primary end point for the overall CARS study was composite of reinfarction, nonfatal ischemic stroke, or cardiovascular death. The incidence of death/MI/unstable angina was 41% among new users vs 28% among never users (p=0.001). This was mainly due to a higher incidence of unstable angina at 39% among new users vs 20% among non-users (p=0.001). New users were more likely to undergo PTCA (23%) than never users (10%; p=0.001). New users were less likely to experience reinfarction (4%) vs never users (9%; p=0.03). The incidence of death was 0% in new users vs 6% (p=0.001) among never users. After adjustment for baseline variables the hazard ratio for likelihood of death/unstable angina/myocardial infarction among new users remained higher than never users (RR 1.44; 95% CI=1.05-1.99) but was not increased among prior users. Patients on estrogen/progestin had a lower incidence of death/myocardial infarction/unstable angina vs users of estrogen only (RR 0.56; 95% CI=0.37-0.85).
Concl.	Postmenopausal women that started hormone replacement therapy after a recent MI had an increased risk of unstable angina during follow-up.

CHAMP

Combination Hemotherapy and Mortality Prevention

Title	Department of veterans affairs cooperative studies program clinical trial comparing combined warfarin and aspirin with aspirin alone in survivors of acute myocardial infarction. Primary results of the CHAMP Study.
Authors	Fiore LD, Ezekowitz MD, Brophy MT, et al.
Reference	Circulation 2002;105:557-563.
Disease	Acute myocardial infarction (MI).
Purpose	To determine whether combined aspirin and warfarin was more effective in reducing death and vascular events than aspirin alone in acute MI patients.
Design	Randomized, open-label, multicenter.
Patients	5059 patients with qualifying acute MI within the preceding 14 days prior to randomization.
Follow-up	Median of 2.7 years.
Regimen	Warfarin (target international normalized ratio [INR] of 1.5-2.5 IU) + aspirin (81 mg/d; n=2522) vs aspirin monotherapy (162 mg/d; n=2537) within 14 days of MI.
Results	Primary outcome was all-cause mortality and secondary outcomes were recurrent MI and stroke, and major hemorrhage. 17.3% of the aspirin monotherapy group and 17.6% of the combination therapy group died (p=NS). Recurrent MI occurred in 13.1% on aspirin and 13.3% on combination therapy (p=NS). Stroke occurred in 3.5% on aspirin and 3.1% on combination (p=NS). Combination therapy was associated with more major bleeding (1.28 events per 100 person-years) than aspirin alone (0.72 events per 100 person-years). Intracranial hemorrhage occurred in 15 patients in the aspirin and 14 patients in the combination group (p=NS). The median INR value was 1.8 U (for warfarin group).
Concl.	Adding warfarin at a median INR of 1.8 to low-dose aspirin did not improve clinical outcome compared to aspirin alone in patients with acute MI.

JAMIS

Japanese Antiplatelet Myocardial Infarction Study

Title	Effects of aspirin and trapidil on cardiovascular events after acute myocardial infarction.
Authors	Yasue H, Ogawa H, Tanaka H, et al.
Reference	Am J Cardiol 1999;83:1308-1313.
Disease	Acute myocardial infarction.
Purpose	To compare the effects of aspirin 81 mg/d, trapidil 300 mg/d, and no antiplatelet therapy, started within 1 month after an acute MI.
Design	Randomized, open-label, multicenter.
Patients	723 patients within 1 month of an acute MI. Patients with congestive heart failure, severe angina, serious ventricular arrhythmia, coexisting severe illness, and hypersensitivity to aspirin or trapidil were excluded.
Follow-up	An average of 475 days.
Regimen	Randomization to aspirin 81 mg/d (n=250), trapidil 100 mg tid (n=243), and no antiplatelet medications (n=230).
Add'l Tx	Nitrates, calcium antagonists, β-blockers and ACE inhibitors were permitted. Patients who underwent percutaneous coronary intervention were withdrawn from the study, because antiplatelet drugs were administered.

Results	Reinfarction occurred in 5 patients in the aspirin group, 9 in the trapidil group, and 17 in the control group. The RR of reinfarction with aspirin compared to control was 0.271 (95% CI=0.101 to 0.722; p=0.0045). The RR of reinfarction with trapidil compared with control was 0.501 (95% CI=0.228 to 1.101; p=0.081). 6 patients in the aspirin group, 4 in the trapidil group and 5 in the control group died because of cardiovascular reasons (RR of aspirin compared with control 1.104; p=0.92; RR of trapidil compared with control 0.757; p=0.70. Cardiovascular events occurred in 36 patients in the aspirin group, 22 patients in the trapidil group and in 42 patients in the control group (RR of aspirin compared with control 0.789; 95% CI=0.525-1.185; p=0.20; RR of trapidil vs control 0.496; 95% CI=0.306-0.804; p=0.0039. Adverse effects were observed in 7 patients in the aspirin group vs 16 in the trapidil group. The study was discontinued because of PCI in 16 patients in the aspirin group, 8 in the trapidil group and 7 in the control group.
Concl.	Long-term aspirin 81 mg/d significantly reduced the risk of reinfarction compared with control. Trapidil was associated with a statistically insignificant reduction of the risk of reinfarction, compared with control. However, compared with no antiplatelet therapy, trapidil, but not aspirin, was associated with a significant reduction of the incidence of cardiovascular events (including cardiovascular mortality, reinfarction, uncontrolled unstable angina and nonfatal ischemic stroke).

STAMI

Study of Ticlopidine vs Aspirin in Myocardial Infarction

Title	Ticlopidine vs aspirin after myocardial infarction (STAMI) Trial.
Authors	Scrutinio D, Cimminiello C, Marubini E, et al.
Reference	J Am Coll Cardiol 2001;37:1259-1265.
Disease	Acute myocardial infarction.
Purpose	To compare efficacy of ticlopidine to aspirin in survivors of acute myocardial infarction who had been treated with thrombolytic therapy.
Design	Randomized, double-blind, multicenter trial.
Patients	1470 patients with acute myocardial infarction who received thrombolytic therapy and survived hospitalization.
Follow-up	6 months.
Regimen	Ticlopidine (250 mg tablets; n=734) vs plain aspirin (80 mg tablets; n=736) bid after meals.
Add'l Tx	Use of anticoagulants or additional antiplatelet agents was forbidden.
Results	Primary end point was first occurrence during 6 month period of fatal and nonfatal MI, fatal and nonfatal stroke, angina with objective evidence of myocardial ischemia, vascular death, or mortality due to any cause. A primary end point occurred in 59 (8.0%) of the ticlopidine patients and 59 (8.0%) of the aspirin patients (p=0.966). There was no difference in incidence of vascular death between ticlopidine patients (0.8%) vs aspirin patients (0.7%; p=NS). Nonfatal acute MI occurred in 8 (1.1%) ticlopidine patients and 18 (2.4%) aspirin patients; p=0.049. There was no significant difference in incidence of nonfatal stroke (0.5 vs 0.4%; p=NS) or angina (5.4% vs 4.4%; p=NS) between ticlopidine vs aspirin groups, respectively. 12.3% in the ticlopidine group vs 9.8% in the aspirin group reported drug related adverse events (p=NS).

Concl.   There was no significant difference in the rate of primary combined end point of death, recurrent acute MI, stroke, and angina between ticlopidine vs aspirin therapy in hospital survivors of acute MI who received thrombolysis. There was a trend toward a lower nonfatal reinfarction rate with ticlopidine.

TIM

Triflusal in Myocardial Infarction

Title	Randomized comparative trial of triflusal and aspirin following acute myocardial infarction.
Authors	Cruz-Fernandez JM, Lopez-Bescos L, Garcia-Dorado D, et al.
Reference	Eur Heart J 2000;21:457-465.
Disease	Acute myocardial infarction (AMI).
Purpose	To assess the efficacy and tolerability of triflusal, a selective platelet cyclooxygenase blocker, in the prevention of cardiovascular events following acute myocardial infarction.
Design	A randomized, double-blind, sequential, parallel group, multicenter.
Patients	2275 patients, 18-80 years old, <24 hours after onset of acute myocardial infarction were included. Patients who were taking antiplatelet drugs in the 15 days prior to enrollment, peptic disease, hepatic or renal disease, history of cerebrovascular hemorrhage, uncontrolled hypertension, AIDS or other severe illness were excluded.
Follow-up	35 days.
Regimen	Randomization to triflusal 600 mg/d or aspirin 300 mg/d.
Add'l Tx	Thrombolytic agents, and all other agents routinely administered for patients following acute myocardial infarction were permitted. Use of antiplatelet agents or nonsteroidal anti-inflammatory drugs was prohibited.

Results	Of 6615 patients screened, 2275 patients were included. 1140 patients were randomized to aspirin and 1135 to triflusal. 2124 patients were included in the final analysis of primary and secondary end points. A total of 441 patients did not complete the 35 day treatment phase for reasons other than death (44.4% due to revascularization, 14.3% due to use of prohibited medications, 13.2% due to adverse events, 11.8% due to non-compliance and 16.3% due to other reasons). The primary end point of death, nonfatal myocardial infarction, or nonfatal cerebrovascular events within 35 days occurred in 105 of the 1068 patients receiving aspirin and in 99 of the 1056 patients receiving triflusal (OR 0.882; 95% CI=0.634-1.227; p=0.582). Death occurred in 79 vs 69 patients in the aspirin and triflusal groups, respectively (OR 0.816; 95% CI=0.564-1.179; p=0.278). Nonfatal myocardial infarction occurred in 18 and 30 patients, respectively, (OR 1.577; 95% CI=0.873-2.848; p=0.131) and nonfatal cerebrovascular event in 14 and 5 patients, respectively, (OR 0.364; 95% CI=0.146-0.908; p=0.030). Adverse events occurred in 33.9% of the aspirin group vs 34.0% of the triflusal group. Triflusal was associated with a significantly less central nervous system associated bleeding (0.27% vs 0.97%; p=0.03) and a trend towards less overall bleeding (2.4% vs 3.6%; p=NS).
Concl.	Patients treated with triflusal had similar event rates as those treated with aspirin. Triflusal and aspirin have comparable efficacy in secondary prevention of cardiovascular events after acute myocardial infarction. Triflusal had better safety profile than aspirin and was associated with reduced rate of nonfatal cerebrovascular events.

ESTEEM

Efficacy and Safety of the Oral Direct Thrombin Inhibitor Ximelagatran in Patients with Recent Myocardial Damage

Title	Oral ximelagatran for secondary prophylaxis after myocardial infarction: the ESTEEM randomised controlled trial.
Authors	Wallentin L, Wilcox RG, Weaver WD, et al.
Reference	Lancet 2003;362:789-797.
Disease	Acute myocardial infarction (ST-elevation or non ST-elevation).
Purpose	To determine the effect of the oral direct thrombin inhibitor, ximelagatran, on clinical outcomes in patients who had recent ST-elevation or non ST-elevation acute myocardial infarctions.
Design	Randomized, placebocontrolled, doubleblind, multicenter.
Patients	1883 patients with recent ST-elevation or non ST-elevation myocardial infarction.
Follow-up	6 months.
Regimen	Within 14 days of myocardial infarction, patients were randomized to 1 of 4 doses of ximelagatran in proportions of 1:1:1:1:2 to 24 mg, 36 mg, 48 mg, 60 mg bid or placebo for 6 months.
Add'l Tx	All patients also received acetylsalicylic acid 160 mg qd.

Results   Primary outcome was dose response of ximelagatran vs placebo for the occurrence of the composite clinical end point of death, nonfatal MI, and severe recurrent ischemia. The risk of achieving the primary end point was 16.3% in the placebo group vs 12.7% in the ximelagatran group (hazard ratio=0.76; 95% CI=0.59-0.98; p=0.036) for combined ximelagatran vs placebo. The efficacy did not differ among the individual ximelagatran doses (12.1%-13.7%). All doses of ximelagatran were more effective than placebo for a number of secondary end points as well, including cardiovascular death, nonfatal MI, ischemic stroke, severe recurrent ischemia and death, or nonfatal MI. Ximelagatran significantly decreased the cumulative risk of death, nonfatal MI, or nonfatal stroke (11.1% vs 7.4%). Major bleeding was rare in the combined ximelagatran groups (1.8%) vs the placebo groups (0.9%).

Concl.   Oral ximelagatran prevented major cardiovascular events during the 6 months of treatment following a recent MI.

LoWASA

Low-Dose Warfarin and Aspirin

Title	Effect of fixed low-dose warfarin added to aspirin in the long term after acute myocardial infarction. The LoWASA study.
Authors	Herlitz J, Holm J, Peterson M, et al.
Reference	Eur Heart J 2004;25:232-239.
Disease	Coronary artery disease, myocardial infarction.
Purpose	To compare the safety and efficacy of low-dose warfarin (1.25 mg/d) added to aspirin 75 mg/d vs aspirin 75 mg/d alone in patients after an acute myocardial infarction.
Design	Prospective, open treatment with blinded end point evaluation, multicenter.
Patients	3300 patients within 42 days of admission for an acute myocardial infarction. Patients with indication for full-dose anticoagulation, contraindications to aspirin and/or anticoagulation, expected survival <1 month, cancer, severe renal failure, and treatment with nonsteroidal anti-inflammatory agents were excluded.
Follow-up	Median follow-up 5.0 years (range 1.7-6.7 years).
Regimen	Randomization to aspirin 75 mg/d alone (n=1641) or to aspirin 75 mg/d with warfarin 1.25 mg/d (n=1659).

Results	Overall, 5.5% of the patients in the aspirin group and 6.8% in the aspirin + warfarin group temporarily withdrew from the study, and 14.0% vs 30.2%, respectively, permanently withdrew from the study (p<0.0001). Termination of the study treatment due to uncomplicated bleeding occurred in 1.8% of the patients in the aspirin group and in 5.5% in the combination group (p<0.0001), and due to complicated bleeding occurred in 0.6% and 1.2% of the patients, respectively. Serious bleeding occurred in 1.0% and 2.2% of the patients, respectively (p=0.0006). 8% of the patients in the aspirin group and 6.8% in the combination group needed full-dose warfarin (p=0.15). Cardiovascular death, reinfarction, or stroke occurred in 28.8% of the patients in the aspirin group and in 28.1% in the combination group (p=0.67). Cardiovascular mortality was 15.7% and 14.2%, respectively (p=0.27). Total mortality was comparable between the aspirin (19.7%) and the combination group (18.8%; p=0.52). There was no difference between the aspirin and the combination group in the rates of reinfarction (16.3% vs 17.1%; p=0.54), or the need for CABG (20.7% vs 18.8%; p=0.15) or PTCA (8.6% vs 9.3%; p=0.39); however, there were less strokes in the combination group (4.7%) than in the aspirin group (7.1%; p=0.004). There was no difference in the rate of hemorrhagic stroke between the combination group and aspirin group (0.6% vs 0.3%); however, there were less nonhemorrhagic strokes (3.4% vs 5.0%; p=0.016) and strokes of undetermined etiology (0.8% vs 1.8%; p=0.016) in the combination group. Rehospitalization for cardiovascular etiology occurred less frequently in the combination group (57.4% vs 60.9%; p=0.048). There was no difference in the primary end point in any of the predefined 7 subgroups (patients who received or did not receive thrombolysis, patients with and without diabetes, patients with and without β-blockers, patients younger or older than 75 years, patients with or without CHF, patients with or without residual ischemia, and patients with or without atrial fibrillation.
Concl.	A fixed low-dose of warfarin (1.25 mg/d) added to aspirin 75 mg/d after an acute MI did not reduce the risk of cardiovascular mortality and reinfarction; however, the combination therapy reduced the risk of nonhemorrhagic strokes and strokes of undetermined etiology without significantly increasing the risk of hemorrhagic strokes. The combination therapy was associated with an increased risk of bleeding complications.

1. Acute Myocardial Infarction
e. Early vs Late Intervention After Acute Myocardial Infarction

1.Acute Myocardial Infarction — e. Early vs. Late Intervention After Acute
Myocardial Infarction

153

Early Revascularization in 14-Day Survivors of Acute Myocardial Infarction

Title	Early revascularization and 1-year survival in 14-day survivors of acute myocardial infarction: a prospective cohort study.
Authors	Stenestrand U, Wallentin L.
Reference	Lancet 2002:359:1805-1811.
Disease	Acute myocardial infarction.
Purpose	To evaluate the effect of revascularization within 14 days after an acute myocardial infarction on 1-year survival.
Design	Prospective registry, multicenter.
Patients	All patients, <80 years old, admitted to the coronary care units of the 61 participating centers in Sweden between 1995-1998, had a first acute myocardial infarction and were alive 14 days after onset of infarction (n=21,912) were included in this analysis of the Register of Information and Knowledge about Swedish Heart Intensive care Admissions (RIKS-HIA).
Follow-up	1 year.
Regimen	This study compared outcome of those who underwent (n=2554) and those who did not (n=19,358) undergo revascularization within 14 days.

| Results | 49% of the patients in each group had ST elevation or left bundle branch block (LBBB) on admission. Patients who underwent revascularization were younger (mean age 62.3±10.5 vs 66.0±10.0 years; p<0.001) and more often received oral anticoagulants, aspirin, β-blockers, statins, and long-term nitrates before entry. 26% of the patients who underwent revascularization and 38% of those who did not received thrombolytic therapy (p<0.001), and 29% vs zero, respectively, underwent primary angioplasty (p<0.001). Overall, 55% of the patients in the revascularization group vs 38% in the non-revascularization group received acute reperfusion therapy (p<0.001). 86% of the patients in the revascularization group vs zero in the non-revascularization group underwent revascularization before discharge (p<0.001). 93% of the patients in the revascularization group vs only 85% in the non-revascularization group received aspirin on discharge (p<0.001), and 84% vs 81%, respectively, received β-blockers upon discharge (p<0.001). 33% and 28% of the patients, respectively, received statins upon discharge (p<0.001). The unadjusted 1-year mortality was 3.3% in the revascularization group and 9.0% in the conservative group (relative risk 0.47; 95% CI=0.37-0.60; p<0.001). The beneficial effect of revascularization on 1-year mortality was apparent in all subgroups irrespective of gender, age, baseline characteristics, or treatment. For patients with ST elevation or LBBB, 1-year mortality was 4% and 8% in the revascularization and non-revascularization groups (RR 0.64; 95% CI=0.46-0.91; p=0.012). For patients with non-ST elevation 1-year mortality was 3% and 10% in the revascularization and non-revascularization groups (RR 0.35; 95% CI=0.24-0.50; p<0.001). |

| Concl. | Revascularization within 2 weeks after first acute myocardial infarction was associated with marked improvement in 1-year survival. |

SIAM III

Southwest German Interventional Study in Acute Myocardial Infarction

Title	Beneficial effects of immediate stenting after thrombolysis in acute myocardial infarction.
Authors	Scheller B, Hennen B, Hammer B, et al.
Reference	J Am Coll Cardiol 2003;42:634-641.
Disease	Acute myocardial infarction.
Purpose	To determine the beneficial effects of immediate stenting following thrombolysis vs delayed (elective) stenting of the infarct related artery.
Design	Randomized, prospective, controlled, multicenter.
Patients	197 patients with acute myocardial infarction with ST elevation or new left bundle-branch block. Patients had to be eligible for thrombolytic therapy.
Follow-up	6 months.
Regimen	Reteplase given in 2 boluses of 10 MU 30 minutes apart, 250 mg aspirin, a bolus of 5000 IU heparin which was then continued as an infusion. Patients were randomized to immediate stenting or elective stenting after 2 weeks (or earlier if there was evidence of continued ischemia). Glycoprotein IIb/IIIa inhibitors were given at the discretion of the physician. The stent used was the MultiLink Stent (Guidant Corporation, Indianapolis, IN).

Results	The primary end point was combined end point of death, reinfarction, ischemic events, and target lesion revascularization at 6 months. A total of 163 patients met full inclusion criteria. The primary end point was reached in 25.6% of the immediate stenting patients vs 50.6% of the delayed stenting patients (p=0.001). 5 patients in the delayed stenting group died within 48 hours of thrombolysis; 0 in the immediate stenting group died in the acute phase. There was a reduction in ischemic events in the patients with immediate stenting (4.9% vs 28.4%, p=0.01). LVEF was improved at 2 weeks in the immediate stenting group at 56.7±11.5% vs the elective stenting group (52.5±13.1%; p=0.037). Further improvement in LVEF was observed at 6 months in the immediate stenting group 61.5%±12.0% but not the elective group.
Concl.	Immediate stenting following thrombolysis reduced cardiac events and better improved LV function vs elective (delayed) stenting.

1. Acute Myocardial Infarction — e. Early vs. Late Intervention After Acute Myocardial Infarction

157

1. Acute Myocardial Infarction
f. Remodeling After Infarction

CAPRICORN

Carvedilol Post-Infarct Survival Control in LV Dysfunction

Title	Effect of carvedilol on outcome after myocardial infarction in patients with left ventricular dysfunction: the CAPRICORN randomised trial.
Authors	Dargie HJ.
Reference	Lancet 2001;357:1385-1390.
Disease	Myocardial infarction, congestive heart failure.
Purpose	To assess whether carvedilol, added to standard therapy, will be beneficial in patients with left ventricular dysfunction after acute myocardial infarction.
Design	Randomized, double-blind, placebo-controlled, multicenter.
Patients	1959 patients, ≥18 years old, 3-21 days after acute myocardial infarction, left ventricular ejection fraction ≤40% or wall motion score index of ≤1.3. All patients received ACE inhibitors for ≥48 hours, unless they were intolerant to ACE inhibitors. Patients who were hemodynamically unstable and those with uncontrolled heart failure, unstable angina, hypotension, uncontrolled hypertension, bradycardia, or unstable insulin-dependent diabetes mellitus were excluded. Patients with an indication for β-blocker agents other than heart failure and those who needed ongoing therapy with β-2 agonists or steroids were not included.
Follow-up	A mean of 1.3 years.
Regimen	Randomization to carvedilol (6.25 mg bid, titrated up to 25 mg bid) (n=975) or placebo (n=984).
Add'l Tx	All patients received ACE inhibitors, unless they were intolerant to ACE inhibitors.

Results	74% of the patients in the carvedilol group reached the target dose of 25 mg bid, and 11% the dose of 12.5 mg bid. Excluding death, 20% of the patients in the carvedilol group vs 18% of the patients in the placebo group were withdrawn permanently from the study. 98% of the patients in the carvedilol group, and 97% in the placebo group received ACE inhibitors and 86% and 86%, respectively, received aspirin. All-cause mortality was 12% in the carvedilol group and 15% in the placebo group (hazard ratio 0.77; 95% CI=0.60-0.98; p=0.031). The primary end point of death or cardiovascular hospitalization was reached by 35% of the carvedilol vs 37% of the placebo group (hazard ratio 0.92; 95% CI=0.80-1.07; p=0.296). Sudden death occurred in 5% and 7%, respectively (p=0.098) and hospitalization because of heart failure in 12% and 14%, respectively (p=0.215). Cardiovascular mortality was 11% and 14% in the carvedilol and placebo group, respectively (hazard ratio 0.75; 95% CI=0.58-0.96; p=0.024). Death due to heart failure occurred in 2% and 3%, respectively (p=0.083). Nonfatal MI occurred in 3% and 6%, respectively (hazard ratio 0.59; 95% CI=0.39-0.90; p=0.014) and death or acute myocardial infarction in 14% and 20%, respectively (hazard ratio 0.71; 95% CI=0.57-0.89; p=0.002).
Concl.	Long-term therapy with carvedilol, in addition to ACE inhibitors and standard therapy, reduced the frequency of death and recurrent myocardial infarction in stable patients with left ventricular systolic dysfunction after an acute myocardial infarction.

GISSI-3 Substudy

Gruppo Italiano per lo Studio della Sopravvivenza nell'Infarto Miocardico-3

Title	Aspirin does not interact with ACE inhibitors when both are given early after acute myocardial infarction. Results of the GISSI-3 Trial.
Authors	Latini R, Santoro E, Masson S, et al.
Reference	Heart Disease 2000;2:185-190.
Disease	Acute myocardial infarction.
Purpose	To determine if there was a possible negative interaction between aspirin and the ACE inhibitor lisinopril following MI.
Design	Randomized, multicenter, 2 x 2 factorial design.
Patients	Subanalysis of 18,895 patients who were part of GISSI-3.
Follow-up	42 days.
Regimen	Patients were randomized within 24 hours of MI to receive lisinopril, nitrates, both, or neither. 15,841 patients received aspirin, 3054 did not receive aspirin.
Results	Primary end point of subanalysis was total mortality up to day 42. Secondary analysis included other clinical events during hospitalization or during 42 day follow-up. Lisinopril decreased 42-day mortality from 7.1% to 6.3%. Mortality was lower in patients on aspirin (5.7%) than those not on aspirin (11.8%). In patients taking aspirin, lisinopril still reduced morality (6.0% to 5.4%) and in those not on aspirin from 13.0% to 10.8%. Proportional reductions of mortality were not significantly different between the 2 groups (9.9% vs 19.1%; p=0.41) suggesting no interaction between aspirin and lisinopril. The early 7-day mortality reduction benefit by lisinopril also was not affected by aspirin. Analysis of in-hospital major clinical events and reinfarction rates at 42 days did not reveal a negative interaction between aspirin and lisinopril.
Concl.	Aspirin did not decrease the mortality benefit of lisinopril after MI or increase the risk of adverse clinical events.

OPTIMAAL

Optimal Trial in Myocardial Infarction with the Angiotensin II Antagonist Losartan

Title	a. Comparison of baseline data, initial course, and management: losartan vs captopril following acute myocardial infarction (the OPTIMAAL Trial). b. Effects of losartan and captopril on mortality and morbidity in high-risk patients after acute myocardial infarction: the OPTIMAAL randomized trial.
Authors	Dickstein K, Kjekshus J, and the OPTIMAAL Steering Committee.
Reference	a. Am J Cardiol 2001;87:766-770. b. Lancet 2002;360:752-760.
Disease	Acute myocardial infarction, heart failure.
Purpose	To compare the outcome of ACE inhibitor captopril vs angiotensin II receptor antagonist, losartan, in patients with acute myocardial infarction and evidence of heart failure or left ventricular dysfunction.
Design	Randomized, double-blind, multicenter.
Patients	5477 patients, ≥50 years old, with documented acute myocardial infarction and signs or symptoms of congestive heart failure, left ventricular ejection fraction <35% or end-diastolic diameter >65 mm and/or new Q-wave anterior myocardial infarction, new LBBB, or patients with any reinfarction and previous pathologic Q-waves in the anterior wall. Patients were enrolled within 10 days of onset of symptoms. Patients with supine systolic blood pressure <100 mm Hg, current on therapy with an ACE inhibitor or angiotensin receptor blocker, unstable angina, significant stenotic valvular disease, significant arrhythmia, and planned coronary revascularization were excluded.
Follow-up	Mean follow-up 2.7±0.9 years. 14,866 patient-years of follow-up.

Regimen	Within 10 days of symptoms' onset, patients were randomized to captopril (n=2733) 12.5 mg tid or losartan (n=2744) 12.5 mg qd and titrated to target of captopril 50 mg tid or losartan 50 mg qd as tolerated.
Results	At the end of the trial 83% of the patients in the losartan group and 81% in the captopril group were still on the target dose of the study medication. All-cause mortality was 18.2% in the losartan group and 16.4% in the captopril group (relative risk [RR] 1.13; 95% CI=0.99-1.28; p=0.069). Sudden cardiac death or resuscitated cardiac arrest occurred in 8.7% and 7.4% of the patients in the losartan and captopril group (RR 1.19; 95% CI=0.99-1.43; p=0.072). Reinfarction occurred in 14.0% and 13.9%, respectively (p=0.722). Cardiovascular mortality was higher in the losartan group (15.3% vs 13.3%; RR 1.17; 95% CI=1.01-1.34; p=0.032). First admission for heart failure occurred in 11.2% and 9.7%, respectively (RR 1.16; 95% CI=0.98-1.37; p=0.072). Cardiovascular admission rate was 53.9% in the losartan and 52.0% in the captopril group (p=0.108). Non-cardiovascular admission rate was 32.3% and 33.1%, respectively (p=0.719). Subgroup analysis stratified by b-blocker use before enrollment did not show a significant interaction between β-blocker use and the study drug (p=0.88 for interaction with β-blockers). Losartan was better tolerated than captopril. 7% of the patients in the losartan group vs 14% in the captopril group discontinued study drug due to adverse effects (p<0.0001). Cough was reported by 9.3% of patients randomized to losartan and 18.7% of the patients in the captopril group (p<0.001). Angioedema was reported in 0.4% and 0.8% of the patients, respectively (p=0.034).
Concl.	Captopril was associated with non-significant lower all-cause mortality (the primary end point of the study) and a significant lower cardiovascular mortality compared to losartan. However, losartan was better tolerated than captopril.

SMILE-2

Survival of Myocardial Infarction Long-Term Evaluation-2

Title	Double-blind comparison between zofenopril and lisinopril in patients with acute myocardial infarction: results of the SMILE-2 study.
Authors	Borghi C, Ambrosioni E, for the Survival of Myocardial Infarction Long-Term Evaluation-2 Working Party.
Reference	Am Heart J 2003;145:80-87.
Disease	Acute myocardial infarction.
Purpose	To compare the safety and efficacy of 2 ACE-inhibitors (zofenopril and lisinopril) in patients with ST-elevation acute myocardial infarction undergoing thrombolytic therapy.
Design	Randomized, double-blind, multicenter.
Patients	1024 patients, 18-75 years, with a confirmed acute myocardial infarction that was treated with intravenous thrombolytic therapy within 12 hours of onset of symptoms, and a systolic blood pressure >100 mm Hg. Patients with Killip class IV, diastolic blood pressure >115 mm Hg, systolic blood pressure >200 mm Hg, bilateral renal artery stenosis, prolonged CPR, coronary artery bypass graft within the preceding 3 months, significant valvular disease, current treatment with ACE-inhibitors or angiotensin II receptor blockers, hypersensitivity to ACE-inhibitors, renal failure, proteinuria, leukopenia, and those who received high doses of diuretics in the preceding 24 hours were excluded.
Follow-up	6 weeks.
Regimen	Within 90 minutes to 12 hours after completion of thrombolytic therapy, patients were randomized to zofenopril (7.5 mg bid; n=504) or lisinopril (2.5 mg/d; n=520). The dose was increased during day 1-5 up to 30 mg bid of zofenopril and 10 mg/d of lisinopril.
Add'l Tx	Standard therapy, excluding other ACE inhibitors or angiotensin II receptor blockers, was permitted.

Results	Treatment was discontinued prematurely in 22.4% of the patients in the zofenopril and 24.8% in the lisinopril group. Severe hypotension was noted in 10.9% and 11.7% of the patients, respectively (p=0.38). Both agents decreased BP. The effect of lisinopril was more persistent. The incidence of drug-related severe hypotension was higher with lisinopril (9.8% vs 6.7%; p=0.048). 6-week mortality was 3.2% in the zofenopril and 4.0% in the lisinopril group (p=0.38). Severe heart failure was noted in 0.8% and 0.6% of the patients, respectively (p=NS). Mean LVEF was comparable (51.9% vs 52.0%, respectively; p=NS). Reinfarction occurred in 4.2% and 3.8% of the patients, respectively (p=NS). Renal function deterioration was noted in 2.6% and 2.7% of the patients, respectively (p=NS). During the 6-week follow-up, discontinuation of the study drug due to adverse events occurred in 16.5% of the patients in the zofenopril group and in 19.0% in the lisinopril group (p=NS).
Concl.	Both lisinopril and zofenopril were safe when started early after thrombolytic therapy for acute MI. The incidence of severe hypotension was low with both drugs. There were no significant differences in outcome between lisinopril and zofenopril.

1.Acute Myocardial Infarction — f. Remodeling After Infarction

TRACE (Diabetic Substudy)

Trandolapril Cardiac Evaluation Study

Title	Effect of the ACE inhibitor trandolapril on mortality and morbidity in diabetic patients with left ventricular dysfunction after acute myocardial infarction.
Authors	Gustafsson I, Torp-Pedersen C, Kober L, et al.
Reference	J Am Coll Cardiol 1999;34:83-89.
Disease	Myocardial infarction, left ventricular dysfunction.
Purpose	To determine the long-term efficacy of treatment with the ACE inhibitor trandolapril in post myocardial infarction diabetic patients with left ventricular dysfunction.
Design	Retrospective analysis of a randomized, double-blind, placebo-controlled trial.
Patients	237 (14%) diabetic patients that were among the 1749 patients that participated in the TRACE study (original reference: N Engl J Med 1995;333:1670-1676). Patients had myocardial infarcts and LVEF ≤35%.
Follow-up	26 months.
Regimen	As per TRACE study. Study medicine started 3-7 days post infarction.
Add'l Tx	As per TRACE study.

Results	126 patients (53%) in the diabetic group died, vs 547 (36%) in the nondiabetic group. Death occurred in 51 (45%) of diabetic patients randomized to trandolapril vs 75 (61%) of diabetics randomized to placebo (RR 0.64; 95% CI=0.45-0.91). Among nondiabetics, death occurred in 253 (33%) of patients on trandolapril vs 294 (39%) of patients on placebo (RR 0.82; 95% CI=0.69-0.97). Trandolapril decreased the risk of progression to severe heart failure (RR 0.38; 95% CI=0.21-0.67), but this end point was not significantly reduced by trandolapril in nondiabetic patients. In diabetic patients trandolapril also decreased the incidence of cardiovascular death, sudden death, and reinfarction. In nondiabetic patients trandolapril significantly decreased the incidence of cardiovascular death, but not sudden death or reinfarction
Concl.	Trandolapril reduced death and other major cardiovascular complications in diabetics with post infarction LV dysfunction.

TRACE (Update)

Trandolapril Cardiac Evaluation

Title	Effect of ACE inhibitor trandolapril on life expectancy of patients with reduced left ventricular function after acute myocardial infarction.
Authors	Torp-Pedersen C, Kober L, for the TRACE Study Group.
Reference	Lancet 1999;354:9-12.
Disease	Congestive heart failure, left ventricular dysfunction, myocardial infarction.
Purpose	To calculate the long-term effect of trandolapril on life expectancy in patients with left ventricular dysfunction after myocardial infarction.
Design	Randomized, double-blind, placebo-controlled, multicenter.
Patients	Same as above.
Follow-up	Up to 7 years.
Regimen	3-7 days after myocardial infarction patients were randomized to placebo or trandolapril up to 4 mg/d. Therapy was continued for 2 years.
Add'l Tx	After termination of the study, ACE inhibitors were prescribed to patients who would be expected to benefit from the therapy.
Results	The life expectancy of patients was significantly longer with trandolapril than placebo (6.2 years vs 4.6 years). The 50% mortality was reached after 55.2 months in the placebo group vs after 70.5 months in the trandolapril group. Therefore, the median lifetime was increased by 15.3 months or 27% increase in median lifetime (95% CI=7-51%). After 1, 2, 3, 4, 5, and 6 years, 32, 55, 87, 66, 64, and 64 lives, respectively, were saved per 1000 patients treated after each year.
Concl.	In patients with left ventricular dysfunction after acute myocardial infarction, long-term treatment with trandolapril for 2 years after myocardial infarction was associated with a significant prolongation of life expectancy.

VALIANT

The Valsartan in Acute Myocardial Infarction Trial

Title	Valsartan, captopril, or both in myocardial infarction complicated by heart failure, left ventricular dysfunction, or both.
Authors	Pfeffer MA, McMurray JJV, Velazques EJ, et al.
Reference	N Engl J Med 2003;349:1893-1906.
Disease	Acute myocardial infarction, congestive heart failure.
Purpose	To compare the effect of valsartan, an angiotensin receptor blocker, to captopril, an angiotensin-converting enzyme inhibitor, or to the combination of the 2 agents on mortality in patients with myocardial infarction complicated by left ventricular dysfunction.
Design	Randomized, double-blind, multicenter.
Patients	14,808 patients, 18 years or older with an acute myocardial infarction between 0.5 and 10 days prior to entry with clinical or radiologic evidence of heart failure, an ejection fraction ≤0.35 by echocardiography or left ventricular angiography and ≤0.40 on radionuclide ventriculography or both. Systolic blood pressure had to be greater than 100 mm Hg.
Follow-up	Median follow-up 24.7 months.
Regimen	Patients randomized to valsartan (4909 patients), valsartan + captopril (4885 patients), or captopril (4909 patients). Starting doses were 20 mg valsartan; 20 mg valsartan and 6.25 mg captopril; or 6.25 mg captopril. Doses were gradually increased to 160 mg valsartan bid; 80 mg valsartan bid + 50 mg captopril tid; or 50 mg captopril tid, by the 3-month visit. About 70% of patients in all 3 groups were also on β-blockade.

Results	The primary end point was death from any cause. At 24.7 months, 979 (19.9%), 941 (19.3%), and 958 (19.5%) patients died in the valsartan, valsartan + captopril, and captopril groups, respectively. There was no significant difference in hazard ratio for the primary end point among the 3 groups. Valsartan was noninferior with regard to mortality and the composite end point of fatal and nonfatal cardiovascular events compared to captopril. Death from cardiovascular causes occurred in 16.8% of the valsartan group, 16.9% of the valsartan and captopril group, and 16.9% of the captopril group (p=NS). Death from cardiovascular causes, MI, or heart failure occurred in 31.1%, 31.1%, and 31.9% among the 3 groups respectively (p=NS). The drug-related adverse events of hypotension and renal dysfunction occurred more commonly in the valsartan group; cough, rash, and taste disturbance were more common in patients in the captopril group; and the most drug-related adverse events occurred with combination therapy.
Concl.	Valsartan did not differ from captopril in its effect on mortality in patients with acute MI and LV dysfunction. There was no advantage to combining valsartan with captopril in this patient population.

1.Acute Myocardial Infarction — f. Remodeling After Infarction

1. Acute Myocardial Infarction
g. Miscellaneous and Adjunctive Therapy

HALT-MI

Hu23F2G Anti-Adhesion to Limit Cytotoxic Injury Following AMI

Title	The effect of blockade of the CD11/CD18 integrin receptor on infarct size in patients with acute myocardial infarction treated with direct angioplasty: the results of the HALT-MI study.
Authors	Faxon DP, Gibbons RJ, Chronos NA, et al.
Reference	J Am Coll Cardiol 2002;40:1199-1204.
Disease	Acute myocardial infarction.
Purpose	To evaluate the safety and efficacy of Hu23F2G, an antibody to the CD11/CD18 integrin receptors, in reducing infarct size in patients with ST-elevation acute myocardial infarction undergoing primary percutaneous coronary interventions.
Design	Randomized, double-blind, placebo-controlled, multicenter.
Patients	420 patients, 18-85 years old, within 6 hours of onset of symptoms of ST-elevation acute myocardial infarction and were candidates for primary PCI. Patients with a history and ECG evidence of previous Q-wave myocardial infarction or an ECG pattern that made the diagnosis of myocardial infarction difficult were excluded. Patients in cardiogenic shock, those who received thrombolytic therapy and those with creatinine >2 mg/dL, evidence of ongoing bacterial infection, pregnancy, and the presence of other serious medical conditions were not included.
Follow-up	Patients underwent technetium-99m sestamibi SPECT imaging 5-9 days after enrollment. Clinical follow-up for 6 months.
Regimen	The patients were taken to the catheterization laboratory after randomization. Only patients with TIMI 0-1 flow grade were included. Patients with TIMI 2-3 flow grade did not receive the study drug. Patients were randomized to receive either 0.3 mg/kg or 1 mg/kg of Hu23F2G or placebo as an intravenous bolus.

Add'l Tx	All patients received aspirin and intravenous heparin (target ACT 250-300 sec). The use of GP IIb/IIIa inhibitors was permitted. Stents and the use of clopidogrel or ticlopidine were also permitted. Only the infarct-related artery was treated.
Results	128 patients received Hu23F2G 0.3 mg/kg, 139 received Hu23F2G 1 mg/kg, and 153 patients received placebo. 88%, 86%, and 89% of the patients in the Hu23F2G 0.3 mg/kg, Hu23F2G 1 mg/kg, and placebo group, respectively, had successful PCI. Stents were implanted in 85% of the patients. TIMI 3 grade flow was achieved by 81%, 86%, and 86% of the patients, respectively. The myocardial perfusion defect was 16% of the LV for the placebo group (n=128), 17.2% for the Hu23F2G 0.3 mg/kg group (n=139), and 16.6% for the Hu23F2G 1 mg/kg group (n=153) (p=NS). In patients with anterior MI, there was no significant difference in infarct size among the 3 treatment groups. There were no significant differences in infarct size among the groups in those patients treated within 2 hours of onset of symptoms. The CK-MB area under the curve for 24 hours was comparable among the 3 groups (175%, 175%, and 184%/h for the placebo, 0.3 mg/kg, and 1 mg/kg groups, respectively). The corrected TIMI frame counts were 21.3%, 23.2%, and 22.3%, respectively. 30-day morality was 3.3% in the placebo, 0.8%, and 1.4% in the Hu23F2G 0.3 and 1 mg/kg groups, respectively (p=0.20). Reinfarction occurred in 3.9%, 0.8%, and 2.9%, respectively. There was no difference in bleeding or major infection among the 3 groups. However, minor infections occurred more frequently in the 0.3 mg/kg and 1 mg/kg Hu23F2G groups (5% and 9%) than in the placebo group (2%).
Concl.	Hu23F2G, an antibody against CD11/CD18 integrin receptor did not reduce infarct size or affect clinical outcomes in patients with ST-elevation acute MI undergoing primary angioplasty.

GISSI-Prevenzione

Gruppo Italiano per lo Studio della Sopravvivenza nell'Infarto Miocardico—Prevenzione

Title	Early protection against sudden death by n-3 polyunsaturated fatty acids after myocardial infarction. Time-course analysis of the results of the GISSI-Prevenzione.
Authors	Marchioli R, Barzi F, Bomba E, et al.
Reference	Circulation 2002;105:1897-1903.
Disease	Myocardial infarction (MI).
Purpose	To determine the time course of benefit of n-3 polyunsaturated fatty acids (PUFAs) on mortality in the GISSI-Prevenzione trial in patients with a recent (<3 months) MI.
Design	Open-label, parallel, multicenter.
Patients	11,323 patients with recent (<3 months) MI.
Follow-up	3.5 years.
Regimen	Patients were randomized to n-3 PUFAs 1 g/d, vitamin E 300 mg/d, a combination of the 2, or control.
Add'l Tx	Lifestyle modification and other preventive interventions.

Results   Primary composite end points were cumulative rate of death, nonfatal MI, nonfatal stroke, cumulative rate of cardiovascular death, nonfatal MI, and nonfatal stroke. Total mortality was significantly lower after 3 months of n-3 PUFA therapy vs control (RR 0.59; 95% CI=0.36-0.97; p=0.037). This lower mortality rate was confirmed at the trial's end at 8.4% vs 9.8%; RR 0.79; 95% CI=0.66-0.93; p=0.006. At 42 months the composite of death, nonfatal MI, and nonfatal stroke was reduced by n-3 PUFA (RR 0.85 [0.74-0.98]; p<0.05). At 42 months the composite of cardiovascular death, nonfatal MI, and nonfatal stroke, was reduced by n-3 PUFA (RR 0.80 [0.68-0.94]; p<0.01). By 4 months reduction in risk of sudden death was significantly lower among patients on n-3 PUFA (RR 0.47; 95% CI=0.219-0.995; p=0.048). Cardiac death became significantly lower with n-3 PUFA therapy at 6 months and coronary death lower at 8 months. n-3 PUFA had no overall effect on total cholesterol, LDL cholesterol, or HDL cholesterol. They did appear to moderately lower triglyceride levels.

Concl.   Early effect of 1 g/d n-3 PUFAs on sudden death and total mortality supports the hypothesis that this therapy has anantiarrhythmic effect.

GISSI-Prevenzione Trial

Gruppo Italiano per lo Studio della Sopravvivenza nell'Infarto Miocardico

Title	Dietary supplementation with n-3 polyunsaturated fatty acids and vitamin E after myocardial infarction: results of the GISSI-Prevenzione trial.
Authors	GISSI-Prevenzione Investigators.
Reference	Lancet 1999;354:447-455.
Disease	Acute myocardial infarction.
Purpose	To evaluate the effects of n-3 polyunsaturated fatty acids (n-3 PUFA), vitamin E, and their combination on mortality and morbidity after acute myocardial infarction.
Design	Randomized, 2 × 2 factorial, open-label, multicenter.
Patients	11,324 patients, ≤3 months after myocardial infarction, with no contraindications to dietary supplements, overt heart failure, severe systemic disease, and congenital coagulation disorder.
Follow-up	42 months.
Regimen	Randomization to n-3 PUFA (850 to 882 mg/d of eicosapentaenoic acid and docasahexenoic acid as ethyl esters) and to vitamin E 300 mg/d.
Add'l Tx	Aspirin, β-blockers, and ACE inhibitors were recommended.

Results   2836 patients were randomized to n-3 PUFA alone, 2830 patients
               to vitamin E alone, 2830 to 3-n PUFA, and vitamin E, and 2828
               patients to no supplement. The primary end point of death,
               nonfatal myocardial infarction or nonfatal stroke was reached
               by 12.6% of the patients assigned to 3-n PUFA vs 13.9% of the
               patients not receiving n-3 PUFA (relative risk [RR] 0.90; 95%
               CI=0.82-0.99; p=0.048). The combined end point of cardiovas-
               cular death, nonfatal myocardial infarction, and nonfatal stroke
               was reached by 9.7% and 10.8% of the patients receiving and
               not receiving n-3 PUFA, respectively (RR 0.89; 95% CI=0.80-
               1.01; p=0.053). Total mortality was 5.1% and 6.2% in patients
               receiving and not receiving n-3 PUFA (RR 0.86; 95% CI=0.76-
               0.97). Vitamin E was not effective. The primary end point of
               death, nonfatal myocardial infarction, and nonfatal stroke
               occurred in 12.9% and 13.6% of the patients receiving and not
               receiving vitamin E, respectively (RR 0.95; 95% CI=0.86-1.05),
               whereas the combined end point of cardiovascular death, nonfa-
               tal myocardial infarction, and nonfatal stroke occurred in 10.1%
               vs 10.3%, respectively (RR 0.98; 95% CI=0.87-1.10). However,
               using 4-way analysis, it was found that vitamin E was associated
               with lower cardiac death rate (RR 0.77; 95% CI=0.61-0.97),
               coronary death (RR 0.75; 95% CI=0.59-0.96), and sudden
               death (RR 0.65; 95% CI=0.48-0.89). Vitamin E did not have
               an additional benefit in patients receiving n-3 PUFA. At the end
               of the study 28.5% of the patients assigned to n-3 PUFA and
               26.2% of the patients assigned to vitamin E had permanently
               stopped taking the study medication.

Concl.   N-3 PUFA treatment for 3.5 years decreased the rates of death,
               nonfatal myocardial infarction, and nonfatal stroke in patients
               with recent myocardial infarction. In contrast, vitamin E was
               not effective in either patients not receiving or receiving n-3
               PUFA. The effects of vitamin E on fatal cardiovascular events
               should be further investigated.

Cariporide in Patients with Acute Anterior Myocardial Infarction

Title	Cardioprotective effects of the Na+/H+ exchange inhibitor cariporide in patients with acute anterior myocardial infarction undergoing direct PTCA.
Authors	Rupprecht HJ, vom Dahl J, Terres W, et al.
Reference	Circulation 2000;101:2902-2908.
Disease	Acute myocardial infarction.
Purpose	To determine whether the Na+/H+ exchange inhibitor, cariporide, limits myocardial infarct size and improves left ventricular function in patients with acute mycardial infarction treated with percutaneous transluminal coronary angioplasty.
Design	Randomized, placebo-controlled, double-blind, multicenter.
Patients	100 patients with acute anterior wall MI (≥30 minutes chest pain, ST elevation of ≥0.2 mV in ≥3 chest leads, occluded left anterior descending coronary artery who could undergo direct PTCA within 6 hours.
Follow-up	3 weeks. Pretreatment and 3-week follow-up LV angiograms were performed.
Regimen	40 mg cariporide or placebo IV given over 10 minutes followed by PTCA.
Add'l Tx	Heparin, IV nitroglycerin as needed.

Results	3 patients in the placebo group died vs 4 in the cariporide group, during hospitalization. End-systolic volume increased over 3 weeks in the placebo group (80.3±6.9 to 97.0±10.3 mL) but decreased in the cariporide group (76.7±5.4 to 69±5.6 mL; p=0.048). There was a trend toward the same pattern in end-diastolic volume. Ejection fraction was unchanged over 3 weeks in the placebo group (40±2% to 40±3%) but increased in the cariporide group (44±2% to 50±2%; p<0.045). The percentage of LV circumference with hypokinesis <-1 SD below the normal mean was unchanged in the placebo group over 3 weeks (70.9% to 70%) whereas this percentage was reduced over 3 weeks in the cariporide group (65.4 to 55.2%; p=0.082). Severity of hypokinesis at the border zone of the infarct improved better in the treated group (p=0.052). Area under the curve for CK-MB was lower in the cariporide group compared to the placebo group (p=0.047).
Concl.	Cariporide attenuated infarct size and improved LV function when administered as adjunctive therapy to reperfusion by PTCA of acute anterior wall MIs.

Does Angina Pectoris the Week Before Protect Against First Acute Myocardial Infarction in Patients with Diabetes Mellitus?

Title	Does angina pectoris the week before protect against first acute myocardial infarction in patients with diabetes mellitus?
Authors	Jiménez-Navarro M, Gómez-Doblas JJ, García JMH, et al.
Reference	Am J Cardiol 2002;90:160-162.
Disease	Acute myocardial infarction.
Purpose	To determine the effect of preinfarction angina on cardiovascular outcomes and left ventricular function in diabetic patients after acute myocardial infarction (AMI).
Design	Retrospective.
Patients	290 consecutive patients who were admitted with a first AMI. 68 (23.4%) were diabetic and 222 (76.6%) were nondiabetic. Only patients who were experiencing their first MI were included. Other inclusion criteria were no history of angina for >1 week before the MI and no evidence of previous structural cardiopathy. Onset of MI was defined as the persistence of cardiac symptoms beyond 30 minutes. Antecedent angina was defined as cardiac symptoms lasting less than 30 minutes before onset.
Follow-up	Mean 19 months.
Regimen	Patients were admitted with MI and received the standard care. LVEF was determined between 6-8 days after the MI, or earlier as clinically necessary.

Results	The end points of the study were death, CHF (defined as rales in >50% of the lung field which persisted after cough and radiographic evidence of pulmonary congestion) and cardiogenic shock, residual ischemia, and occurrence of malignant arrhythmias (ie, ventricular fibrillation and complete heart block). Diabetic patients were more likely to be women (44% vs 18%; p<0.001), have hypercholesterolemia (40% vs 25%; p<0.01), and not as likely to smoke (40% vs 68%; p<0.001). No differences were found between diabetics and nondiabetics with respect to prodromal angina, AMI localization, impaired post-MI ventricular function, and therapy with fibrinolysis. Preinfarction angina was present in 39.7% and 36% in diabetics and nondiabetics, respectively. There was no relationship of presence of preinfarction angina and characteristics such as age, cardiovascular risk factors, AMI localization, and use of or time to thrombolysis. Among the patients with diabetes (n=68), 27 (39.7%) had prodromal angina, and 41 (60.3%) did not. The end point of death was reduced in diabetic patients who had preinfarction angina vs diabetics who did not (0% vs 17%; p=0.03). Arrhythmia was also significantly reduced in the preinfarction angina group (0% vs 22%, p=0.01), as were the combined numbers of death and heart failure (7% vs 29%; p=0.03). There were no significant differences according to the presence of preinfarction angina for heart failure/shock, residual ischemia, peak creatinine kinase, or follow-up complications. Also, there was no difference in depressed AMI ventricular function (defined as ejection fraction <40%) according to the presence of preinfarction angina.
Concl.	Preinfarction angina in diabetics appeared to be effective in reducing death, arrhythmia, and the combined end point of death and heart failure after acute MI, but did not have significant effect on other measures such as ejection fraction, residual ischemia, infarct size, or complications.

AMISTAD

Acute Myocardial Infarction Study of Adenosine Trial

Title	Adenosine as an adjunct to thrombolytic therapy for acute myocardial infarction: results of multicenter, randomized, placebo-controlled trial: the acute myocardial infarction study of adenosine (AMISTAD) Trial.
Authors	Mahaffey KW, Puma JA, Barbagelata A, et al.
Reference	J Am Coll Cardiol 1999;34:1711-1720.
Disease	Acute myocardial infarction.
Purpose	To determine whether adenosine administered as an adjuvant to thrombolytic therapy would further reduce myocardial infarct size.
Design	Prospective, randomized, placebo-controlled, open-label, multicenter.
Patients	236 patients with acute ST segment elevation myocardial infarction who presented within 6 hours of chest pain slated for thrombolytic therapy.
Follow-up	6-day infarct size determination, in-hospital outcomes.
Regimen	Adenosine IV at 70 µg/kg/min for 3 hours or placebo infusion (normal saline). Adenosine was to begin prior to thrombolytic therapy (accelerated alteplase or streptokinase).
Add'l Tx	Lidocaine prior to thrombolytic therapy (1 experimental study suggested adenosine only reduced infarct size given with lidocaine).

Results	Primary end point was infarct size determined with Tc-99 m sestamibi SPECT (single photon emission computed tomography) myocardial perfusion imaging 5-7 days after enrollment. Secondary end points included a myocardial salvage index and composite in-hospital clinical outcomes (death, reinfarction, shock, congestive heart failure, or stroke). Adenosine was associated with a 33% relative reduction in myocardial infarct size (p=0.03). Final infarct size for anterior infarcts was 45.5% of the LV in placebo patients, vs 15% for adenosine patients (p=0.014). For nonanterior myocardial infarcts, infarct size was 11.5% in both adenosine and placebo groups (p=NS). Myocardial salvage index (myocardium at risk minus final infarct size/myocardium at risk) in patients with anterior infarcts was 0.62 in adenosine patients and was 0.15 in placebo patients. There was no difference in this index between groups in the nonanterior infarcts. There were no significant differences in clinical outcomes between adenosine and placebo, and event rates were small. However, there was a nonsignificant increase in deaths (10 vs 6), reinfarctions (7 vs 3), CHF (13 vs 8) and cardiogenic shock (6 vs 4) in adenosine vs placebo patients. This excess of adverse events tended to occur in the nonanterior MI group.
Concl.	Adenosine decreased myocardial infarct size in anterior wall MIs; there was a nonsignificant trend toward increased adverse events in patients with nonanterior wall MIs who received adenosine. A large clinical outcome trial is warranted.

DECREASE

Dutch Echocardiographic Cardiac Risk Evaluation Applying Stress Echocardiography Study Group

Title	The effect of biosoprolol on perioperative mortality and myocardial infarction in high risk patients undergoing vascular surgery.
Authors	Poldermans D, Boersma E, Bax JJ, et al.
Reference	N Engl J Med 1999;341:1789-1794.
Disease	Cardiac death and myocardial infarction in patients undergoing major vascular surgery.
Purpose	To determine the effects of perioperative β-adrenergic receptor blockade on outcomes in patients at high risk who were undergoing major vascular surgery.
Design	Randomized, multicenter.
Patients	846 patients with 1 or more cardiac risk factors undergoing elective abdominal aortic or infrainguinal arterial reconstruction underwent dobutamine echocardiography. Of these patients, 173 had positive results for ischemia on dobutamine echo and were considered high risk.
Follow-up	30 days after surgery.
Regimen	Standard perioperative care (n=53) or standard care plus bisoprolol (n=59). Bisoprolol was started at least 1 week before surgery. Initial dose of bisoprolol was 5 mg orally once-a-day and increased to 10 mg once-a-day if heart rate remained >60 bpm.
Add'l Tx	Standard perioperative care.
Results	9 patients (17%) in the standard care group died of cardiac causes vs 2 in the bisoprolol group (3.4%; p=0.02). 9 patients (17%) in the standard care group and 0 in the bisoprolol group developed a nonfatal myocardial infarction (p<0.001). The primary end point of death from cardiac causes or nonfatal myocardial infarction was reached in 18 patients in the standard care group (34%) and 2 patients in the bisoprolol group (3.4%; p<0.001).

Concl.   Bisoprolol reduced perioperative mortality and myocardial infarction in high risk patients who were undergoing vascular surgery.

EMIP-FR

European Myocardial Infarction Project—Free Radicals

Title	Effect of 48-h intravenous trimetazidine on short- and long-term outcomes of patients with acute myocardial infarction, with and without thrombolytic therapy. A double-blind, placebo-controlled, randomized trial.
Authors	The EMIP-FR Group.
Reference	Eur Heart J 2000;21:1537-1546.
Disease	Acute myocardial infarction.
Purpose	To assess the effects of trimetazidine, an antioxidant, on short- and long-term mortality in patients with acute myocardial infarction.
Design	Randomized, double-blind, stratified, multicenter.
Patients	19,725 patients within 24 hours of onset of symptoms suggesting acute myocardial infarction. Patients who had taken trimetazidine within the previous 48 hours or had received a fibrinolytic drug within the last 24 hours, and patients with a serious renal or liver disease were excluded. In this trial patients in whom thrombolysis was planned, as well as patients in whom it was not planned.
Follow-up	35 days and up to 3 years.
Regimen	Patients were randomized to trimetazidine or placebo. Trimetazidine was administered as a 40 mg IV bolus followed by a continuous infusion of 60 mg/24 hours for 48 hours. Treatment was to be started before or up to 15 minutes after initiation of thrombolytic therapy in patients for whom thrombolysis was planned.

Results	The average length of follow-up was 12 months, ranging from 35 days to 39 months. Intention-to-treat analysis revealed that 35-day mortality was comparable between the trimetazidine (12.5%) and the placebo (12.5%) groups (p=0.98). Among patients receiving thrombolytic therapy 35 day mortality was 11.3% in the trimetazidine group and 10.5% in the placebo group (p=0.15). Among patients not receiving thrombolytic therapy 35-day mortality was 14.0% and 15.1%, respectively (p=0.14). Survival curves at 35 days adjusted for age and sex did not show differences between the 2 groups. Cardiovascular mortality was also comparable between the trimetazidine (10.96%) and the placebo (11.14%) (p=0.70). In a per-protocol analysis the beneficial effect of trimetazidine in patients not undergoing thrombolytic therapy became statistically significant (13.3% vs 15.1%; p=0.027). Long-term mortality was 21.54% in the trimetazidine group and 21.07% in the placebo group (p=0.42).
Concl.	Trimetazidine did not reduce mortality in patients undergoing thrombolytic therapy. It might have some beneficial effects in patients not receiving reperfusion therapy.

ESCAMI

Evaluation of the Safety and Cardioprotective Effects of Eniporide in Acute Myocardial Infarction

Title	The Na+/H+ exchange inhibitor eniporide as an adjunct to early reperfusion therapy for acute myocardial infarction. Results of the Evaluation of the Safety and Cardioprotective effects of eniporide in Acute Myocardial Infarction (ESCAMI) Trial.
Authors	Zeymer U, Suryapranata H, Monassier JP, et al.
Reference	J Am Coll Cardiol 2001;38:1644-1650.
Disease	Acute myocardial infarction.
Purpose	To assess the efficacy on reducing infarct size and safety of eniporide as an adjunct to reperfusion therapy (thrombolysis or primary angioplasty) in patients with ST elevation acute myocardial infarction.
Design	Randomized, double-blind, placebo-controlled, phase II, multicenter.
Patients	1389 patients, 18-75 years old, with ST elevation acute myocardial infarction who would have been receiving reperfusion therapy (thrombolysis or PCI) within 6 hours of onset of symptoms. Patients who received prehospital thrombolysis and those who were in cardiogenic shock on admission were not included. Patients with renal failure, history of severe allergic reaction, autoimmune diseases, pregnancy, and severe concurrent disease were excluded.
Follow-up	6 weeks.
Regimen	Stage 1: Patients were randomized to 4 doses of eniporide (50 mg, 100 mg, 150 mg, and 200 mg) (n=433). Stage 2: Comparison of the most effective doses in the first stage (150 and 100 mg) with placebo (n=978). The study drug should be infused over 10 minutes, completing at least 15 minutes after beginning of thrombolytic therapy or 10 minutes before the start of PCI.

1.Acute Myocardial Infarction —g. Miscellaneous and Adjunctive Therapy

Results	There were 410 patients in the placebo group, and 86, 412, 390, and 91 in the eniporide 50, 100, 150, and 200 mg, respectively. 38.0% of the patients underwent primary PCI and 61.3% thrombolysis (streptokinase or alteplase). Stage 1: The cumulative release of alpha-hydroxybutyrate dehydrogenase (alpha-HBDH) (area under the curve in the first 72 hours) was 44.2±26.0 U/mL/h in the placebo group and 45.3±31.8, 40.2±22.5, 33.9±20.5, and 43.9±27.0 U/mL/h in the eniporide 50, 100, 150, and 200 mg, respectively (p=0.12). When the 100 and 150 mg eniporide groups were compared with placebo there was a statistically significant reduction in alpha-HBDH, creatine kinase (CK) and CK-MB release. The effect was most striking in patients who underwent primary PCI (50.7 U/mL/h in the placebo vs 37.7 and 29.6 U/mL/h in the 100 and 150 mg eniporide, respectively. Stage 2: There was no difference in alpha-HBDH release among the placebo, and the 100 and 150 eniporide groups (41.2±28.5, 43.0±26.1, and 41.5±25.9 U/mL/h, respectively). There were no differences in the area under the curve of CK and CK-MB and the peak troponin I and troponin T values. Analysis of subgroups, including patients undergoing thrombolysis, patients undergoing primary PCI, anterior infarction, inferior infarction, etc., showed no difference among the placebo and either the 100 or 150 mg eniporide groups. 42-day mortality tended to be higher in the eniporide (6.9%, 4.6%, 5.1%, and 8.8% in the 50, 100, 150, and 200 mg groups) than in the placebo group (3.7%). 6-month mortality was 4.4% in the placebo group and 6.9%, 6.1%, 7.4%, and 12.1% in the 4 eniporide groups, respectively (p=NS). Cardiogenic shock occurred in 3.2% of the patients in the placebo group and in 5.8%, 1.9%, 2.8%, and 6.6% in the 4 eniporide groups (p=NS). Similarly, there was no significant difference in the rate of reinfarction or the combined end point of death, sustained ventricular arrhythmia, cardiogenic shock, and heart failure among the groups. Stroke tended to occur more often in the eniporide groups (0, 0.7%, 1.8%, and 2.2%, respectively) than in the placebo group (0.2%); however, the difference was not statistically significant.
Concl.	The Na+/H+ exchange inhibitor eniporide was not effective in limiting infarct size or improving clinical outcome in patients with ST elevation acute myocardial infarction.

FLORIDA

Fluvastatin on Risk Diminishment After Acute Myocardial Infarction

Title	Effect of fluvastatin on ischaemia following acute myocardial infarction: a randomized trial.
Authors	Liem AH, van Boven AJ, Veeger NJ, et al.
Reference	Eur Heart J 2002;23:1931-1937.
Disease	Coronary artery disease, myocardial infarction.
Purpose	To determine whether early administration of fluvastatin after acute myocardial infarction decreases the incidence of residual myocardial ischemia at 1 year.
Design	Randomized, double-blind, placebo-controlled, multicenter.
Patients	540 patients, ≥18 years old, with an acute myocardial infarction and serum cholesterol ≤6.5 mmol/L and triglycerides ≤4.5 mmol/L. Patients using lipid-lowering drugs, patients treated with digoxin, quinidine or tricyclic antidepressants, known familial dyslipidemia, severe renal insufficiency, hepatic disease, severe (NYHA class IV) heart failure, scheduled PCI or CABG, atrial fibrillation, WPW syndrome, LBBB, known baseline ST deviation before the myocardial infarction, ECG signs of left ventricular hypertrophy with repolarization changes, and permanent pacemaker were excluded.
Follow-up	1 year.
Regimen	Randomization to placebo (n=275) or fluvastatin 40 mg bid (n=265) within 14 days of MI (at least 1 day before hospital discharge). Therapy was continued for 1 year.

Add'l Tx	Aspirin, β-blockers, and ACE-inhibitors were permitted.
Results	The median time from onset of infarction to initiation of study treatment was 8 days. 11.3% of the patients in the fluvastatin vs 13.5% in the placebo group discontinued study medications permanently, and 6.0% and 5.8%, respectively discontinued their medications temporarily. Fluvastatin decreased LDL cholesterol by 21%, whereas LDL cholesterol increased by 9% in the placebo group (p<0.001). Total cholesterol decreased by 13% in the fluvastatin group and increased by 9% in the placebo group (p<0.001). HDL cholesterol increased by 7% and 3%, respectively (p=0.38), and triglycerides increased by 22% and 44%, respectively (p<0.001). Major clinical events occurred in 62 patients in the fluvastatin group and in 68 patients in the placebo group (p=0.764). All-cause mortality was 2.6% in the fluvastatin group and 4.0% in the placebo group (p=NS). The primary end point (detection of residual myocardial ischemia on 48-hour ambulatory ECG after 1 year) was not affected by fluvastatin (7% of the patients in the fluvastatin group and 9% of the patients in the placebo group [p=NS]. The composite end point of either ischemia detected by ambulatory ECG or major clinical events occurred in 33% of the patients in the fluvastatin vs 36% in the placebo group (p=0.24). Residual ischemia on the baseline ambulatory ECG was predictive for the occurrence of any major clinical event (relative risk [RR] 2.35; 95% CI=1.39-3.72; p=0.0003). Post-hoc analysis in patients with the most pronounced ischemia at baseline showed a trend for a benefit from fluvastatin (p=0.084).
Concl.	Fluvastatin therapy, started early after an acute MI did not reduce the frequency of ambulatory ECG monitoring ischemia at 1 year and did not alter adverse clinical events. Patients with residual ischemia at baseline were more likely to have clinical events.

INTERCEPT

Incomplete Infarction Trial of European Research Collaborators Evaluating Progress Post-Thrombolysis

Title	Diltiazem in acute myocardial infarction treated with thrombolytic agents: a randomized placebo-controlled trial.
Authors	Boden WE, van Gilst WH, Scheldewaert RG, et al.
Reference	Lancet 2000;355:1751-1756.
Disease	Coronary artery disease, acute myocardial infarction.
Purpose	To assess the role of long acting diltiazem in the secondary prevention of recurrent events after acute myocardial infarction.
Design	Randomized, placebo-controlled, double-blind, multicenter.
Patients	874 patients, ≤75 years old, who had received thrombolytic therapy and aspirin within 12 hours of onset of symptoms of an ST elevation acute myocardial infarction. Only patients with cardiac enzyme elevation were included. Patients were randomized within 36-96 hours of onset of myocardial infarction. Patients with congestive heart failure, bradycardia, atrioventricular block, sick sinus syndrome, hypotension, severe hypertension, hemodynamic instability, ongoing myocardial ischemia, current therapy with calcium antagonists, or intolerance to diltiazem or aspirin were excluded.
Follow-up	6 months.
Regimen	Randomization to diltiazem 300 mg once a day (n=430) or placebo (n=444). Therapy was continued for 6 months.
Add'l Tx	All patients received aspirin. β-blockers and nitrates were administered to patients who developed recurrent ischemia after randomization. ACE inhibitors and diuretics were recommended for hypertension. However, routine prophylactic use of ACE inhibitors and β-blockers was prohibited.

Results	The primary end point of the study (cardiac death, nonfatal myocardial reinfarction, or refractory angina) occurred in 30% in the placebo group vs 23% in the diltiazem group (hazard ratio [HR] 0.79; 95% CI=0.61-1.02; p=0.07). Cardiac mortality was 1.4% in the placebo group vs 1.6% in the diltiazem group (HR 1.26; 95% CI=0.42-3.76; p=0.67). Nonfatal reinfarction occurred in 5% and 4% in the placebo and diltiazem groups, respectively (HR 0.79; 95% CI=0.41-1.50; p=0.47). Refractory ischemia occurred in 23% and 17%, respectively (HR 0.76; 95% CI=0.56-1.02; p=0.07). Nonfatal myocardial reinfarction or refractory ischemia occurred in 28% in the placebo group vs 21% in the diltiazem group (HR 0.76; 95% CI=0.58-1.00; p=0.05). Nonfatal myocardial reinfarction or revascularization occurred in 17% vs 11% (HR 0.67; 95% CI=0.46-0.96; p=0.03). 12% vs 7% in the placebo and diltiazem groups underwent revascularization (HR 0.61; 95% CI=0.39-0.96; p=0.03). Diltiazem was not associated with an increase in cancer, bleeding, strokes, or congestive heart failure.
Concl.	Diltiazem was not associated with a reduction in the cumulative occurrence of cardiac death, myocardial reinfarction, or refractory ischemia during 6 month follow-up. Diltiazem reduced the occurrence of nonfatal cardiac events, especially the rates of revascularization.

LIMIT AMI

Limitation of Myocardial Infarction Following Thrombolysis in Acute Myocardial Infarction Study

Title	Double-blind, randomized trial of an anti-CD18 antibody in conjunction with recombinant tissue plasminogen activator for acute myocardial infarction.
Authors	Baran KW, Nguyen M, McKendall GR, et al.
Reference	Circulation 2001;104:2778-2783.
Disease	Acute myocardial infarction.
Purpose	To assess the ability of a recombinant monoclonal antibody to CD18 subunit of β2 integrin adhesion receptors (rhuMAb CD18) to reduce myocardial infarct size in patients receiving thrombolytic therapy.
Design	Randomized, double-blind, placebo-controlled, multicenter.
Patients	394 patients presenting within 12 hours of chest pain with ST elevation.
Follow-up	90 days.
Regimen	0.5 or 2.0 mg/kg rhuMAb CD18 or placebo as an IV bolus.
Add'l Tx	Recombinant tissue plasminogen activator. Adjunctive angioplasty, glycoprotein IIb/IIIa inhibitor as per investigators' discretion.

Results	Primary end point was corrected TIMI frame count at 90 minutes; secondary end points were percent of patients achieving grade 3 flow at 90 minute angiogram, single-photon-emission computed tomography (SPECT)-determined myocardial infarct size at ≥120 hours, and ST-segment elevation resolution. Corrected TIMI frame count was 46, 51, and 45 in the placebo, 0.5 mg/kg and 2.0 mg/kg CD18 dose, respectively (p=NS). Percent achieving TIMI grade 3 flow was 66%, 58%, 63%, respectively (p=NS). Myocardial infarct size by SPECT, as a median percent LV defect size was 10%, 13%, and 13%, respectively. Myocardial infarct size also was similar among the 3 groups when assessed by creatine kinase-MB. There was no difference in ECG ST-segment elevation resolution ≥70% at 90 or 180 minutes among groups. There was a trend, although not statistically significant, toward more bacterial infections in the treated group.
Concl.	RhuMAb CD18 did not improve coronary blood flow assessed by TIMI grade or TIMI frame count, nor did it reduce myocardial infarct size.

MAGIC

Magnesium in Coronaries

Title	Early administration of intravenous magnesium to high-risk patients with acute myocardial infarction in the Magnesium in Coronaries (MAGIC) trial: a randomised controlled trial.
Authors	The Magnesium in Coronaries (MAGIC) Trial Investigators.
Reference	Lancet 2002;360:1189-1196.
Disease	Acute myocardial infarction.
Purpose	To investigate whether early IV administration of magnesium reduces mortality of high-risk patients with ST-elevation acute myocardial infarction.
Design	Randomized, double-blind, placebo-controlled, multicenter.
Patients	6213 patients with ischemic discomfort and ≥0.1 mV ST elevation in ≥2 limb leads, ≥0.2 mV ST elevation in ≥2 precordial leads, or presumably new LBBB that could receive the tested drug within 6 hours of onset of symptoms. High-risk was defined either as age ≥65 years for patients who were candidates for reperfusion therapy (thrombolysis or primary PCI) or patients of any age not scheduled for reperfusion therapy. Patients who received reperfusion therapy in the preceding 7 days, systolic blood pressure <90 mm Hg despite treatment with pressors, heart rate <50 bpm, advanced atrioventricular block, and chronic renal failure were not included.
Follow-up	30 days.
Regimen	Within 6 hours of onset of symptoms, patients were randomized to IV magnesium (2 g IV bolus over 15 minutes followed by a 17 g infusion for 24 hours) (n=3113) or placebo (n=3100).

Results	Therapy was started at a median of 3.8 hours from onset of symptoms. The study drug bolus was administered to 3107 patients randomized to magnesium and to 3095 patients randomized to placebo, and the infusion was given to 3085 and 3079 patients, respectively. Magnesium was well tolerated. Sustained hypotension and bradycardia occurred with similar proportions in the 2 groups. 30-day mortality was 15.2% in the placebo group and 15.3% in the magnesium group (OR 1.0; 95% CI= 0.9-1.2; p=0.96). Magnesium had no effect on mortality in the 8 prespecified subgroup analyses. Including patients undergoing reperfusion therapy (17% vs 18% in the placebo and magnesium group, respectively; OR 1.1; 95% CI=0.9-1.4); patients without reperfusion therapy (15% vs 14%, respectively; OR 1.0; 95% CI=0.8-1.1); patients treated within 1 hour, 1-3 hours, 3-6 hours, or >6 hours of onset of symptoms; patients with and without diabetes; patients with or without previous MI; patients with and without chest pain at randomization; the type of reperfusion therapy (thrombolysis vs angioplasty); and age above or below 65 years. Multivariate regression analysis failed to show any advantage of magnesium (OR 0.95; 95% CI=0.82-1.10; p=0.53). Heart failure occurred in 18% of the patients randomized to placebo and in 19% of the patients randomized to magnesium (p=0.28). Defibrillation for ventricular fibrillation or tachycardia was performed in 5% of the patients in each group (p=0.93). 2 percent of the patients in each group needed a temporary pacemaker (p=0.52).
Concl.	Early intravenous administration of magnesium did not affect 30-day mortality in high-risk patients with ST-elevation acute MI.

NEHDP

National Exercise and Heart Disease Project

Title	Results of multicenter randomized clinical trial of exercise and long-term survival in myocardial infarction patients. The NEHDP.
Authors	Dorn J, Naughton J, Imamura D, et al.
Reference	Circulation 1999;100:1764-1769.
Disease	Myocardial infarction.
Purpose	To determine whether a supervised exercise program improved survival in male myocardial infarct patients.
Design	Randomized, multicenter.
Patients	651 men ages 30-64 with documented MI ≥8 weeks but <3 years before being enrolled. Had to be able to exercise ≥3 metabolic equivalents.
Follow-up	19 years.
Regimen	Following completion of a low level exercise program of 6 weeks duration patients were assigned to exercise group (n=323) or nonexercise group (n=328). Exercise prescription based on patient's performance on ECG monitored treadmill testing. Included various forms of physical activity. Initially they exercised for 8 weeks in a laboratory. After this, they jogged, cycled, or swam guided by target heart rate.
Add'l Tx	As per physician.

Results	All cause mortality risk estimates in the exercise group vs controls was 0.69 (95% CI=0.39-1.25) after 3 years follow-up; 0.84 (0.55-1.28) at 5 years; 0.95 (0.71-1.29) at 10 years; 1.02 (0.79-1.32) at 15 years; and 1.09 (0.87-1.36) at 19 years. Thus, the nonsignificant lower mortality estimates in the exercise group continued for up to 10 years but the reduction in risk was attenuated over time, especially by 15-19 years. A trend toward reduction in death due to cardiovascular disease was only detected during the earliest years of the study (a benefit in favor of exercise RR 0.73; 95% CI=0.37-1.43 at 3 years) and by 5 years relative risk approached unity. Thereafter there was a nonsignificant increased risk for cardiovascular death associated with exercise (RR 1.21, 1.14, and 1.16 at 10, 15, and 19 years, respectively). Men who were younger, smoked cigarettes, and had a low initial physical work capacity, benefited more from exercise than men who were older, nonsmokers, or had a high initial physical work capacity. Each 1 metabolic equivalent increase in work capacity from baseline to end of the trial was associated with a decrease in all cause mortality risk of 8%-14%.
Concl.	Exercise program resulted in a nonsignificant decrease in mortality during the first 5 years of follow-up that then diminished over time.

SADHART

Sertraline Antidepressant Heart Attack Randomized Trial

Title	Sertraline treatment of major depression in patients with acute MI or unstable angina.
Authors	Glassman AH, O'Connor CM, Califf RM, et al.
Reference	JAMA 2002;288:701-709.
Disease	Acute myocardial infarction.
Purpose	To determine whether the antidepressant sertraline, a selective serotonin reuptake inhibitor, is safe and effective in the treatment of major depressive disorder (MDD) in patients hospitalized with acute myocardial infarction or unstable angina.
Design	Randomized, double-blind, placebo-controlled, multicenter.
Patients	369 patients, randomized to sertraline (n=186) or placebo (n=183). Patients were eligible if they were hospitalized with unstable angina or had had an acute MI in the 30 days before study entry, and were currently experiencing an episode of MDD based on criteria in the Diagnostic and Statistical Manual, 4th Edition (DSM-IV). Diagnosis of acute MI was based on having at least 1 criterion from 2 categories: the first category consisted of 1) creatine kinase isoenzyme MB (CK-MB) level greater than the upper limit of normal; 2) CK or troponin T or troponin I level greater than 2 times the upper limit of normal; or 3) total lactate dehydrogenase (LDH) level that was more than 1.5 times the upper limit of normal (and LDH 1>LDH 2). Criteria in the second category were: 1) characteristic ischemic symptoms (chest pain or shortness of breath) lasting >10 minutes; or 2) electrocardiographic changes of ST-segment depression or elevation, or new pathologic Q waves. Patients were also eligible for study entry if they satisfied criteria for unstable angina, including: 1) angina or anginal

equivalent symptoms at rest and episodes lasting >10 minutes and resulting in hospitalization, with ST-segment elevation or depression >0.5 mm, or T-wave inversion >1 mm within 12 hours of chest pain episode; or 2) hospitalization for symptoms of unstable angina and known coronary artery disease with history of previous MI, previous revascularization, or documented coronary stenosis >75% in 1 or more major epicardial vessels. There were numerous exclusion criteria; among these were: uncontrolled hypertension (systolic blood pressure >180 mm Hg or diastolic blood pressure >100 mm Hg); anticipated cardiac surgery during the next 6 months; MI or unstable angina that occurred less than 3 months after a coronary artery bypass graft procedure; resting heart rate <40 bpm (or <50/min if symptomatic or daytime sinus pauses of >3.5 sec); MI or unstable angina not of atherosclerotic origin; Killip class III or IV status, and use of any of the following medications: class I antiarrhythmic medications; reserpine, guanethidine, clonidine, or methyldopa; anticonvulsants or neuroleptics; antidepressants; benzodiazepine; or psychotherapy within 3 months prior to study entry, and other medical conditions such as significant renal or hepatic dysfunction.

Follow-up	24 weeks.
Regimen	Enrolled patients received placebo in a single-blind fashion for 14 days to undergo prestudy cardiovascular assessments (multiple gated acquisition scans and Holter recording) and to establish the presence of depressive symptoms for at least 2 weeks. Patients then received 50 mg/d of either sertraline or placebo for 6 weeks. According to patient response and tolerability, dosages were increased to 2 tablets (100 mg/d or matching placebo) at week 6, to 3 tablets (150 mg/d or matching placebo) at week 10, and no more than 4 tablets (200 mg/d or matching placebo) at week 12. Dosages could be decreased by 50 mg at a time if there were adverse events, with a minimum dose of 50 mg daily. The only psychotropic medication that was permitted was chloral hydrate, which was allowed for sleep at a maximum of 1 g.

Results	The primary safety end point of the study was change of LVEF from baseline. Secondary safety end points were: heart rate, BP, standard ECG, runs of ventricular premature complexes and heart rate variability, and the occurrence of cardiovascular events, MI, stroke, severe angina, CHF, and death. The efficacy end point was depression severity as determined by the Beck Depression Inventory (BDI), the 17-item Hamilton Depression scale (HAM-D), and the Clinical Global Impression, Severity (CGI-S) and Improvement (CGI-I) scales. There were no significant differences in baseline characteristics between the 2 groups. 24% of the patients were classified in the severe subgroup characterized by greater depression severity (HAM-D score ≥ 18) and multiple previous episodes of depression. The primary safety end point, LVEF, was similar between the 2 groups at baseline and at the end of week 16, with little change within the groups from study start to finish (patients with >5-point decrease in LVEF, 6/135 vs 5/125, sertraline vs placebo). At week 16, 20/135 in the sertraline group had an LVEF <30% and 24/125 in the placebo group had an LVEF <30%; both values were identical to values at study start. Similarly, secondary parameters (systolic and diastolic BPs; heart rate, PR interval, QRS duration, QTc, runs of ventricular premature complexes (VPC) were unchanged between study start and finish for both groups. There were no significant differences in incidence of death, MI, CHF, stroke, or angina between the groups. The composite risk of these events was slightly lower in the sertraline group; this was not significant (RR 0.77; 95% CI=0.51-1.16). Depression was significantly improved in patients treated with sertraline on the CGI-S scale at 24 weeks, across all baseline severities. Patients with recurrent MDD and more severe MDD demonstrated benefit from sertraline as assessed by the CGI-I and HAM-D scores (p values <0.02). At study completion, the number of patients who responded with a CGI-I score of 1 or 2 (very much or much improved) was significantly higher in the sertraline group compared to placebo (p<0.01), regardless of baseline severity or number of recurrent episodes.
Concl.	Sertraline was safe and effective for treating major depression in patients with unstable angina or acute MI.

Glucose Insulin Potassium Study

Title	Glucose insulin potassium infusion in patients treated with primary angioplasty for acute myocardial infarction. The Glucose Insulin Potassium Study: a randomized trial.
Authors	van der Horst IC, Zijlstra F, van't Hof AW, et al.
Reference	J Am Coll Cardiol 2003;42:784-791.
Disease	Acute myocardial infarction.
Purpose	To determine whether therapy with glucose, insulin, and potassium as adjunctive therapy to primary coronary transluminal angioplasty further reduces mortality.
Design	Randomized, open-label.
Patients	940 patients with acute myocardial infarction with ST-segment elevation of >1 mm in 2 or more contiguous leads on the electrocardiogram or a new left bundle-branch block. Patients were slated for percutaneous transluminal coronary angioplasty of the infarct artery.
Follow-up	30 days.
Regimen	The glucose, insulin, and potassium group received a continuous infusion of 80 mmol potassium chloride in 500 mL 20% glucose with a rate of 3 mL/kg body weight/hour over 8-12 hours plus a continuous infusion of short-acting insulin (50 units) in 50 mL 0.9% sodium chloride. Infusion could be adjusted depending on blood glucose levels. After the infusion was started or no infusion patients proceeded to the catheterization laboratory for coronary angiography and percutaneous transluminal coronary angioplasty.

1g

Add'l Tx	IV heparin, nitroglycerin, aspirin.
Results	The primary end point was 30-day mortality. Of 940 patients, 476 were randomized to glucose, insulin, and potassium (GIK) and 464 to the control group. At 30 days, mortality was 23 of 476 (4.8%) in the GIK group vs 27 of 464 (5.8%) in the control group (relative risk [RR] 0.82; 95% CI=0.46-1.46). However, there were differences in outcome depending upon whether the patients were in heart failure. Of 856 patients without signs of heart failure, mortality was 5 of 426 (1.2%) in the GIK group vs 18 of 430 (4.2%) in the control group (RR 0.28; 95% CI=0.1-0.75; p=0.01). In contrast, in the 84 patients with signs of heart failure (Killip class ≥2), mortality was 18 of 50 (36%) in the GIK group vs 9 of 34 (26.5%) in the control group (RR 1.44; 95% CI=0.65-3.22). The authors postulated that in some patients with underlying heart failure, a potential positive effect of GIK on cardiac metabolism was overcome by a volume load.
Concl.	GIK did not reduce mortality in the total cohort of acute MI patients undergoing angioplasty. In a subgroup of patients without signs of heart failure, it appeared to decrease mortality.

ADMIRE

AmP579 Delivery for Myocardial Infarction Reduction

Title	A randomized, double-blinded, placebo-controlled, dose-ranging study measuring the effect of an adenosine agonist on infarct size reduction in patients undergoing primary percutaneous transluminal coronary angioplasty: the ADMIRE (AmP579 Delivery for Myocardial Infarction REduction) study.
Authors	Kopecky SL, Aviles RJ, Bell MR, et al.
Reference	Am Heart J 2003;146:146-152.
Disease	Acute myocardial infarction.
Purpose	To investigate the effect of AMP579, an adenosine A1 and A2 receptor agonist, on infarct size in patients with acute myocardial infarction undergoing primary coronary balloon angioplasty.
Design	Randomized, double-blind, placebo-controlled, dose-ranging, multicenter.
Patients	311 patients, 18-85 years old, within 6 hours of onset of symptoms of acute ST elevation myocardial infarction (or new left bundle-branch block) referred for primary percutaneous coronary angioplasty. Pregnant or lactating women were not included. Patients with electrocardiogram evidence of prior Q-wave infarction, old left bundle-branch block, Wolf-Parkinson-White syndrome, or paced rhythm were not included. Patients treated with thrombolytic therapy, those with cardiogenic shock, serum creatinine >2.0 mg/dL, theophylline treatment, or unavailability for follow-up were excluded.
Follow-up	Technetium-99m sestamibi single-photon emission computed tomography 5-9 days after enrollment. Left ventricular ejection fraction by multiple gated acquisition at 4 weeks. Clinical follow-up for 180 days.
Regimen	Randomization to 6-hour infusion of placebo or AMP579 15 µg/kg, 30 µg/kg or 60 µg/kg, started before angioplasty.

Add'l Tx	All patients underwent primary angioplasty. The use of glyco-protein IIb/IIIa inhibitors and coronary stents was permitted. The use of rotational atherectomy was prohibited.
Results	Heart rate and BP after infusion were comparable among the 4 groups. Infarct size was comparable among groups. The median infarct size for anterior infarction was 18.3% in the placebo group and 21.1% (p=0.44 vs placebo), 14.0% (p=0.74 vs placebo), and 13.5% (p=0.42 vs placebo) in the AMP579 15, 30, and 60 μg/kg groups. For non-anterior infarction, infarct size was 9.9% in the placebo and 10.0% (p=0.65 vs placebo), 8.0% (p=0.36 vs placebo), and 10.5% (p=0.28 vs placebo) in the 3 AMP579 groups, respectively. In a subset of patients with anterior infarction (n=45) who underwent sestamibi imaging before angioplasty and predischarge, there was a trend toward increased myocardial salvage with higher doses of AMP579 (p=0.384). There was no difference between the groups in the duration of hospitalization or duration of stay in the intensive care unit. 4-week ejection fraction was comparable among the groups. Clinical outcomes, including death, MI, recurrent angina, and heart failure were comparable between the groups.
Concl.	AMP579 was safe, but did not reduce infarct size, LVEF, or affected clinical outcomes.

ALIVE

Azimilide Post-Infarct Survival Evaluation

Title	Mortality in patients after a recent myocardial infarction: a randomized, placebo-controlled trial of azimilide using heart rate variability for risk stratification.
Authors	Camm AJ, Pratt CM, Schwartz PJ, et al.
Reference	Circulation 2004;109:990-996.
Disease	Acute myocardial infarction.
Purpose	Azimilide, a class III antiarrhythmic drug, was investigated for its effects on mortality in patients with depressed left ventricular function after a recent myocardial infarction and in a subpopulation of patients with low heart rate variability (>20 U).
Design	International, multicenter, randomized, placebo-controlled, double-blind study.
Patients	3381 postmyocardial infarction patients with depressed left ventricular function.
Follow-up	12 months.
Regimen	Azimilide 100 mg or placebo. Treatment was initiated within 5-21 days of myocardial infarction.

Results	Placebo patients with low heart variability (HRV) (n=642) had a significantly higher 1-year mortality rate than those with high HRV (n=1048) (15% vs 9.5%; p<0.0005) despite nearly identical ejection fractions. There were no significant differences between patients receiving azimilide or placebo for all-cause mortality, either among those in the "at risk" population identified by depressed LV function (12% in both groups), in the subpopulation of "high-risk" patients identified by low HRV (14% vs 15%), or for total cardiac or arrhythmic mortality. Fewer patients receiving azimilide had atrial fibrillation than did patients receiving placebo (0.5% vs 1.2%; p<0.04). The incidence of torsade de pointes was slightly higher in the azimilide group (0.3%) than in the placebo group (0.1%). Severe neutropenia with an absolute neutrophil count of ≤500 cells/μL was also slightly higher in the azimilide patients (0.9%) vs controls (0.2%).
Concl.	Depressed LV function is associated with increased all-cause mortality after MI. Reduced HRV is associated with increased sudden cardiac mortality risk after MI. Azimilide did not affect mortality in these patients. Low HRV independently identified a subpopulation at particularly high risk of death.

ATTACC

Attenuation by Adenosine of Cardiac Complications

Title	Left ventricular function and cardiovascular events following adjuvant therapy with adenosine in acute myocardial infarction treated with thrombolysis.
Authors	Quintana M, Hjemdahl P, Sollevi A, et al.
Reference	Eur J Clin Pharmacol 2003;59:1-9.
Disease	Acute myocardial infarction.
Purpose	To assess whether low-dose adenosine infusion will improve left ventricular function in patients with acute myocardial infarction receiving thrombolytic therapy.
Design	Randomized, double-blind, placebo-controlled, multicenter.
Patients	608 patients, 18-80 years old, within 12 hours of onset of symptoms of ST elevation acute myocardial infarction who were candidates for thrombolytic therapy. Patients who could not receive β blockers were excluded. Pregnant or lactating women were not included. Patients with second degree atrioventricular block without permanent pacemaker were not enrolled.
Follow-up	Predischarge echocardiography. 1-year clinical follow-up.
Regimen	Randomization to placebo or adenosine (10 µg/kg/min) infusion for 6 hours, started before or simultaneously with the infusion of thrombolytic agent.
Add'l Tx	All patients received thrombolytic therapy (tissue-type plasminogen activator or streptokinase). Other cardiac medications or revascularizations were left to the discretion of the treating physician. None of the patients underwent rescue percutaneous coronary intervention due to failure of thrombolysis.

Results	Hypotension (systolic BP <100 mm Hg) was noted in 86 of the 302 patients in the placebo group and in 79 of the 302 patients in the adenosine group. Bradycardia (<50 bpm) was noted in 86 and 79 patients, respectively. Atrioventricular block was detected in 5 and 3 patients, respectively, and recurrent chest pain in 13 and 10 patients, respectively. 2 patients in the placebo and 4 in the adenosine group died during treatment. At discharge, 13 patients in the placebo group and 14 in the adenosine group died, and 14 patients in each group had CHF. There was no difference between the placebo and adenosine groups in LV end diastolic diameter (27 ± 4 vs 28 ± 4 mm/m^2), LV end systolic diameter (19 ± 4 vs 19 ± 4 mm/m^2), fractional shortening ($31\%\pm9\%$ vs $32\%\pm8\%$), LVEF ($45\%\pm11\%$ vs $44\%\pm10\%$), and wall motion score index (1.50 ± 0.43 vs 1.53 ± 0.40). 1-year mortality was 12.7% in the placebo group and 10.6% in the adenosine group (p=0.4). Cardiovascular mortality was 12.1% vs 8.9%, respectively (p=0.2). There was no difference in the rate of nonfatal MI (12.4% vs 11.6%; p=0.7) or cardiovascular mortality and MI (21.0% vs 20.2%; p=0.8) between the placebo and adenosine groups. However, when data were analyzed for anterior and inferior infarction separately, 1-year mortality tended to be lower in the adenosine group (8.4%) vs the placebo group (15.3%) for anterior infarction. There was no such difference among patients with inferior infarction (12.5% and 10.3%, respectively; p=0.5). Among patients with anterior infarction, cardiovascular mortality was 8.4% in the adenosine group and 14.6% in the placebo group (p=0.09). Among patients with inferior infarction, cardiovascular mortality was 9.3% and 9.6%, respectively (p=0.9).
Concl.	Low-dose adenosine infusion did not improve the predischarge echocardiographic indices of LV function. There was a trend towards lower 1-year all-cause mortality and cardiovascular mortality with adenosine among patients with anterior MI; however, the differences did not reach statistical significance.

COMMA

The Complement Inhibition in Myocardial Infarction Treated with Angioplasty Trial

Title	Pexelizumab, an anti-C5 complement antibody, as adjunctive therapy to primary percutaneous coronary intervention in acute myocardial infarction. The COMMA trial.
Authors	Granger CB, Mahaffey KW, Weaver D, et al.
Reference	Circulation 2003;108:1184-1190.
Disease	Acute myocardial infarction.
Purpose	To determine the effect of pexelizumab, a C5 complement inhibitor on myocardial infarct size in patients with ST-segment elevation myocardial infarctions undergoing percutaneous coronary interventions.
Design	Randomized, multicenter.
Patients	960 patients with acute ST-elevation myocardial infarction within 6 hours of symptoms or new left bundle-branch block undergoing primary percutaneous coronary intervention.
Follow-up	6 months.
Regimen	Patients were randomized to 1) placebo bolus and infusion; 2) 2.0 mg/kg bolus of pexelizumab and placebo infusion; or 3) 2.0 mg/kg bolus and 0.05 mg/kg/h infusion of pexelizumab for 20 hours.

Results	The primary outcome was creatine kinase-MB area under the curve, or enzymatic myocardial infarct size. The end point did not differ among the 3 groups: 4393 ng/mL in the placebo group (median value); 4526 in the pexelizumab bolus-alone group; and 4713 in the pexelizumab bolus + infusion group. There was no difference among the 3 groups in a composite clinical outcome of 90-day death, new or worsening heart failure, shock or stroke (11.1%, 10.7%, 8.5% in the placebo, bolus-pexelizumab, or bolus + infusion pexelizumab groups); however, 90-day mortality was lower with the pexelizumab bolus + infusion (1.8%) vs in the placebo group (5.9%; p=0.014); while the pexelizumab bolus-only group had an intermediate mortality rate of 4.2%. Adverse events were not increased in the pexelizumab group.
Concl.	Pexelizumab did not reduce myocardial infarct size in patients undergoing PCI for acute MI. The reduction in the mortality in the pexelizumab bolus + infusion group suggests that the agent may benefit patients through an as yet unidentified novel mechanism.

COMPLY

The Complement Inhibition in Myocardial Infarction Treated with Thrombolytics Trial

Title	Effect of pexelizumab, an anti-C5 complement antibody, as adjunctive therapy to fibrinolysis in acute myocardial infarction: the Complement inhibition in myocardial infarction treated with thrombolytics (COMPLY) trial.
Authors	Mahaffey KW, Granger CB, Nicolau JC, et al.
Reference	Circulation 2003;108:1176-1183.
Disease	Acute ST-segment elevation, acute myocardial infarction.
Purpose	To determine whether pexelizumab, a novel C5 complement monoclonal antibody fragment, reduces myocardial infarct size in patients reperfused with thrombolytic therapy.
Design	Parallel, double-blind, placebo-controlled, multicenter trial.
Patients	943 patients with acute ST-segment elevation acute myocardial infarction reperfused with thrombolytic therapy. The choice of thrombolytic therapy was up to the physician.
Follow-up	6 months.
Regimen	Patients (N=943) were randomized to 1) placebo bolus + placebo infusion; 2) 2.0 mg/kg pexelizumab bolus followed by placebo infusion for 20 hours; or 3) 2.0 mg/kg pexelizumab bolus and 0.05 mg/kg/h pexelizumab infusion for 20 hours. Patients were assigned to therapy within 6 hours of onset of symptoms.

Results	The primary end point was infarct size measured by creatine kinase-MB area under the curve. Median infarct size was 5230 ng/mL in the placebo group; 4952 in the pexelizumab bolus + placebo infusion and 5557 in the pexelizumab bolus + infusion group (p=NS). There was no difference in resolution of ST-segment abnormality or QRS scores among the 3 groups. The clinical composite end point at 90 days of death, new or worsening CHF, shock, or stroke did not differ among the 3 groups: 18.6%, 18.4%, and 19.7% in the placebo, bolus, and bolus + infusion groups, respectively. The drug did inhibit complement for 4 hours in the bolus-only dose and for 20-24 hours in the bolus + infusion group. Infections were infrequent, occurring in 6 placebo, 4 bolus, and 2 bolus + infusion patients; most common infection was pneumonia.
Concl.	Pexelizumab, an anti-C5 complement antibody, did not reduce MI size, nor did it reduce adverse cardiovascular events.

WIZARD

Weekly Intervention with Zithromax for Atherosclerosis and Its Related Disorders

Title	Azithromycin for the secondary prevention of coronary heart disease events: the WIZARD study: a randomized controlled trial.
Authors	O'Connor CM, Dunne MW, Pfeffer MA, et al.
Reference	JAMA 2003;290:1459-1466.
Disease	Coronary artery disease, postmyocardial infarction.
Purpose	To determine whether antibiotic therapy with azithromycin had any effect on cardiac events in patients with stable coronary artery disease and known exposure to Chlamydia pneumoniae.
Design	Randomized, placebo-controlled, blinded, multicenter.
Patients	7747 patients had to have had a history of myocardial infarction more than 6 weeks before screening and an immunoglobulin G titer to C pneumoniae of 1:16 or greater. Patients could not have had coronary artery bypass graft or percutaneous coronary intervention in the preceding 6 months.
Follow-up	Median of 14 months.
Regimen	Azithromycin 600 mg or matched placebo qd for 3 days, then once weekly for 11 weeks.

Results   A primary end point was death from any cause; recurrent MI, CABG, or PCI; or hospitalization for angina, whichever occurred first. There was no significant risk reduction in developing a primary event with azithromycin vs placebo (7% risk reduction; 95% CI=-5% to 17%; p=0.23). There were no significant risk reductions of the individual components of the primary end point, including: death (8%); recurrent MI (7%); CABG or PTCA (5%); or hospitalizations for angina (-1%). Results were similar after adjusting for cardiac risk factors. There was no significant correlation between C pneumoniae titers and treatment effect. Side effects of study drug included diarrhea resulting in drug discontinuation in 1.6% vs 0.4% of placebo patients.

Concl.   A 3-month course of the antibiotic azithromycin did not significantly reduce cardiac events in patients with a previous MI and stable CAD.

2. Acute Treatment of Stroke

Title	Aptiganel hydrochloride in acute ischemic stroke. A randomized controlled trial.
Authors	Albers GW, Goldstein LB, Hall D, et al.
Reference	JAMA 2001;286:2673-2682.
Disease	Acute ischemic cerebrovascular accident.
Purpose	To determine whether aptiganel hydrochloride, a selective ligand for ion-channel site of N-methyl-D-aspartate receptor channel complex—an agent that showed neuroprotection in animal models—improves clinical outcome in patients with acute strokes.
Design	Nested Phase 2/Phase 3 randomized, controlled, multicenter study.
Patients	628 patients with hemispheric ischemic strokes. Average age 72 years.
Follow-up	90-120 days.
Regimen	Patients were randomized to 1 of 3 regimens within 6 hours of stroke: High-dose aptiganel (5 mg bolus followed by infusion of 0.75 mg/h for 12 hours; n=214); low-dose aptiganel (3 mg bolus followed by infusion of 0.5 mg/h for 12 hours; n=200); vs placebo (n=214).
Add'l Tx	Use of heparin, aspirin, ticlopidine, and warfarin allowed. Use of fibrinolytic, thrombolytic agents not allowed.

Results Primary end point was modified Rankin scale score at 90 days. Trial suspended because of lack of efficacy and imbalance in mortality. There was no difference in the median modified Rankin scale score which was equal to 3 in all 3 treatment groups. Placebo patients showed slightly greater neurologic improvement on a National Institutes of Health (NIH) stroke scale (-0.8 points) vs high-dose aptiganel patients (0.9 points; p=0.04). At 120 days, mortality rate in high-dose aptiganel group (26.3%) was higher than in the placebo group (19.2%; p=0.06). In the low-dose group mortality was 22.5% (p=0.39 vs placebo). Mortality rate was 3.1% in the placebo group during the first week vs 8.6% and 9.9% in the low- and high-dose aptiganel groups, respectively (p=0.03 for placebo vs combined 2 doses of drug).

Concl. Aptiganel was not effective in reducing clinical outcome following acute stroke and may be harmful.

ATLANTIS

Alteplase Thrombolysis for Acute Noninterventional Therapy in Ischemic Stroke

Title	Recombinant tissue type plasminogen activator (alteplase) for ischemic stroke 3-5 hours after symptom onset. The ATLANTIS study: A randomized controlled trial.
Authors	Clark WM, Wissman S, Albers GW.
Reference	JAMA 1999;282:2019-2026.
Disease	Ischemic stroke.
Purpose	To assess whether rt-PA administration to patients with acute ischemic stroke, presenting 3-5 hours after onset of symptoms, is effective and safe.
Design	Randomized, double-blind, placebo-controlled, multicenter.
Patients	613 patients, 18-79 years old, who presented within 3-5 hours of onset of symptoms of ischemic stroke. All patients underwent CT scan to exclude intracerebral hemorrhage before enrollment. Patients with signs of cerebral ischemia in >1/3 of the territory of the middle cerebral artery were excluded.
Follow-up	90 days.
Regimen	Randomization to placebo or to rt-PA 0.09 mg/kg as a bolus, followed by a 60 minute infusion of 0.81 mg/kg.
Add'l Tx	Administration of heparin, oral anticoagulants, other hemorrheologic agents, and antiplatelet agents was not permitted during the initial 24 hours.

Results	547 patients received study medication between 3-5 hours of onset of symptoms. Mean time to treatment was 4.40 hours in the placebo group and 4.47 hours in the rt-PA group. 32% of the placebo group vs 34% of the rt-PA group had an excellent recovery at 90 days (p=0.65). All secondary functional outcome measures were comparable between the 2 groups. Infarct volume at 30 days was 47±74% in the placebo group vs 46±66% in the rt-PA group (p=0.95). Symptomatic intracerebral hemorrhage occurred in 1.1% of the placebo vs 7.0% of the rt-PA group (p<0.001), whereas asymptomatic intracerebral hemorrhage occurred in 4.7% vs 11.4%, respectively (p=0.004), and fatal intracerebral hemorrhage in 0.3% vs 3.0%, respectively (p<0.001). 30-day mortality was 4.4% in the placebo group vs 7.0% in the rt-PA group (p=0.18), whereas 90-day mortality was 6.9% vs 11.0%, respectively (p=0.09).
Concl.	rt-PA was associated with increased risk of intracerebral hemorrhage but was not associated with clinical benefits when administered to patients within 3-5 hours after onset of symptoms of stroke.

NINDS

Neurological Disorders and Stroke Recombinant Tissue Plasminogen Activator Stroke Study

Title	Effects of tissue plasminogen activator for acute ischemic stroke at one year.
Authors	Kwiatkowski TG, Libman RB, Frankel M, et al.
Reference	N Engl J Med 1999;340:1781-1787.
Disease	Ischemic stroke.
Purpose	Previously, this group showed that patients treated with tPA within 3 hours of symptoms of acute ischemic stroke were at least 30% more likely than patients treated with placebo to have minimal or no disability at 3 months. This study analyzed data on outcomes from this study at 6 and 12 months.
Design	Randomized, multicenter.
Patients	624 patients with stroke who could be treated within 3 hours of onset of symptoms.
Follow-up	12 months.
Regimen	tPA vs placebo.
Results	Primary outcome was "favorable outcome" which was defined as minimal or no disability using various neurologic indices and scales (Barthel index, modified Rankin scale, Glasgow outcome scale), and using a global statistic. Favorable effects of tPA on the global statistic were observed in the tPA group. At 6 months, the odds ratios for a favorable outcome with tPA vs placebo was 1.7 (95% CI=1.3-2.3) and at 12 months was 1.7 (95% CI=1.2-2.3). Patients that received tPA were at least 30% more likely to have minimal or no disability at 12 months than placebo patients. Mortality at 12 months was similar between the tPA group (24%) vs the placebo group (28%; p=0.29). There was no difference in rates of recurrent strokes between groups.

Concl.   Patients with acute ischemic stroke who were treated with tPA within 3 hours after symptom onset were more likely to have minimal or no disability than patients receiving placebo at 6 and 12 months.

PROCAT II

Prolyse in Acute Cerebral Thromboembolism II

Title	Intra-arterial prourokinase for acute ischemic stroke. The PROCAT II study: A randomized controlled trial.
Authors	Furlan A, Higashida R, Wechsler L, et al.
Reference	JAMA 1999;282:2003-2011.
Disease	Ischemic stroke.
Purpose	To evaluate the efficacy and safety of intra-arterial administration of recombinant prourokinase in patients with acute ischemic stroke of <6 hours, caused by middle cerebral artery occlusion.
Design	Randomized, open-label with blinded follow-up, multicenter.
Patients	180 patients, 18-85 years old, with new focal neurological signs related to the middle cerebral artery territory that could have been treated within 6 hours of onset of symptoms. Patients with a National Institutes of Health Stroke Scale (NIHSS) >30, coma, rapid improving neurological signs, clinical suspicion of subarachnoid hemorrhage, seizures, history of intracerebral bleeding, uncontrolled hypertension, and contraindications to thrombolytic therapy were excluded. All patients underwent CT scan before enrollment to exclude intracranial tumors and hemorrhage. Patients with acute hypodense parenchymal lesion or effacement of cerebral sulci in >1/3 of the middle cerebral artery territory were excluded. Then patients underwent cerebral angiography and only patients with complete occlusion of the middle cerebral artery were further included.
Follow-up	90 days.
Regimen	After cerebral angiography patients were randomized to selective intra-arterial administration of r-prourokinase 9 mg over 2 hours through an infusion microcatheter placed in the proximal 1 third of the middle cerebral artery thrombus + IV heparin (n=121) or to IV heparin alone (n=59).
Add'l Tx	All patients received IV heparin (2000 U bolus followed by 500 U/h for 4 hours).

Results   12323 patients with acute ischemic stroke were screened, 474 (4%) underwent cerebral angiography at a median of 4.5 hours after onset of symptoms. 180 patients were finally randomized. The median time to initiation of prourokinase infusion was 5.3 hours. 40% of the prourokinase and 25% of the control patients had slight or no neurological disability (a modified Rankin score of ≤2) at 90 days (odds ratio 2.13; 95% CI=1.02-4.42; p=0.04). NIHSS stratum adjusted 90-day mortality was 25% in the prourokinase group vs 27% in the control group (p=0.80). Systemic hemorrhage (mainly minor) occurred in 7% of the prourokinase group vs 17% of the control group, whereas worsening of neurological symptoms occurred in 1% vs 0%, and anaphylaxis in 1% vs 0%, respectively. Intracranial hemorrhage within the first 24 hours occurred in 35% of the prourokinase group vs 13% of the control group (p=0.003). However, after 10 days, the rates of intracerebral hemorrhage were 68% and 57%, respectively (p=0.23). Intracranial hemorrhage with neurological deterioration within 24 hours of treatment occurred in 10% and 2% of the prourokinase and control groups, respectively (p=0.06). All symptomatic intracranial hemorrhages occurred in patients with large baseline stroke (NIHSS >11). Recanalization of the occluded middle cerebral artery within 2 hours of therapy occurred in 66% of the prourokinase group and in 18% of the control group (p<0.001). Complete reperfusion (TIMI flow grade 3) was found in 19% of the prourokinase group vs 2% of the control group (p<0.003).

Concl.   Selective intra-arterial prourokinase infusion within 6 hours of onset of acute ischemic stroke caused by occlusion of the middle cerebral artery was associated with improved recovery of neurological function, and recanalization of the occluded middle cerebral artery, however, there was a slight increased risk of early intracerebral hemorrhage with neurological deterioration.

STAT

Stroke Treatment with Ancord Trial

Title	Intravenous ancord for treatment of acute ischemic stroke. The STAT study: A randomized controlled trial.
Authors	Sherman DG, Atkinson MP, Chippendale T, et al.
Reference	JAMA 2000;283:2395-2403.
Disease	Stroke.
Purpose	To assess the safety and efficacy of the defibrinogenating agent ancord in patients with acute ischemic stroke.
Design	Randomized, double-blind, placebo-controlled, multicenter.
Patients	500 patients, ≥18 years old, within 30 minutes to 3 hours after onset of symptoms of an acute or progressing ischemic neurological deficit. Patients with rapidly improving neurologic deficits were excluded. Patients with intracranial hemorrhage, neoplasm, very mild stroke, coma, prior stroke within 6 weeks, hypertension or hypotension, coagulation disorder or recent thrombolytic therapy were excluded.
Follow-up	3 months.
Regimen	Randomization to placebo (n=252) or ancord (n=248) infusion for 72 hours, followed by infusions lasting 1 hour, given at 90-102 hours and 114-126 hours after the beginning of therapy. The target fibrinogen level in the ancord treated patients was 1.18 to 2.03 µmol/L.
Add'l Tx	During the study drug infusion aspirin, anticoagulants, dextran, and thrombolytic agents were prohibited.

Results   102 patients in the ancord group (41.1%) achieved favorable functional status vs only 89 patients in the placebo group (35.3%; odds ratio 1.55; 95% CI=1.02-2.36). The covariate adjusted proportion of patients reaching favorable functional status was 42.2% vs 34.4%, respectively (p=0.04). Ancord therapy reduced the proportion of severely disabled patients. The covariate adjusted proportion of severely disabled patients was 11.8% in the ancord group vs 19.8% in the placebo group (40.4% relative risk reduction; p=0.01). The covariate adjusted proportion of patients with complete recovery was 36.1% in the ancord group vs 28.4% in the placebo group (27.1% relative increase; p=0.02). 7 day mortality was 8.9% in the ancord group vs 9.5% in the placebo group. 90-day mortality was 25.4% and 23.0%, respectively (p=0.62). Adverse events occurred in 98.4% in the ancord group vs 99.2% in the placebo group (p=NS). Symptomatic intracranial bleeding occurred in 5.2% in the ancord group vs 2% in the placebo group (odds ratio 2.58; 95% CI=0.95-8.21; p=0.06). Asymptomatic intracranial hemorrhage occurred in 19.0% in the ancord group vs 10.7% in the placebo group (odds ratio 1.92; 95% CI=1.14-3.27; p=0.01). The beneficial effect of ancord was observed in all predefined subgroups of age, stroke severity, gender, pre-stroke disability, and time to treatment (≤3 or >3 hours after onset of symptoms). Achievement of early defibrinogenation state was related to treatment success with ancord. Treatment success was noted in 45.8% of the patients with 6 hour fibrinogen levels of ≤3.82 µmol/L vs only 34.6% of the patients with >3.82 µmol/L at 6 hours of therapy.

Concl.   Ancord infusion, started 30 minutes to 3 hours after onset of acute ischemic stroke was associated with better functional status at 3 months compared with placebo. However, ancord therapy resulted in an increase in the rate of asymptomatic intracranial hemorrhage and a trend towards an increase in the rate of symptomatic intracranial hemorrhage, without affecting total mortality. Patients who achieved early controlled defibrinogenation had greater benefit from therapy.

WARSS

Warfarin Aspirin Recurrent Stroke Study

Title	A comparison of warfarin and aspirin for the prevention of recurrent ischemic stroke.
Authors	Mohr JP, Thompson JLP, Levin B, et al.
Reference	N Engl J Med 2001;345:1444-1451.
Disease	Noncardioembolic ischemic stroke.
Purpose	To compare aspirin and warfarin for the prevention of recurrent ischemic stroke in patients with noncardioembolic ischemic stroke.
Design	Randomized, double-blind, multicenter.
Patients	2206 patients, 30-85 years old, who had an ischemic stroke within the previous 30 days, and had ≥3 on the Glasgow Outcome Scale. Patients with contraindications to anticoagulant therapy, baseline international normalized ratio (INR) >1.4, stroke related to a procedure, high-grade carotid stenosis, cardioembolic stroke or atrial fibrillation were excluded.
Follow-up	2 years ± 1 month (maximum 761 days).
Regimen	Patients were randomized to aspirin 325 mg/d (n=1103) or to warfarin (target INR 1.4-2.8) (n=1103).
Results	The mean daily INR for the warfarin group was 2.1. After 2 years, death or recurrent ischemic stroke occurred in 17.8% of the patients in the warfarin group vs 16.0% in the aspirin group (hazard ratio 1.13; 95% CI=0.92-1.38; p=0.25). The combined end point of death, recurrent stroke, or major hemorrhage occurred in 20.0% and 17.8%, respectively (p=0.16). Mortality was 4.3% in the warfarin group and 4.8% in the aspirin group (p=0.61). Major hemorrhage occurred at a rate of 2.2 per 100 patient-years for the warfarin group and 1.49 per 100 patient-years in the aspirin group (p=0.10). Minor hemorrhage occurred more frequently in the warfarin group (20.8 vs 12 events per 100 patient-years; p<0.001). There was no significant difference in the time to primary event (death or recurrent stroke) between the 2 groups.

Concl.	There were no differences in outcome, including mortality, recurrent stroke, or major hemorrhage between patients treated with warfarin and aspirin after ischemic noncardio-embolic stroke. Both aspirin and warfarin are acceptable therapeutic alternatives.

AAASPS

African American Antiplatelet Stroke Prevention Study

Title	Aspirin and ticlopidine for prevention of recurrent stroke in black patients: a randomized trial.
Authors	Gorelick PB, Richardson D, Kelly M, et al.
Reference	JAMA 2003;289:2947-2957.
Disease	Stroke.
Purpose	To determine the efficacy and safety of aspirin vs ticlopidine to prevent recurrent stroke in black patients.
Design	Randomized, double-blind, investigator-initiated, multicenter trial.
Patients	1809 black men and women who recently had a noncardioembolic ischemic stroke.
Follow-up	2 years.
Regimen	Ticlopidine 500 mg/d (n=902) or aspirin 650 mg/d (n=907).
Results	Recurrent stroke, MI, or vascular death was the composite primary end point (according to intent-to-treat analysis). The secondary end point was fatal or nonfatal stroke. The blinded phase of the study was halted after about 6.5 years when futility analysis revealed a <1% probability of ticlopidine being shown superior to aspirin for prevention of the primary outcome end point. Futility analysis also indicated a 40%-50% likelihood of aspirin being significantly better than ticlopidine in reducing the risk of recurrent fatal or nonfatal stroke if the trial were to continue to completion. The primary outcome was reached by 133 (14.7%) of the ticlopidine-treated patients and 112 (12.3%) of the aspirin-treated patients (hazard ratio 1.22; 95% CI=0.94-1.57). Time to event for primary outcome did not differ between groups. Time to event for the secondary outcome tended to favor aspirin. The frequency of serious adverse events was similar between the 2 groups (29.9% for ticlopidine and 28.9% for aspirin). Other adverse events were slightly but not significantly more common in ticlopidine-treated patients (diarrhea 0.3% vs 0.2%; neutropenia 3.4% vs 2.2%; thrombocytopenia 0.3% vs 0.2%).

Concl.   Over 2 years of follow-up, ticlopidine and aspirin yielded similar results in terms of prevention of recurrent stroke, MI, or vascular death. There was a trend toward a reduction of fatal or nonfatal stroke among patients receiving aspirin. Given these results, and the risk of serious adverse events with ticlopidine, aspirin may be regarded as a better treatment for aspirin-tolerant black patients with noncardioembolic ischemic stroke.

ACST

Asymptomatic Carotid Surgery Trial

Title	Prevention of disabling and fatal strokes by successful carotid endarterectomy in patients without recent neurological symptoms: randomised controlled trial.
Authors	MRC Asymptomatic Carotid Surgery Trial (ACST) Collaborative Group.
Reference	Lancet 2004;363:1491-1502.
Disease	Carotid stenosis, stroke.
Purpose	To evaluate the long-term results of carotid endarterectomy on overall stroke risk in asymptomatic patients with significant carotid artery narrowing.
Design	Randomized, open-label, multicenter.
Patients	3120 patients with unilateral or bilateral carotid stenosis (≥60% diameter stenosis per ultrasound) and without stroke, transient ischemic attack, or other relevant neurological symptoms in the preceding 6 months. Patients who had known circumstances or conditions likely to preclude long-term follow-up were excluded. Patients with prior carotid endarterectomy, recent myocardial infarction, potential cardiac source of emboli, or any major life-threatening illness were not included.
Follow-up	5 years.
Regimen	Randomization to immediate carotid endarterectomy vs deferral of intervention until a definite indication was thought to have occurred.
Add'l Tx	All patients received appropriate medical care, including antiplatelet therapy, antihypertensive treatment, and lipid-lowering therapy, as needed.

Results	A total of 1560 patients were randomized to each group. Among the patients randomized to immediate carotid endarterectomy (CEA), 1348 patients underwent a total of 1405 CEA procedures (about half of the patients within 1 month, 88% within 1 year of randomization, and 91% within 5 years). Among the deferral group, 229 patients underwent 245 CEA procedures (6% within 1 year and 18% within 5 years). In the immediate group, perioperative death or stroke occurred in 10 patients (2.8%). Among the deferral patients who underwent CEA, perioperative stroke or death occurred in 2 patients (4.5%; p=NS). The overall risk of perioperative death or stroke was 3.1%. Over the 5 years of follow-up, any stroke or perioperative death occurred in 6.42% of the patients in the immediate group vs 11.78% in the deferred group (5.35% difference; 95% CI=2.96%-7.75%; p<0.0001). Fatal or disabling stroke or perioperative death occurred in 3.53% vs 6.07% of the patients, respectively (2.54% difference; 95% CI=0.77%-4.32%; p=0.004). Any type of nonperioperative stroke occurred in 3.77% of the patients in the immediate group vs 10.94% in the deferral group (7.17% difference; 95% CI=4.95%-9.39%; p<0.0001). Nonoperative fatal or disabling stroke occurred in 1.93% vs 5.78%, respectively (3.84% difference; 95% CI=2.20%-5.48%; p<0.0001). Nonperioperative carotid territory ischemic stroke occurred in 2.73% in the immediate group and 9.52% in the deferral group (6.78% difference; 95% CI=4.75%-8.82%; p<0.0001). Nonperioperative fatal or disabling carotid artery territory ischemic stroke occurred in 1.59% vs 5.26% of the patients, respectively (3.67% difference; 95% CI=2.12%-5.22%; p<0.0001). Subgroup analyses found no significant heterogeneity in the efficacy of early CEA among the different subgroups, although the difference between the immediate and deferral groups was not statistically significant among patients ≥75 years old.
Concl.	Immediate CEA reduced the risk of stroke during 5 years of follow-up by 50% in asymptomatic patients <75 years old with ≥70% carotid stenosis.

VISP

Vitamin Intervention for Stroke Prevention

Title	Lowering homocysteine in patients with ischemic stroke to prevent recurrent stroke, myocardial infarction, and death. The Vitamin Intervention for Stroke Prevention randomized controlled trial.
Authors	Toole JF, Malinow MR, Chambless LE, et al.
Reference	JAMA 2004;291:565-575.
Disease	Atherosclerosis, stroke.
Purpose	To determine whether large doses of folic acid, pyridoxine (vitamin B_6), and cobalamin (vitamin B_{12}) reduce the risk of stroke over a 2-year period compared with low doses of these vitamins.
Design	Multicenter, international, randomized, double-blind, controlled trial.
Patients	3680 adults with nondisabling stroke.
Follow-up	2 years.
Regimen	High-dose formulation (n=1827) containing pyridoxine 25 mg, cobalamin 0.4 mg and folic acid 2.5 mg, or low-dose formulation (n=1853) containing pyridoxine 200 µg, cobalamin 6 µg, and folic acid 20 µg.
Add'l Tx	Best medical and surgical care plus a multivitamin containing the United States Food and Drug Administration's reference daily intakes of other vitamins.

Results   The mean reduction in total homocysteine level was 2 μmol greater in patients receiving the high-dose formulation; however, this did not yield a change in the incidence of any end point event (recurrent cerebral infarction [primary outcome], coronary heart disease (CHD) events and death [secondary outcomes]). The unadjusted risk ratio for any stroke, CHD event, or death was 1.0 (95% CI=0.8-1.1); risk of an event within 2 years was 18% in those receiving the high-dose formulation and 18.6% in those receiving the low-dose formulation. The risk of ischemic stroke within 2 years was 9.2% for the high-dose and 8.8% for the low-dose formulation (p=NS). There was an association between baseline total homocysteine level and outcomes: a lower total homocysteine level was associated with lower rates of stroke, CHD, and death in the low-dose group with NS trends in the same directions for the high-dose group.

Concl.   Although a moderate reduction in total homocysteine level after ischemic stroke did not affect vascular outcomes after 2 years, the association of total homocysteine with vascular risk suggests that further exploration of the hypothesis is appropriate.

2. Acute Treatment of Stroke

3. Unstable Angina/Non-Q-Wave Infarction/Non-ST-Elevation Myocardial Infarction or Acute Coronary Syndrome

Randomized Trial Comparing IV Nitroglycerin and Heparin for Treatment of Unstable Angina Secondary to Restenosis After Coronary Artery Angioplasty

Title	Randomized trial comparing IV nitroglycerin and heparin for treatment of unstable angina secondary to restenosis after coronary artery angioplasty.
Authors	Doucet S, Malekianpour M, Théroux P, et al.
Reference	Circulation 2000;101:955-961.
Disease	Unstable angina, coronary artery disease.
Purpose	To determine the efficacy of IV nitroglycerin vs heparin for the treatment of unstable angina pectoris secondary to restenosis.
Design	Double-blind, placebo-controlled, randomized, single-center.
Patients	200 patients with unstable angina hospitalized within 2-6 months of coronary angioplasty.
Follow-up	48-96 hours after randomization at which time coronary angiography was performed.
Regimen	1) IV nitroglycerin infusion plus placebo heparin; 2) IV heparin 5000 U bolus plus 1000-1200 U/hour infusion plus placebo nitroglycerin; 3) IV nitroglycerin plus heparin; 4) placebo.
Add'l Tx	Aspirin, β-blockers, or calcium blockers allowed.
Results	75% of patients in the placebo group and heparin alone group developed recurrent angina vs 42.6% of patients in the nitroglycerin alone and 41.7% in the nitroglycerin plus heparin group (p<0.003). Refractory angina requiring angiography occurred in 22.9% of the placebo patients, 29.2% of the heparin patients, 4.3% of the nitroglycerin patients, and 4.2% of the combined patients (p<0.002). There was no interaction detected between heparin and nitroglycerin. Multivariate logistic regression analysis, that took into account the severity of restenosis, showed that the use of nitroglycerin highly predicted the absence of angina.

Concl.   Nitroglycerin but not heparin prevented recurrent angina in patients with unstable angina secondary to restenosis.

Efegatran in Unstable Angina

Title	Anticoagulant properties, clinical efficacy and safety of efegatran, a direct thrombin inhibitor, in patients with unstable angina.
Authors	Klootwijk P, Lenderink T, Meij S, et al.
Reference	Eur Heart J 1999;20:1101-1111.
Disease	Unstable angina, acute coronary syndrome.
Purpose	To assess the efficacy and safety of efegatran sulphate, a direct thrombin inhibitor, in patients with unstable angina.
Design	Randomized, single-blind, dose-ranging, multicenter.
Patients	432 patients, 21-75 years old, with unstable angina. Patients with suspected acute myocardial infarction or recent myocardial infarction, baseline EKG abnormalities, heparin therapy, current use of anticoagulants, recent administration of thrombolytic therapy and high risk for bleeding were excluded.
Follow-up	48 hours continuous EKG monitoring, clinical follow-up for 30 days.
Regimen	In the dose ranging phase, patients were randomized to 5 doses of efegatran: the first 4 groups received an IV bolus of 0.1 mg/kg over 15 minutes, followed by continuous infusion over 0.105, 0.32, 0.63, or 0.84 mg/kg/h. Patients in the 5th group received a bolus of 0.3 mg/kg over 1 minute, followed by continuous infusion of 1.2 mg/kg/h. The study drug infusion was continued for 48±10 hours. In the parallel phase of the study patients were randomized to 3 groups: 1) efegatran 0.1 mg/kg bolus and 0.63 mg/kg/h infusion; 2) efegatran 0.3 mg/kg bolus and 1.2 mg/kg/h infusion; and 3) IV unfractionated heparin (5000 U bolus followed by a continuous infusion of 1000 U/h for 48±10 hours).
Add'l Tx	Heparin was prohibited during efegatran infusion. After termination of the study drug infusion, nonstudy heparin could be initiated. All patients received aspirin 80 mg/d.

Results	There were 132 patients in the dose ranging phase and 300 in the parallel phase. Efegatran induced a dose dependent prolongation of the activated partial thromboplastin time (aPTT), with the highest dose of 1.2 mg/kg/h resulting in a steady state mean aPTT comparable to that of heparin. The aPTT was more stable with efegatran than with heparin. Prothrombin time (PT) was mildly increased with efegatran. Thrombin time was prolonged with a dose dependent manner by efegatran, whereas heparin did not affect thrombin time. Fibrinogen levels decreased with efegatran but not with heparin. All coagulation tests rapidly returned to normal range after discontinuation of efegatran. With continuous EKG monitoring, there was no significant difference between the number of patients with recurrent ischemia or the number or duration of ischemic episodes between the heparin group and the various efegatran groups. However, there was a trend towards less ≥30 minute ischemia with the highest doses of efegatran (11% and 23% in the 0.84 and 1.2 mg/kg/h groups) than with heparin (33%; p=0.068). Kaplan-Meier estimates of the probability of remaining free of recurrent ischemia during EKG monitoring were comparable among groups. At 7 days, the primary end point of recurrent angina, myocardial infarction, death or coronary intervention occurred in 71% in the heparin group vs 52%-71% in the various efegatran groups (p=NS), although the need for percutaneous interventions was slightly higher in the efegatran groups (8%-9%) than in the heparin group (4%). At 30 days 73%-81% of the patients in the efegatran groups reached a primary end point vs 81% in the heparin group, and death or acute myocardial infarction occurred in 3.2% in the efegatran groups vs 2.1% in the heparin group. Minor bleeding (p=0.001) and thrombophlebitis (p=0.0001) occurred more often with efegatran than with heparin, although there was no significant difference in the incidence of major bleeding (0.8% with efegatran vs 1.6% with heparin). No strokes occurred in this study.
Concl.	Efegatran sulphate infusion provided a more stable anticoagulation effect than heparin. However, efegatran was not associated with better clinical outcomes and was associated with more thrombophlebitis and minor bleeding episodes.

Title	Angiotensin-converting enzyme inhibition is associated with reduced troponin release in non-ST elevation acute coronary syndromes.
Authors	Kennon S, Barakat K, Hitman GA, et al.
Reference	J Am Coll Cardiol 2001;38:724-728.
Disease	Acute coronary syndrome.
Purpose	To assess the effects of ACE inhibitors on troponin release in non-ST elevation acute coronary syndrome.
Design	Prospective cohort.
Patients	301 consecutive patients with non-ST elevation acute coronary syndrome (Braunwald class 3B). Patients who developed Q-waves and patients with recent myocardial infarction (≤ 21 days) were excluded. In addition, patients who underwent percutaneous coronary intervention in the preceding 6 months and patients with congestive heart failure (New York Heart Association class III-IV) were excluded.
Results	93 patients (31%) had troponin I levels >0.1 µg/L. Patients with positive troponin I were older (64.5±10.6 vs 58.8±10.9 years; p<0.0001). Pretreatment with aspirin (48.4% vs 61.8%; p=0.03) and ACE inhibitors (7.5% vs 22.2%; p=0.002) was recorded less frequently in patients with positive troponin I. 18.3% of the patients with positive troponin vs 28.0% of the troponin I negative patients were pretreated with β-blockers (p=0.07). There was no difference in the percentage of patients treated with statins (12.9% vs 18.4%; p=0.24) or calcium channel blockers (37.6% vs 37.2%; p=0.94) between the positive and negative troponin I groups. Logistic regression analysis revealed that pretreatment with ACE inhibitors was independently associated with reduced rates of troponin I release (OR 0.25; 95% CI=0.10-0.64; p=0.004), whereas pretreatment with aspirin was not. However, maximum troponin I levels were lower in patients pretreated with aspirin (2.31 µg/L vs 5.85 µg/L; p=0.05). There was no association between ACE genotype and troponin I release.

| Concl. | Pretreatment with ACE inhibitors reduces troponin I release in patients with non-ST elevation acute coronary syndrome. |

***Women Do Have an Improved Long-Term Outcome After Non-
ST-Elevation Acute Coronary Syndromes Treated Very Early
and Predominantly with Percutaneous Coronary Intervention***

Title	Women do have an improved long-term outcome after non-ST-elevation acute coronary syndromes treated very early and predominantly with percutaneous coronary intervention.
Authors	Mueller C, Neumann F-J, Roskamm H, et al.
Reference	J Am Coll Cardiol 2002;40:245-250.
Disease	Unstable angina/non-Q-wave myocardial infarction.
Purpose	To determine if there is differential long-term outcome according to gender after very early aggressive intervention in patients who have non-ST-elevation acute coronary syndrome.
Design	Prospective, cohort.
Patients	1450 consecutive patients with non-ST-elevation acute coronary syndrome, with ischemic symptoms at rest (generally Braunwald class IIIB unstable angina). Exclusion criteria were new angina on exertion or worsening angina during exertion only (Braunwald class 1A to 1C), persistent ST-elevation, and postinfarction angina (Braunwald class 1C, 2C, 3C).
Follow-up	Mean 20 months.

Regimen	All symptomatic patients underwent immediate coronary angiography. Patients who were asymptomatic on medical therapy underwent angiography within 24 hours. Coronary stenting was performed immediately after angiography whenever possible. In the event that PCI was not possible but revascularization was still deemed necessary, urgent coronary artery bypass grafting was performed.
Results	The composite primary end point was death from all causes or nonfatal MI. There were 417 women and 1033 men in the study. There were significant differences in baseline characteristics between the men and women: women were older, less likely to have had prior MI or CABG, and more likely to be hypertensive. Rates of ST-segment depression were similar, but women more often had T-wave inversion. Women were less likely to have a high-grade coronary lesion or 3-vessel disease, which resulted in more frequent CABG in men (15% vs 11%; p=0.02) and more frequent medical therapy in women (36% vs 28%; p=0.01). The primary end point of all-cause death or nonfatal MI occurred in 29 (7.0%) women and 108 (10.5%) men (hazard ratio (HR) 0.65; 95% CI=0.42-0.99; p=0.045). All-cause death was 4.1% in women and 6.4 % in men (HR 0.62; 95% CI=.23-1.66; p=0.346). Nonfatal MI occurred in 3.1% of women and 4.5% of men (HR 0.66; 95% CI=0.34-1.28; p=0.219). A multivariate Cox regression analysis including baseline characteristics, ECG findings, inflammatory markers, myocardial necrosis, and angiographic extent of CAD showed female gender to be an independent predictor of death or nonfatal MI (HR 0.51; 95% CI=0.28-0.92; p=0.024).
Concl.	Women with non-ST-elevation acute coronary syndromes who undergo early coronary angiography with aggressive early revascularization have a reduced risk of death or nonfatal MI vs men.

2nd SYMPHONY

Sibrafiban vs Aspirin to Yield Maximum Protection From Ischemic Heart Events Post-Acute Coronary Syndromes

Title	Randomized trial of aspirin, sibrafiban, or both for secondary prevention after acute coronary syndromes.
Authors	Second SYMPHONY Investigators.
Reference	Circulation 2001;103:1727-1733.
Disease	Acute coronary syndromes, coronary artery disease.
Purpose	To determine whether longer treatment (12-18 months) with low-dose sibrafiban (a potent oral glycoprotein IIb/IIIa inhibitor) plus background aspirin or high-dose sibrafiban alone is more effective than aspirin alone (also see first SYMPHONY trial).
Design	Randomized, blinded, multicenter.
Patients	6671 patients.
Follow-up	Study was stopped prematurely when the first SYMPHONY results became known. Patients were treated for a median of 90 days; median duration follow-up was 95 days.
Regimen	Patients randomized to high-dose sibrafiban, low-dose sibrafiban plus aspirin, or aspirin alone. Sibrafiban (3.0, 4.5, or 6.0 mg) depending upon weight and serum creatinine. Aspirin dose was 80 mg given twice daily in low-dose plus aspirin arm.
Add'l Tx	Ticlopidine for 2-4 weeks in patients undergoing stenting.

Results	Primary end point was time to all cause mortality, MI, or severe recurrent ischemia. There was no difference in the primary end point between aspirin (9.3%) and low-dose sibrafiban (9.2%) or high-dose sibrafiban (10.5%). There was a nonsignificant (31%) increase in mortality and 12% increase in death or MI with low-dose sibrafiban plus aspirin. High-dose sibrafiban was associated with a significantly greater rate of death (2.4%), MI (6.9%), and their composite (8.6%) vs aspirin (at 1.3%, 5.3%, and 6.1%, respectively). Major bleeding was more common in low-dose sibrafiban plus aspirin (5.7%) vs aspirin alone (4.0%); high-dose sibrafiban alone (4.6%) did not cause more bleeding than aspirin alone. Rates of rehospitalization were significantly higher in both sibrafiban arms.
Concl.	There was a higher rate of mortality or MI in high-dose sibrafiban group. Combining low-dose sibrafiban with aspirin did not improve outcome and caused more bleeding than aspirin alone.

3

ACUTE 2

Antithrombolic Combination Using Tirofiban and Enoxaparin

Title	Randomized double-blind safety study of enoxaparin vs unfractionated heparin in patients with non-ST-segment elevation acute coronary syndromes treated with tirofiban and aspirin: the ACUTE 2 study.
Authors	Cohen M, Theroux P, Borzak S, et al.
Reference	Am Heart J 2002;22:470-477.
Disease	Acute coronary syndrome.
Purpose	To compare the efficacy and safety of the combination of tirofiban and aspirin with enoxaparin or unfractionated heparin in patients with non-ST-elevation acute coronary syndromes.
Design	Randomized, double-blind, multicenter.
Patients	525 patients with non-ST-elevation acute coronary syndromes and either ECG signs of myocardial ischemia or abnormal cardiac markers. Patients with ST-elevation acute MI within the preceding 48 hours, contraindications to anticoagulation therapy, thrombocytopenia, intolerance or allergy to aspirin, heparin or tirofiban, need for immediate revascularization, and renal failure were excluded.
Follow-up	30 days.
Regimen	Patients were randomized to unfractionated heparin (5000 U as a bolus followed by 1000 U/h (target aPTT 1.5-2.5 times control) (n=210), or enoxaparin (1.0 mg/kg bid) (n=315). Enoxaparin and heparin were administered for 24-96 hours.
Add'l Tx	All patients received aspirin 160-325 mg/d and IV tirofiban (0.4 µg/kg/min for 30 minutes, followed by 0.1 µg/kg/min for 47.5-107.5 hours). Coronary angiography and PCI were allowed after the study drugs had been administered for ≥24 hours.

Results   Bleeding (according to TIMI trial criteria) occurred in 4.8% of the patients in the unfractionated heparin (UFH) group and in 3.5% in the enoxaparin group (OR 1.4; 95% CI=0.6-3.4; p=NS). TIMI-major bleeding occurred in 1.0% vs 0.3%, respectively (p=0.57), and TIMI-minor bleeding in 4.3% vs 2.5%, respectively (p=0.11). 4.3% of the patients in the UFH group vs 2.5% in the enoxaparin group received blood transfusion. Cutaneous bleeding (11.4% vs 30.8%; p<0.001) and oral bleeding (0 vs 2.5%; p=0.02) occurred less often in the UFH group. The duration of hospitalization was comparable. 60.0% vs 59.4% of the patients in the UFH and enoxaparin group underwent coronary angiography. 30-day mortality was 1.9% in the UFH and 2.5% in the enoxaparin group (p=0.77). Myocardial infarction occurred in 7.1% vs 6.7%, respectively (p=0.86). Refractory ischemia requiring urgent revascularization occurred in 4.3% of the patients in the UFH and in 0.6% in the enoxaparin group (p=0.01), and rehospitalization due to unstable angina in 7.1% vs 1.6% of the patients, respectively (p=0.02).

Concl.   The safety of the combination of aspirin and tirofiban with enoxaparin appears to be comparable to that of aspirin and tirofiban with unfractionated heparin. Enoxaparin, added to aspirin and tirofiban was associated with fewer episodes of refractory angina and hospitalization for unstable angina than unfractionated heparin.

APLAUD

Antiplatelet Useful Dose

Title	Dose-finding, safety, tolerability study of an oral platelet glyco-protein IIb/IIIa inhibitor, lotrafiban, in patients with coronary or cerebral atherosclerotic disease.
Authors	Harrington RA, Armstrong PW, Graffagnino C, et al.
Reference	Circulation 2000;102:728-735.
Disease	Coronary, cerebrovascular disease.
Purpose	To determine the safety, tolerability, and pharmacodynamics of lotrafiban, an oral glycoprotein IIb/IIIa inhibitor in patients with cerebrovascular or cardiovascular disease.
Design	Randomized, double-blind, multicenter, dose-finding, safety, tolerability study.
Patients	451 patients with recent cerebrovascular or cardiovascular acute ischemic events.
Follow-up	13 weeks.
Regimen	Patients randomized in a double-blind fashion to 1 of 5 treatments: placebo twice daily or 5, 20, 50 or 100 mg lotrafiban twice daily.
Add'l Tx	Aspirin 300-325 mg/d.

Results	Primary end point was incidence and tolerability of major and minor bleeding. Pharmacodynamic-inhibition of platelet aggregation, thrombocytopenia also monitored. Placebo and lotrafiban 5 mg groups had similar low rates of minor and major bleeding. There was a dose-dependent increase in minor bleeding. Major bleeding (0.9-2.9%) and packed red blood cell transfusions (0-1%) were infrequent in the placebo 5, 20, 50 mg arms but higher in the 100 mg arm (12.1% major bleeding; 11.8% packed red cell transfusion). The 100 mg arm was terminated early because of this excess of major bleeding. Thrombocytopenia (<100,000 platelets/ µL) occurred in 5 lotrafiban-treated patients (1.4%; 95% CI=0.2%-2.7%) and 1 placebo patient (1.1%; 95% CI=0%-3.1%). 3 lotrafiban-treated patients developed a nadir platelet count <20,000. Lotrafiban caused a dose-dependent inhibition of platelet aggregation. Effects of 5 mg dose were similar to placebo; the 100 mg dose inhibited platelet aggregation by nearly 100%. Composite end point of death, MI, or readmission for cardiac or neurologic events occurred in 10% in combined lotrafiban patients (excluding 100 mg group) vs 13.8% of placebo patients (p=0.29).
Concl.	Lotrafiban provided dose-dependent platelet inhibition. Level of platelet inhibition appeared to correlate with bleeding risk.

AZACS

Azithromycin in Acute Coronary Syndrome

Title	Effect of short-term treatment with azithromycin on recurrent ischaemic events in patients with acute coronary syndrome in the Azithromycin in Acute Coronary Syndrome (AZACS) trial: a randomised controlled trial.
Authors	Cercek B, Shah PK, Noc M, et al.
Reference	Lancet 2003;361:809-813.
Disease	Acute coronary syndrome.
Purpose	To study whether short-term azithromycin, initiated shortly after acute coronary syndrome, will reduce the risk of recurrent ischemic events and death in the following 6 months.
Design	Randomized, double-blind, placebo-controlled, multicenter.
Patients	1439 patients, ≥18 years old, within 28 days of admission for unstable angina or acute myocardial infarction. Patients who had had a Q-wave myocardial infarction within the preceding 28 days of current admission, pregnant or breastfeeding women, known hypersensitivity to macrolide antibiotics, or those with significant comorbidity were excluded.
Follow-up	6 months.
Regimen	Randomization to azithromycin (500 mg on the first day, 250 mg/d for 4 days) (n=716) or placebo (n=723).

Results   6-month mortality was 3% in the azithromycin and 4% in the placebo group (hazard ratio [HR] 0.80; 95% CI=0.46-1.38; p=0.42). Nonfatal MI occurred in 2% and 3%, respectively (HR 0.78; 95% CI=0.42-1.47; p=0.448). 9% of the patients in the azithromycin vs 8% in the placebo underwent revascularization (HR 1.10; 95% CI=0.77-1.56; p=0.606). The primary end point of the study (death, acute MI, or need for revascularization) was reached by 14% of the patients in the azithromycin and 15% in the placebo group (HR 0.94; 95% CI=0.72-1.24; p=0.664). Azithromycin also did not affect events in the subgroup of patients who had MI at enrollment or those with positive serological test for Chlamydia pneumoniae.

Concl.   4-day treatment with azithromycin did not affect recurrent ischemic events in patients with acute coronary syndrome.

CURE

Clopidogrel in Unstable Angina to Prevent Recurrent Events

Title	Effects of clopidogrel in addition to aspirin in patients with acute coronary syndromes without ST-segment elevation.
Authors	CURE Trial Investigators.
Reference	N Engl J Med 2001;345:494-502.
Disease	Coronary artery disease, acute coronary syndrome.
Purpose	To assess the efficacy and safety of clopidogrel in addition to aspirin in patients with acute coronary syndromes without ST elevation.
Design	Randomized, double-blind, placebo-controlled, multicenter.
Patients	12,562 patients hospitalized within 24 hours of onset of non-ST elevation acute coronary syndromes. After the first 3000 patients, only patients with ECG changes or above normal levels of cardiac enzymes or markers were included. Patients with ST elevation, contraindications to antithrombotic or antiplatelet therapy, at increased risk of bleeding, and with severe heart failure were excluded. In addition, patients who received IV glycoprotein IIb/IIIa receptor antagonists in the 3 days preceding enrollment, those who were on oral anticoagulants and those who underwent coronary revascularization in the 3 months preceding enrollment were not included.
Follow-up	3-12 months, mean duration: 9 months.
Regimen	Randomization to placebo or clopidogrel (300 mg loading dose, followed by 75 mg/d).
Add'l Tx	All patients received aspirin 75-325 mg/d.

Results	The primary end point of the study (cardiovascular mortality, nonfatal MI, or stroke) occurred in 9.3% in the clopidogrel group vs 11.4% in the placebo group (relative risk [RR] 0.80; 95% CI=0.72-0.90; p<0.001). Cardiovascular mortality, nonfatal MI, stroke, or refractory ischemia occurred in 16.5% vs 18.8%, respectively (RR 0.86; 95% CI=0.79-0.94; p<0.001). Cardiovascular mortality was 5.1% in the clopidogrel group vs 5.5% in the placebo group (RR 0.93; 95% CI=0.79-1.08). In contrast, there was no difference in noncardiovascular mortality (0.7% vs 0.7%, respectively). MI occurred in 5.2% vs 6.7%, respectively (RR 0.77; 95% CI=0.67-0.89). Stroke occurred in 1.2% vs 1.4%, respectively. Refractory ischemia during the initial hospitalization occurred in 1.4% in the clopidogrel group vs 2.0% in the placebo group (RR 0.68; 95% CI=0.52-0.90; p=0.007). In contrast, there was no difference in the rates of refractory ischemia after discharge (7.6% in each group). 36.0% of the patients in the clopidogrel vs 36.9% in the placebo underwent revascularization (20.8% vs 22.7% during the initial hospitalization [p=0.03]). Radiologic evidence of heart failure was found in 3.7% vs 4.4%, respectively (p=0.026). The benefit of clopidogrel was evident within the first few hours of therapy. 1.4% of the patients in the clopidogrel vs 2.1% in the placebo group had cardiovascular death, MI, or stroke within the first 24 hours after randomization (RR 0.66; 95% CI=0.51-0.86). Major bleeding occurred in 3.7% of the patients in the clopidogrel vs 2.7% in the placebo group (RR 1.38; 95% CI=1.13-1.67; p=0.001). Minor bleeding occurred in 5.1% vs 2.4% (RR 2.12; 95% CI=1.75-2.56; p<0.001). 21.1% of the patients in the clopidogrel vs 18.8% in the placebo group discontinued the study drug permanently. 1.1% and 2.0% of the patients in the clopidogrel and placebo group, respectively, received thrombolytic therapy (p<0.001), and 5.9% vs 7.2%, respectively, received a glycoprotein IIb/IIIa inhibitor (p=0.003).
Concl.	Long-term use of clopidogrel, in addition to aspirin, reduced the risk of clinical events in patients with non-ST elevation acute coronary syndromes. However, clopidogrel was associated with an increased risk of bleeding.

CURE

Clopidogrel in Unstable Angina to Prevent Recurrent Events (Substudy)

Title	Benefit of clopidogrel in patients with acute coronary syndromes without ST-segment elevation in various risk groups.
Authors	Budaj A, Yusuf S, Mehta S, et al.
Reference	Circulation 2002;106:1622-1626.
Disease	Acute coronary syndrome.
Purpose	To determine the treatment effects of clopidogrel in patients categorized according to their TIMI (Thrombolysis in Myocardial Infarction) risk score.
Design	Randomized, double-blind, placebo-controlled, multicenter.
Patients	12,562 patients who were hospitalized within 24 hours after symptoms began and demonstrated ECG changes but not ST-segment elevation, or already had elevated cardiac enzymes or markers greater than or equal to twice the upper limit of normal. Exclusion criteria included contraindication to antiplatelet/antithrombotic therapy, high bleeding risk, requirement for long-term anticoagulation, coronary revascularization in the past 3 months, or glycoprotein IIb/IIIa inhibitors in the past 3 days.
Follow-up	9 months.
Regimen	Patients were randomized to either clopidogrel (loading dose of 300 mg followed by 75 mg daily) or placebo. Aspirin was given (75 mg to 325 mg) to all patients.

Results	The primary study end point was the composite of cardiovascular death, nonfatal MI, or stroke. The co-primary outcome was the composite of the primary end point or refractory angina. The 2 groups were well matched with respect to the TIMI risk factors. The primary end point was seen increasingly as the TIMI risk score increased. In the low risk group (TIMI score 0-2), the rate of the primary end point was 4.1% in the clopidogrel group and 5.7% in the placebo group (relative risk [RR] 0.71; 95% CI=0.52-0.97; p<0.04). In the intermediate-risk group (TIMI score 3-4) the rate of the primary end point was 9.8% vs 11.4% in the clopidogrel and placebo groups (RR 0.85; 95% CI=0.74-0.98; p<0.03). In the high-risk group (TIMI score 5-7) the rate of the primary end point was 15.9% vs 20.7% in the clopidogrel and placebo groups (RR 0.73; 95% CI=0.60-0.90; p<0.004). The relative risk of major bleeding complications was increased in the clopidogrel group compared to placebo; in the low-risk group, the relative risk was 1.34 (95% CI=0.85-2.11; p=0.21), in the intermediate-risk group, RR 1.44 (95% CI=1.12-1.86; p=0.005), and in the high-risk group, RR 1.24 (95% CI=0.83-1.86; p=0.30).
Concl.	Clopidogrel had a significant benefit compared to placebo on the composite outcome of cardiovascular death, MI, and stroke in low, intermediate, and high-risk subgroups.

CURE

Clopidogrel in Unstable Angina to Prevent Recurrent Events (Substudy)

Title	Early and late effects of clopidogrel in patients with acute coronary syndromes.
Authors	Yusuf S, Mehta SR, Gersh BJ, et al.
Reference	Circulation 2003;107:966-972.
Disease	Acute coronary syndrome.
Purpose	To determine how quickly benefit was seen in patients who received clopidogrel in addition to aspirin after an acute coronary syndrome, and to determine if the beneficial effects were sustained during 1 year.
Design	Randomized, double-blind, placebo-controlled, multicenter.
Patients	12, 562 patients. See CURE trial.
Follow-up	Minimum 3 months, maximum 12 months, mean 9 months.
Regimen	Patients started treatment within 24 hours of symptom onset. Patients were randomized to clopidogrel at an initial dose of 300 mg followed by 75 mg/d orally or matching placebo. Aspirin was given at doses between 75 mg and 325 mg/d according to the treating physician.
Results	The primary study outcome was the combined end point of cardiovascular death, myocardial infarction, or stroke. The secondary study outcome was the primary end point plus refractory ischemia. Refractory ischemia had differing definitions according to whether it occurred in hospital or after discharge. During hospitalization, refractory ischemia was the recurrence of angina with new changes on ECG despite maximal antianginal and antithrombotic therapy, requiring immediate intervention or transfer for intervention within 24 hours. After discharge from the hospital, refractory ischemia meant rehospitalization for unstable angina with changes on ECG. Another secondary outcome was severe ischemia (recurrent angina with new changes on ECG while on optimal medical therapy). Characteristics of

the 2 groups at baseline were similar. Aspirin was used in over 93% of patients during the entire study period. Unfractionated or low-molecular weight heparin was used in 91.4% of patients in hospital. During the entire follow-up, 9.3% of patients in the clopidogrel group experienced the primary end point vs 11.4% in the placebo group (relative risk [RR] 0.80; 95% CI=0.72-0.90; p<0.0001). The result was similar and significant both in the first 30 days (RR 0.79; p<0.004), and after 30 days (RR 0.82; p<0.01). In the first 30 days, 5.4% of patients in the placebo group had a primary end point event vs 4.3% in the clopidogrel group (RR 0.79; 95% CI=0.67-0.92; p<0.004). Inclusion of refractory ischemia in the primary outcome also showed a difference between the placebo (9.2%) and clopidogrel (7.7%) groups (RR 0.83; 95% CI=0.73-0.93; p<0.002). Inclusion of severe ischemia to the primary outcome also showed a benefit for clopidogrel (11.7% vs 9.6%; RR 0.81; 95% CI=0.73-0.90; p<0.0001). In the first 7 days, there was a relative risk of major bleeding of 1.18 associated with clopidogrel (95% CI=0.80-1.75; absolute excess 0.13%), and from 8-30 days, the relative risk was 1.43 (95% CI=1.00-2.04; absolute excess 0.35%). In the period of 30 days through 12 months, there was a 18% RR reduction in the primary outcome for clopidogrel (p<0.01). 1.18% of placebo patients and 1.75% of clopidogrel patients had a major bleed in this time period (RR 1.48; 95% CI=1.1-1.99; absolute excess 0.57%). The rate of life-threatening bleeds was similar in the 2 groups during this time period (RR 1.09; 95% CI=0.75-1.59; absolute excess 0.08%).

| Concl. | Clopidogrel reduces the risk of ischemic events in patients who have had an acute coronary syndrome. Its effects begin immediately after initiation and are maintained for up to 12 months when patients are kept on clopidogrel. |

ESSENCE (1-Year Results)

Efficacy and Safety of Subcutaneous Enoxaparin in Non-Q-Wave Coronary Events

Title	Randomized trial of low-molecular-weight heparin (enoxaparin) vs unfractionated heparin for unstable coronary artery disease. 1-year results of the ESSENCE study.
Authors	Goodman SG, Cohen M, Bigonzi F, et al.
Reference	J Am Coll Cardiol 2000;36:693-698.
Disease	Coronary artery disease.
Purpose	To assess whether the short-term beneficial effects of enoxaparin were maintained after 1 year of follow-up.
Patients	Of the 3171 patients enrolled, 87 (2.7%) died within the first 30 days. Complete 1-year follow-up was available for 2915 (91.9%) patients, and complete 1-year vital status in 2992 (94.4%) patients.
Follow-up	1 year.
Regimen	As per ESSENCE.
Results	By intention-to-treat analysis, the composite end point of death, acute myocardial infarction or recurrent angina occurred in 32.0% of the patients in the enoxaparin group vs 35.7% in the unfractionated heparin group (hazard ratio 0.87; 95% CI=0.77-0.98; p=0.022). Death or myocardial infarction occurred in 11.5% of the enoxaparin group vs 13.5% of the unfractionated heparin group (hazard ratio 0.84; 95% CI=0.69-1.02; p=0.082). During the first 30 days after enrollment, 47.9% of the patients in the enoxaparin vs 51.9% of the patients in the unfractionated heparin group underwent diagnostic cardiac catheterization (p=0.024) and 27.0% vs 32.2%, respectively, underwent coronary revascularization (p=0.001). After 1 year, 55.8% of the patients in the enoxaparin group vs 59.4% of the patients in the unfractionated heparin group underwent diagnostic cardiac catheterization (hazard ratio 0.91; 95% CI=0.83-0.99; p=0.036), and 35.9% vs 41.2%, respectively, underwent revascularization (hazard ratio 0.84; 95% CI=0.75-0.94; p=0.002).

Concl.   In patients with non-ST-elevation acute coronary syndrome, enoxaparin was associated with less recurrent ischemic events and need for repeat cardiac catheterization and revascularization. The beneficial effects of enoxaparin were present at 30 days and maintained at 1 year after enrollment.

ESSENCE (ST Segment Monitoring Substudy)

Efficacy and Safety of Subcutaneous Enoxaparin in Non-Q-Wave Coronary Events

Title	Low-molecular-weight heparin decreases rebound ischemia in unstable angina or non-Q-wave myocardial infarction: The Canadian ESSENCE (ST Segment Monitoring Substudy).
Authors	Goodman SG, Barr A, Sobtchouk A, et al.
Reference	J Am Coll Cardiol 2000;36:1507-1513.
Disease	Unstable angina, non-Q-wave MI.
Purpose	To determine whether low-molecular-weight heparin, enoxaparin was more effective than heparin in reducing recurrent ischemic episodes.
Design	Randomized, double-blind, multicenter.
Patients	A substudy of 288 patients from the ESSENCE main trial. Patients with rest angina occurring within 24 hours and evidence of underlying coronary disease.
Follow-up	ST segment monitoring performed on patients for first 48 hours after randomization (n=220) and an additional 48 hours (n=174) after IV drug was discontinued.
Regimen	As per ESSENCE, patients randomized to unfractionated heparin vs enoxaparin over a mean of 3.4 days.
Add'l Tx	Aspirin.

Results	During the first 48 hours of ECG monitoring the time to first episode of ischemia was earlier in heparin-treated patients (11±11 minutes) vs enoxaparin patients (25±18 minutes; p=0.001). The number of patients experiencing at least 1 ischemic episode was 27.2% for heparin-treated patients and 22.6% for enoxaparin-treated patients (p=0.44). During follow-up 48 hours ST monitoring 44.6% of heparin and 25.6% of enoxaparin patients experienced at least 1 ischemic episode (p=0.009). Time to first ischemic episode was shorter in the heparin group (13.9± 23.3) vs enoxaparin group (23.8±21.1 minutes; p=0.03). The mean number of episodes (1.5±3.0 vs 0.4±0.9 episodes per 24 hours; p=0.005) and duration of episodes (18.0±39.2 vs 4.6±12.4 minutes of ischemia per 24 hours; p=0.005) was greater in the heparin group than the enoxaparin group. Recurrent ischemia after drug discontinuation occurred more frequently in the heparin group. Patients with ischemia were more likely to die or have a recurrent MI at 1 year (18.4% vs 8.3% p=0.023).
Concl.	Enoxaparin was more effective than unfractionated heparin in reducing rebound ischemia.

FRAX.I.S

Fraxiparine in Ischemic Syndrome

Title	Comparison of two treatment durations (6 days and 14 days) of a low molecular weight heparin with a 6 day treatment of unfractionated heparin in the initial management of unstable angina or non-Q-wave myocardial infarction: FRAX.I.S. (FRAxiparine in Ischaemic Syndrome).
Authors	The FRAX.I.S. Study Group.
Reference	Eur Heart J 1999;20:1553-1562.
Disease	Unstable angina, non-Q-wave myocardial infarction.
Purpose	To compare the efficacy of 2 regimens (6 days and 14 days) of low molecular weight heparin (nadroparin) with that of unfractionated heparin in non ST elevation acute coronary syndromes.
Design	Randomized, double-blind, multicenter.
Patients	3468 patients, >18 years old, weighing 40-110 kg, with suspected unstable angina or non-Q-wave myocardial infarction (anginal pain within the preceding 48 hours + ST depression, T wave inversion, or ST elevation not justifying thrombolysis). Patients with renal or hepatic failure, bleeding diathesis, thrombocytopenia, those with a need for long-term treatment with oral anticoagulants, and those who underwent PTCA, CABG, acute myocardial infarction, unstable angina, or stroke in the preceding 6 months were excluded.
Follow-up	3 months clinical follow-up.
Regimen	After randomization, patients received either nadoparin (IV bolus 86 anti Xa IU/kg followed by SC injections of 86 anti Xa IU/kg bid) or unfractionated heparin (IV bolus of 5000 IU, followed by an infusion of 1250 IU/h). IV unfractionated heparin was administered for 6±2 days, and subcutaneous nadoparin for 6 or 14 days. The unfractionated heparin group received subcutaneous injections of placebo and the nadoparin groups received IV infusion of placebo.

Add'l Tx	All patients received up to 325 mg/d aspirin for 3 months. Nonstudy unfractionated heparin and low molecular weight heparin, oral anticoagulants, antiplatelet agents, antithrombin agents, and fibrinolytic drugs were prohibited during the study period. In case of coronary angiography or PTCA during the study treatment phase, open-label heparin could be administered.
Results	1151 patients received unfractionated heparin, 1166 nadoparin for 6 days, and 1151 nadoparin for 14 days. The primary end point of the study (cardiac mortality, myocardial infarction, refractory angina, and recurrence of unstable angina at day 14) occurred in 18.1% of the unfractionated heparin group, 17.8% in the nadoparin 6 days group, and 20.0% in the nadoparin 14 days group (p=NS). The absolute differences between the 3 groups with respect to the occurrence of the primary end point were -0.3% (95% CI=-3.5%-2.8%; p=0.85) for the nadoparin 6 days vs the unfractionated heparin groups and +1.9% (95% CI=-1.3%-5.1%; p=0.24) for the nadoparin 14 days group vs unfractionated heparin group. There were no statistically significant differences among the groups in the occurrence of any of the secondary end points (total mortality, cardiac mortality, myocardial infarction, refractory angina, recurrent angina, or the rates of PTCA + CABG) either at day 6, day 14, or at 3 months. At 3 months, recurrent angina occurred more often in the nadoparin 14 days group (19.9%) than in the nadoparin 6 days group (16.9%) or unfractionated heparin group (17.7%) (adjusted p value=0.09). The risk of major hemorrhage at day 14 was 1.6% in the unfractionated heparin, 1.5% in the nadoparin 6 days group, and 3.5% in the nadoparin 14 days group.
Concl.	Nadoparin therapy for 6±2 days was comparable to IV infusion of unfractionated heparin for the same period of time in patients with unstable angina or non-Q-wave myocardial infarction. A prolonged regimen of nadoparin for 14 days was not associated with additional benefit and was associated with an increased risk of major hemorrhage.

FRISC II

Fragmin and Fast Revascularisation During Instability in Coronary Artery Disease II

Title	a. Long-term low-molecular-mass heparin in unstable coronary artery disease: FRISC II prospective randomized multicenter study. b. Invasive compared with noninvasive treatment in unstable coronary artery disease: FRISC II prospective randomized multicenter study. c. Outcome at 1 year after an invasive compared with a noninvasive strategy in unstable coronary artery disease: the FRISC II invasive randomised trial.
Authors	a. + b. Fragmin and Fast Revascularisation During Instability in Coronary Artery Disease (FRISC II) investigators. c. Wallentin L, Lagerqvist B, Husted S, et al.
Reference	a. Lancet 1999;354:701-707. b. Lancet 1999;354:708-715. c. Lancet 2000;356:9-16.
Disease	Unstable angina, non-Q-wave myocardial infarction.
Purpose	a. To evaluate whether long-term dalteparin therapy will be associated with better outcome than placebo in patients with unstable acute coronary syndromes undergoing a noninvasive treatment strategy. b. To compare an invasive strategy of early coronary angiography and revascularization with a conservative approach. c. To report outcomes at 1 year of the invasive vs noninvasive strategy.
Design	Randomized, multicenter (the comparison between dalteparin treatment and placebo was double-blind, and the comparison between the invasive vs noninvasive strategies was open).

Patients	a. 2267 patients.
	b. + c. 2457 patients. Patients, ≤75 years old, within 48 hours of episode of ischemia at rest or suspected acute MI accompanied by ST depression or T wave inversion or by raised creatine kinase or troponin-T levels. Patients at high-risk of bleeding, anemia, indication for a treatment within the preceding 24 hours with thrombolytic agents, angioplasty within the preceding 6 months, being on the waiting list for coronary revascularization, renal or hepatic failure, other severe cardiac disease, osteoporosis, previous open heart surgery and with other severe illness were excluded.
Follow-up	a. + b. 6 months.
	c. 12 months.
Regimen	a. After randomization, all patients received dalteparin 120 IU/kg bid for ≥5 days. Then patients were randomized to double-blind therapy with subcutaneous injections of dalteparin or placebo bid for 3 months.
	b. Within 72 hours of open-label therapy, patients were randomized to 1 of 4 groups: 1) long-term dalteparin + noninvasive strategy; 2) long-term placebo + noninvasive strategy; 3) long-term dalteparin + invasive strategy; or 4) long-term placebo + invasive strategy.
Add'l Tx	All patients initially received subcutaneous dalteparin or intravenous standard heparin before randomization. a. All patients for this study were treated with a noninvasive strategy. Coronary angiography or intervention was recommended only in patients with recurrent or refractory angina or with severe ischemia on exercise test. All patients received oral aspirin 75-320 mg/d. β-Blockers were recommended.

3

Results   a. 2267 patients were randomized into the noninvasive arm of
the trial, 2105 of them actually entered the double-blind treatment period. At 1 month, death or acute MI occurred in 6.2%
of the dalteparin group vs 8.4% of the placebo group (relative
risk [RR] 0.73; 95% CI=0.54-0.99; p=0.048). Death, MI, or
revascularization occurred in 19.5% vs 25.7% of the dalteparin
and placebo group, respectively (RR 0.76; 95% CI=0.65-0.89;
p=0.001). At 3 months, the difference between the groups in
the rate of death or MI was statistically insignificant (10.0% vs
11.2%, respectively [RR 0.89; 95% CI=0.70-1.13; p=0.34]).
However, there was still a statistically significant difference in
favor of the dalteparin group in the rates of death, MI, or revascularization (29.1% vs 33.4% [RR 0.87; 95% CI=0.77-0.99;
p=0.031]). At 6 months, there was no difference in the occurrence of either death or MI (13.3% vs 13.1%; p=0.93) or death,
MI, or revascularization (38.4% vs 39.9%; p=0.50) between the
groups. Patients with elevated troponin-T concentrations had
a 30.0% relative decrease in the incidence of death or MI at 3
months (2.7% absolute decrease; p=0.07) with dalteparin. In
contrast, patients without troponin-T elevation had no apparent benefit from dalteparin. Dalteparin had no beneficial effects
on symptoms of angina. There were 3.3% major and 23.0%
minor bleeding episodes in the dalteparin group vs 1.5% and
8.4% in the placebo group. The rate of strokes was 1.0% in
the dalteparin group vs 0.8% in the placebo group. Long-term
therapy with dalteparin was not associated with higher rates
of thrombocytopenia, allergic reactions or fractures.

b. 1222 patients were randomized to the invasive regimen and
1235 to the noninvasive regimen. 96% vs 10% of the invasive and noninvasive group underwent coronary angiography
within 7 days of enrollment. Overall, during follow-up 98% vs
47% of the patients, respectively, underwent coronary angiography. Revascularization procedures were done within 10 days
of enrollment in 71% of the invasive group vs 9% in the noninvasive group. Within 6 months, 77% vs 37%, respectively,
underwent revascularization procedures. After follow-up of 6
months, death or MI occurred in 9.4% of the invasive regimen
vs 12.1% of the noninvasive regimen (RR 0.78; 95% CI=0.62-
0.98; p=0.031). MI occurred in 7.8% vs 10.1% of the invasive and noninvasive groups (RR 0.77; 95% CI=0.60-0.99;
p=0.045), whereas death occurred in 1.9% vs 2.9%, respectively (RR 0.65; 95% CI=0.39-1.09; p=0.10). The percentages of
patients with angina and the Canadian Cardiovascular Society
angina class were significantly lower in the invasive compared

to the noninvasive group, at 6 week, 3 month and 6 month visits. Re-admissions during the 6 months of follow-up occurred in 31% of the patients in the invasive strategy vs 49% of the noninvasive strategy (RR 0.62; 95% CI=0.60-0.69; p<0.001). The event rates during the first months of follow-up were lower in the noninvasive dalteparin group. However, after 6 months, the event rates were lower in the invasive approach (both in the dalteparin and placebo groups) than in the noninvasive regimen. Invasive approach was effective especially at older age, in men, and in patients with longer duration of angina, symptoms at rest, and those with ST segment depression.c. 99% of the patients in the invasive group vs 52% in the noninvasive group underwent coronary angiography within 12 months; 78% vs 43%, respectively, underwent revascularization (44% vs 21% underwent percutaneous coronary interventions and 38% vs 23% underwent CABG). 1-year mortality was 2.2% in the invasive group vs 3.9% in the noninvasive group (RR 0.57; 95% CI=0.36-0.90; p=0.016). Acute MI occurred in 8.6% and 11.6% of the patients in the invasive and noninvasive groups, respectively (RR 0.74; 95% CI=0.59 to 0.94; p=0.015). The composite end point of death or MI occurred in 10.4% vs 14.1%, respectively (RR 0.74; 95% CI=0.60-0.92; p=0.005). During the 12 months, 37% of the patients in the invasive arm vs 57% of the patients in the noninvasive arm were rehospitalized (RR 0.67; 95% CI=0.62-0.72; p<0.001), and 7.5% vs 31%, respectively, underwent revascularization after the initial admission (RR 0.24; 95% CI=0.20-0.30).

| Concl. | a. 3-month therapy with low-molecular-weight heparin (dalteparin) resulted in lower rates of death, MI, and need for revascularization in patients with acute coronary syndrome treated conservatively. This effect lasted for at least 1 month and vanished over the next 2 months of therapy and after an additional 3 months of follow-up. Initial therapy with dalteparin could be used to decrease the risk of cardiac events in patients waiting for revascularization procedures. |

b. Early invasive approach is preferred over noninvasive strategy in most patients with acute coronary syndromes. Early invasive approach resulted in lower rates of MI and a trend toward lower mortality rate over 6 months of follow-up and marked improvement in the prevalence and severity of angina and lower rates of readmission.

c. The invasive strategy was associated with significantly lower mortality, lower incidence of MI, and lower rehospitalization rate at 1 year.

FRISC II (Substudy)

Fragmin and Fast Revascularization During Instability in Coronary Artery Disease II

Title	Is early invasive treatment of unstable coronary artery disease equally effective for both women and men?
Authors	Lagerqvist B, Säfström K, Ståhle F, et al.
Reference	J Am Coll Cardiol 2001;38:41-48.
Disease	Coronary artery disease (CAD), unstable coronary disease, myocardial infarction (MI).
Purpose	To determine gender differences in early invasive vs noninvasive strategies in treating unstable CAD.
Design	As per FRISC II.
Patients	749 patients and 1708 men randomized to early invasive or non-invasive strategies for symptoms of ischemia that were increasing or occurring at rest or if symptoms suggested acute MI.
Follow-up	≈360 days.
Regimen	As per FRISC II. Coronary angiography within first 7 days in 96% of invasive groups and 10% of noninvasive groups. Revascularization within first 10 days of 71% of invasive group and 9% of noninvasive group.
Add'l Tx	As per FRISC II.

Results	Women were older (68±8 years) than the men (64±10 years). More women had previous angina treated with antianginal medicine. More men had previous MIs and pathologic Q-waves on admission. Left ventricular dysfunction and elevated tropinin T levels were more common in men. Angiographic coronary stenoses were less common in women. 24.6% had no coronary stenoses vs 9.5% in men. At 12 months incidence of MI or death among women in the invasive group was 12.4% vs women in the noninvasive group at 10.5% (p=NS). However, in men invasive treatment reduced the risk of MI or death (9.6%) vs noninvasive treatment (15.8%; p<0.001). Effect of early invasive strategy differed in its effect for the 2 genders by an interaction analysis (p=0.008).
Concl.	In men, with unstable CAD, an early invasive strategy benefited risk of future events. In women, an early invasive strategy did not reduce future risk. Overall, women had a better prognosis than men.

FROST

Fibrinogen Receptor Occupancy Study

Title	Safety and preliminary efficacy of one month glycoprotein IIb/IIIa inhibition with lefradafiban in patients with acute coronary syndromes without ST elevation. A phase II study.
Authors	Akkerhuis KM, Neuhaus KL, Wilcox RG, et al.
Reference	Eur Heart J 2000;21:2042-2055.
Disease	Acute coronary syndrome, unstable angina, non-Q-wave myocardial infarction.
Purpose	To assess the safety and efficacy of 3 doses of lefradafiban, an oral GP IIb/IIIa inhibitor, for patients with non-ST elevation acute coronary syndromes.
Design	Randomized, double-blind, placebo-controlled, dose-escalation, multicenter, phase II.
Patients	531 patients, 18-80 years old, with unstable angina or non-ST elevation acute myocardial infarction, within 24 hours of onset of symptoms and with ECG changes. Patients with concomitant serious illness, history of stroke, epilepsy, cranial surgery, active bleeding, peptic ulcer, recent major surgery, uncontrolled hypertension, thrombocytopenia, current therapy with anticoagulants, recent myocardial infarction or receipt of fibrinolytic therapy, abnormal baseline ECG interfering with a reliable interpretation of the ST segment, and planned revascularization within 24 hours of enrollment were excluded.
Follow-up	30 days.
Regimen	All patients received aspirin and unfractionated or low-molecular weight heparin for 2-5 days.
Add'l Tx	Patients were randomized to placebo (n=130) or lefradafiban 20 (n=218), 30 (n=136), or 45 mg (n=47) × 3/d. Ticlopidine was not permitted.

Results	The Data and Safety Monitoring Board terminated the study prematurely because the 45 mg × 3/d group had a high rate of major bleeding complications (11%). 60% of the patients in the lefradafiban 45 mg × 3/d discontinued study medication (excluding those who discontinued the drug due to termination of the trial), whereas the discontinuation rate was 58% in the lefradafiban 30 mg × 3/d, 55% in the lefradafiban 20 mg × 3/d and 51% with the placebo. Event rates were determined from start of therapy up to 72 hours of study drug discontinuation. Death or myocardial infarction occurred in 3.1% of the placebo, and in 3.2%, 2.2%, and 4.3% in the lefradafiban 20, 30 and 45 mg groups (p=0.72). Death, myocardial infarction or revascularization occurred in 31.5%, 30.7%, 22.1%, and 25.5%, respectively (p=0.096). Death, myocardial infarction or recurrent angina occurred in 17.7%, 17.0%, 4.4%, and 12.8%, respectively (p<0.001). At 30 days the incidence of death or myocardial infarction was 3.1% in the placebo and 4.1%, 4.4%, and 4.3%, respectively (p=0.75), whereas death, myocardial infarction, or revascularization occurred in 43.1%, 35.9%, 32.6%, and 40.4%, respectively (p=0.077). The dose-dependent reduction in event rate with lefradafiban 20 and 30 mg was greater in patients with a positive (15% and 30%) vs negative (10% and 13%) baseline troponin-I test. The incidence of major or minor bleedings was 1% in the placebo group and 5%, 7%, and 15% with lefradafiban 20, 30, and 45 mg × 3/d. 1%, 2%, 4% and 9% of the patients, respectively, needed transfusion. Lefradafiban was associated with leukopenia (5.7% vs 2.3% in the placebo group) and neutropenia (5.2% vs 1.5% in the placebo group). Thrombocytopenia was detected in 0.5% of the lefradafiban treated patients vs zero of the placebo-treated patients.
Concl.	Administration of lefradafiban for 1 month in patients with non-ST elevation acute coronary syndromes resulted in a decrease in cardiac events (with a dose of 30 mg × 3/d). The favorable effect was especially noted in patients with a positive troponin-I test on enrollment. However, lefradafiban was associated with an increased risk of bleeding.

GUARDIAN

Guard During Ischemia Against Necrosis

Title	Inhibition of the sodium-hydrogen exchanger with cariporide to prevent myocardial infarction in high-risk ischemic situations. Main results of the GUARDIAN trial.
Authors	Théroux P, Chaitman BR, Danchin N, et al.
Reference	Circulation 2000;102:3032-3038.
Disease	Unstable angina, non-ST elevation MI, high-risk percutaneous or surgical revascularization.
Purpose	To determine whether inhibition of the sodium-hydrogen exchanger with cariporide could prevent ischemic necrosis in high-risk ischemic situations.
Design	Randomized, multicenter.
Patients	11,590 patients with unstable angina, non-ST elevation MI or undergoing high-risk percutaneous or surgical revascularization.
Follow-up	6 months.
Regimen	Placebo vs doses of 20, 80, or 120 mg of cariporide as a 60 minute infusion in 50 mL of normal saline. Therapy began as soon as possible on unstable angina and non-ST-elevation MI patients and between 15 minutes and 2 hours before intervention or surgery.

Results	Primary end point was all-cause mortality or MI between randomization and 36 days. Secondary end points were primary end points at day 10, events secondary to LV dysfunction (cardiac mortality, MI, cardiogenic shock, overt congestive heart failure, life-threatening arrhythmia) at 6 months, and size of myocardial infarction determined by peak CK-MB elevation. At 36 days, the rate of death or MI showed a nonsignificant 10% risk reduction at the 120 mg cariporide dose (p=0.122) with no difference between placebo and 20 and 80 mg cariporide dose. At the 120 mg dose, the benefit was limited to patients undergoing coronary artery bypass surgery (risk reduction 25%; 95% CI=3.1%-41.5%; p=0.03) and was maintained after 6 months. No effect was seen on mortality alone. Overall CK-MB scores were similar among the 4 groups. Ratio of peak CK-MB elevation to upper limit of normal tended to be lower with increasing doses of cariporide in the surgery patients. Rate of Q-wave MI was reduced by 32% across all entry diagnoses (2.6% vs 1.8%; p=0.005) whereas rate of non-Q-wave MI was decreased only in patients undergoing CABG (7.1% vs 3.8%; p=0.005). Cariporide did not cause an increase in serious adverse events.
Concl.	While cariporide did not result in a significant decrease in the primary end point of death or MI in a wide range of high-risk ischemic situations, high doses did appear to have a protective effect in preventing cell necrosis, especially in patients undergoing CABG.

3

GUSTO IV

Global Use of Strategies to Open Occluded Coronary Arteries IV—Acute Coronary Syndrome (1-Year Follow-Up)

Title	Long-term results after the glycoprotein IIb/IIIa inhibitor abciximab in unstable angina.
Authors	Ottervanger JP, Armstrong P, Barnathan ES, et al.
Reference	Circulation 2003;107:437-442.
Disease	Unstable angina/non-Q-wave infarction.
Purpose	To determine the 1-year outcome of abciximab vs placebo in patients with non-ST-elevation acute coronary syndrome, not scheduled for percutaneous coronary intervention.
Design	Multicenter, randomized, prospective.
Patients	7800 patients with acute coronary syndrome without persisting ST-segment elevation, which included non-ST-elevation myocardial infarction and unstable angina. Patients were eligible if they were at least 21 years of age and had at least 1 episode of angina lasting at least 5 minutes within 24 hours of admission. Patients also had either abnormal levels of cardiac troponin T or I, or at least 0.5 mm of ST-segment depression.
Follow-up	1 year.
Regimen	As per GUSTO-IV.

Results	The primary study end point was the occurrence of all-cause mortality or MI at 30 days after study entry. 1-year follow-up data were obtained for 99.3% of initial study patients. The mortality at 1 year was similar between the 3 groups: 7.8% in the placebo group, 8.2% in the 24-hour abciximab group, and 9.0% in the 48-hour abciximab group. In comparison to placebo, the hazard ratio (HR) for the 24-hour abciximab infusion was 1.1 (95% CI=0.86-1.29), and for the 48-hour infusion was 1.2 (95% CI=0.95-1.41). Increasing age was predictive of 1-year mortality. Patients who had body weight ≤75 kg had a 1-year mortality of 9.6% vs 7.4% for patients who had body weight between 75 and 90 kg, and 6.6% in patients who were ≥90 kg (p<0.001). Patients who had a positive troponin had a 1-year mortality of 9.1% vs 6.9% in patients who had a negative troponin (p<0.001). Patients who had an elevated C-reactive protein (CRP) had a 1-year mortality of 13.9% vs 6.5% in those who did not have an elevated CRP. The effect of abciximab was investigated in different subgroups (sex, age, diabetes, body weight, troponin T, CRP). There were no subgroups in which abciximab treatment led to significantly reduced 1-year mortality. Patients who had a negative troponin and received abciximab had a greater mortality risk than those who received placebo (5.8% in the placebo group vs 8.5% in the 48-hour infusion group, HR 1.5; 95% CI=1.1-2.1). Patients who had an elevated CRP level and received abciximab also had a worse 1-year mortality outcome (12.1% in the placebo group vs 16.3% in the 48-hour infusion group, HR 1.4; 95% CI=1.0-2.0).
Concl.	In patients with acute coronary syndrome with ST depression or elevated troponin, abciximab did not produce a survival benefit at 1 year vs placebo in patients who did not undergo early coronary revascularization.

GUSTO-IV-ACS

Global Utilization of Strategies to Open Occluded Coronary Arteries-IV—Acute Coronary Syndromes

Title	Effect of glycoprotein IIb/IIIa receptor blocker abciximab on outcome in patients with acute coronary syndromes without early coronary revascularisation: the GUSTO-IV-ACS randomised trial.
Authors	The GUSTO-IV-ACS Investigators.
Reference	Lancet 2001;357:1915-1924.
Disease	Acute coronary syndromes, coronary artery disease.
Purpose	To assess the effect of abciximab, a GP IIb/IIIa inhibitor, on outcome of patients with non-ST-elevation acute coronary syndromes who were not undergoing early revascularization.
Design	Randomized, double-blind, placebo-controlled, multicenter.
Patients	7800 patients, ≥21 years old, with ≥1 episodes of angina lasting ≥5 minutes within the preceding 24 hours, and either a positive troponin T or I test or ≥0.5 mm ST depression. Patients with secondary forms of myocardial ischemia, persistent ST elevation myocardial infarction or new left bundle branch block were excluded. In addition, patients who underwent percutaneous coronary intervention within the preceding 14 days, those scheduled for PCI or coronary artery bypass graft surgery within 30 days after enrollment, patients with active bleeding, high risk for bleeding, intracranial neoplasm or aneurysm, atrioventricular malformation, stroke within the preceding 2 years or stroke at any time with residual neurological deficit, thrombocytopenia, international normalized ratio >1.4, blood pressure >180/100 mm Hg, weight more than 120 kg, history of vasculitis and allergy to abciximab were excluded.
Follow-up	30 days.
Regimen	Randomization to: 1) abciximab for 24 hours (0.25 mg/kg bolus followed by 0.125 μg/kg/min up to 10 μg/min) followed by 24 hours of placebo infusion (n=2590); 2) abciximab for 48 hours (0.25 mg/kg bolus followed by 0.125 μg/kg/min up to 10 μg/kg/min) (n=2612); or 3) placebo infusion for 48 hours (n=2598).

Add'l Tx	All patients received aspirin and heparin (70 U/kg bolus followed by 10 U/kg/h with a target activated partial thromboplastin time 50-70 seconds) for 48 hours. In a substudy, patients received dalteparin (120 IU/kg ×2/d subcutaneously) for 5-7 days instead of unfractionated heparin. β-blockers were recommended. Coronary angiography was not to be done within the first 60 hours of enrollment, unless the patient had recurrent or continuing ischemia at rest. If PCI was performed during placebo study-drug infusion, masked active abciximab was administered. The use of GP IIb/IIIa inhibitors after completion of study-drug administration was permitted.
Results	30% of the patients underwent revascularization within 30 days after enrollment (19% underwent PCI and 11% CABG). 48-hr mortality was 0.3% in the placebo, 0.7% in the abciximab 24 hr and 0.9% in the abciximab 48 hr (the OR of abciximab 24 hr vs placebo was 2.3 [95% CI=0.98-5.22] and for abciximab 48 hr vs placebo 2.9 [95% CI=1.28-6.44]; p=0.008). 7-day mortality was 1.8% in the placebo, 1.5% in the abciximab 24 hr and 2.0% in the abciximab 48 hr (the OR of abciximab 24 hr vs placebo was 0.9 [95% CI=0.55-1.30] and for abciximab 48 hr vs placebo 1.1 [95% CI=0.77-1.71]; p=0.574). 30-day mortality was 3.9% in the placebo, 3.4% in the abciximab 24 hr and 4.3% in the abciximab 48 hr (the OR of abciximab 24 hr vs placebo was 0.9 [95% CI=0.64-1.50] and for abciximab 48 hr vs placebo 1.1 [95% CI=0.83-1.43]; p=0.664). Death or MI at 30 days occurred in 8.0% in the placebo, 8.2% in the abciximab 24 hr, and 9.1% in the abciximab 48 hr (the OR of abciximab 24 hr vs placebo was 1.0 [95% CI=0.83-1.24] and for abciximab 48 hr vs placebo 1.1 [95% CI=0.94-1.39]; p=0.190). No subgroup of patients had a significant treatment advantage with abciximab. Major non-CABG bleeding occurred in 0.3% in the placebo group, 0.6% in the abciximab 24 hr, and in 1% in the abciximab 48 hr group (p<0.05). Minor bleeding occurred in 2%, 3%, and 4%, respectively (p<0.05). Thrombocytopenia (<50,000 cells/μL) occurred in 1 patient in the placebo group, 2% in the abciximab 24 hr and in 1% in the abciximab 48 hr group (p<0.05).
Concl.	Abciximab was not beneficial, when added to aspirin and heparin, in patients with non-ST-elevation acute coronary syndromes who were not undergoing early revascularization.

HASI (Update)

Bivalirudin Angioplasty Study (Hirulog Angioplasty Study)

Title	Bivalirudin vs heparin during coronary angioplasty for unstable or postinfarction angina: final report reanalysis of the bivalirudin angioplasty study.
Authors	Bittl JA, Chaitman BR, Feit F, et al.
Reference	Am Heart J 2001;142:952-959.
Disease	Unstable angina, percutaneous coronary intervention (PCI).
Purpose	Re-analysis (intention-to-treat) of the data comparing the efficacy of bivalirudin (hirulog) and heparin as an adjunctive therapy after angioplasty for unstable or post-infarction angina.
Design	Randomized, double-blind, multicenter.
Patients	4312 patients, >21 years old, with unstable angina or post-infarction angina <2 weeks after myocardial infarction scheduled for coronary angioplasty. Patients with renal failure; thrombolytic therapy within the preceding 24 h; planned coronary atherectomy, stent or laser; planned staged PTCA procedure; possible pregnancy; and intolerance to heparin or aspirin were excluded.
Follow-up	6 months.
Regimen	Randomization to bivalirudin (n=2161) or unfractionated heparin (n=2151). See HASI.
Add'l Tx	See HASI.

Results	7-day mortality was 0.2% in each group (OR 0.99; 95% CI=0.28-3.46; p=0.987). 7-day myocardial infarction occurred in 3.3% in the bivalirudin and 4.2% in the heparin group (OR 0.78; 95% CI=0.57-1.07; p=0.126). Fewer patients in the bivalirudin group needed revascularization in the first 7 days (4.2% vs 5.6%; OR 0.74; 95% CI=0.56-0.97; p=0.030). The combined end point of death, myocardial infarction, or revascularization occurred in 6.2% vs 7.9% (OR 0.78; 95% CI=0.62-0.99; p=0.039). Among the subgroup of patients with post-infarction angina the 7-day combined end point occurred in 4.9% in the bivalirudin group and in 9.9% in the heparin group (OR 0.47; 95% CI=0.26-0.84; p=0.009). 90-day mortality was 1.1% and 0.9% of the bivalirudin and heparin patients, respectively (p=0.487). Myocardial infarction at 90 days occurred in 4.6% and 5.4%, respectively (OR 0.84; 95% CI=0.64-1.11; p=0.221), and 13.2% in the bivalirudin vs 15.8% in the heparin group underwent revascularization at 90 days (OR 0.81; 95% CI=0.68-0.96; p=0.015). The 90-day combined end point occurred less often in the bivalirudin group (15.7% vs 18.5%; OR 0.82; 95% CI=0.70-0.96; p=0.012). At 180 days mortality was 1.7% in the bivalirudin and 1.2% in the heparin group (p=0.194). There was no significant difference in the 180-day rates of myocardial infarction (5.3% vs 6.1%; p=0.252), or revascularization (19.9% vs 21.8%; p=0.131). The combined end point occurred at 180 days in 23.0% in the bivalirudin vs 24.7% in the heparin group (OR 0.90; 95% CI=0.78-1.04; p=0.153). Among the subgroup of patients with post-infarction angina the 180-day rate of the combined end point was 18.7% in the bivalirudin and 25.3% in the heparin group (OR 0.70; 95% CI=0.49-1.00; p=0.049). Clinically significant bleeding occurred less often with bivalirudin (3.5% vs 9.3% at 7 days; OR 0.34; 95% CI=0.26-0.45; p<0.001). At 90 days major hemorrhages occurred less often with bivalirudin (3.7% vs 9.3%; p<0.001).
Concl.	Bivalirudin was better than unfractionated heparin in reducing the combined end point of death, myocardial infarction, and revascularization and bleeding complications in patients with unstable angina or postinfarction angina undergoing balloon angioplasty. The differences were mainly due to reduction in the rates of revascularization in the bivalirudin group.

INTERACT

Integrilin and Enoxaparin Randomized Assessment of Acute Coronary Syndrome Treatment

Title	Randomized evaluation of the safety and efficacy of enoxaparin versus unfractionated heparin in high-risk patients with non-ST-segment elevation acute coronary syndromes receiving the glycoprotein IIb/IIIa inhibitor eptifibatide.
Authors	Goodman SG, Fitchett D, Armstrong PW, et al.
Reference	Circulation 2003;107:238-244.
Disease	Unstable angina/non-Q-wave infarction.
Purpose	To determine the safety and efficacy of combined glycoprotein IIb/IIIa inhibitor therapy with low-molecular-weight-heparin therapy.
Design	Prospective, randomized, multicenter.
Patients	746 patients, ≥18 years of age, hospitalized for ischemic chest symptoms of at least 10 minutes duration at rest and no more than 24 hours before study entry. Patients needed to have ST-segment depression ≥0.1 mV or transient ST-segment elevation ≥0.1 mV in ≥2 contiguous ECG leads, and/or elevated levels of troponin I or T at least 3 times the upper limit of normal, or creatine kinase (CK-MB) greater than normal. Exclusion criteria were numerous and were related to cardiovascular (ie, left bundle branch block, ischemia due to a precipitating cause such as heart failure, recent coronary artery bypass surgery or percutaneous coronary intervention, others), risk of bleeding (uncontrolled blood pressure, anemia, recent stroke, others), recent or ongoing therapy with abciximab, tirofiban, eptifibatide, or anticoagulants, and general (renal failure, other serious disease). Study protocol was changed after enrollment of 265 patients to include patients who had received unfractionated heparin or enoxaprin ≤12 hours before study entry.
Follow-up	30 days.

Regimen	Patients received either eptifibatide in a 180-µg/kg bolus followed by a 2.0 $\mu g^{-1} \times kg^{-1} \times min^{-1}$ infusion over 48 hours. All patients received at least 160 mg of aspirin initially and then 80 to 325 mg daily. Patients were then randomized to receive either enoxaparin (1 mg/kg of body weight, subcutaneously every 12 hours for 48 hours) or unfractionated heparin (70-U/kg IV bolus followed by a $15\text{-U} \times kg^{-1} \times h^{-1}$ infusion, adjusted to achieve a partial-thromboplastin time [aPTT] of 1.5-2 times control for 48 hours).
Results	The primary outcome of safety was the occurrence of 96-hour major bleeding not related to coronary artery bypass surgery. Major bleeding was defined to include a bleed resulting in death, retroperitoneal hemorrhage, or bleeding at a specific site together with a decrease in hemoglobin of at least 3 g/dL. Minor bleeding was any overt bleeding that did not meet the criteria for major bleeding. The primary outcome for efficacy was the rate of recurrent ischemia as measured by continuous ECG monitoring. Evaluation was made in the first 48 hours and from 48-96 hours after randomization. Other clinical outcomes were the 30-day composite of either death or nonfatal MI or death, MI, or recurrent angina. The primary safety outcome was lower in the eptifibatide and enoxaparin group compared with the eptifibatide and unfractionated-heparin group (1.8% vs 4.6%, respectively; p=0.03). A difference was detected in the first 48 hours (1.1% vs 3.8%; p=0.014). At 96 hours, there were lower rates of major hemorrhage in the enoxaparin group compared with the unfractionated heparin group (2.1% vs 5.5%; p=0.016) as well as at 30 days (5.3% vs 8.7%; p=0.062). The incidence of minor bleeding was more frequent in the enoxaparin group vs the unfractionated heparin group at 96 hours (30.3% vs 20.8%; p=0.003), which was mostly due to increased ecchymoses at the injection site and oropharyngeal bleeding (mostly epistaxis). Patients in the enoxaparin group had lower rates of ischemia during the first 48 hours (14.3% vs 25.4%; p=0.0002), and during 48-96 hours (12.7% vs 25.9%; p<0.0001). The 30-day combined end point of death or MI was significantly lower in the enoxaparin group vs the unfractionated heparin group (5% vs 9%; p=0.031). The combined end point of death, MI, or recurrent angina was lower in the enoxaparin group (9% vs 12.6%; p=0.11).
Concl.	In high-risk patients with non-ST-segment elevation acute coronary syndrome using aspirin and eptifibatide (a glycoprotein IIb/IIIa inhibitor), usage of enoxaparin improves safety and efficacy outcomes vs usage of unfractionated heparin.

NUT-2

The Nonsteroidal Anti-Inflammatory Drugs in Unstable Angina Treatment-2 Pilot Study

Title	Efficacy assessment of meloxicam, a preferential cyclooxygenase-2 inhibitor, in acute coronary syndromes without ST-segment elevation: The Nonsteroidal Anti-Inflammatory Drugs in Unstable Angina Treatment-2 (NUT-2) pilot study.
Authors	Altman R, Luciardi HL, Muntaner J, et al.
Reference	Circulation 2002;106:191-195.
Disease	Unstable angina/non-Q-wave myocardial infarction.
Purpose	To determine whether meloxicam, a nonsteroidal anti-inflammatory drug that selectively inhibits cyclooxygenase isoform 2 (COX-2), when added to heparin and aspirin, is more effective in reducing recurrent cardiovascular thrombotic events than heparin and aspirin in patients with non-ST-segment elevation acute coronary syndromes.
Design	Open-label, randomized, single-blind, prospective.
Patients	120 patients, randomized to aspirin plus heparin (n=60), or aspirin, heparin, and meloxicam (n=60). Patients were eligible if they had chest pain associated with ST-segment depression (≥0.5 mm) within the 24 hours prior to study enrollment and either evidence of ischemia on electrocardiography or previously documented coronary artery disease. Exclusion criteria included persistent ST-segment elevation and increased levels of creatine kinase muscle-brain isoform (CK-MB) consistent with acute MI, revascularization within the previous 6 months, malignancy, pregnancy, renal or hepatic disease, anticoagulant use, treatment with anti-inflammatory medications, or contraindication to study drugs.
Follow-up	90 days.

Regimen	Patients were randomized to receive either: aspirin and heparin; or aspirin, heparin, and meloxicam. Immediately after randomization, patients in the active treatment group received 15 mg of meloxicam intravenously followed by 15 mg orally qd during hospitalization and 30 days after discharge. All patients received aspirin 100-300 mg/d for 30 days dosed at the discretion of the patient's physician. All patients also received SC low-molecular-weight heparin (either nadroparin 87 IU/kg bid or enoxaparin 1 mg/kg bid) or IV unfractionated heparin as a 5000 IU initial bolus followed by infusion at 1000 IU/h for 7 days or until hospital discharge. The activated partial thromboplastin time was maintained between 45-87 seconds (normal: 30±5 seconds).
Results	The primary outcome of the study was a composite of recurrent angina, MI, or death during stay at the coronary care unit and at 90 days of follow-up. The secondary outcome was a composite of MI, death, and all revascularization procedures (PTCA or CABG surgery). During the coronary care unit stay, a composite event occurred less frequently in the meloxicam group (9/60, 15%) vs the control group (23/60, 38.3%), a relative risk reduction (RRR) of 60.8% (95% CI=23-80; p=0.007). Recurrent angina was less frequent in the meloxicam group (9 vs 21 patients; RRR 57.1%; 95% CI=14-79; p=0.02). There were 2 MIs and 1 vascular death in the 60 patients of the control group; there were no MIs or vascular deaths in the meloxicam group. The secondary outcome occurred in 6/60 (10%) patients in the meloxicam group and 16/60 (26.7%) in the control group. This difference was also significant (RRR 62.5%; 95% CI=11-84; p=0.034). At 90 days follow-up, the primary outcome had occurred in 13 patients (21.7%) in the meloxicam group and in 29 patients (48.3%) in the control group, a statistically significant difference (RRR 55.1%; 95% CI=22-74; p=0.004). There were no MIs or vascular deaths in the meloxicam group; there were 3 MIs and 2 vascular deaths in the placebo group. In the meloxicam group, the frequency of recurrent angina was reduced (12 vs 26 patients; 20% vs 43.3%; RRR 53.8%; 95% CI=17-74; p=0.011) and the secondary end point occurred much less frequently (13.3 % vs 33.3%; RRR 60.1%; 95% CI=16-81; p=0.015). Meloxicam was not associated with adverse events such as bleeding or impairment of renal function.
Concl.	Meloxicam, a selective COX-2 inhibitor, when added to heparin and aspirin, was effective in reducing the risk of cardiovascular thrombotic events in patients with a non-ST-segment elevation acute coronary syndrome.

OPUS-TIMI-16

Oral Glycoprotein IIb/IIIa Inhibition with Orbofiban in Patients with Unstable Coronary Syndromes

Title	Oral glycoprotein IIb/IIIa inhibition with orbofiban in patients with unstable coronary syndromes (OPUS-TIMI-16) trial.
Authors	Cannon CP, McCabe CH, Wilcox RG, et al.
Reference	Circulation 2000;102:149-156.
Disease	Coronary artery disease; unstable coronary syndromes.
Purpose	To determine whether chronic oral IIb/IIIa inhibition provides additional reduction in recurrent ischemic events.
Design	Randomized, placebo-controlled, multicenter.
Patients	10,288 patients with acute coronary syndromes defined by ischemic pain at rest within 72 hours of randomization with new ST-T ischemic changes, positive cardiac markers, history of myocardial infarction, percutaneous intervention, or coronary artery bypass graft surgery, angiographic evidence of CAD, age ≥65 years, plus angina or a positive exercise test, prior peripheral vascular, cerebrovascular disease or diabetes.
Follow-up	1 year.
Regimen	Randomized to 1) 50 mg orbofiban twice daily (50/50 group); 2) 50 mg twice daily for 30 days followed by 30 mg twice daily (50/30 group); or 3) placebo.
Add'l Tx	All patients received 150-162 mg of aspirin daily. Patients with stents were given double-blinded stent medication for 2-4 weeks, those in the placebo group received 250 mg of ticlopidine twice daily, those in orbofiban received matching placebo for ticlopidine (plus orbofiban).

Results	Primary end point was composite of death, MI, recurrent ischemia at rest requiring rehospitalization, or stroke. At 30 days composite end point was 9.9% for orbofiban (both treatment groups combined since dose was the same for both for first 30 days) vs 10.8% for placebo, p=0.12. However, death occurred in 2.0% of orbofiban groups vs 1.4% of the placebo group (p=0.02). While ischemia requiring urgent revascularization was decreased by orbofiban compared to placebo (2.7% vs 4.4%; p<0.0001) treatment did not improve recurrent MI, stroke and recurrent ischemia requiring rehospitalization. At 10 months, the composite end point was not decreased by either orbofiban 50/50 or 50/30. Death rates were 3.7%, 5.1%, and 4.5% for placebo, orbofiban 50/30 and orbofiban 50/50, respectively (p=0.009 for 50/30 vs placebo and 0.12 for 50/50 vs placebo). The greater mortality with treatment was explained by the difference observed at 30 days—no significant further increase in mortality occurred after 30 days. New thrombotic events occurred at 24%, 30%, and 33.9% of the placebo, orbofiban 50/30 and orbofiban 50/50 groups, respectively. Major or severe bleeding was more frequent with orbofiban at 3.7% (50/30), 4.5% (50/50) vs 2.0% of placebo patients. 1 subgroup—those that underwent PCI, had a lower mortality and decrease in end point with orbofiban (27.5% placebo, 23.9% for 50/30 [p=0.01] and 21.8% for 50/50 p=[0.002]).
Concl.	Chronic oral therapy with orbofiban failed to decrease major cardiovascular events and increased mortality in patients with acute coronary syndromes.

PARAGON B

Platelet IIb/IIIa Antagonist for the Reduction of Acute Coronary Syndrome Events in a Global Organization Network B

Title	Randomized, placebo-controlled trial of titrated intravenous lamifiban for acute coronary syndromes.
Authors	PARAGON B Investigators.
Reference	Circulation 2002;105:316-321.
Disease	Coronary artery disease. Acute coronary syndrome without persistent ST-segment elevation.
Purpose	To determine whether adding lamifiban (a highly specific inhibitor of platelet glycoprotein IIb/IIIa) could improve clinical outcomes in patients with acute coronary syndromes without persistent ST-segment elevation when the drug was titrated to target plasma concentrations.
Design	Randomized, double-blind, placebo-controlled, multicenter.
Patients	5225 patients with acute coronary syndromes including unstable angina and myocardial infarction (MI) without persistent ST elevation.
Follow-up	30 days-primary end point; 1 year.
Regimen	500-mg IV lamifiban bolus or placebo; then adjusted-dose infusion for ≤72 hours or until discharge. Infusion titrated to target plasma lamifiban concentration of 18-42 ng/mL and adjusted to renal function.
Add'l Tx	150-325 mg aspirin per day. IV unfractionated heparin given with study drug that could be stopped after successful percutaneous coronary intervention. Low-molecular-weight heparin could be substituted.

Results	Primary end point was 30-day composite incidence of death, MI, or severe recurrent ischemia. The primary end point was reached in 12.8% of placebo patients and 11.8% of lamifiban patients (OR 0.914; 95% CI=0.769-1.087; p=0.329). There was no difference in survival curves for the composite of death or MI to 6 months, between the 2 groups. 15 (0.6%) placebo patients developed stroke vs 28 (1.1%) lamifiban patients (p=0.05). Intracranial hemorrhage occurred in 2 patients in each group. Bleeding was more common in the lamifiban group. In patients who had plasma lamifiban concentrations measured, 91% had a concentration >18 ng/mL. Outcomes did not differ in these patients vs those that achieved a lower concentration.
Concl.	Lamifiban bolus and infusion, despite achieving adequate plasma concentrations had no significant clinical benefits in patients with non-ST elevation acute coronary syndromes.

PARAGON B (Troponin T Substudy)

Platelet IIb/IIIa Antagonism for the Reduction of Acute Coronary Syndrome Events in a Global Organization Network

Title	Benefit of glycoprotein IIb/IIIa inhibition in patients with acute coronary syndromes and troponin T-positive status.
Authors	Newly LK, Ohman EM, Christenson RH, et al.
Reference	Circulation 2001;103:2891-2896.
Disease	Non-ST-segment elevation acute coronary syndromes.
Purpose	To determine the interaction between baseline Troponin T (TnT) levels and treatment in patients with non-ST-segment elevation acute coronary syndromes.
Design	Double-blind, randomized, placebo-controlled, multicenter. TnT levels obtained before study treatment and at 24 and 72 hours later.
Patients	1160 patients with non-ST-segment elevation acute coronary syndromes as part of the PARAGON B study.
Follow-up	30 days.
Regimen	Lamifiban (a short-acting, nonpeptide, small-molecule GP IIb/IIIa antagonist) as a 500 µg bolus, followed by an infusion adjusted for renal function in targeting a steady state plasma concentration of 18-42 ng/mL. Drug continued for 72 hours vs placebo.
Add'l Tx	Aspirin, IV heparin (unfractionated or low molecular weight). Percutaneous coronary intervention as needed.

Results	Primary end point was 30-day composite of death, MI, or severe recurrent ischemia requiring urgent intervention. 40.2% of patients were TnT positive (≥0.1 ng/mL) and positive patients were more often male, older, or smokers. Patients who were TnT positive at baseline had a greater rate of the primary end point (OR=1.5; 95% CI=1.1-2.1) vs patients who were TnT negative. Among TnT positive patients, lamifiban reduced the primary end point (19.4% to 11.0%; p=0.01); but was not effective in those patients who were TnT negative (11.2% for placebo vs 10.8% for lamifiban; p=0.86).
Concl.	Lamifiban benefited TnT-positive patients, but not TnT-negative patients. TnT predicted poor short-term outcomes in these patients.

PCI-CURE

Clopidogrel in Unstable Angina to Prevent Recurrent Events—Percutaneous Coronary Intervention Substudy

Title	Effects of pretreatment with clopidogrel and aspirin followed by long-term therapy in patients undergoing percutaneous coronary intervention: the PCI-CURE study.
Authors	Mehta SR, Yusuf S, Peters RJG, et al.
Reference	Lancet 2001;358:527-533.
Disease	Coronary artery disease, acute coronary syndrome, percutaneous coronary intervention.
Purpose	To assess whether pretreatment with clopidogrel followed by long-term therapy after PCI will reduce adverse events compared with 4-week clopidogrel therapy following PCI in patients with non-ST elevation acute coronary syndromes.
Design	Randomized, double-blind, placebo-controlled, multicenter.
Patients	2658 patients hospitalized within 24 hours of onset of non-ST elevation acute coronary syndromes and who were undergoing PCI. This study was part of the CURE study. Only patients with ECG changes or above normal levels of cardiac enzymes or markers were included. Patients with ST elevation, contraindications to antithrombotic or antiplatelet therapy, at increased risk of bleeding, and with severe heart failure (New York Heart Association class IV) were excluded. In addition, patients who received IV glycoprotein IIb/IIIa receptor antagonists in the 3 days preceding enrollment, those who were on oral anticoagulants, and those who underwent coronary revascularization in the 3 months preceding enrollment were not included.
Follow-up	3-12 months, average 8 months.
Regimen	Randomization to placebo (n=1345) or clopidogrel (300 mg loading dose, followed by 75 mg/d)(n=1313).

Add'l Tx	All patients received aspirin 75-325 mg/d. All patients participating in this study underwent PCI at the discretion of the local investigator. In patients who underwent stent implantation, the study medication was stopped after PCI and the patients received open-label clopidogrel or ticlopidine for 2-4 weeks. Thereafter, the study medication was resumed.
Results	1730 PCIs were performed during the initial hospital stay and 928 after discharge. The median number of days before PCI was 10 days in both groups (6 days for procedures done during the initial hospitalization). 24.7% of the patients in the placebo group and 26.4% in the clopidogrel group received open-label clopidogrel or ticlopidine before PCI, and 84.1% and 82.9%, respectively, received it after PCI for a median of 30 days (interquartile range 19-33 days). Before PCI, MI or refractory angina occurred in 15.3% of the patients in the placebo group vs 12.1% in the clopidogrel group (relative risk [RR] 0.76; 95% CI=0.62-0.93; p=0.008). MI before PCI occurred in 5.1% vs 3.6% (RR 0.68; 95% CI=0.47-0.99; p=0.04). From PCI to 30 days, cardiovascular death, MI, or urgent revascularization occurred in 6.4% vs 4.5%, respectively (RR 0.70; 95% CI=0.50-0.97; p=0.03), whereas cardiovascular death or MI occurred in 4.4% vs 2.9% (RR 0.66; 95% CI=0.44-0.99; p=0.04). Cardiovascular death occurred in 1.0% and 1.1%, respectively, and MI in 3.8% vs 2.1% (RR 0.56; 95% CI=0.35-0.89). 2.8% of the patients in the placebo group vs 1.9% in the clopidogrel group had urgent revascularization from PCI until day 30 (RR 0.67; 95% CI=0.41-1.11). Cardiovascular death or MI from PCI to the end of the follow-up occurred in 8.0% of the patients in the placebo group and 6.0% in the clopidogrel group (RR 0.75; 95% CI=0.56-1.00; p=0.047), and cardiovascular death, MI or revascularization at that time period occurred in 21.7% vs 18.3% (RR 0.83; 95% CI=0.70-0.99; p=0.03). The difference was due to less MI (4.5% vs 6.4%) and revascularization (14.2% vs 17.1%) in the clopidogrel group, but there was no difference in cardiovascular mortality (2.4% vs 2.3%, respectively). Less patients in the clopidogrel group received IV glycoprotein IIb/IIIa during PCI (20.9% vs 26.6%; p=0.001). Major bleeding from PCI to 30 days occurred in 1.4% of the patients in the placebo group vs 1.6% in the clopidogrel group (p=0.69). Major bleeding from PCI to the end of follow-up occurred in 2.5% vs 2.7%, respectively (p=0.64), whereas minor bleeding occurred in 2.1% vs 3.5%, respectively (p=0.03).

3

Concl.   Pretreatment with clopidogrel followed by long-term treatment
          resulted in reduction in clinical events, mainly MI and repeat
          revascularization in patients with non-ST elevation acute coro-
          nary syndromes who underwent PCI and received long-term
          aspirin therapy. Pretreatment with clopidogrel, in addition to
          aspirin, was associated with fewer clinical events before PCI in
          patients with non-ST elevation acute coronary syndrome.

PRISM-PLUS

Platelet Receptor Inhibition in Ischemic Syndrome Management in Patients Limited by Unstable Signs and Symptoms

Title	Inhibition of the platelet glycoprotein IIb/IIIa receptor with tirofiban in unstable angina and non-Q-wave myocardial infarction.
Authors	PRISM-PLUS Investigators.
Reference	N Engl J Med 1998; 338:1488-1497.
Disease	Coronary artery disease, unstable angina, non-Q-wave myocardial infarction.
Purpose	To evaluate the effectiveness of tirofiban in treating unstable angina and non-Q-wave infarctions.
Design	Randomized, double-blind, multicenter.
Patients	1915 patients with unstable angina or non-Q-wave infarcts.
Follow-up	6 months.
Regimen	All patients received aspirin. They were randomized to tirofiban, heparin, or tirofiban plus heparin. Study drugs were infused for a mean of 71 h. Coronary angiography and angioplasty performed when indicated after 48 h.
Results	Tirofiban alone was associated with an excess of mortality at 7 days (4.6%) compared with patients on heparin alone (1.1%). The incidence of the composite end point (death, myocardial infarction, or refractory ischemia) was lower among patients on tirofiban plus heparin (12.9%) compared to patients on heparin alone (17.9%, risk ratio 0.68; 95% CI=0.53-0.88; p=0.004). This benefit persisted at 30 days (18.5% vs 22.3%; p=0.03) and 6 months (27.7% vs 32.1%; p=0.02) Tirofiban plus heparin was also associated with a lower rate of death or myocardial infarction at 7, 30, and 60 days. Major bleeding was present in 3% of heparin group and 4% in combination group.
Concl.	Tirofiban alone (without heparin) caused excess mortality early. However, when administered with heparin it was associated with a better clinical outcome than patients who received heparin.

PRISM-PLUS (Angiographic Results)

Platelet Receptor Inhibition for Ischemic Syndrome Management in Patients Limited by Unstable Signs and Symptoms

Title	Intracoronary thrombus and platelet glycoprotein IIb/IIIa receptor blockade with tirofiban in unstable angina or non-Q-wave myocardial infarction. Angiographic results from the PRISM-PLUS Trial.
Authors	Zhao X-Q, Theroux P, Snapinn SM, et al.
Reference	Circulation 1999;100:1609-1615.
Disease	Unstable angina, non-Q-wave myocardial infarction.
Purpose	To describe the angiographic substudy results of the PRISM-PLUS study. To assess the effects of tirofiban on the characteristics of the culprit lesion in patients with unstable angina and non-Q-wave MI.
Design	As per PRISM-PLUS.
Patients	1491 patients with readable coronary angiograms obtained at a median of 65 hours after randomization.
Follow-up	Angiograms done at about 65 hours following randomization.
Regimen	As per PRISM-PLUS.
Add'l Tx	As per PRISM-PLUS.

Results	Angiograms were analyzed by a core laboratory. The primary end point was the intracoronary thrombus burden and secondary end points were TIMI flow grade distribution and severity of the obstruction and underlying atherosclerotic lesion. Compared to heparin alone, tirofiban plus heparin reduced the frequency and severity of thrombus. Tirofiban plus heparin decreased the intracoronary thrombus burden compared to heparin alone (odds ratio [OR] 0.65; p=0.002) and reduced the severity of obstruction (p=0.037). Small thrombus, medium thrombus, and large thrombus were seen in 9.0%, 15.8%, and 3.0% of heparin alone patients, respectively, vs 11.4%, 11.4%, and 2.1% of tirofiban plus heparin patients, respectively. TIMI grade 3 was present in 74% of heparin alone patients vs 82% of patients on tirofiban plus heparin. As expected tirofiban plus heparin did not alter the severity of underlying atherosclerotic plaque. Persistence of thrombus increased the odds of death and myocardial infarction.
Concl.	Tirofiban plus heparin decreased thrombus burden of the culprit lesion and improved coronary perfusion in patients with unstable angina and non-Q-wave myocardial infarction.

PRISM-PLUS (Diabetic Substudy)

Platelet Receptor Inhibition in Ischemic Syndrome Management in Patients Limited by Unstable Signs and Symptoms

Title	Glycoprotein IIb/IIIa receptor blockade improves outcomes in diabetic patients presenting with unstable angina/non-ST-elevation myocardial infarction. Results from the PRISM-PLUS Study.
Authors	Théroux P, Alexander J Jr, Pharand C, et al.
Reference	Circulation 2000;102:2466-2472.
Disease	Unstable angina, non-ST-elevation MI.
Purpose	To determine whether diabetic patients in the PRISM-PLUS study benefited from platelet glycoprotein IIb/IIIa receptor-mediated inhibition by tirofiban.
Design	As per PRISM-PLUS.
Patients	23% of 1915 patients with unstable angina, non ST elevation MI.
Follow-up	180 days.
Regimen	Data from diabetics in the tirofiban plus heparin group (n=169) vs heparin control arm (n=193) presented in this analysis.
Add'l Tx	Aspirin as per PRISM-PLUS.
Results	Primary end point was composite of death from any cause, new MI, or refractory ischemia within 7 days of randomization. There was a nonstatistically significant lower incidence of the composite primary end point in patients who received tirofiban plus heparin vs those who received heparin alone at 2, 7, 30 and 180 days (7.7% vs 8.3%, 14.8% vs 21.8%, 20.1% vs 29.0% and 32.0% vs 39.9%, respectively (p=NS). There were significant differences in the rate of MI or death in those diabetic patients favoring tirofiban plus heparin, at 2, 7, 30 and 180 days: (0.0% vs 3.1%, p=0.03; 1.2% vs 9.3%, p=0.005; 4.7% vs 15.5%, p=0.002; and 11.2% vs 19.2%, p=0.03). The effect of tirofiban was stronger among diabetics than nondiabetics in reducing the incidence of MI/death. There was a small but not statistically significant increase in risk of bleeding with combination of tirofiban plus heparin.

Concl.   In diabetic patients presenting with unstable angina or non-ST-elevation MI, the addition of tirofiban to heparin and aspirin was effective in preventing MI or death.

PURSUIT

Platelet Glycoprotein IIb/IIIa in Unstable Angina:
Receptor Suppression Using Integrilin Therapy

Title	Inhibition of platelet glycoprotein IIb/IIIa with eptifibatide in patients with acute coronary syndromes.
Authors	The PURSUIT Trial Investigators
Reference	N Engl J Med 1998;339:436-443.
Disease	Acute coronary syndromes.
Purpose	To test the hypothesis that inhibition of platelets with eptifibatide would have benefit beyond heparin in decreasing adverse outcomes in patients with acute coronary syndromes.
Design	Randomized, double-blind, multicenter.
Patients	10,948 patients. Patients had to present with ischemic chest pain within 24 hours and transient ST T changes compatible with ischemia (but not persistent ST elevation) or high CK-MB.
Follow-up	30 days.
Regimen	Eptifibatide (bolus of 180 µg per kg body weight, followed by infusion of 1.3 µg per kg per minute; or bolus of 180 µg per kg followed by an infusion of 2.0 µg per kg per minute). Infusion lasted until hospital discharge or 72 hours, whichever came first.
Add'l Tx	All patients could receive aspirin and IV or subcutaneous heparin. During infusion of eptifibatide, thrombolytic therapy was not allowed.

Results	45%-46% of patients were admitted with myocardial infarction. About 65% had angina at rest. Patient enrollment occurred at a median of 11 hours of symptoms. The frequency of the composite end point (death from any cause or nonfatal myocardial infarction at 30 days) was 7.6% in eptifibatide group and 9.1% in placebo group at 96 hours (p=0.01); 10.1% vs 11.6% at 7 days, (p=0.02); and 14.2% vs 15.7% at day 30 (p=0.04). Thus at 30 days there was a 1.5% absolute reduction of primary end points with treatment. The effect was less consistent in women. Bleeding was more common in the treatment group and tended to be mild involving vascular access sites. There was no increase in hemorrhagic stroke in the treatment group.
Concl.	Eptifibatide reduced the composite end point of death from any cause and nonfatal myocardial infarction in patients with acute coronary syndromes without persistent ST segment elevation on the electrocardiogram.

PURSUIT (Subanalysis)

Platelet Glycoprotein IIb/IIIa in Unstable Angina: Receptor Suppression Using Integrilin Therapy

Title	Attenuation of rebound ischemia after discontinuation of heparin therapy by glycoprotein IIb/IIIa inhibition with eptifibatide in patients with acute coronary syndromes. Observations from the PURSUIT trial.
Authors	Lauer MA, Houghtaling PL, Peterson JG, et al.
Reference	Circulation 2001;104:2772-2777.
Disease	Acute coronary syndromes, unstable angina.
Purpose	To determine effect of glycoprotein IIb/IIIa inhibition on heparin rebound (reactivation of ischemia after discontinuation of heparin) in acute coronary syndromes.
Design	Randomized, double-blind, placebo-controlled, multicenter.
Patients	6186 patients in the PURSUIT study who presented within 24 hours of symptoms of ischemia at rest with ST segment depression, transient ST elevation, T wave inversion, or creatine kinase-MB level above upper limit of normal.
Follow-up	For this study, 48 hours after heparin discontinuation.
Regimen	High dose eptifibatide as a 180 µg/kg bolus followed by 2.0 µg/kg/min infusion to hospital discharge or 72 hours.
Add'l Tx	Aspirin. IV or subcutaneous heparin. IV heparin given as a bolus dose of 5000 U followed by infusion at 1000 U/hour.

Results	End point for this analysis was death or MI occurring either with heparin infusion or in 48 hours after heparin discontinuation. There was no difference in events during heparin infusion in eptifibatide group (0.82% per 12 hours) vs placebo (0.90% per 12 hours). The event rate increased in both groups 0-12 hours after heparin discontinuation. The event rate was 1.68% in the eptifibatide group vs 2.53% in the placebo group (p=0.03). Death rate was 0.77% in the placebo group and 0.21% in the eptifibatide group (p=0.002). Event rate in the 2 groups returned to near on-heparin rate in the 12-24 hour period and below on-heparin rate after 24 hours. Multivariate predictors of heparin rebound included duration of heparin infusion, age, lack of eptifibatide treatment and study site in North America.
Concl.	In patients with acute coronary syndromes, withdrawal of heparin is associated with a 12-hour period of an increase in death or MI that is attenuated with eptifibatide.

PURSUIT (Substudy)

Platelet Glycoprotein IIb/IIIa in Unstable Angina: Receptor Suppression Using Integrilin Therapy

Title	Outcomes of patients with acute coronary syndromes and prior coronary artery bypass grafting. Results from the PURSUIT trial.
Authors	Labinaz M, Kilaru R, Pieper K, et al.
Reference	Circulation 2002;105:322-327.
Disease	Non-ST-segment elevation acute coronary syndromes.
Purpose	To determine the baseline characteristics and outcomes in patients with acute coronary syndromes without ST-segment elevation who have had prior coronary artery bypass grafting (CABG) and assess the effects of eptifibatide (a glycoprotein IIb/IIIa antagonist) on their outcomes.
Design	Double-blind, placebo-controlled, randomized, multicenter.
Patients	In PURSUIT, 1134 (12%) had a history of prior CABG while 8321 did not. In patients who had histories of prior CABG, half received eptifibatide and half did not.
Follow-up	Primarily 30 days; also 180 days.
Regimen	Eptifibatide (bolus of 180 mg/kg IV followed by infusion of 2 mg/kg per minute) or a bolus plus infusion of placebo. Infusion continued for 72 hours of hospital discharge.
Add'l Tx	Aspirin. IV or subcutaneous heparin was recommended. Percutaneous coronary intervention at discretion of treating physician.

Results	Primary and secondary end points were composite of death from any cause or nonfatal myocardial infarction (MI) at 30 days. Patients with prior CABG had more adverse baseline characteristics including older age, more men, more diabetes, more prior MI, more smokers, hypertensives, and more patients with hypercholesterolemia. After adjusting for baseline characteristics and treatment, those in the subgroup with prior CABG had a higher 30-day mortality rate (hazard ratio [HR] 1.45; 95% CI=1.06-1.98; p=0.019] and a higher 180 day mortality rate [HR 1.32; 95% CI=1.04-1.67; p=0.02]. Death or MI at 30 days in the prior CABG cohort was 15.0% with eptifibatide vs 16.5% with placebo (HR 0.90; 95% CI=0.67-1.20). In the non-prior CABG patients this primary end point occurred in 14.1% of eptifibatide treated patients vs 15.5% of placebo patients (HR 0.89; 95% CI=0.80-0.99). There was no significant interaction between treatment and prior CABG.
Concl.	Patients with acute coronary syndromes with non-ST-segment elevation have a worse outcome if they have a history of a prior CABG. Treatment effect of eptifibatide in these patients was similar in those with or without prior CABG.

3

PURSUIT (Substudy)

Platelet Glycoprotein IIb/IIIa in Unstable Angina: Receptor Suppression Using Integrilin Therapy

Title	Enhanced efficacy of eptifibatide administration in patients with acute coronary syndrome requiring in-hospital coronary artery bypass grafting.
Authors	Marso SP, Bhatt DL, Roe MT, et al.
Reference	Circulation 2000;102:2952-2958.
Disease	Coronary artery disease.
Purpose	To determine whether pretreatment with eptifibatide in patients with ischemic syndromes who required CABG was associated with decreased rates of death and nonfatal myocardial infarction in the PURSUIT trial.
Design	As per PURSUIT.
Patients	1558 participants in PURSUIT trial that underwent in-hospital CABG. Patients had to have non-ST segment elevation acute coronary syndromes.
Follow-up	6 months.
Regimen	As per PURSUIT. Eptifibatide infusion (n=866) vs placebo infusion (n=692).
Add'l Tx	As per PURSUIT.
Results	Primary end point was death or MI rates at 6 months. At 30 days, death or MI was 30.8% in the placebo group and 26.1% in the eptifibatide group (p=0.041). At 6 months these rates were 32.7% in the placebo group and 27.6% in the eptifibatide group (p=0.029). Reduction in 6-month death or MI rate was greater for those patients that received eptifibatide within 72 hours of the CABG. Major bleeding occurred in 56.6% of placebo patients and 58% of eptifibatide patients (p=0.7).
Concl.	Eptifibatide reduced death or MI in patients admitted with non-ST segment elevation acute coronary syndrome who went on to in-hospital CABG.

PURSUIT (Substudy)

Platelet Glycoprotein IIb/IIIa in Unstable Angina: Receptor Suppression Using Integrilin Therapy

Title	Early, percutaneous coronary intervention, platelet inhibition with eptifibatide, and clinical outcomes in patients with acute coronary syndromes.
Authors	Kleiman NS, Lincoff AM, Flaker GC, et al.
Reference	Circulation 2000;101:751-757.
Disease	Acute coronary syndromes.
Purpose	To determine the effects of GP IIb/IIIa platelet antagonist eptifibatide in patients with acute coronary syndromes in those with percutaneous coronary interventions vs those managed conservatively.
Design	As per PURSUIT.
Patients	1228 patients had early (<72 hours) percutaneous coronary intervention; 8233 did not.
Follow-up	30 days.
Regimen	As per PURSUIT.
Add'l Tx	As per PURSUIT.
Results	Primary end point was composite of death or MI within first 30 days; secondary end point was death or MI among patients who had percutaneous coronary intervention within the first 72 hours. Myocardial infarction preceded early percutaneous coronary intervention in 34 placebo patients (5.5%) vs 10 eptifibatide patients (1.7%; p=0.001). There was a reduction in primary composite end point in eptifibatide patients (p=0.035) when patients were censored for percutaneous coronary intervention over a 30-day period. In patients with early percutaneous coronary intervention, eptifibatide decreased 30-day event rates (11.6% vs 16.7%; p=0.01), and there was a trend for this benefit in patients who did not undergo early intervention (14.6% vs 15.6%; p=0.23). Following adjustment for intervention propensity, eptifibatide treatment did not appear to differ between patients who had vs those that did not have early intervention.

Concl.   "Eptifibatide reduced the composite rates of death or myocardial infarction in patients receiving percutaneous coronary interventions and those managed conservatively."

RITA 3

Randomized Intervention Trial of Unstable Angina

Title	Interventional versus conservative treatment for patients with unstable angina or non-ST-elevation myocardial infarction: the British Heart Foundation RITA 3 randomised trial.
Authors	Fox KA, Poole-Wilson PA, Henderson RA, et al.
Reference	Lancet 2002;360:743-751.
Disease	Acute coronary syndrome.
Purpose	To study whether an interventional strategy (routine early angiography with revascularization, if indicated) is better than a conservative approach (optimum medical therapy with angiography and revascularization only in symptomatic patients or in those with positive stress test) in patients with acute coronary syndrome.
Design	Randomized, open-label, multicenter.
Patients	1810 patients with unstable angina or non-ST-elevation acute myocardial infarction. Patients with probable evolving acute myocardial infarction, including candidates for reperfusion therapy, were excluded. Patients with new pathological Q waves or CK or CK-MB ′2 the upper limit of normal before randomization were not included. Patients with myocardial infarction in the preceding 1 month, PCI in the preceding 1 year or previous CABG were not included. Patients scheduled for coronary angiography within 72 hours of admission could not be enrolled. In addition, patients with known cardiomyopathy or significant valvular disease, and those in whom ischemia was precipitated by arrhythmia, anemia, or non-coronary causes were excluded.
Follow-up	Planned 5 years. Median follow-up was 2.0 years, 97% of the patients had >1 year of follow-up.

Regimen	Patients were randomized to a conservative approach (n=915) or interventional approach (n=895) within 48 hours of the index episode of chest pain. The conservative approach included aspirin, enoxaparin 1 mg/kg bid for 2-8 days and antianginal medications including β-blockers. Patients with recurrent ischemia or positive exercise tests were referred for coronary angiography. The interventional approach included medical therapy similar to the conservative approach with coronary angiography within 72 hours of randomization.
Add'l Tx	GP IIb/IIIa inhibitors and other antiplatelet agents could be prescribed. There were no protocol restrictions in the use of stents, other interventional devices, or pharmacological agents during interventions.
Results	97% of the patients in the interventional arm underwent cardiac catheterization, with a median of 2 days after enrollment. ≥1 significantly narrowed coronary artery was found in 78% of the patients (33%, 24%, and 22% having 1-, 2-, and 3-vessel disease, respectively). 36% of the patients were planned to undergo PCI and 22% CABG. In the conservative arm 10% underwent revascularization during the index admission and an additional 17% during the first year. The overall 1-year revascularization rate was 57% in the interventional arm and 28% in the conservative arm. The primary end point of the study (death, MI, or refractory angina) occurred at 4 months in 9.6% of the patients in the interventional arm and in 14.5% in the conservative arm (risk ratio [RR] 0.66; 95% CI=0.51-0.85; p=0.001). 4-month mortality was 2.9% in the interventional arm and 2.5% in the conservative arm (p=0.61). At 4 months, MI occurred in 3.4% and 3.7% of the patients, respectively (p=0.68). In contrast, refractory angina occurred less often at 4 months in the interventional arm (4.4% vs 9.3%; RR 0.47; 95% CI=0.32-0.68; p<0.0001). At 1 year there was no difference in mortality (4.6% and 3.9% in the interventional and conservative arms, respectively [p=0.50]), or MI rate (3.8% and 4.8%, respectively [p=0.29]). However, refractory angina occurred less often in the interventional arm (6.5% and 11.6%, respectively; RR 0.56; 95% CI=0.41-0.76; p=0.0002). Death or MI at 1 year occurred in 7.6% and 8.3% of the patients, respectively (RR 0.91; 95% CI=0.67-1.25; p=0.58). For men, the incidence of the primary end point at 4 months was lower in the interventional arm (8.8% vs 17.3%). However, for women the incidence was comparable (10.9% and 9.6%, respectively)

(interaction test p=0.004). Interventional strategy was associated with reduction in the prevalence of angina (CCS grade ≥2) (26.3% vs 36.3% at 4 month; p<0.0001). At 1 year 23.8% of the patients in the intervention group vs only 14.8% in the conservative group were not taking any anti-anginal medications (p<0.0001).

Concl.	After admission for unstable angina or acute non-ST-elevation MI, an early interventional approach resulted in significant reduction in refractory angina or severe angina without an increased risk of death or MI.

ROXIS Pilot Study

Randomization Trial of Roxithromycin in Non-Q-Wave Coronary Syndromes

Title	Randomized trial of roxithromycin in non-Q-wave coronary syndromes: ROXIS pilot study.
Authors	Gurfinkel E, Bozovich A, Daroca A, et al.
Reference	Lancet 1997; 350:404-407.
Disease	Coronary artery disease, unstable angina or non-Q-wave myocardial infarction.
Purpose	To determine the effectiveness of the antibiotic roxithromycin for reducing severe recurrent angina, acute myocardial infarction, and death in patients with unstable angina or non-Q-wave infarction.
Design	Randomized, double-blind, placebo-controlled study.
Patients	202 patients with unstable angina or non-Q-wave infarction.
Follow-up	31 days.
Regimen	Oral roxithromycin, 150 mg × 2/d for 30 days vs placebo. All patients received, aspirin, IV nitroglycerin, heparin.
Results	No difference between groups for individual outcomes of angina, myocardial infarction, or death. There was a trend (p=0.06) for reduced triple end point of angina plus infarction plus death.
Concl.	Nonsignificant trend toward improvement with antibiotic when examined in an intention-to-treat analysis.

SYMPHONY

Sibrafiban vs Aspirin to Yield Maximum Protection From Ischemic Heart Events Post-Acute Coronary Syndromes

Title	Comparison of sibrafiban with aspirin for prevention of cardiovascular events after acute coronary syndromes: A randomized trial.
Authors	The SYMPHONY Investigators.
Reference	Lancet 2000;355:337-345.
Disease	Acute coronary syndrome.
Purpose	To investigate whether sibrafiban, an oral glycoprotein IIb/IIIa receptor antagonist, would be more effective than aspirin in preventing cardiovascular events in patients with acute coronary syndromes.
Design	Randomized, double-blind, multicenter.
Patients	9233 patients within 7 days of an acute coronary syndrome. All patients had to be clinically stable for 12 hours before enrollment, with Killip class ≤2. Patients at high risk for bleeding; previous stroke or intracerebral hemorrhage; anemia, thrombocytopenia; treatment with oral anticoagulants, antiplatelet agents or nonsteroidal anti-inflammatory agents; or renal failure were excluded.
Follow-up	90 days.
Regimen	Randomization to aspirin 80 mg bid (n=3089), high dose sibrafiban (n=3039) or low dose sibrafiban (n=3105). The sibrafiban dose was between 3-6 mg bid, adjusted to body weight and serum creatinine.
Add'l Tx	Other oral antiplatelet agents were prohibited, except for open-label aspirin on the day of and the day after PCI. In case of stent implantation patients received a stent kit containing either ticlopidine (for the aspirin group) or placebo (for the sibrafiban groups).

Results   Premature discontinuation of the study drug occurred in 19.2% in the aspirin group, 22.3% in the low dose sibrafiban group and 23.8% in the high dose sibrafiban group. The primary end point of the study (death, myocardial [re]infarction, or severe recurrent ischemia at 90 days) occurred in 9.8% in the aspirin group, 10.1% in the low dose sibrafiban group and 10.1% in the high dose sibrafiban group (odds ratio for aspirin vs both the low- and high-dose sibrafiban 1.03; 95% CI=0.87-1.21). Death or myocardial (re)infarction occurred in 7.0%, 7.4%, and 7.9%, respectively. There were no differences among the 3 groups concerning the predefined secondary end points of either all cause mortality, myocardial (re)infarction, severe recurrent ischemia, readmission, reversible coronary ischemia, or any revascularization. Large myocardial infarctions (CKMB >5 × the upper limit of normal) occurred less often in the aspirin group (37.4%) than in the low (45.3%) or high dose (49.7%) sibrafiban groups. Treatment effects were comparable among the various subgroups. Bleedings occurred in 13.0% in the aspirin group vs 18.7% and 25.4% in the low and high dose sibrafiban groups. Major bleedings occurred in 3.9%, 5.2%, and 5.7%, respectively. Thrombocytopenia was infrequent and did not differ among the treatment groups.

Concl.   Sibrafiban had no advantage over aspirin for prevention of major ischemic events in stable patients after an acute coronary syndrome and was associated with higher bleeding rates than aspirin.

TACTICS-TIMI-18

Treat Angina with Aggrastat and Determine Cost of Therapy with an Invasive or Conservative Strategy—Thrombolysis in Myocardial Infarction-18

Title	Comparison of early invasive and conservative strategies in patients with unstable coronary syndromes treated with the glycoprotein IIb/IIIa inhibitor tirofiban.
Authors	Cannon CP, Weintraub WS, Demopoulos LA, et al.
Reference	N Engl J Med 2001;344:1879-1887.
Disease	Acute coronary syndrome.
Purpose	To compare the effectiveness and costs of an early invasive strategy with conservative treatment for patients with non-ST-elevation acute coronary syndromes.
Design	Randomized, open-label, multicenter.
Patients	2220 patients, ≥18 years old, with acute coronary syndromes who were eligible for coronary revascularization. Patients with persistent ST elevation, secondary angina, a history of revascularization in the preceding 6 months, increased risk of bleeding, left bundle branch block or paced rhythm, severe heart failure, cardiogenic shock, severe non-cardiac disease, serum creatinine >2.5 mg/dL, and those taking oral anticoagulation therapy, ticlopidine or clopidogrel for >3 days before enrollment, were excluded.
Follow-up	6 months.
Regimen	Randomization to early invasive strategy (coronary angiography 4-48 hours after enrollment and revascularization when appropriate) or an early conservative strategy (if stable—predischarge exercise tolerance test. Only patients with prolonged or recurrent angina at rest with changes in cardiac enzyme levels or ECG changes, hemodynamic instability, documented ischemia before the end of the second stage of the standard Bruce protocol, or at any time during a pharmacologic stress test, unstable angina requiring hospitalization, Canadian Cardiovascular Society class III or IV angina, or a new myocardial infarction were referred for coronary angiography).

Add'l Tx	All patients received aspirin 325 mg/d, intravenous heparin (5000 U bolus followed by 1000 U/h for 48 hours), and tirofiban (0.4 µg/kg/min in 30 minutes and then, 0.1 µg/kg/min for 48 hours or 12 hours after percutaneous coronary intervention if performed.
Results	97% of the patients in the invasive strategy group underwent coronary angiography during the index admission (a median of 22 hours after enrollment), and 60% underwent PCI or CABG. In contrast, only 51% of the patients in the conservative strategy underwent coronary angiography (a median of 79 hours after enrollment) and 36% underwent revascularization during the index hospitalization. After 6 months, 98% of the patients in the invasive strategy vs 61% in the conservative strategy underwent coronary angiography, 42% vs 29%, respectively, underwent PCI, and 22% vs 16% underwent CABG. Tirofiban was used in 94% of the PCIs in the invasive strategy group vs 59% in the conservative strategy group. 30-day mortality was 2.2% in the invasive strategy and 1.6% in the conservative strategy (OR 1.40; 95% CI=0.76-2.59; p=0.29). Fatal or nonfatal MI occurred in 3.1% and 5.8%, respectively (OR 0.51; 95% CI=0.33-0.77; p=0.002). Rehospitalization for acute coronary syndrome occurred in 3.4% and 5.5%, respectively (OR 0.61; 95% CI=0.40-0.92; p=0.018). Death, nonfatal MI or rehospitalization for an acute coronary syndrome at 30 days occurred in 7.4% of the patients in the invasive strategy vs 10.5% in the conservative strategy (OR 0.67; 95% CI=0.50-0.91; p=0.009). Death, nonfatal MI or rehospitalization for an acute coronary syndrome at 6 months occurred in 15.9% of the patients in the invasive strategy vs 19.4% of the patients in the conservative strategy (OR 0.78; 95% CI=0.62-0.97; p=0.025). 6-month mortality was 3.3% and 3.5%, respectively (OR 0.93; 95% CI=0.58-1.47; p=0.74). MI within the first 6 months occurred in 4.8% of the patients in the invasive strategy vs 6.9% in the conservative strategy (OR 0.67; 95% CI=0.46-0.96; p=0.029). 11.0% of the patients in the invasive strategy vs 13.7% in the

conservative strategy were rehospitalized during the first 6 months because of acute coronary syndrome (OR 0.78; 95% CI=0.60-1.00; p=0.054). The rate of death or MI during the 6 month follow-up was 7.3% vs 9.5%, in the invasive vs conservative strategy, respectively (OR 0.74; 95% CI=0.54-1.00; p<0.05). The benefit of an early invasive strategy was consistent among the subgroups tested (age <65 years and ≥65 years; men and women; patients with and without prior MI; patients with or without diabetes, and patients with or without troponin T elevation). The beneficial effect of the early invasive strategy was especially apparent in patients without prior use of aspirin and in patients with ST segment deviation at baseline.

| Concl. | In patients with non-ST-elevation acute coronary syndromes who were treated with tirofiban, the strategy of early catheterization and revascularization was associated with less major cardiac events than the conservative strategy. |

TACTICS-TIMI-18 (Substudy)

Treat Angina with Aggrastat and Determine Cost of Therapy with an Invasive or Conservative Strategy—Thrombolysis in Myocardial Infarction-18

Title	Cost and cost-effectiveness of an early invasive vs conservative strategy for the treatment of unstable angina and non-ST-segment elevation myocardial infarction.
Authors	Mahoney EM, Jurkovitz CT, Chu H, et al.
Reference	JAMA 2002;288:1851-1858.
Disease	Acute coronary syndrome.
Purpose	To compare total 6-month costs and cost-effectiveness of the invasive and the conservative arms in the TACTICS-TIMI-18 trial.
Design	Randomized, open-label, multicenter.
Patients	1722 patients recruited for the TACTICS-TIMI-18 trial at US non-Veterans Affairs hospitals. Inclusion and exclusion criteria as above.
Follow-up	6 months.
Regimen	As above.
Add'l Tx	As above.
Results	For patients assigned for the invasive strategy, the initial hospitalization costs averaged $15,714, whereas for those assigned for the conservative arm it was $14,047 (an average difference of $1667; 95% CI=$387-$3091). At 6 months, the average costs from discharge were $6098 and $7180 in the invasive and conservative arms, respectively (an average difference of $1082; 95% CI= -$2051 to $76). The average total costs at 6 months were $19,780 and $19,111, respectively (an average difference of $670; 95% CI= -$1035 to $2321). The average total costs (including productivity costs) at 6 months were $21,813 and $21,227, respectively (an average difference of $586; 95% CI= -$1087 to $2486). The estimated cost per life saved with the invasive strategy was $12,739 for the base case (range $8371-$25,769).

Concl.   In patients with non-ST-elevation acute coronary syndromes
         treated with glycoprotein IIb/IIIa inhibitor, the benefit of early
         invasive strategy was associated with only a small increase in
         cost, supporting the broader use of an early invasive strategy in
         patients with acute coronary syndromes.

TIMI-11B

Thrombolysis in Myocardial Infarction-11B

Title	Enoxaparin prevents death and cardiac ischemic events in unstable angina/non-Q-wave myocardial infarction. Results of the TIMI 11B Trial.
Authors	Antman EM, McCabe CH, Gurfinkel EP, et al.
Reference	Circulation 1999;100:1593-1601.
Disease	Unstable angina/non-Q-wave myocardial infarction.
Purpose	To test the benefits of an extended course of antithrombotic therapy with uninterrupted enoxaparin with standard unfractionated heparin treatment for preventing death and cardiac events in patients with unstable angina or non-Q-wave myocardial infarction.
Design	Randomized, double-blind, multicenter. Study had 2 phases: an acute phase and an outpatient phase.
Patients	3910 patients with unstable angina or non-Q-wave myocardial infarction.
Follow-up	43 days.
Regimen	All patients received both an IV infusion (unfractionated heparin or placebo) and subcutaneous injections (enoxaparin or matched placebo). Unfractionated heparin was given in a weight adjusted fashion for a minimum of 3 days starting as a bolus of 70 U/kg and infusion of 15 U/kg/hour. Target aPTT was 1.5-2.5 times control. Enoxaparin was given as an initial IV bolus of 30 mg followed by subcutaneous injection of 1 mg/kg (100 anti-factor Xa units per kg) every 12 hours. Injections were continued until hospital discharge or day 8. For the chronic phase those originally assigned to enoxaparin received enoxaparin given as 40 mg subcutaneously every 12 hours if patients weighed <65 kg and 60 mg if they weighed ≥65 kg for 43 days; patients that had been originally assigned to IV unfractionated heparin received placebo subcutaneous injections, twice daily.
Add'l Tx	Aspirin.

Results	The primary end point was the composite of all cause mortality, recurrent myocardial infarction, or urgent revascularization. This end point was achieved by 8 days in 14.5% of patients in the unfractionated heparin group and 12.4% in the enoxaparin group (OR=0.83; 95% CI=0.69-1.00; p=0.048). By 43 days the composite end point was reached in 19.7% of the unfractionated heparin group and 17.3% in the enoxaparin group (OR=0.85; 95% CI=0.72-1.00; p=0.048). The event rates for each element of the composite end point were also lower in the enoxaparin group through 14 days and there was no evidence of a rebound after discontinuing the study drugs. Benefits of enoxaparin were most evident during the acute phase without further relative decrease in events during the outpatient phase. Rates of major hemorrhage during hospitalization did not differ between groups. During the outpatient phase, major hemorrhage was more common in the enoxaparin group (2.9%) vs the group receiving placebo (1.5%; p=0.021).
Concl.	Enoxaparin was superior to unfractionated heparin for decreasing the composite end point of death, myocardial infarction, and urgent revascularization in patients with unstable angina or non-Q-wave myocardial infarction.

VANQWISH Trial (Non-Q-Wave Myocardial Infarction Following Thrombolysis)

Veterans Affairs Non-Q-Wave Infarction Strategies In-Hospital

Title	Non-Q-wave myocardial infarction following thrombolytic therapy: A comparison of outcomes in patients randomized to invasive or conservative post-infarct assessment strategies in the Veterans Affairs non-Q-Wave infarction strategies in-hospital (VANQWISH) Trial.
Authors	Wexler LF, Blaustein AS, Lavori PW, et al.
Reference	J Am Coll Cardiol 2001;37:19-25.
Disease	Non-Q-wave MI following thrombolytic therapy.
Purpose	To determine effect of post-infarct management strategy on event rate in patients who evolved non-Q-wave MI following thrombolytic therapy as part of the VANQWISH trial.
Design	As per VANQWISH.
Patients	115 patients who evolved non-Q-wave MI following thrombolytic therapy.
Follow-up	Average of 23 months.
Regimen	Randomized to routine early coronary angiography or conservative strategy of noninvasive functional assessment with angiography reserved for patients with spontaneous or induced ischemia.
Add'l Tx	Aspirin, diltiazem, other medicines as needed.

Results   19 of 58 patients (33%) randomized to invasive management died or developed recurrent nonfatal MI vs 11 of 57 patients (19%) randomized to conservative therapy (p=0.152). Death rate among post-thrombolytic patients was 11 of 58 patients (19%) in invasive strategy group vs only 2 of 57 (3.5%) among conservative strategy group (p=0.02). Excess death rate in invasive group was not due to periprocedural mortality. Revascularization (PTCA or CABG) occurred in 47% of invasive patients vs 28% of conservative patients (p=0.064). PTCA occurred in 36% of invasive patients vs 18% of conservative patients (p=0.041).

Concl.   Death or recurrent nonfatal MI were comparable between conservative vs invasive strategies in patients who evolved non-Q-wave MIs following thrombolytic therapy. Mortality rate was low in patients receiving conservative therapy (3.5%) while routine invasive management was associated with increased risk of death.

VINO

Value of First Day Coronary Angiography/Angioplasty in Evolving Non-ST-Segment Elevation Myocardial Infarction. An Open Multicenter Randomized Trial

Title	Value of first day angiography/angioplasty in evolving non-ST-segment elevation myocardial infarction: an open multicenter randomized trial. The VINO study.
Authors	Spacek R, Widimsky P, Straka Z, et al.
Reference	Eur Heart J 2002;23:230-238.
Disease	Non-ST elevation myocardial infarction.
Purpose	To compare outcome after invasive strategy on the first day of admission and early conservative approach in patients with evolving myocardial infarction without persistent ST elevation.
Design	Randomized, open-label, multicenter.
Patients	131 patients with chest pain of >20 minutes, within the last 24 hours before enrollment and ST depression and/or negative T waves without ST elevation. Patients had to have creatine kinase-MB >1.5 the upper limit of normal or positive troponin I. Patients with unstable post-infarction angina resistant to maximal medical therapy in whom urgent angiography was indicated were not included. Patients with cardiogenic shock, Q-wave myocardial infarction, or thrombolytic therapy in the preceding month, revascularization in the preceding 6 months, and serious concomitant disease that might influence 1-year survival were excluded.
Follow-up	6 months.
Regimen	Randomization to angiography and revascularization on the first day (n=64) or to early conservative approach (n=67). In the conservative group, coronary angiography was performed only in the presence of recurrent ischemia or positive exercise stress test.

Add'l Tx	All patients received IV aspirin 250 mg and heparin 5000 IU. Subsequently, all patients received heparin for ≥3 days and oral aspirin 200 mg/d. After stenting, patients received ticlopidine 250 mg bid for 1 month.
Results	All patients in the invasive group vs 55% in the conservative group underwent coronary angiography within 6 months (p=0.0001). 73% and 39%, respectively, underwent revascularization (p=0.0001). 47% vs 3% of patients underwent PCI on the first day (p=0.0001), 5% vs 10% underwent elective PTCA (p=NS), and 35% vs 30% underwent CABG (p=NS). 30-day mortality was 1.6% in the invasive group and 7.5% in the conservative group (p=NS). However, at 6 months the difference in mortality became significant (3.1% vs 13.4%; p<0.03). Recurrent nonfatal myocardial infarction occurred in 1.6% of the patients in the invasive group and in 7.5% in the conservative group (p=NS) at 30 days, and in 3.1% and 14.9%, respectively at 6 months (p<0.02). The primary end point of death or myocardial infarction occurred in 3.1% in the invasive group and in 10.4% in the conservative group at 30 days (p<0.165), and in 6.3% vs 22.4%, respectively at 6 months (relative risk of conservative vs invasive approach 3.34; 95% CI=1.2-9.6; p<0.001). Length of hospitalization was longer for the conservative group (10.4±3.1 days vs 8.2±2.9 days; p<0.0001).
Concl.	The invasive approach of angiography and subsequent revascularization on the first day of admission for non-ST elevation acute myocardial infarction reduced mortality and morbidity compared to the classical approach of early conservative management.

Title	Evaluation of prolonged antithrombotic pretreatment ("cooling-off" strategy) before intervention in patients with unstable coronary syndromes. A randomized controlled trial.
Authors	Neumann FJ, Kastrati A, Pogatsa-Murray G, et al.
Reference	JAMA 2003;290:1593-1599.
Disease	Unstable coronary syndromes. Unstable angina plus either ST-segment depression or elevation of cardiac troponin T.
Purpose	To determine whether prolonged antithrombotic pretreatment is better than early catheter intervention for unstable coronary syndromes.
Design	Randomized, controlled trial.
Patients	410 patients with angina pectoris at rest or minimal exertion within 24 hours of study entry. Myocardial ischemia verified by ST-segment depression of ≥0.1 mV and/or cardiac troponin T elevation.
Follow-up	30 days.
Regimen	Patients were randomized to early intervention (n=203) or prolonged antithrombotic pretreatment (n=207). Early intervention included coronary angiography within at least 6 hours during which time antithrombotic pretreatment was given. Prolonged antithrombotic pretreatment included pretreatment for 3-5 days, after which patients had coronary angiography. After coronary angiography, immediate revascularization with percutaneous catheter intervention was the goal. Antithrombotic pretreatment (prior to coronary angiography) was the same in both groups except for the duration of therapy and included: unfractionated heparin (60 U/kg IV bolus followed by infusion, aspirin (500 mg IV followed by 100 mg bid oral dose), oral clopidogrel (600 mg, followed by 75 mg bid), and IV tirofiban (10 µg/kg bolus followed by infusion of 0.1 µg/kg/min).

Results   The primary end point was the composite 30-day incidence of large nonfatal MI or death from any cause. This end point was reached in 11.6% (3 deaths, 21 MIs) of the prolonged antithrombotic treatment vs 5.9% (0 deaths, 12 MIs) in the early intervention group (relative risk=1.96; 95% CI=1.01-3.82; p=0.04). Findings were similar in patients with ST-segment depression or elevated levels of cardiac troponin T. Median time to catheterization in the prolonged group was 86 hours; it was 2.4 hours in the early intervention group. Benefits of early intervention were attributable to events occurring prior to catheterization. The event rate following catheterization was similar between the 2 groups.

Concl.   Delaying intervention in order to follow prolonged antithrombotic pretreatment did not improve outcome compared to immediate intervention.

4. Stable Angina Pectoris and Silent Ischemia—Medical Therapy

Dutch Echocardiographic Cardiac Risk Evaluation Applying Stress Echocardiography

Title	Bisoprolol reduces cardiac death and myocardial infarction in high-risk patients as long as 2 years after successful major vascular surgery.
Authors	Poldermans D, Boersma E, Bax JJ, et al.
Reference	Eur Heart J 2001;22:1353-1358.
Disease	Coronary artery disease.
Purpose	To evaluate the long-term effects of bisoprolol on cardioprotection after successful major vascular surgery in high-risk patients.
Design	Randomized, multicenter.
Patients	Patients >70 years old, undergoing elective abdominal aortic or infra-inguinal arterial reconstruction and with angina pectoris, previous myocardial infarction, congestive heart failure, treated diabetes mellitus, current treatment with anti-arrhythmic drugs or limited exercise capacity. Eligible patients underwent dobutamine echocardiography. Those with dobutamine-induced new or worsening wall motion abnormalities were included in the study. Patients who were taking β-blockers were excluded. Of the 1351 patients screened, 112 were included in the study. 11 patients died within the first 30 days of surgery. Finally, 57 patients in the bisoprolol and 44 in the standard care groups were followed for 2 years.
Follow-up	11-30 months after surgery (median 22 months).
Regimen	Patients were randomized to bisoprolol 5-10 mg/d (n=59) or standard care (n=53).

Results	The maintenance dose of bisoprolol was 5 mg/d in 32 patients and 10 mg/d in 25 patients. Cardiac mortality was 11% in the bisoprolol group vs 20% in the standard care group (p=0.259). Nonfatal myocardial infarction occurred in 2% vs 11%, respectively (p=0.083). The combined end point of cardiac death or nonfatal myocardial infarction occurred in 12% vs 32% in the bisoprolol and standard care groups, respectively (OR 0.3; 95% CI=0.11-0.83; p=0.025). 2 patients in the bisoprolol and 5 in the standard care underwent repeated surgery for leg ischemia (p=NS).
Concl.	Bisoprolol reduced long-term cardiac death and myocardial infarction in patients with positive dobutamine echocardiography for ischemia who underwent elective major noncardiac vascular surgery.

Antianginal and Anti-Ischemic Effects of Ivabradine, an I_f Inhibitor, in Stable Angina

Title	Antianginal and anti-ischemic effects of ivabradine, an I_f inhibitor, in stable angina: a randomized, double-blind, multicentered, placebo-controlled trial.
Authors	Borer JS, Fox K, Jaillon P, et al.
Reference	Circulation 2003;107:817-823.
Disease	Stable angina.
Purpose	To determine if ivabradine, a selective heart rate-lowering medication that acts on the sinoatrial node, was safe and effective in reducing angina and ischemic symptoms in patients with stable angina.
Design	Randomized, double-blind, placebo-controlled, parallel-arm.
Patients	360 patients, age ≥18 years, ≥3-month history of chronic, stable angina, induced by exercise, without any history of previous mechanical therapy or >3 months after coronary artery bypass graft surgery or >6 months after percutaneous intervention. Angina was relieved by rest or nitroglycerin. Patients should have had coronary artery disease documented by catheterization or a myocardial infarction at least 3 months before study entry. All patients had to have a positive exercise tolerance test (ETT) (consisting of both limiting angina and ST-segment depression ≥1 mm vs rest) at study entry. Repeat performance on the ETT on placebo could not differ by more than 20% or more than 1 minute to 1 mm ST-segment depression. Exclusion criteria were: unstable angina, Prinzmetal angina/"microvascular angina", valve disease, atrial fibrillation/flutter, pacemaker, 2°/3° atrioventricular block, or inability to do ETT.
Follow-up	3-4 months.

Regimen   Randomization to 2.5, 5, or 10 mg bid of ivabradine, or placebo.
           Treatment was started with a wash-out period for antianginal
           medications (b-blockers, calcium channel blockers, long-act-
           ing nitrates) that lasted 2-7 days. Patients then underwent an
           ETT and received study medication or placebo for 2 weeks in
           a double-blind fashion. After the 2-week period, there was a 2-
           3-month open-label phase in which all patients received 10 mg
           bid of ivabradine and only short-acting nitrates as antianginal
           medication. After the open-label phase, there was a double-blind
           phase in which patients were randomized to 10 mg bid of ivabra-
           dine or placebo, followed by an ETT.

Results   The primary efficacy outcome of the study was change in time to 1 mm horizontal or downsloping ST-segment depression ≥0.08 seconds after the J point and time to limiting angina during the ETT, performed at the trough of drug activity (12 hours after the last administration of the medication). Other outcome measures were change in ETT at time of maximal medication activity (4 hours after administration) and frequency of angina attacks according to patients' diaries. The safety end points were adverse events, vital signs, BP during ETT, rest ECG, and 24-hour Holter monitoring. During the double-blind phase, the resting heart rate at the trough of drug activity decreased vs placebo at all 3 doses of ivabradine ($p<0.05$). The heart rate was found to vary inversely with the dose at rest and during exercise ($p<0.0001$ for both). The time to 1 mm ST-segment depression during ETT increased significantly in the 5 mg and 10 mg groups (change from study start to finish was 44.1 seconds in the 5 mg group, 46.2 seconds in the 10 mg group, and 9.0 seconds in placebo group). The time to onset of angina and to limiting angina was increased at all doses but was only significant relative to placebo in the 10 mg group. There were significant reductions in the rate-pressure product (heart rate × systolic BP) during peak exercise ($p=0.011$) and an increase in total work performed during the ETT ($p=0.019$) for patients on ivabradine. There was a significant dose-dependent relationship for both ($p=0.002$). Changes were significant relative to placebo only for the 10 mg group. Improvements seen in the double-blind phase were maintained during the open-label phase, and patients who were previously on placebo and switched to ivabradine during the open-label phase had reduced ischemia and angina. There was no hypotension seen at any dose, and the average BP changed a small amount relative to placebo. Frequency of angina attacks and use of short-acting nitrates was reduced in the ivabradine groups in the double-blind phase but the reduction was not significant. Patients continuing on ivabradine during the open-label phase had a significant reduction in angina attacks vs baseline (4.14±5.59 attacks/week at baseline vs 0.95±2.24 attacks/week at the end of the open-label phase; $p<0.001$). Use of short-acting nitrates decreased from 2.28±3.74 U/week to 0.50±1.14 U/week (p<0.001). The principal adverse event observed was visual symptoms, which were not reported in the placebo group but were reported by 1 patient in the 2.5 mg and 5 mg ivabradine groups each and 13 patients (14.8%) in the 10 mg ivabradine group. Symptoms included photopsia (n=10), stroboscopic effect (n=4), and non-typical blurred vision (n=1). All symptoms resolved after discontinuation or withdrawal of medication. There were no serious cardiac events after withdrawal of treatment.

| Concl. | Ivabradine was safe and effective for producing dose-dependent improvement in exercise tolerance and time to ischemia during exercise. |

Effects of Oral Magnesium Therapy on Exercise Tolerance, Exercise-Induced Chest Pain, and Quality of Life in Patients with Coronary Artery Disease

Title	Effects of oral magnesium therapy on exercise tolerance, exercise-induced chest pain, and quality of life in patients with coronary artery disease.
Authors	Shechter M, Merz NB, Stuehlinger H-G, et al.
Reference	Am J Cardiol 2003;91:517-521.
Disease	Coronary artery disease.
Purpose	To compare the effect of oral magnesium therapy to placebo on exercise tolerance, exercise-induced ischemia, and quality of life in patients with known coronary artery disease.
Design	Randomized, prospective, multicenter, double-blind, placebo-controlled.
Patients	187 patients, greater than 20 years of age, with known coronary artery disease from previous myocardial infarction, coronary artery bypass surgery, or coronary angiography or angioplasty. Exclusion criteria included unstable angina, congestive heart failure greater than New York Heart Association class III, chronic diarrhea, renal failure, acute myocardial infarction in the past 3 months, thyroid disease, insulin-dependent diabetes mellitus, peripheral vascular disease, history of drug or alcohol abuse, or chronic liver disease.
Follow-up	6 months.
Regimen	Magnesium 15 mmol bid (365 mg total) or placebo bid. Patients underwent maximum symptom-limited exercise testing after an overnight fast and 24-hour withdrawal of β-blockers, calcium channel blockers, and ACE inhibitors.

Results	The 2 groups had similar characteristics at baseline. The efficacy analysis included 73 patients (78%) in the magnesium group and 84 patients (90%) in the placebo group. The primary end points of the study were the effect of the magnesium therapy on exercise tolerance, exercise-induced ischemia, and quality of life, all at 6 months. The duration of exercise was significantly greater in the magnesium group vs the placebo group at 6 months (8.7 ± 2.1 vs 7.8 ± 2.9 minutes; $p=0.0075$). At 6 months, there were significantly fewer patients with exercise-induced chest pain in the magnesium group vs placebo (8% vs 21%; $p=0.0237$). Fewer patients in the magnesium group had to discontinue their exercise test due to angina (7% vs 17%; $p=0.0522$). There were no significant differences in resting and exercise heart rate, BP, or percent target heart rate achieved between the groups. Most of the quality-of-life measures were significantly improved in the magnesium group vs the placebo group; criteria on the Seattle Angina Questionnaire such as physical limitation, anginal stability, anginal frequency, treatment satisfaction, and disease perception were significantly improved in the magnesium group at 6 months ($p<0.02$ for all), but fewer were changed in the placebo group. At 6 months, there were more patients in the placebo group that answered yes to the question: "Did the present medication improve your condition?" (66% vs 47%; $p=0.0165$). The number of adverse events was greater in the placebo group at 6 months vs magnesium; (61% vs 32%; $p=0.0054$).
Concl.	Supplementation with oral magnesium for 6 months in patients with CAD resulted in a significant improvement in exercise tolerance, exercise-induced chest pain, and quality of life vs placebo.

CAPE II Trial

Circadian Anti-Ischemic Program in Europe II

Title	Medical treatment of myocardial ischemia in coronary artery disease: effect of drug regime and irregular dosing in the CAPE II trial.
Authors	Deanfield JE, Detry J-M, Sellier P, et al.
Reference	J Am Coll Cardiol 2002;40:917-925.
Disease	Coronary artery disease.
Purpose	To determine the efficacy of amlodipine and diltiazem in preventing ischemia when an irregular dosing pattern is used.
Design	Double-blind, randomized, multicenter.
Patients	250 patients, 128 in the amlodipine group, 122 in diltiazem group. Patients age 21-80 years were eligible if they had a history of stable angina (≥2 attacks/week and no change in symptoms for ≥1 month), positive exercise test, and at least 1 other objective finding of coronary artery disease. Exclusion criteria were: congestive heart failure, uncontrolled arrhythmia or hypertension, standing systolic blood pressure <100 mm Hg, heart rate <50 bpm, heart block greater than 1 ° AV-block, or abnormal ECG that would potentially impair the interpretation of study findings.
Follow-up	14 weeks.

Regimen	The study began with a 2-week placebo run-in period during which patients underwent ambulatory ECG monitoring and exercise testing. Patients were then randomized to 6 weeks of treatment with 5 mg amlodipine or 180 mg diltiazem once a day. 2 weeks later, the dosages were increased to 10 mg and 300 mg, respectively. 72-hour ambulatory ECG monitoring and exercise testing were performed 2 weeks after the dosage increase. Both groups were given a placebo pill on the third day of ECG monitoring to simulate a missed dose, with exercise testing performed again thereafter. Atenolol, 50 mg once a day, was then added to patients in the amlodipine group and isosorbide 5-mononitrate, 50 mg once a day, was added to patients in the diltiazem group. After 2 weeks of this combined treatment, the dosages of atenolol and isosorbide were each increased to 100 mg daily. At 14 weeks, (total 6 weeks combined treatment) patients underwent 72-hour ambulatory ECG monitoring and exercise testing, with a placebo pill again given for the last 24 hours.
Results	Age, gender, angina history, incidence of previous MI or revascularization, heart rate, or BP were not significantly different between the 2 groups. Many of the patients were already being treated with aspirin and ACEIs, and use of lipid-lowering drugs was common. The primary outcome measures determined by the ECG records were: total number of ST-segment episodes, total duration of such episodes, and peak ST-segment depression, all recorded during the 48-hour monitoring period while on active drug therapy. Secondary outcome measures were: ECG records from the 24-hour off-medication period, exercise test results, and daily angina diary data. Ischemic events at baseline were similar between the 2 groups. Among the primary outcome measures, there was a significant reduction in transient ST-segment depression events in both groups when compared with baseline, and there was no significant difference between the 2 groups. During the medication-free period, ischemic suppression was maintained in the amlodipine group; patients in the diltiazem group showed a significantly higher number ($p<0.0001$), duration ($p=0.0002$), and peak ST depression ($p<0.0001$) of ischemic episodes than patients in the amlodipine group. Outcome measures of ischemia determined by ECG were reduced further with the addition of atenolol to amlodipine ($p<0.0001$) for number, duration, and peak ST depression of ischemic episodes. The combination of isosorbide 5-mononitrate and diltiazem resulted in a

nonsignificant reduction in these measures. During the drug holiday, the amlodipine/atenolol group showed less ischemia than the diltiazem/isosorbide 5-mononitrate group, demonstrated by fewer episodes of ST segment depression (p=0.02) and peak ST segment depression (p=0.02). The atenolol/amlodipine combination resulted in a significant reduction in ischemia in the 24-hour drug holiday period (p<0.001). However, the addition of isosorbide to diltiazem resulted in only a small benefit vs monotherapy. There was significant improvement in ischemia during exercise testing for both amlodipine and diltiazem (time to 1 mm ST depression, amlodipine [477 seconds] vs baseline [430 seconds] and diltiazem [477 seconds] vs baseline [428 seconds]; p<0.01 for both). However, diltiazem was much less effective during the medication-free period; (474 seconds for amlodipine vs 443 seconds for diltiazem; p=0.03). During active therapy, the amlodipine/atenolol group showed a significantly increased total exercise time, time to angina onset, and 1 mm ST-segment depression vs the diltiazem/isosorbide group (time to 1mm ST-segment depression 520 seconds on amlodipine/atenolol vs 478 seconds on diltiazem/isosorbide; p<0.05). The drug-free day produced the same results (502 seconds vs 434 seconds; p<0.002). Both monotherapies were highly effective in reducing angina attacks and nitroglycerin consumption (p<0.0001), and combination therapy was more effective than monotherapy in reducing both of these (p<0.0001). Frequently reported adverse effects were edema (12.5% in the amlodipine group, 4.1% in diltiazem), and headache (7.0% and 20.5%, respectively).

Concl.   Amlodipine and diltiazem are effective in reducing ischemic episodes when used as monotherapy. The addition of atenolol and isosorbide 5-mononitrate, respectively, further augments this effect. Amlodipine, alone or in combination therapy, is more likely than diltiazem to be beneficial in patients who miss doses, or dose irregularly.

EMIT

European Mivazerol Trial

Title	Effect of mivazerol on perioperative cardiac complications during noncardiac surgery in patients with coronary heart disease.
Authors	Oliver MF, Goldman L, Julian DG, et al.
Reference	Anesthesiology 1999; 99:951-961.
Disease	Coronary heart disease.
Purpose	To determine whether mivazerol (has alpha2 agonist properties that decreases post ganglionic noradrenaline availability and sympathetic output) reduced cardiac events in patients with known coronary heart disease or patients at risk for coronary heart disease undergoing noncardiac surgery.
Design	Double-blind, randomized, placebo-controlled, multicenter.
Patients	1897 patients with known coronary artery disease undergoing vascular surgery (48%), nonvascular thoracic or abdominal surgery (32%), or orthopedic surgery (20%).
Follow-up	30 days.
Regimen	Saline or mivazerol given as an infusion starting 20 minutes prior to induction of anesthesia and for 72 hours postoperatively.
Results	The primary end point was the incidence of acute myocardial infarction or death during the intra and postoperative hospitalization period (up to 30 days post surgery). In the total cohort of 1897 patients, myocardial infarction and/or death occurred in 100 (10.6%) of placebo patients and in 91 (9.5%) of mivazerol patients (p=NS). However, in a subgroup of 904 patients with known coronary heart disease who had vascular surgery there were fewer myocardial infarctions and/or deaths in the mivazerol group (44; 9.7%) vs the placebo group (64; 14.2%; risk ratio = 0.67; 95% CI=0.45-0.98; p=0.039). All cause death in coronary patients undergoing vascular surgery was also lower in the mivazerol group (8; 1.8%) vs the placebo group (20; 4.4%; risk ratio=0.37; 95% CI=0.16-0.82; p=0.014).

Concl.   Mivazerol did not reduce overall rate of myocardial infarction and death in patients with coronary disease undergoing non-cardiac surgery, but may protect those patients with coronary disease who have vascular surgery.

FIRST

FGF Initiating Revascularization Trial

Title	Pharmacological treatment of coronary artery disease with recombinant fibroblast growth factor-2. Double-blind, randomized, controlled clinical trial.
Authors	Simons M, Annex BH, Laham RJ, et al.
Reference	Circulation 2002;105:788-793.
Disease	Coronary artery disease (CAD).
Purpose	To evaluate the safety and efficacy of intracoronary administration of fibroblast growth factor (FGF)-2 in patients with CAD.
Design	Randomized, double-blind, placebo-controlled, multicenter.
Patients	337 patients with advanced CAD who were suboptimal candidates for coronary artery bypass graft surgery or standard percutaneous coronary intervention.
Follow-up	180 days.
Regimen	Patients received a single intracoronary infusion of fibroblast growth factor-2 (rFGF-2) at 0.3, 3, or 30 mg/kg vs placebo.
Add'l Tx	Heparin.
Results	Primary end point was change in exercise tolerance test duration from baseline to 90-day follow-up. At 90 days exercise tolerance was increased in all groups and did not differ between placebo and FGF-treatment. rFGF-2 therapy was not superior at exercise testing at either 90 or 180 days. rFGF-2 therapy was not superior at exercise testing at either 90 or 180 days. rFGF-2 did decrease anginal frequency score as determined by the Seattle Angina Questionnaire (p=0.035) and a physical component summary scale of the Medical Outcomes Study Short Form 36 (p=0.033). However these differences were not significant by 180 days as there was continued improvement in angina in the placebo group. Hypotension occurred more frequently in the 30 mg/kg rFGF-2 group, but other adverse events were similar across groups. Nuclear perfusion imaging showed no difference in rest or stress perfusion between groups.

Concl.   Intracoronary infusion of rFGF-2 showed a trend toward improved symptoms of angina at day 90 but not day 180 and did not improve exercise tolerance nor improve myocardial perfusion.

IONA

Impact of Nicorandil in Angina

Title	Effect of nicorandil on coronary events in patients with stable angina: the Impact of Nicorandil in Angina (IONA) randomised trial.
Authors	The IONA Study Group.
Reference	Lancet 2002;359:1269-1275.
Disease	Stable angina.
Purpose	To assess the cardioprotective effects of nicorandil, an adenosine triphosphate-sensitive potassium channel opener, in patients with stable angina.
Design	Randomized, double-blind, placebo-controlled, multicenter.
Patients	5126 patients with established coronary artery disease (history of myocardial infarction, revascularization, documented by coronary angiography, or positive exercise test with high-risk features), stable angina on optimal medical therapy (as determined by the investigator) (men >45 years old, women >55 years old). Patients with unstable angina or sulphonylurea treatment were excluded.
Follow-up	1-3 years (mean 1.6±0.5 years).
Regimen	Randomized to nicorandil (10 mg bid for 2 weeks and then 20 mg bid) (n=2565) or placebo (n=2561).
Add'l Tx	All other antianginal medications were permitted. Sulphonylurea agents were prohibited.

Results	Coronary heart disease mortality was 2.3% with nicorandil and 2.9% with placebo. Nonfatal myocardial infarction occurred in 2.1% in the nicorandil and in 2.8% in the placebo. Unstable angina occurred in 2.1% and 2.9%, respectively, and stroke or transient ischemic attack in 1.4% and 1.6%, respectively. The primary combined end point of coronary heart disease mortality, myocardial infarction, or hospital admission for cardiac chest pain occurred in 13.1% in the nicorandil group vs 15.5% in the placebo group (hazard ratio [HR] 0.83; 95% CI=0.72-0.97; p=0.014). Coronary heart disease mortality or myocardial infarction occurred in 4.2% vs 5.2%, respectively (HR 0.79; 95% CI=0.61-1.02; p=0.068). Coronary heart disease mortality, myocardial infarction, or unstable angina occurred in 6.1% with nicorandil vs 7.6% with placebo (HR 0.79; 95% CI=0.64-0.98; p=0.028). Cardiovascular events occurred in 14.7% and 17.0%, respectively (HR 0.86; 95% CI=0.75-0.98; p=0.027). All-cause mortality was 4.3% and 5.0%, respectively (HR 0.85; 95% CI=0.66-1.10; p=0.222).
Concl.	Nicorandil was effective in reducing the rates of the combined end point of coronary heart disease mortality, myocardial infarction, or admission for chest pain and the secondary end point of coronary heart disease mortality, myocardial infarction, or unstable angina, as well as the rates of cardiovascular events in patients with stable angina.

MUST-EECP

Multicenter Study of Enhanced External Counterpulsation

Title	The multicenter study of enhanced external counterpulsation (MUST-EECP): Effect of EECP on exercise induced myocardial ischemia and anginal episodes.
Authors	Arora RR, Chou TM, Jain D, et al.
Reference	J Am Coll Cardiol 1999;33:1833-1840.
Disease	Coronary artery disease; stable angina pectoris.
Purpose	To determine the safety and efficacy of enhanced external counterpulsation.
Design	Randomized, placebo (sham) controlled, multicenter.
Patients	139 patients with chronic stable angina. Patients of I-III Canadian Cardiovascular Society Classification of angina were eligible with documented CAD and positive exercise tolerance test.
Follow-up	4-7 weeks.
Regimen	Enhanced external counterpulsation (35 hours) or sham over 4-7 weeks. Cuffs were wrapped around the patient's legs. The cuffs were inflated with compressed air in sequence synchronized with the cardiac cycle. The technique increases retrograde aortic blood flow during diastole and decreases vascular impedance.
Add'l Tx	Nitrates, aspirin, other antianginal agents.

Results   Primary end point was exercise duration and time to develop-
             ment of ≥1 mm ST segment depression. In the active coun-
             terpulsation group exercise duration increased from 426±20
             seconds at baseline to 470±20 seconds post-treatment. In the
             sham group exercise duration was 432±22 seconds at baseline
             and increased to 464±22 seconds post treatment (p=NS between
             groups). Change in time to ≥1 mm ST segment depression
             increased in the active counterpulsation group by 37±11 seconds
             whereas it decreased in the sham group (-4±12 sec; p=0.01). In
             patients who finished ≥34 sessions of active counterpulsation,
             angina counts (self reported episodes of angina per 24 hours)
             were 0.72±0.14 at baseline and 0.57±0.38 post treatment; in
             the sham group, angina counts were 0.77±0.14 at baseline and
             0.76±0.22 post treatment. Difference between groups in change
             in angina counts was significant (p<0.035). There was a nonsig-
             nificant trend toward a reduction in sublingual nitroglycerin use
             in treated patients.

Concl.   Enhanced external counterpulsation decreased angina frequen-
             cy and improved time to exercise induced ischemia.

PATCH

Program to Assess Alternative Treatment Strategies to Achieve Cardiac Health

Title	Chelation therapy for ischemic heart disease. A randomized controlled trial.
Authors	Knudtson ML, Wyse DG, Galbraith PD, et al.
Reference	JAMA 2002;287:481-486.
Disease	Coronary artery disease (CAD), stable angina.
Purpose	To determine whether chelation therapy with EDTA has a beneficial effect on exercise tolerance and quality of life in patients with stable CAD.
Design	Randomized, double-blind, placebo-controlled, multicenter.
Patients	84 patients with CAD proven by angiography or documented myocardial infarction and stable angina on optimal medical therapy. Patients had to demonstrate at least 1 mm ST depression on an exercise treadmill test.
Follow-up	27 weeks exercise test; 1-year follow-up of clinical events.
Regimen	Weight adjusted (40 mg/kg) EDTA chelation therapy (n=41) vs placebo (n=43). Treatment was 3 hours per session, twice weekly for 15 weeks; once a month for additional 3 months.
Add'l Tx	Multivitamin.

Results   Primary end point was change in time to reach at least 1 mm of ST-segment depression at 27-week exercise test. Other end point was quality of life questionnaires. At baseline, mean exercise time on treadmill to ischemic ST changes were 572 seconds in the placebo group and 589 in the chelation group. At 27 weeks time to ischemia had increased compared to baseline in both placebo groups (54 seconds) and chelation group (63 seconds) with no significant difference between groups. Absolute time to ischemia was 626 seconds in the placebo group vs 652 in the chelation group. There was no difference in increase in Vo2 max between the 2 groups. There were modest increases in quality-of-life scores in both the placebo and chelation groups with no significant differences between groups. Over the course of a year, 1 patient in the placebo group and 1 patient in the chelation group suffered an acute myocardial infarction. 6 patients in the placebo group and 9 in the chelation group were admitted at least once for worsening angina. 1 patient in the chelation group was withdrawn secondary to transient increase in serum creatinine.

Concl.   There was no evidence supporting a beneficial effect of chelation therapy in patients with stable CAD.

PISA

Persantin in Stable Angina

Title	Dipyridamole in chronic stable angina pectoris. A randomized, double-blind, placebo-controlled, parallel group study.
Authors	Picano E, on behalf of the PISA study group.
Reference	Eur Heart J 2001;22:1785-1793.
Disease	Coronary artery disease, stable angina pectoris.
Purpose	To evaluate the efficacy and safety of dipyridamole in patients with stable chronic angina pectoris.
Design	Randomized, placebo-controlled, double-blind, multicenter.
Patients	400 patients, 35-78 years old, with ≥3 month history of stable effort induced angina pectoris. Only patients with interpretable electrocardiographic exercise stress test and ST depression during exercise were included.
Follow-up	28 weeks with repeated exercise tests.
Regimen	After a 2-week eligibility phase, patients were randomized to placebo (n=202) or dipyridamole 200 mg bid (n=198) in addition to the patients' conventional antianginal medications for 24 weeks. Thereafter, the conventional antianginal medications were withdrawn and the patients continued with the study medication for an additional 4 weeks.
Add'l Tx	During the second phase, all antianginal medications were permitted, including calcium channel blockers, β-blockers, and nitrates. During the third phase only short-acting nitrates were permitted.

Results	134 patients in the dipyridamole and 162 in the placebo group completed the add-on phase. Adverse events leading to withdrawal from the study occurred in 41 vs 24 patients in the dipyridamole and placebo groups, respectively (p=0.063). Serious adverse events occurred in 7.6% and 6.0% of the patients, respectively (p>0.05). Only 40 patients entered the third phase of the study. Overall, adverse events occurred in 70.2% of the patients in the dipyridamole group vs 62.7% in the placebo group (p>0.05). Headache leading to discontinuation of drug therapy occurred in 9.1% vs 0%, respectively (p<0.001). The percentages of patients reporting chest pain and angina pectoris were comparable between groups. The total treadmill exercise time change from baseline was comparable between the dipyridamole and placebo group at week 8, 24, and 28. At week 8, the time to >0.1 mV ST depression was 21 seconds longer in the dipyridamole group than in the placebo group (p=0.024). However, at week 24, the time to first anginal pain was 13 seconds longer in the placebo than the dipyridamole group (p=0.040). Otherwise, the exercise parameters were comparable between the groups.
Concl.	Oral dipyridamole, added to conventional antianginal medications, was safe and well tolerated. However, it was not associated with augmentation of exercise capacity.

QUO VADIS

Quinapril on Vascular ACE and Determinants of Ischemia

Title	Effects of quinapril on clinical outcome after coronary artery bypass grafting (The QUO VADIS Study).
Authors	Oosterga M, Voors AA, Pinto YM, et al.
Reference	Am J Cardiology 2000;87:542-546.
Disease	Coronary artery disease.
Purpose	To determine the effect of 1-year therapy with quinapril on ischemia during exercise testing and 48-hour ambulatory ECG monitoring as well as clinical ischemic events in patients that had CABG.
Design	Randomized, double-blind, placebo-controlled.
Patients	149 coronary artery disease patients scheduled for elective CABG.
Follow-up	1 year.
Regimen	Quinapril (40 mg/d) on placebo begun 4 weeks prior to surgery and then for 1 year.
Add'l Tx	Other ACE inhibitors not allowed. Diuretics, antiarrhythmics, digitalis, tricyclic antidepressants not allowed.
Results	Symptom—limited bicycle exercise test obtained at randomization and 1 year after CABG. Total exercise time increased in both groups after 1 year (+79 seconds for placebo and +72 seconds for quinapril; p=NS). All patients had ischemic ST change on exercise at baseline. At 1 year 29% in the placebo group and 37% in quinapril group demonstrated ST change during exercise (p=NS). At 1 year ambulatory ECG monitoring revealed equal number of patients experiencing ≥1 ischemic episode. Clinical ischemic events included death, repeat CABG, PCI, MI, recurrent angina, ischemic stroke or transient ischemic attack. At 1 year 15% of placebo patients experienced a clinical event vs 4% of quinapril patients (hazard ratio 0.23; 95% CI=0.067-0.87; p=0.02).

Concl.   Following CABG, chronic therapy with quinapril reduced clinical ischemic events but did not change ischemia with exercise
testing or ischemia detected on ambulatory ECG monitoring.

TIME

Trial of Invasive vs Medical Therapy in Elderly Patients

Title	Trial of invasive vs medical therapy in elderly patients with chronic symptomatic coronary-artery disease (TIME): a randomised trial.
Authors	The TIME Investigators.
Reference	Lancet 2001;358:951-957.
Disease	Coronary artery disease, stable angina.
Purpose	To compare outcome of patients ≥75 years old (average 80.0±3.7 years) with stable angina pectoris randomized to either an invasive strategy of coronary angiography and revascularization or to a conservative strategy of optimizing medical therapy.
Design	Randomized, open-label, multicenter.
Patients	305 patients, ≥75 years old, with stable angina pectoris despite ≥2 antianginal drugs. Patients with acute myocardial infarction within the preceding 10 days, concomitant valvular or other heart disease, congestive heart failure, life-limiting comorbid disease, severe renal failure, unwillingness to undergo revascularization, or inability to increase medical therapy were excluded.
Follow-up	6 months.
Regimen	Patients were randomized to optimization of medical therapy (n=150) or an invasive strategy (n=155).

Results   Of 305 patients initially randomized, 3 were excluded by the Critical Event Committee. 147 (96%) of the 153 patients in the invasive group underwent coronary angiography and 109 (74%) underwent revascularization. The remaining 38 (26%) were treated medically because they could not be revascularized, refused revascularization, or did not have significant coronary artery disease. In the conservative group, antianginal medication was increased by a mean of 0.8 ± 0.6 drugs per patient, with additional increases in drug dosages in 55% of the patients (n=81). Angina severity decreased, and all indices of quality of life improved significantly during follow-up in both groups. However, the improvements in angina severity and health status were greater in patients in the invasive strategy than in the conservative strategy. Angina pectoris class decreased by 2.0 ± 1.3 in the invasive group vs only 1.6 ± 1.4 in the conservative group (p=0.01). The general health score (Medical Outcomes Study Short Form 36) increased by 11.4 ± 20.0 and 3.8 ± 18.7, respectively (p= 0.008). Major adverse cardiac events (death, documented nonfatal myocardial infarction, and hospital admission for increasing or unstable angina) occurred in 19% of the patients in the invasive group vs 49% in the conservative group (p<0.0001). However, death occurred in 8.5% vs 4.1%, respectively (p=0.15). Patients in the invasive group had a trend toward less nonfatal myocardial infarction (7.8% vs 11.5%; p=0.46), and significantly less hospitalization for acute coronary syndromes, both without (3.3% vs 12.2%; p=0.006) and with (6.5% vs 37.2%; p<0.001) revascularization.

Concl.   A strategy of early coronary angiography and revascularization resulted in reduction of the risk for major adverse cardiac events and improvement in quality of life, compared to a conservative strategy of optimization of medical therapy in elderly patients with stable angina pectoris. However, the invasive strategy was associated with a trend toward an increased mortality.

TRIMPOL II

Trimetazidine in Poland II

Title	Combination treatment in stable effort angina using trimeta-zidine and metoprolol. Results of a randomized, double-blind, multicentre study (TRIMPOL II).
Authors	Szwed H, Sadowski Z, Elikowski W, et al.
Reference	Eur Heart J 2001;22:2267-2274.
Disease	Coronary artery disease; stable angina pectoris.
Purpose	To study the safety and efficacy of trimetazidine, an inhibitor of long-chain 3-ketoacyl coenzyme A thiolase that reduces fatty acid metabolism and increases myocardial glucose oxidation, in patients with stable angina pectoris.
Design	Randomized, double-blind, placebo-controlled, multicenter.
Patients	426 patients, 18-70 years old, with stable angina pectoris for ≥3 months and documented coronary artery disease. Patients with recent myocardial infarction or unstable angina, cardiac surgery, percutaneous coronary intervention (PCI), stroke or transient ischemic attack in the previous 6 months were excluded. In addition, patients with Prinzmetal angina, blood pressure >160/95 mm Hg; New York Heart Association class III or IV heart failure, inability to perform exercise test, sig-nificant cardiac abnormalities, baseline ECG abnormalities, severe renal failure or hepatic disease, and drug or alcohol abuse were not included.
Follow-up	12 weeks with clinical follow-up and repeated exercise tests (ini-tial assessment, baseline, and after 4 and 12 weeks of therapy).
Regimen	After 1 week on metoprolol 50 mg bid, patients were random-ized to placebo or trimetazidine 20 mg tid.
Add'l Tx	All patients received metoprolol 50 mg bid. Amiodarone, guani-dine, monoamine oxidase inhibitors, calcium channel blockers, long-acting nitrates, molsidomine, other β-blockers, and digi-talis were prohibited.

Results	347 patients (179 trimetazidine and 168 placebo) completed the study. After 12 weeks of treatment, time to 1 mm ST depression was 381±148 seconds in the placebo group and 427±134 seconds in the trimetazidine group (p<0.001). Total exercise time was 458±134 seconds vs 485±122 seconds, respectively (p<0.05). Time to onset of angina was 423±150 seconds vs 465±124 seconds, respectively (p<0.01). The mean weekly angina attacks were significantly lower in the trimetazidine treated patients (2.1±2.4 vs 3.3±4.2; p<0.01). There was no evidence of development of tolerance to trimetazidine. There were a total of 4 adverse events in each group. These adverse events were minor. In the trimetazidine group the adverse events were headache in 1 patient, nausea in 1 patient, epigastric pain in 1 patient and other gastrointestinal disorders in 1 patient.
Concl.	The combination of trimetazidine + metoprolol resulted in greater improvement in exercise performance and severity of angina than metoprolol alone in patients with stable effort induced angina. Trimetazidine was safe and well tolerated.

AGENT-2

Angiogenic Gene Therapy

Title	A randomized, double-blind, placebo-controlled trial of Ad5FGF-4 gene therapy and its effect on myocardial perfusion in patients with stable angina.
Authors	Grines CL, Watkins MW, Mahmarian JJ, et al.
Reference	J Am Coll Cardiol 2003;42:1339-1347.
Disease	Stable angina pectoris.
Purpose	To determine whether intracoronary administration of the adenoviral gene for fibroblast growth factor (Ad5FGF-4) can improve myocardial perfusion compared with placebo.
Design	Multicenter, randomized, double-blind, placebo-controlled trial.
Patients	52 patients with stable angina and reversible ischemia comprising >90% of the left ventricle on single photon emission computed tomography.
Follow-up	8 weeks.
Regimen	Gene therapy (n=35) or placebo (n=17).
Results	Overall, the mean total perfusion defect size at baseline was 32.4% of the left ventricle, with 20% reversible ischemia and 12.5% scar. At 8 weeks, injection of Ad5FGF-4 caused a significant reduction in ischemic defect size (4.2% absolute, 21% relative; p<0.001). Placebo-treated patients showed no improvement. The change in reversible perfusion defect size between Ad5FGF-4 and placebo was not significant (4.2% vs 1.6%). When a single outlier was excluded, the difference became significant (4.2% vs 0.8%; p<0.05). Gene therapy was well tolerated. In the treated group, 30% of patients were free of angina vs 13% of the placebo group. In the treated group, 43% of the patients were not taking nitroglycerin 8 weeks after treatment, compared with 17% of the placebo group.

Concl.	AGENT-2 is the first randomized, placebo-controlled trial to test the effect of gene therapy on myocardial perfusion in humans. The findings of a significant reduction in defect size after treatment with Ad5FGF-4, the trend toward a greater reduction than with placebo, and significantly fewer patients with worsening of ischemic defect size suggest efficacy of the treatment. Larger trials exploring the effect of AD5FGF-4 on clinical outcomes are warranted.

CARISA

Combination Assessment of Ranolazine in Stable Angina

Title	Effects of ranolazine with atenolol, amlodipine, or diltiazem on exercise tolerance and angina frequency in patients with severe chronic angina: a randomized controlled trial.
Authors	Chaitman BR, Pepine CJ, Parker JO, et al.
Reference	JAMA 2004;291:309-316.
Disease	Angina, coronary artery disease.
Purpose	To determine whether ranolazine improves total exercise time in patients with chronic angina and ischemia at low workloads despite standard doses of atenolol, amlodipine, or diltiazem; and to determine times to angina onset and to myocardial ischemia, effect on angina attacks and nitroglycerin use, and effect on long-term survival.
Design	Randomized, 3-group, parallel, double-blind, placebo-controlled trial.
Patients	823 adults with symptomatic chronic angina.
Follow-up	2 years.
Regimen	Placebo or 750 mg or 1000 mg of ranolazine bid.

Results   Main outcome measures were change in exercise duration, time
to onset of angina, time to onset of ischemia, nitroglycerin
use, and number of angina attacks. Trough exercise duration
increased by 115.6 seconds in both ranolazine groups vs 91.7
seconds in the placebo group (p=0.01). Times to angina and
ECG ischemia also increased in the ranolazine groups, at peak
more than at trough. The increases did not depend on changes
in BP, heart rate, or background antianginal therapy and persisted throughout 12 weeks. Patients receiving ranolazine had
fewer angina attacks and used less nitroglycerin compared with
placebo (p<0.02). Survival of 750 patients taking ranolazine
during the trial or the associated long-term open-label study
was 98.4% in the first year and 95.9% in the second year. These
survival rates are superior to those previously reported (4%-
13%) in patients with severe chronic angina. Adverse events
were reported in 26.4% of patients receiving placebo, 31.2%
of patients receiving ranolazine 750 mg, and 32.7% receiving
ranolazine 1000 mg. The most common were constipation, diz-
ziness, nausea, and asthenia.

Concl.   Twice-daily ranolazine increased exercise capacity and provided additional antianginal relief in patients with severe chronic
angina taking standard doses of atenolol, amlodipine, or diltiazem, without adverse effects on survival over 1-2 years of
therapy. This therapy may be useful in patients who cannot
tolerate the initiation or upward titration of currently available antianginal drugs because of their depressive effects on
BP and heart rate.

IEPR

International EECP Patient Registry

Title	Two-year outcomes after enhanced external counterpulsation for stable angina pectoris (from the International EECP Patient Registry [IEPR]).
Authors	Michaels AD, Linnemeier G, Soran O, et al.
Reference	Am J Cardiol 2004;93:461-464.
Disease	Stable angina pectoris.
Purpose	To assess the long-term efficacy of enhanced external counterpulsation in improving quality of life and angina score in patients with chronic stable angina pectoris.
Design	Registry, multicenter.
Patients	1097 patients (mean age 65.8±10.9 years) with chronic stable angina pectoris who had ≥1 hour of enhanced external counterpulsation treatment.
Follow-up	2 years.
Regimen	Enhanced external counterpulsation.

Results   82% of the patients completed the 35-hour course of enhanced external counterpulsation (EECP). 10% discontinued EECP because of clinical events, and 8% of the patients did not want to continue the course. Mortality was 0.3% during EECP and 8.5% during the 2-year follow-up. MI occurred in 0.9% of the patients during EECP and in 8.9% during the follow-up. 2-year event-free survival was 40.8%. Immediately after the EECP course there was a significant decrease in the Canadian Cardiovascular Society Classification (CCSC) ($p < 0.001$). 73% of the patients reported improvement in angina class ≥ 1, 26% had no change, and 1% had worsening in angina class. The average number of anginal episodes per week decreased by 7.8 ± 12.3; $p < 0.001$. In addition, 53.2% of the patients reported an improvement in their quality of life immediately after the EECP course, and 57.8% reported that their satisfaction improved. At the end of the 2-year follow-up, 74.9% of the patients had an improvement in their CCSC compared to baseline and 46.8% reported that their quality of life improved. Nitroglycerin therapy decreased from 10.3 ± 13.5 times/wk at baseline to 8.1 ± 13.0 at 2 years ($p < 0.01$). In addition, less patients at follow-up were taking aspirin or antiplatelet agents ($p < 0.001$).

Concl.   This nonrandomized trial showed an improvement in angina score and quality of life among patients with stable angina treated with EECP. The effect was sustained for 2 years after completing the EECP course.

JMIC-M

Japan Multicenter Investigation for Cardiovascular Diseases-Mochida

Title	Effect of trapidil on cardiovascular events in patients with coronary artery disease (results from the Japan Multicenter Investigation for Cardiovascular Diseases-Mochida [JMIC-M]).
Authors	Hirayama A, Kodama K, Yui Y, et al.
Reference	Am J Cardiol 2003;92:789-793.
Disease	Coronary artery disease.
Purpose	To assess whether trapidil is effective in reducing morbidity and mortality in patients with coronary artery disease.
Design	Randomized, open-label, multicenter.
Patients	1748 patients, ≤70 years old, with angiographic evidence of coronary artery disease. Only patients who had ≥1 coronary artery without any coronary intervention and no plan to undergo revascularization were included. Patients with recent acute coronary syndrome or myocardial infarction, bleeding disorders, and severe renal or hepatic insufficiency were excluded.
Follow-up	3 years.
Regimen	Randomization to trapidil 300 mg/d (n=875) or control (n=873).
Add'l Tx	All other medications were permitted.

Results 5 patients did not complete the study. More patients in the control group (56%) than in the trapidil group (48%) received antiplatelet drugs (p=0.001). Cardiovascular events occurred in 11.1% of the patients in the trapidil group and in 14.9% in the control group (relative risk [RR] 0.75; 95% CI=0.58-0.98; p=0.036). CAD mortality was 0.3% and 1.1%, respectively (RR 0.31; 95% CI=0.09-1.12; p=0.059). Nonfatal MI occurred in 2% in each group. 7.3% of the patients in the trapidil group vs 9.9% in the control group were admitted for angina (RR 0.76; 95% CI=0.55-1.04; p=0.088). 5.8% and 8.3% of the patients in the trapidil and control groups, respectively, underwent revascularization (RR 0.72; 95% CI=0.47-1.11; p=0.133). Less patients in the trapidil group had a stroke (0.8% vs 2.1%; RR 0.40; 95% CI=0.17-0.95; p=0.032). Overall, cardiac events occurred in 10.6% in the trapidil group vs 16.4% in the control group (RR 0.65; 95% CI=0.44-0.94; p=0.023). Subgroup analysis showed that trapidil was more beneficial in women, patients ≥60 years, and in those with previous MI. Trapidil did not show significant benefit in patients with a history of PCI or those who did not receive antiplatelet therapy. Trapidil was safe and adverse effects were mild and transient.

Concl. Long-term administration of trapidil reduced the incidence of cardiovascular events in patients with CAD.

MARISA

Monotherapy Assessment of Ranolazine in Stable Angina

Title	Anti-ischemic effects and long-term survival during ranolazine monotherapy in patients with chronic severe angina.
Authors	Chaitman BR, Skettino SL, Parker JO, et al.
Reference	J Am Coll Cardiol 2004;43:1375-1382.
Disease	Coronary artery disease.
Purpose	To determine the dose-response relationship of ranolazine, an antianginal compound believed to act by inhibiting fatty acid oxidation, shifting metabolism toward carbohydrate oxidation, and increasing the efficiency of oxygen use, on symptom-limited exercise duration.
Design	Randomized, double-blind, 4-period crossover study.
Patients	191 patients with angina-limited exercise.
Follow-up	1 week.
Regimen	Sustained-release ranolazine 500, 1000, or 1500 mg or placebo, each administered bid for 1 week.
Results	Exercise duration at trough increased with ranolazine 500, 1000, and 1500 mg bid by 94, 103, and 116 seconds, respectively, vs a 70-second increase with placebo (p<0.005). There were dose-related increases in exercise duration at peak and in times to 1 mm of ST-segment depression at trough and peak and to angina at trough and peak (p<0.005). The effects on heart rate and BP were minor. The 1-year survival rate, combining data from the MARISA trial and its open-label follow-on study, was 96.3%±1.7%. Fewer than 8% of patients discontinued ranolazine because of adverse effects; three fourths of these withdrawals were at the 1500-mg dose. There were dose-related complaints of dizziness, nausea, asthenia, and constipation.

Concl. In patients with chronic stable angina, ranolazine was well tolerated and increased exercise performance at all doses studied, without clinically important hemodynamic effects. 1-year survival was what would be expected in this high-risk population. Ranolazine represents a novel metabolic approach to treating chronic angina.

QUASAR

The Quinapril Anti-Ischemia and Symptoms of Angina Reduction Trial

Title	Effects of angiotensinconverting enzyme inhibition on transient ischemia: the Quinapril Anti-Ischemia and Symptoms of Angina Reduction (QUASAR) trial.
Authors	Pepine CJ, Rouleau J-L, Annis K, et al.
Reference	J Am Coll Cardiol 2003;42:2049-2059.
Disease	Coronary artery disease.
Purpose	To determine whether angiotensin-converting enzyme inhibition prevents exertional and spontaneous transient myocardial ischemia in patients with coronary artery disease.
Design	Randomized, doubleblind, placebo-controlled, multicenter.
Patients	336 coronary artery disease patients with stable angina. Coronary artery disease documented by: ≥60% diameter stenosis of 1 or more major coronary arteries, Q-wave myocardial infarction, abnormal stress test. Patients had to then have an abnormal exercise treadmill test limited by angina and accompanied by an ischemic ST-segment response within 8 minutes of exercise. Patients could not have uncontrolled hypertension, left ventricular dysfunction, or recent myocardial infarction.
Follow-up	Up to 20 weeks.
Regimen	There were 3 study periods. There was a 2-4 week, single-blinded, placebobaseline period. Then there was an 8-week double-blinded period in which patients were randomized to placebo (group 1; n=159), or quinapril 40 mg/d (group 2; n=177) for 8 weeks. They then entered a third phase in which group 1 patients received 80 mg/d of quinapril and group 2 continued the 40 mg/d dose. Patients underwent an exercise treadmill test at the end of the baseline period (single-blind placebo), at the end of the second phase (8 weeks of double-blind treatment) and at the end of the third phase (16 weeks). 48-hour ambulatory electrocardiogram and angina questionnaire were filled out at 4, 8, and 16 weeks.

Add'l Tx	Aspirin or other antiplatelet agents, nitrates, calcium blockers, β-blockers.
Results	At the end of phase 2 there was no difference in time to ST-segment depression in the placebo group (4.7±0.2) vs the quinapril 40-mg dose (4.8±0.2 minutes) on exercise testing. Time to angina (6.1±0.2 minutes vs 6.6±0.2 minutes) was the same in the placebo vs the quinapril 40-mg dose. Total exercise time was 6.4±0.2 minutes and 6.7±0.2 minutes in the placebo vs quinapril group respectively. There was no difference between the 80 vs 40 mg dose of quinapril in exercise parameters at 16 weeks and these did not appear better than placebo at 8 weeks. By ambulatory monitoring, the number of ischemic episodes per 24 hours was 1.3±2.3 at the end of the second phase in the placebo group vs 0.9±1.3 in the quinapril 40 mg group (p=NS). The number of patients with ischemia was 62 in the placebo group vs 73 in the quinapril group. With 80 mg of quinapril, the number of ischemic episodes was 0.9±1.5 and number with ischemia was 58. There were no differences in the angina questionnaire between groups.
Concl.	Short-term therapy with ACE inhibition in CAD patients without hypertension, LV dysfunction, or acute MI did not significantly affect transient spontaneously induced or exerciseinduced myocardial ischemia.

RITA-2

Second Randomized Intervention Treatment of Angina

Title	Seven-year outcome in the RITA-2 trial: coronary angioplasty vs medical therapy.
Authors	Henderson RA, Pocock SJ, Clayton TC, et al.
Reference	J Am Coll Cardiol 2003;42:1161-1170.
Disease	Stable angina pectoris.
Purpose	To compare the long-term consequences of percutaneous transluminal coronary angioplasty (PTCA) and continued medical treatment.
Design	International, multicenter, randomized trial.
Patients	1018 patients considered suitable for either PTCA or conservative (medical) care.
Follow-up	Median 7 years.
Regimen	PTCA (n=504) or medical management (n=514).
Results	The rate of death or MI, the primary trial end point, was 14.5% (n=73) in the PTCA patients and 12.3% (n=63) in the medical patients (95% CI=-2% to 6.4%; p=0.21). 43 patients died in each group; 41% were cardiac-related. 12.7% of PTCA patients subsequently underwent CABG surgery, and 14.5% required additional nonrandomized PTCA. Most repeat interventions occurred within 1 year of randomization; after 2 years the repeat intervention rate was 2.3% per year. In the medically treated group, 35.4% required myocardial revascularization: 15% in the first year and 3.6% per year after 2 years. An initial policy of PTCA was associated with an improvement in angina and exercise times. Treatment differences narrowed over time, mainly because of coronary interventions in medical patients with severe symptoms.

Concl.   The RITA-2 trial provides the only available randomized evidence comparing the long-term results of PTCA and medical treatment in patients with angina. Initial PTCA did not reduce the risk of death or MI but did result in improved angina symptoms and exercise tolerance. Patients who are candidates for either PTCA or medical therapy can be safely managed with continued medical therapy; PTCA may be appropriate if symptoms are not controlled with medical therapy.

New Pharmacological Treatment for Intermittent Claudication: Results of a Randomized, Multicenter Trial

Title	A new pharmacological treatment for intermittent claudication: Results of a randomized, multicenter trial.
Authors	Beebe HG, Dawson DL, Cutler BS, et al.
Reference	Arch Intern Med 1999;159:2041-2050.
Disease	Claudication, peripheral vascular disease.
Purpose	To evaluate safety and efficacy of cilostazol, an inhibitor of platelet aggregation with vasodilating effects in patients with intermittent claudication.
Design	Multicenter, randomized, double-blind, placebo-controlled.
Patients	516 men and women age ≥40 years with a history of at least 6 months of stable, intermittent claudication with reproducible walking distances on screening treadmill tests.
Follow-up	24 weeks.
Regimen	Cilostazol 100 mg or 50 mg orally twice a day.

Results	End points included exercise treadmill pain free and maximal walking distances, Doppler measured peripheral limb pressures, quality of life, and functional status questionnaires. 93% of patients had a history of smoking; more than one third were current smokers. At 24 weeks, improvement in pain free walking distance was 59% in the 100 mg cilostazol group and 48% in the 50 mg group vs 20% with placebo (p<0.001 vs 100 mg and 50 mg.) Maximal walking distance improved by 51% in the 100 mg cilostazol group, 38% in the 50 mg group, and 15% in the placebo group (p<0.001 vs both treatment groups). The arithmetic mean increase was from 129.7 m at baseline to 259 m at 24 weeks for cilostazol 100 mg and from 131.5 at baseline to 198.8 m with cilostazol 50 mg. Improvements in treadmill times were observed as early as 4 weeks. Cilostazol also was associated with improvements in quality of life and functional status (which asked various questions about pain and discomfort with physical activities). There were no differences among the 3 groups in combined cardiovascular morbidity or all cause mortality. The most common side effects were headache, loose or soft stools, diarrhea, dizziness, and palpitation.
Concl.	Cilostazol improved walking distance (both maximal and pain free) in patients with intermittent claudication.

5. Interventional Cardiology

a. Percutaneous Transluminal Coronary Angioplasty (and/or Stenting) vs Coronary Artery Bypass Graft Surgery; Off- vs On-Pump Coronary Artery Bypass Graft

Cognitive Outcome After Off-Pump and On-Pump Coronary Artery Bypass Graft Surgery. A Randomized Trial

Title	Cognitive outcome after off-pump and on-pump coronary artery bypass graft surgery. A randomized trial.
Authors	Van Dijk D, Jansen EWL, Hijman R, et al., for the Octopus Study Group.
Reference	JAMA 2002;287:1405-1412.
Disease	Coronary artery disease (patients undergoing CABG).
Purpose	To determine cognitive outcome in patients with CABG surgery on-pump vs CABG surgery off-pump.
Design	Randomized, controlled.
Patients	Patients who were scheduled for their first CABG; mean age=61; n=281.
Follow-up	3- and 12-month cognitive outcome.
Regimen	Patients randomized to off-pump surgery (n=142) without the use of cardiopulmonary bypass or on-pump (n=139) with cardiopulmonary bypass.
Add'l Tx	Use of cardiopulmonary bypass included full heparinization, IV high-dose opioids for general anesthesia. In off-pump procedure 54% of patients had thoracic epidural anesthesia plus low dose opioids.

Results   Primary outcome was cognitive outcome at 3 months; 12-month testing also performed and compared to neuropsychology tests performed 1-day prior to surgery. These standardized tests assessed motor skills, verbal memory capacity, attention, speed, and capacity of memory, visual-spatial capacity, attention, and others. Cognitive decline occurred in 21% of off-pump group vs 29% of on-pump group (relative risk [RR] 0.65; CI=0.36-1.16; p=0.15) at 3 months. Standardized change score (improvement in cognitive performance) was 0.19 in off-pump vs 0.3 in on-pump patients (p=0.03). However at 12 months cognitive decline occurred in 30.8% and 33.6% of off-pump and on-pump groups respectively (p=NS) and overall standardized change score did not differ between the 2 groups (0.19 off-pump vs 0.12 on-pump; p=0.09). There were no statistically significant differences between groups in stroke rate, all-cause mortality, or quality of life at 3 and 12 months.

Concl.   While at 3 months patients who received their first CABG without cardiopulmonary bypass had improved cognitive outcomes vs those with cardiopulmonary bypass, the effects were limited and differences disappeared by 12 months.

Octopus Study (Early Outcome)

Title	Early outcome after off-pump vs on-pump coronary bypass surgery. Results from a randomized study.
Authors	Van Dijk D, Nierich AP, Jansen EWL, for the Octopus Study Group.
Reference	Circulation 2001;104:1761-1766.
Disease	Coronary artery disease.
Purpose	To determine cardiac outcome following off-pump surgery using the Octopus device (a device that can immobilize and present all views of the beating heart) vs on-pump coronary artery bypass grafting (CABG).
Design	Randomized, multicenter.
Patients	281 patients scheduled for first CABG.
Follow-up	1 month in this analysis.
Regimen	142 patients randomized to off-pump CABG and 139 patients randomized to on-pump CABG. On pump (cardiopulmonary bypass) included priming with a crystalloid-colloid mixture and then cold crystalloid cardioplegia.
Add'l Tx	Opioids.

Results	Cardiac outcome end point was survival free of stroke, MI, or coronary re-intervention. Completeness of revascularization was deemed similar between groups and mean number of distal anastomoses were similar at 2.4 and 2.6 in the off-pump and on-pump groups, respectively. 13% of the on-pump patients required blood products vs 3% of off-pump patients ($p<0.01$). There was less release of creatine kinase-MB in the off-pump group. All-cause mortality was zero in both groups. Stroke occurred in 1 (0.7%) off-pump and 2 (1.4%) on-pump patients; MI occurred in 7 (4.9%) vs 6 (4.3%) in off and on-pump patients, respectively. PTCA was needed in 2 (1.4%) off-pump vs 0 (0%) on-pump patients. Repeat CABG was not needed in either group by 1 month. Overall survival free of cardiovascular events occurred in 93% of patients off-pump vs 94.2% on-pump (p=NS). Off-pump patients were discharged 1 day earlier than on-pump patients. 4% patients in both groups had recurrent angina.
Concl.	Off-pump CABG is safe in selected patients and at 1 month yields cardiac outcome results similar to on-pump CABG.

Title	A comparison of on-pump and off-pump coronary bypass surgery in low-risk patients.
Authors	Nathoe HN, van Dijk D, Jansen EW, et al.
Reference	New Engl J Med 2003;348:394-402.
Disease	Coronary artery disease.
Purpose	To determine cardiac outcome and cost effectiveness following off-pump surgery using the Octopus device (a device that can immobilize and present all views of the beating heart) vs on-pump coronary artery bypass grafting at 1 year after surgery.
Design	Randomized, multicenter.
Patients	281 patients with unstable angina (Braunwald class IB or IIB) with ventricular function that was normal or moderately impaired who were referred for coronary artery bypass surgery for the first time and for whom an off-pump procedure was judged to be feasible. Exclusion criteria included need for emergency or concomitant major surgery, Q-wave myocardial infarction in the past 6 weeks, or poor left ventricular function.
Follow-up	1 year.
Regimen	139 patients were assigned to on-pump surgery and 142 to off-pump surgery. On-pump surgery involved use of cardiopulmonary bypass and cold crystalloid cardioplegia. Off-pump surgery utilized the Octopus stabilizer, a device which allowed a target area of the heart to be immobilized enough to permit safe anastomosis. The goal of the surgeries was to achieve complete revascularization of the involved arterial segment.

Results	The primary end point was freedom from the composite of all-cause death, stroke, MI, and repeat revascularization (surgery or angioplasty). The secondary end points included freedom from angina and exercise-induced ischemia. Direct medical costs as well as follow-up costs and in-hospital costs were assessed. The health-related quality of life was evaluated using the EuroQol questionnaire and its summary score. 76% of those in the on-pump group and 84% in the off-pump group achieved complete arterial revascularization. At 1 year, 90.6% of the on-pump group and 88.0% of the off-pump group had achieved the primary end point, representing an absolute difference of 2.6% (95% CI=-4.6 to 9.8; p=0.48). There was no significant difference between the groups at 1 year in rates of cardiac and noncardiac death, fatal and nonfatal stroke, fatal or nonfatal MI, and repeat coronary revascularization. The rate of the secondary end point, freedom from angina, was 89.0% in the on-pump group and 89.3% in the off-pump group (absolute difference -0.3 %; 95% CI=-7.7 to 7.0). Exercise testing was performed in 246 patients (87.5%), and the rate of freedom from myocardial ischemia was 79.8% in the on-pump surgery group and 83.1% in the off-pump surgery group (absolute difference -3.3 %; 95% CI=-13.4 to 6.9). The exercise capacity was 9.5 metabolic equivalents (MET) in the on-pump group and 9.0 MET in the off-pump group (absolute difference=0.5 MET; 95% CI=-0.4 to 1.4). The total direct costs at 1 year were $14,908 for the on-pump group and $13,069 for the off-pump group, which was significant (p<0.01). The quality of life improved to a similar degree in both groups: the EuroQol summary scores improved in both groups from 0.65 at baseline to 0.84 3 months after the surgery (increase=0.20; 95% CI=0.17-0.23). Cost-effective ratios indicated that with 95% certainty, off-pump surgery was more cost-effective than on-pump surgery.
Concl.	In this group of low-risk patients, cardiovascular outcomes at 1 year were similar between patients who had on-pump bypass surgery vs those who had off-pump surgery. Off-pump surgery was more cost-effective.

Arterial Revascularization Therapies Study

Title	Comparison of coronary-artery bypass surgery and stenting for the treatment of multivessel disease.
Authors	Serruys PW, Unger F, Sousa JE, et al.
Reference	N Engl J Med 2001;344:1117-1124.
Disease	Coronary artery disease.
Purpose	To compare clinical outcomes and cost of coronary artery bypass surgery vs stenting in patients with multivessel CAD.
Design	Randomized, multicenter.
Patients	1205 patients with angina or silent ischemia and multivessel CAD in whom a cardiac surgeon and interventional cardiologist agreed that the same extent of revascularization could be achieved with coronary artery bypass grafting or angioplasty plus stenting.
Follow-up	1 year.
Regimen	Patients were randomized to CABG (n=605) vs angioplasty plus stenting (n=600).

Results	Primary end point was freedom from major adverse cardiac or cerebrovascular events (death, stroke, transient ischemic attacks, reversible ischemic neurologic deficits, nonfatal MI, repeat revascularization by percutaneous intervention or surgery). Also reported were deaths from all causes. Secondary end points included a number of factors including cost. There was no difference between stenting and CABG for rates of death, stroke, or MI at 1 year. Death occurred in 2.5% of the stenting group and 2.8% of the CABG group. Cerobrovascular accident (worst event) occurred in 1.5% of stenting and 2.0% of CABG group; MI occurred in 5.3% of the stenting group and 4.0% of the surgery group. Repeated revascularization was more common in the stenting group (16%) than the surgery group (3.5%). Rate of event-free survival at 1 year was 73.8% in stenting group and 87.8% in CABG group ($p<0.001$). In patients who survived without a stroke or MI, 16.8% underwent a second revascularization in the stenting group vs 3.5% in the CABG group. At 1 year the cost of stenting was less than CABG (by $2973 per patient).
Concl.	At 1 year coronary stenting offered the same degree of protection against death, stroke, and MI as CABG; stenting was less expensive. Stenting was associated with more repeated revascularization.

5a

Comparison of Stenting with Minimally Invasive Bypass Surgery for Stenosis of the Left Anterior Descending Coronary Artery

Title	Comparison of stenting with minimally invasive bypass surgery for stenosis of the left anterior descending coronary artery.
Authors	Diegeler A, Thiele H, Falk V, et al.
Reference	N Engl J Med 2002;347:561-566.
Disease	Coronary artery disease, percutaneous intervention, coronary artery bypass graft.
Purpose	To compare stenting and minimally invasive bypass surgery with respect to efficacy and clinical outcome.
Design	Randomized, prospective, single-site.
Patients	220 patients with had isolated high-grade lesions (stenosis ≥75%) in the proximal left anterior descending artery, in the area between the origin of the left circumflex coronary artery and the first major septal branch. Exclusion criteria were: acute coronary syndrome that required immediate intervention, additional significant coronary lesions or valve disease that required treatment, stenosis of the first diagonal branch or stenosis that extended over a major diagonal branch, or previous interventional or surgical treatment for coronary artery disease. Lesions that were totally occlusive or a left anterior descending artery that ran an intramyocardial course were also excluded from the study.
Follow-up	6 months.

Regimen	Patients were randomized to treatment with either stenting (n=110) or minimally invasive surgery (n=110). Stent placement using a femoral approach was performed according to accepted clinical practice. On the day before the procedure all patients were started on 350 mg aspirin daily and either 500 mg ticlopidine daily or 300 mg clopidogrel daily. Ticlopidine or clopidogrel were continued for a minimum of 4 weeks, and aspirin was continued indefinitely. At the start of the procedure, a bolus of 10,000 U of heparin was given. Balloon size was based on visual evaluation of the target vessel, with a recommended balloon-to-vessel ratio between 1.1 and 1.2. For minimally invasive bypass surgery, a limited anterolateral thoracotomy was performed through the fourth intercostal space, and the internal thoracic artery was harvested. Heparin was given (100 U/kg). The internal thoracic artery was divided and anastomosed to the appropriate coronary artery with a running 8-0 polypropylene suture. Protamine was administered to neutralize 80% of the heparin dose. Wounds were closed in the usual manner.
Results	The primary end point was termed freedom from major adverse cardiovascular events and was a composite of MI, death from cardiac causes, and repeat revascularization of the original lesion, all within 6 months. The secondary end points were each of these individual components, assessment of clinical status according to the Canadian Cardiovascular Society (CCS) classification, and need for antianginal drugs at follow-up. Adverse events around the time of procedure were also documented. At a 6-month follow-up, a primary end point had occurred in 34/108 (31%) patients in the stenting group vs 16/108 (15%) patients in the surgery group (relative risk [RR] 0.47; 95% CI=0.21-0.89; p=0.02). There were 0 deaths from cardiac causes in the stent group and 2 in the surgery group. There were 3 MIs in the stent group and 5 in the surgery group (RR 1.77; 95% CI=0.41-7.58; p=0.68). There was a significantly increased need for revascularization in the stent group: 31 vs 9 in the surgery group (RR 0.29; 95% CI=0.09-0.65; p=0.003). The mean CCS angina class improved from 2.6±0.9 to 0.3±0.7 (p<0.001) after surgery, with 79% of patients angina-free. In the stenting group, CCS angina class improved from 2.6±0.9 to 0.7±1.0 (p<0.001 vs baseline; p=0.02 vs surgery group), with 62 % of patients angina-free (p=0.03 vs the surgery group). Patients requiring antianginal drug therapy were 6% in the surgery group vs 19% in the stent group (p=0.006).

Concl.   For patients with isolated high-grade lesions of the left anterior descending coronary artery, stenting and minimally invasive bypass surgery are both effective treatments. Stenting is associated with fewer periprocedural adverse events but surgery was more effective in reducing the need for revascularization and keeping patients free of angina.

ARTS

Arterial Revascularization Therapy Study

Title	The effect of completeness of revascularization on event-free survival at 1 year in the ARTS trial.
Authors	van den Brand MJ, Rensing BJ, Morel MA, et al.
Reference	J Am Coll Cardiol 2002;39:559-564.
Disease	Coronary artery disease.
Purpose	To compare the difference in outcomes in patients who undergo coronary artery bypass graft surgery (CABG) vs percutaneous intervention between subgroups that were completely or incompletely revascularized.
Design	Randomized, multicenter.
Patients	1205 patients with stable or unstable angina or objective signs of ischemia and multivessel disease.
Follow-up	400 days.
Regimen	Angiograms were reviewed by surgeon and cardiologist regarding potential for equivalence in revascularization completely either by CABG or stenting. Patients were then randomized to CABG or stented angioplasty.

5a

Results	Primary end point was freedom from major adverse cardiac or cerebrovascular events: death, stroke, nonfatal myocardial infarction, any revascularization after the initial procedure. 1172 patients were treated according to assigned protocol: 593 had stented angioplasty; 579 CABG. 84.1% of CABG patients and 70.5% of stented angioplasty patients had complete revascularization (all lesions of >50% diameter stenosis successfully treated); $p<0.001$. Stented angioplasty patients with incomplete revascularization had a lower 1-year event-free survival than stented patients completely revascularized (69.4% vs 76.6%; $p<0.05$). This difference was primarily due to a need for more subsequent CABG in this group (10.0%) vs the group with complete revascularization (2.0%; $p<0.05$). CABG patients with incomplete revascularization at 1 year had only slightly lower event-free survival vs those with complete revascularization (87.8% vs 89.9%). There were no significant differences in infarct-free and stroke-free survival among the 4 subgroups (CABG—complete, incomplete; percutaneous transluminal coronary angioplasty stenting—complete/incomplete). There was no difference in the incidence of death among the 4 groups.
Concl.	CABG was better at achieving complete revascularization. At 1 year, there was no difference in event-free survival in CABG patients who had complete vs incomplete revascularization. Patients randomized to angioplasty-stenting had less event-free survival if revascularization was incomplete, because they had a need for subsequent CABG.

AWESOME

Angina with Extremely Serious Operative Mortality Evaluation

Title	Percutaneous coronary intervention vs coronary artery bypass graft surgery for patients with medically refractory myocardial ischemia and risk factors for adverse outcomes with bypass: a multicenter, randomized trial.
Authors	Morrison DA, Sethi G, Sacks J, et al.
Reference	J Am Coll Cardiol 2001;38:143-149.
Disease	Coronary artery disease, angina pectoris.
Purpose	To compare the long-term outcome of patients with medically refractory myocardial ischemia and a high risk for coronary artery bypass grafting (CABG) randomly referred to either CABG or PCI strategy.
Design	Randomized, open-label, multicenter.
Patients	454 patients (mean age 67 years) with medically refractory ischemia who were at high risk [≥1 of the following risk factors: 1) prior heart surgery; 2) age >70 years; 3) left ventricular ejection fraction <35%; 4) intra-aortic balloon pump before enrollment; or 5) myocardial infarction within 7 days before enrollment]. Patients with single-vessel circumflex disease, unprotected left main disease, coronary anatomy unsuitable for PCI or CABG, and comorbidity likely to limit life expectancy were excluded. Eligible patients underwent coronary angiography. Patients whose coronary anatomy was suitable for both PCI and CABG were randomized.
Follow-up	60 months.
Regimen	CABG (n=232) vs PCI (n=222).

5a

Results   Of the 22,662 patients screened, 454 met all the inclusion criteria and consented. 98% of the patients in the CABG group and 99.5% in the PCI group underwent revascularization. 94% of the patients in the CABG vs 3.5% in the PCI group underwent CABG, and 5% vs 99%, respectively underwent PCI. The left internal mammary artery was used in 70% and right internal mammary artery in 3.4% of the patients in the CABG group. In 54% of the PCI group stents were deployed. 30-day mortality was 5% in the CABG group and 3% in the PCI group, and 6-month mortality was 10% in the CABG group and 6% in the PCI group. 36-month survival rate was 79% in the CABG and 80% in the PCI group (p=0.46). Stroke occurred in 1% of the patients in each group. Survival free of unstable angina at 60 months was 60% in the CABG group and 56% in the PCI group (p=0.16). Survival free of unstable angina or revascularization was 55% vs 44% in the CABG and PCI group, respectively (p=0.001).

Concl.   Long-term mortality was comparable between patients at high risk for CABG and with medically refractory angina who were randomized to either PCI or CABG, although patients who underwent CABG needed less repeated revascularization procedures during follow-up.

BARI (7-Year Outcome, Diabetics)

Bypass Angioplasty Revascularization Investigation

Title	7-Year outcome in the bypass angioplasty revascularization investigation (BARI) by treatment and diabetic status.
Authors	The BARI Investigators.
Reference	a. N Engl J Med 1996;335:217-225. b. J Am Coll Cardiol 2000;35:1122-1129.
Disease	Coronary artery disease.
Purpose	To assess 7-year survival in coronary artery disease patients randomized to initial therapy with CABG or PTCA.
Design	As per BARI.
Patients	1829 symptomatic coronary artery patients with multivessel coronary artery disease, including diabetic patients.
Follow-up	Average of 7.8 years.
Regimen	Initial PTCA vs CABG.
Add'l Tx	As per BARI.

5a

Results	At 7 years, survival for total population was 84.4% for CABG patients vs 80.9% for PTCA (p=0.043). This treatment difference was secondary to differences in a subgroup of 353 patients who had treated diabetes. At 7 years, among these diabetics 76.4% that received CABG survived vs 55.7% assigned to PTCA (p=0.001). These differences in treatment between CABG and PTCA in treated diabetics were even greater than observed at 5 years. Among 1476 patients without treated diabetes, survival was 86.4% in CABG patients and 86.8% in PTCA patients (p=NS). Subsequent revascularization rates remained higher in the PTCA patients (59.7%) compared to the CABG patients (13.1%; p<0.001). Among diabetic patients who underwent CABG, those who received at least 1 internal mammary artery graft had improved survival (83.2%) compared to those diabetic patients that had only saphenous vein bypass grafts (54.5%—a rate that was actually similar to diabetic patients who received PTCA (55.5%). Among survivors with 7 year follow-up, incidence of angina was 15.1% in PTCA patients vs 11.4% in CABG patients (p=0.075).
Concl.	At 7 years CABG had a significant survival benefit over PTCA which was due to improved survival in diabetic patients who received CABG, especially those that received an internal mammary implant.

BHACAS (1 and 2)

Beating Heart Against Cardioplegic Arrest Studies 1 and 2

Title	Early and midterm outcome after off-pump and on-pump surgery in Beating Heart Against Cardioplegic Arrest Studies (BHACAS 1 and 2): a pooled analysis of two randomized controlled trials.
Authors	Angelini GD, Taylor FC, Reeves BC, et al.
Reference	Lancet 2002:359;1194-1199.
Disease	Coronary artery disease, coronary artery bypass grafting.
Purpose	To compare the short- and mid-term outcome of patients undergoing CABG using either cardiopulmonary bypass (on-pump) or off-pump technique.
Design	Randomized, open-label, single-center.
Patients	Overall, 401 patients were included. The BHACAS 1 was conducted from March 1997 to August 1998 and included 200 patients with left ventricular ejection fraction ≥30%. Patients with recent myocardial infarction, history of supraventricular arrhythmia, renal or respiratory impairment, previous CABG, previous stroke or transient ischemic attack, coagulopathy, and coronary lesions in distal marginal branches of the left circumflex artery were excluded (at that time it was considered technically difficult to anastomose the distal marginal branches using an off-pump technique). The BHACAS 2 was conducted from September 1998 to November 1999 and included 201 patients. In this study, patients with recent myocardial infarction and lesions in the distal marginal branches of the left circumflex artery were not excluded.
Follow-up	Mean follow-up was 25.0±9.1 months in BHACAS 1 and 13.7±5.5 months in BHACAS 2.
Regimen	Randomization to off-pump CABG (n=200) or on-pump (using cardioplegic arrest) surgery (n=201).

Results	2 patients randomized to off-pump CABG underwent on-pump surgery. 2 patients in the on-pump group vs zero in the off-pump group died in-hospital (p=0.50). Fewer patients in the off-pump group had chest infection (risk ratio [RR] 0.39; 95% CI=0.22-0.68; p=0.001) and needed inotropic support (RR 0.27; 95% CI=0.15-0.49; p<0.0001). Fewer patients in the off-pump group had arrhythmia (RR 0.37; 95% CI=0.26-0.53; p<0.0001) or atrial fibrillation (RR 0.34; 95% CI=0.23-0.51; p<0.0001). Patients undergoing off-pump surgery needed packed blood cell transfusion less often (RR 0.36; 95% CI=0.26-0.51; p<0.0001). Fewer patients in the off-pump group needed to stay in-hospital over 7 days (RR 0.54; 95% CI=0.36-0.80; p=0.002). After a mean follow-up of 25 months for BHACAS 1 and 13.7 months for BHACAS 2, 6 patients were lost to follow-up. Between 30 days to the end of the follow-up 3 patients in the on-pump vs 2 in the off-pump died. Pooled survival estimates at 24 months were 96% for the on-pump and 97% for the off-pump group (hazard ratio 0.57; 95% CI=0.17-1.96). In BHACAS 1, death or cardiac event occurred in 27% of the patients in the on-pump group vs 19% in the off-pump group. In the BHACAS 2 death or cardiac event occurred in 15% and 14% of the patients, respectively. When the 2 studies were pooled, the HR for mortality or cardiac event was 0.78 (95% CI=0.49-1.22) for off-pump vs on-pump surgery. Myocardial infarction occurred in 5% vs 2% of the on-pump and off-pump groups in BHACAS 1, and in 3% vs 2%, respectively in BHACAS 2. Recurrent angina was noted in 14% of the patients in the on-pump vs 12% in the off-pump group. 3% of the patients in the on-pump vs 4% in the off-pump needed repeat cardiac catheterization.
Concl.	Pooled data from these 2 randomized trials show that in-hospital and short-term (30 day) morbidity were lower after off-pump CABG than after conventional on-pump technique, without compromising mid-term outcome or increasing the need for repeat heart catheterization and revascularization.

EAST (8-Year Mortality Data)

Emory Angioplasty vs Surgery Trial

Title	8-year mortality in the Emory angioplasty vs surgery trial (EAST).
Authors	King SB, Kosinski AS, Guyton RA, et al.
Reference	a. N Engl J Med 1996;331:1044-1050. b. J Am Coll Cardiol 2000; 35:1116-1121.
Disease	Coronary artery disease.
Purpose	To assess long-term outcome of patients randomized to initial coronary angioplasty vs coronary artery bypass surgery.
Design	Randomized, single-center.
Patients	392 patients with multivessel coronary artery disease as per EAST.
Follow-up	8 years.
Regimen	Initial percutaneous transluminal coronary angioplasty (PTCA; n=198) or coronary artery bypass surgery (CABG; n=194).

5a

Results	Results of the primary EAST trial are in previous editions of this book. In brief, at 3 years follow-up the primary composite end point of death, myocardial infarction, or large ischemic defect, did not differ between groups. Repeat revascularization procedures were more frequent in the angioplasty group. Late follow-up was achieved by annual patient questionnaires, telephone contact, and examination of medical records. Survival at 8 years for the CABG group was 82.7% and for the angioplasty group was 79.3% (p=0.40). There was a small but not statistically significant survival advantage for 3 vessel disease with CABG (81.6%) vs PTCA (75.5%; p=0.35); but this benefit of surgery was not observed in patient with double vessel disease (83.4% with CABG vs 81.8% with PTCA). Patients with proximal left anterior descending coronary stenoses faired slightly but not significantly better with CABG (85.6% survival) vs PTCA (79.6%; p=0.16) as did diabetics (75.5% survival with CABG and 60.1% with PTCA; p=0.23). During the first 3 years after revascularization, additional procedures were more common in the PTCA group; after this time the curves of percent of patients having additional revascularization remained parallel.
Concl.	8 year survival of patients with multivessel coronary artery disease did not differ between PTCA and CABG.

ERACI II

Argentine Randomized Trial of Percutaneous Transluminal Coronary Angioplasty vs Coronary Artery Bypass Surgery in Multivessel Disease II

Title	Argentine randomized study: coronary angioplasty with stenting vs coronary bypass surgery in patients with multiple-vessel disease (ERACI II): 30-day and one-year follow-up results.
Authors	Rodriguez A, Bernardi V, Navia J, et al.
Reference	J Am Coll Cardiol 2001;37:51-58.
Disease	Coronary artery disease.
Purpose	To compare a strategy of percutaneous transluminal coronary revascularization with a free use of stents vs coronary artery bypass surgery in patients with multivessel coronary artery disease.
Design	Randomized, multicenter, open-label.
Patients	Patients with stable angina (Canadian Cardiovascular Society class III-IV) despite maximal medical therapy or with a large area of myocardium at risk identified by exercise testing. All patients should have ≥70% coronary artery stenosis in ≥1 vessel and ≥50% stenosis in ≥1 additional vessel, which was suitable to either percutaneous coronary intervention or CABG. Patients with single-vessel disease, previous CABG, PCI within the last year, previous stenting, acute myocardial infarction within the last 24 hours, left ventricular ejection fraction ≤35%, >2 chronic total occlusions, concomitant severe valvular disease, concomitant illness, and advanced age were excluded. Patients with unprotected left main stenosis could be included if they were amenable to single-stenting.
Follow-up	5 years (this paper reports the 30 days and at an average of 18.5±6.4 months results).
Regimen	Randomization to PCI with a free use of stents (n=225) or to CABG (n=225). Elective stenting was permitted only when the reference arterial diameter was ≥3 mm.

Add'l Tx	Patients who were randomized to PCI received aspirin 325 mg/d and ticlopidine.
Results	Of the 2759 patients who were screened, 1076 met the inclusion criteria and finally, only 450 patients were randomized. PCI was successful without occurrence of death, Q-wave myocardial infarction, or emergent CABG in 98.2% of the patients. Excluding the patients with chronic total occlusion, only 8.8% of the patients in the PCI group had severe residual stenosis in 1 major epicardial artery after revascularization. PCI was not attempted in 52 chronic total occlusions (23.4%) in patients with prior myocardial infarction. 28% of the PCI patients received abciximab. Complete anatomic revascularization was achieved in 85% of the CABG vs 50.2% in the PCI group (p=0.002). In the CABG group, the left internal mammary artery was used in 88.5% of the patients. 1.4 stents per patients were implanted in the PCI group. 30-day mortality was 0.9% in the PCI group and 5.7% in the CABG group (p=0.012). Q-wave myocardial infarction occurred in 0.9% and 5.7%, respectively (p=0.012). 30-day death or Q-wave MI occurred in 1.8% vs 11.4%, respectively (p=0.0001), and major adverse cardiac events in 3.6% vs 12.3%, respectively (p=0.002). Hospital stay was shorter in the PCI group (4.9±4.9 vs 9±4.5 days; p=0.002). The Kaplan-Meier survival curves showed better survival in the PCI group (96.9%) than in the CABG group (92.5%; p<0.017). Kaplan-Meier freedom from myocardial infarction curves was also better for the PCI group (97.7% vs 93.7%; p<0.017). However, the PCI group underwent more repeated revascularization procedures (16.8% vs 4.8%; p<0.001). During follow-up 11 PCI patients underwent CABG. The PCI patients were less often free of angina (84.5% vs 92%; p=0.01). Event-free survival was comparable between the groups. The overall cost per patient, including the repeated revascularization procedures was $12,320 for the PCI group and $11,160 for the CABG group (p=NS).
Concl.	PCI with stenting was associated with better survival and reduced risk of MI than CABG. However, the PCI strategy was associated with more repeated revascularization procedures.

SOS

Stent or Surgery

Title	Coronary artery bypass surgery vs percutaneous coronary intervention with stent implantation in patients with multivessel coronary artery disease (the Stent or Surgery trial): a randomised controlled trial.
Authors	The SOS Investigators.
Reference	Lancet 2002;360:965-970.
Disease	Coronary artery disease.
Purpose	To determine the effect of percutaneous intervention with stenting vs coronary artery bypass grafting surgery in the management of patients with multivessel disease.
Design	Randomized, open-label, multicenter.
Patients	988 patients, randomized to PCI (n=488), or CABG (n=500). Patients had multivessel, symptomatic coronary artery disease in which revascularization was indicated and deemed appropriate by either PCI or CABG. Patients with previous thoracotomy or coronary revascularization were excluded. Patients who required therapy for valvular, great vessel or aorta pathology were also excluded.
Follow-up	Median 2 years, range 1-4 years.
Regimen	Randomization to CABG (m=500) or stent-assisted PCI (m=488). Revascularization was performed according to optimal local practice. Equivalent revascularization was encouraged but not required. There were no restrictions on equipment, method, or medications given. The choice of stent was left to the interventionist.

5a

Results	In the patients who received PCI, 94% of lesions (a mean of 2.7 lesions/patient) were revascularized successfully. Stents were placed in 78% of lesions; the median number of stents per patient was 2. 3% of patients received only balloon angioplasty, and 8% of patients received glycoprotein IIb/IIIa inhibitors during the initial procedure. Among the patients who received CABG, the mean number of bypass grafts was 2.8/patient. An internal mammary vessel was used in 93% of patients. 3% of procedures did not use cardiopulmonary bypass. The primary outcome was the incidence of repeat revascularization. The secondary outcomes were: death or Q-wave MI, all-cause death, angina symptoms, cardiac medication requirements, and left-ventricular function. With a median of 2 years follow-up, 21% (n=101) of patients in the PCI group eventually required 1 or more additional procedures for revascularization, whereas this number was 6% (n=30) in the patients originally assigned to CABG. The frequency of death or non-fatal MI was similar between the groups (hazard ratio (HR) 0.95; 95% CI=0.63-1.42; p=0.80). Death occurred in 5% in the PCI group (n=22) and 2% in the CABG group (n=8) (HR 2.91; 95% CI=1.29-6.53; p=0.01). Q-wave MI occurred less frequently in the PCI group (5%, n=26) vs the CABG group (8%, n=41). A greater number of patients were angina-free at follow-up in the CABG group vs the PCI group (79% vs 66%; p<0.0001), and a greater proportion of patients in the CABG group were taking no anti-anginal medications (35% vs 18%; p<0.0001).There was no significant difference in left-ventricular ejection fraction at 1 year follow-up: PCI vs CABG, 55.3% vs 54.8%, p=0.55.
Concl.	The use of PCI is associated with a significantly higher rate of revascularization vs CABG. There was a significant decrease in mortality risk associated with CABG in this study. The authors note that the use of stents was associated with a lower need for repeat revascularization vs previous studies using balloon angioplasty alone.

Title	Off-pump vs conventional coronary artery bypass grafting: early and 1-year graft patency, cost, and quality-of-life outcomes. A randomized trial.
Authors	Puskas JD, Williams WH, Mahoney EM, et al.
Reference	JAMA 2004;291:1841-1849.
Disease	Coronary artery disease.
Purpose	To assess graft patency, clinical and quality-of-life outcomes, and cost of off-pump vs conventional coronary artery bypass graft (CABG) surgery among patients while in the hospital and at 1-year follow-up.
Design	Single-surgeon, randomized, controlled trial.
Patients	197 patients referred for primary elective CABG surgery, who were unselected for coronary anatomy, ventricular function, or comorbidities between March 10 and August 20, 2001, at an academic center.
Follow-up	1 year.
Regimen	Elective off-pump coronary artery bypass (n=98) or CABG surgery with cardiopulmonary bypass (n=99).
Results	The main outcome measures were angiographically documented graft patency before hospital discharge and at 1 year; health-related quality of life; and cost of the index and subsequent hospitalization(s). Graft patency was similar for the 2 procedures at 30 days (absolute difference 1.3%; 95% CI=-0.66% to 3.31%; p=0.19) and at 1 year (absolute difference=-2.2%; 95% CI=-6.1% to 1.7%; p=0.27). Rates of death, stroke, MI, angina, and repeat intervention were similar at 30 days and 1 year between the 2 groups. Health-related quality of life was similar between the groups. Mean total hospitalization cost per patient at hospital discharge was $2272 less for off-pump coronary artery bypass (OPCAB) (p=0.002) and $1955 less at 1 year (p=0.08).

5a

| Concl. | OPCAB produced similar graft patency in the hospital and at 1 year. Cardiac outcomes and health-related quality of life at 30 days and 1 year were similar and patients incurred a lower cost with OPCAB compared to standard CABG. OPCAB may provide complete and persistent revascularization that is also cost-effective. A larger multicenter trial is needed to compare OBCAB with CABG with cardiopulmonary bypass and to evaluate the generalizability of these results in the routine care of patients with multivessel CAD. |

Title	Randomized comparison between stenting and off-pump bypass surgery in patients referred for angioplasty.
Authors	Eefting F, Nathoe H, van Dijk D, et al.
Reference	Circulation 2003;108:2870-2876.
Disease	Coronary artery disease.
Purpose	To compare cardiac outcome, quality of life, and cost-effectiveness of stenting vs off-pump surgery for coronary artery patients referred for angioplasty.
Design	Randomized, prospective.
Patients	280 patients referred for coronary angioplasty with stable or unstable angina and/or documented ischemia in whom stenting and off-pump surgery were considered feasible and likely to lead to a similar degree of revascularization.
Follow-up	1 year.
Regimen	Stenting was performed with standard techniques and off-pump surgery performed by use of the Octopus stabilizer device.

5a

Results	Patients had single vessel disease in 68 of 138 stent patients and 74 of 142 off-pump patients (p=0.28). Patients had double-vessel disease in 30 of 138 stent patients and 24 of 142 off-pump patients. The primary end point was freedom from all cause death, stroke, acute MI, and repeat revascularization. Secondary end points included quality of life and cost. At 1 year, the primary end point was observed in 85.5% of the stenting patients and 91.5% of the off-pump surgery patients (relative risk 0.93; 95% CI=0.86-1.02). At 1 year, there were 4 deaths in the off-pump group (2.8%) vs 0 in the stent group. 78.3% of the stented patients and 87.0% of the off-pump patients were free of angina (p=0.06). There was no difference in exercise capacity assessed by exercise testing at 1 year. Absence of exercise-induced ischemia was present in 99 patients (74.4%) of the stent group vs 104 (79.4%) of the off-pump group (p=NS). At 1 year, there was no difference in quality of life between the 2 groups. Stenting was associated with lower in-hospital costs and lower costs at 1 year than surgery. Hospital stay was longer in the surgery group (5.77 days) vs the stenting group (1.43 days).
Concl.	Stenting maintained comparable cardiac outcome and quality of life compared to off-pump bypass surgery in patients who were referred for coronary angioplasty. Stenting was more cost-effective and can be recommended as first choice revascularization therapy in selected patients.

Title	A randomized comparison of off-pump and on-pump multivessel coronary artery bypass surgery.
Authors	Khan NE, DeSouza AD, Mister R, et al.
Reference	N Engl J Med 2004;350:21-28.
Disease	Coronary artery disease, coronary artery bypass surgery.
Purpose	To compare graftpatency rates and clinical outcomes in patients receiving conventional "on-pump" coronary artery bypass grafting vs off-pump surgery.
Design	Prospective, randomized, controlled, single-center.
Patients	104 patients referred for first time coronary artery bypass grafting who required at least 3 grafts. Patients could not have recent myocardial infarction or poor left ventricular function.
Follow-up	3 month coronary angiogram.
Regimen	In the on-pump group (n=50) cardiopulmonary bypass performed in a standard fashion with use of a membrane oxygenator and roller pump and antegrade delivery of coldblood cardioplegia. For off-pump surgery (n=54), the octopus stabilizer device (Medtronic, Inc, Minneapolis, MN) was used. Patients in on-pump surgery protocol were cooled to 32°C; those in the off-pump surgery group were warmed to maintain a core temperature not below 35°C. Coronary angiography was performed at 3 months including quantitative analysis.

5a

Results	On-pump group received 3.4 grafts and off-pump group received 3.1 grafts (p=NS). Median postoperative length of stay was 7 days in both groups; there were no deaths. Area under the curve of troponin T levels was higher during the first 72 hours in the on-pump group (31 h · μg/L) vs the off-pump group (19 h · μg/L, p=0.02). However, at 3 months 127 of 130 (98%) grafts were patent in the on-pump group vs 114 of 130 (88%; p=0.002) in the off-pump group. There was a trend toward a higher percentage of stenosis at the site of the left internal thoracic artery graft to the left anterior descending artery in the off-pump group (35%) vs the on-pump group (21%; p=0.06).
Concl.	While off-pump surgery was as safe as on-pump surgery and caused initially less myocardial damage (troponin T levels) at 3 months graft, patency was lower in the off-pump vs on-pump group.

PRAGUE-4

Primary Angioplasty in AMI Patients From General Community Hospitals Transported to PCI Units vs Emergency Thrombolysis-4

Title	Off-pump vs on-pump coronary surgery: final results from a prospective randomized study PRAGUE-4.
Authors	Straka Z, Widimsky P, Jirasek K, et al.
Reference	Ann Thorac Surg 2004;77:789-793.
Disease	Coronary artery disease, coronary artery bypass graft.
Purpose	To compare the results of off-pump and conventional on-pump surgery among unselected patients scheduled for coronary artery bypass graft.
Design	Randomized, open-label, single center.
Patients	400 patients referred for coronary artery bypass graft, including patients with acute coronary syndromes. Patients who needed concomitant valvular or aortic surgery were excluded. Patients who underwent emergency surgery were not included.
Follow-up	30-days.
Regimen	Randomization to on-pump (n=192) or off-pump (n= 208) coronary artery bypass graft. The surgeon could change the technique and switch over any time before or during surgery.

Results	3 patients withdrew the informed consent, 7 underwent PCI, and 2 patients were lost to follow-up before surgery. A total of 184 were randomized to on-pump and 204 to off-pump CABG. 5.4% of the patients in the on-pump group and 5.4% in the off-pump group were crossed over by the surgeon prior to surgery. 1.1% and 9.8% of the patients, respectively, were crossed over during surgery (p<0.001). Finally 173 patients (85%) of those randomized to off-pump underwent off-pump surgery. The number of distal anastomosis per patient was 2.7 for the on-pump group and 2.3 for the off-pump group (p<0.001). Left internal mammary artery was used in 90% of the patients in the on-pump group and in 97% in the off-pump group (p=0.01). The off-pump group had significantly lower blood loss (560 vs 680 mL; p<0.001), but there was no difference in the number of patients receiving transfusion between the groups. Creatine kinase (p<0.001) and creatine kinase MB (p<0.001) levels were significantly lower at 6, 18, and 36 hours after surgery in the off-pump group. 30-day mortality (intention-to-treat analysis) was 1.1% in the on-pump and 2.0% in the off-pump group (p=0.39). Q-wave MI occurred in 1.6% and 2.0%, respectively (p=0.91). Stroke occurred in 1.1% and 0 of the patients, respectively (p=0.22). There was no difference in the percentage of patients needing hemodialysis (1.1% and 1.0%; p=0.65). The combined end point of death, Q-wave MI, stroke and the need for hemodialysis occurred in 4.9% and 2.9% of the patients, respectively (p=0.32). When comparing patients that actually underwent on-pump (n=172) and off-pump (n=173) surgery, the combined end point occurred in 5.2% of the patients in the on-pump and in 1.7% in the off-pump group (p=0.14). The median intensive care unit stay was 24 hours and 23 hours, respectively (p=0.40). The median hospital stay was comparable (5 days in each group). Total hospital cost was €4387 in the on-pump group and €3451 in the off-pump group (p<0.001).
Concl.	Off-pump CABG is feasible in about 85% of unselected patients referred for elective CABG. The 30-day clinical outcomes are comparable to those of traditional on-pump surgery. Off-pump surgery was associated with smaller blood loss, lower creatine kinase values, and lower hospital costs.

5. Interventional Cardiology
b. Percutaneous Transluminal Coronary Angioplasty vs Stenting vs Other Percutaneous Devices, Intravascular Ultrasound-Guided Stenting

Coronary-Artery Stenting Compared with Balloon Angioplasty for Restenosis After Initial Balloon Angioplasty

Title	Coronary-artery stenting compared with balloon angioplasty for restenosis after initial balloon angioplasty.
Authors	Erbel R, Haude M, Höpp HW, et al, for the Restenosis Stent Study Group.
Reference	N Engl J Med 1998;339:1672-1678.
Disease	Coronary artery disease.
Purpose	To determine whether intracoronary stenting vs percutaneous transluminal coronary angioplasty reduces the recurrence of luminal narrowing in lesions with restenosis.
Design	Prospective, randomized, multicenter.
Patients	383 patients who previously had undergone balloon angioplasty and had clinical and angiographic evidence of restenosis.
Follow-up	6 months.
Regimen	Angioplasty alone (192 patients) vs intracoronary stenting with a Palmaz-Schatz stent (191 patients).
Add'l Tx	Aspirin, heparin during procedure. Following stenting heparin followed by coumadin for 3 months. After angioplasty, 300 mg aspirin.

Results	The rate of restenosis (defined as stenosis of more than 50% of the lumen) at 6 months was higher in the angioplasty group (32%) compared to the stent group (18%; p=0.03). Revascularization of the target vessel was necessary in 27% of angioplasty patients but in only 10% of stent patients (p=0.001). There was a smaller mean minimal luminal diameter in the angioplasty vs the stent group. Subacute thrombosis was more common in the stent group (3.9%) compared to the angioplasty group (0.6%). Event-free survival (free of death, myocardial infarction, bypass surgery, revascularization of target vessel after randomization) was present in 72% of angioplasty patients and 84% of stent patients, at 250 days (p=0.04).
Concl.	Coronary artery stenting reduced the rate of recurrent restenosis despite a higher incidence of subacute thrombosis.

5b

Comparison of GR-II Stent and Palmaz-Schatz Stent

Title	Randomized comparison of GR-II Stent and Palmaz-Schatz Stent for elective treatment of coronary stenoses.
Authors	Lansky AJ, Roubin GS, O'Shaughnessy CD, et al.
Reference	Circulation 2000;102:1364-1368.
Disease	Coronary artery disease.
Purpose	To compare the long-term angiographic and clinical outcomes of elective treatment with the Gianturco-Roubin (GR)-II stent and Palmaz-Schatz (PS) stent in patients with coronary stenoses.
Design	Randomized, multicenter.
Patients	755 patients with myocardial ischemia and de novo native coronary stenoses.
Follow-up	12 months.
Regimen	Randomized to PS (n=375) in the GR-II stent (n=380).
Add'l Tx	Aspirin (325 mg daily) and ticlopidine (250 mg twice daily) for 48 hours before procedure. Bolus IV heparin during procedure. After stenting, ticlopidine (250 mg twice daily) for 4 weeks and daily aspirin, indefinitely.
Results	Primary end point was 12-month target lesion revascularization free survival. Secondary end points included procedural success, stent thrombosis, major adverse cardiac events—including death, MI, TLR at 30 days and 12 months. Secondary angiographic end point was restenosis frequency (>50% follow-up diameter stenosis in the stent). GR-II had a lower 12 month TLR-free survival rate (71.7%) vs PS (83.9%, p<0.001). Procedural success rate was similar between GR-II (98.5%) and PS (99.4%; p=0.19). At 30 days, stent thrombosis rate was greater with GR-II (3.9%) than PS (0.3%; p<0.001) and TLR rate was 3.9% for GR-II and 0.5% for PS; p<0.001. GR-II also had a higher follow-up restenosis rate (47.3%) than to PS (20.6%; p<0.001).

Concl.   GR-II stent should be limited to use for acute treatment of abrupt or threatened closure following failed conventional balloon angioplasty procedures.

Stent Implantation in Small Coronary Arteries

Title	Immediate and one-year outcome of intracoronary stent implantation in small coronary arteries with 2.5-mm stents.
Authors	Al Suwaidi J, Garratt KN, Berger PB, et al.
Reference	Am Heart J 2000;140:898-905.
Disease	Coronary artery disease.
Purpose	To compare the immediate and long-term results of 2.5 mm stent implantation vs standard balloon angioplasty in small coronary arteries.
Design	Registry, single-center.
Patients	651 patients with lesions in small coronary arteries who underwent either balloon angioplasty (using 2.5-mm balloons) or 2.5-mm stent implantation.
Follow-up	12 months.
Regimen	Standard balloon angioplasty (using 2.5-mm balloons) percutaneous transluminal coronary angioplasty or implantation of 2.5-m stents.
Add'l Tx	All patients received aspirin 325 mg/d, and either ticlopidine 500 mg or clopidogrel 300 mg before procedure. All patients received intravenous heparin. Abciximab was administered to high-risk patients.

Results	A total of 108 patients underwent stenting and 543 underwent PTCA. The angiographic success rate was 97.2% in the stent group and 90.2% in the PTCA group (p=0.001). Postprocedural residual diameter stenosis was 4.7±12.8% in the stent group and 29.6±21.7% in the PTCA group (p=0.0001). The frequency of in-hospital death (0.9% vs 3.3%; p=0.18), myocardial infarction (4.6% vs 2.4%; p=0.20), coronary artery bypass graft surgery (0.9% vs 1.7%; p=0.57), and abrupt vessel closure in laboratory (2.8% vs 1.1%; p=0.96) were comparable between the stent and the PTCA group. At 1-year after successful hospitalization, the frequency of death (3.8% vs 4.8%; p=0.37), myocardial infarction (10.2% vs 4.0%; p=0.30), and CABG (8.4% vs 6.8%; p=0.89) were comparable between the stent and PTCA group. However, target vessel revascularization (18.9% vs 11.7%; p=0.03), and any cardiovascular event (35.4% vs 22.1%; p=0.05) occurred more frequently in the stent group. The diasadvantages of stenting persisted when only patients who underwent elective stenting were compared with the PTCA group (40.1% vs 22.1%; p=0.06). Multivariate analysis revealed stent use (RR 1.6; 95% CI=1.0-2.5; p=0.05) to be independent predictor of major adverse cardiac events.
Concl.	Although the initial angiographic success rate of stenting small coronary arteries is high, the immediate and 1-year clinical outcome after stenting is not better than after standard PTCA alone.

5b

Title	A randomized comparison of elective high-pressure stenting with balloon angioplasty: six-month angiographic and two-year clinical follow-up.
Authors	Witkowski A, Ruzyllo W, Gil R, et al.
Reference	Am Heart J 2000;140:264-271.
Disease	Coronary artery disease.
Purpose	To compare the 6-month angiographic results and 2-year clinical outcome in patients randomized to high-pressure stenting or standard balloon angioplasty.
Design	Randomized, single-blind, multicenter.
Patients	400 patients with I-IV Canadian Cardiovascular Society Class, single de novo coronary artery lesion >50% in diameter stenosis, <15 mm in length that could be entirely covered by a single Palmaz-Schatz 153 stent, and with a target artery reference diameter ≥2.5 mm. Patients with acute or recent myocardial infarction, or contraindication to heparin, aspirin or ticlopidine were excluded. In addition, patients with treatment of chronic total occlusion, true bifurcation lesion, lesions in a previously grafted artery and left main coronary artery lesions were not included.
Follow-up	6-month angiographic follow-up and 2 years clinical follow-up.
Regimen	Randomization to either balloon angioplasty or Palmaz-Schatz 153 stent implantation using ≥14 atm after predilatation of the target lesion.
Add'l Tx	All patients received aspirin 300 mg/d and ticlopidine 250 mg bid, started for ≥2 days before the procedure. In all patients, ticlopidine was continued for 1 month and aspirin indefinitely. At the time of the percutaneous coronary intervention, all patients received IV 10,000 IU.

Results	4 patients in the PTCA group and 8 patients in the stent group were excluded from further analysis. There were 192 patients in the stent group and 196 patients in the PTCA group. 3 patients in the stent group were switched to PTCA alone and 19 patients in the PTCA group were switched to stent. Angiographic success rate was 98.47% in the PTCA group and 98.44% in the stent group (p=NS). The procedural success rate was 97.45% and 97.92%, respectively (p=NS). Acute or threatened vessel closure occurred in 1.56% of the patients in the stent group vs 7.65% in the PTCA group (p=0.001). No acute or subacute stent thrombosis was observed. Events (death, stroke, myocardial infarction or revascularization) within the first 14 days occurred in 2.55% of the patients in the PTCA group vs 2.08% in the stent group (p=NS). Minimal luminal diameter immediately after procedure was larger in the stent group (3.05±0.56 mm vs 2.51±0.62 mm; p=0.001). Minimal luminal diameter at 6 months was 2.29±0.86 mm in the stent group vs 2.0±0.8 mm in the PTCA group (p=0.001). Restenosis rate was 8.18% and 24.87%, in the stent group vs PTCA group, respectively (p=0.055). At 6 months, 14.44% of the patients in the stent group and 20.21% of the patients in the PTCA group underwent target lesion revascularization (p=0.05). Clinical events occurred in 16.67% and 22.96% of the patients, respectively, at 6 months (p=0.057). At 2 years, target lesion revascularization was performed in 17.19% in the stent group vs 25.51% in the PTCA group (p=0.02). There were no differences in the rates of death or acute myocardial infarction between the stent and PTCA groups. Event-free survival for the stent and PTCA groups was 86.77% and 78.44% at 6 months, 84.13% and 76.70% at 12 months, and 83.07% and 73.54% at 24 months (p=0.0172).
Concl.	Coronary stenting was associated with better 6-month angiographic and 2-year clinical outcomes than standard PTCA. The difference in 2-year event-free survival rate was related to a lower target lesion revascularization rate in the stent group.

5b

Cutting Balloon Angioplasty

Title	Cutting balloon angioplasty for the treatment of in-stent restenosis: a matched comparison with rotational atherectomy, additional stent implantation, and balloon angioplasty.
Authors	Adamian M, Colombo A, Briguori C, et al.
Reference	J Am Coll Cardiol 2001;38:672-679.
Disease	Coronary artery disease.
Purpose	To determine whether cutting balloon angioplasty has advantages over other modalities as therapy for in-stent restenosis.
Design	Randomized, single-center study.
Patients	258 patients, in which 1 lesion per patient was randomized. The lesions were in-stent restenosis and matched per baseline conditions. In-stent restenosis was defined as >50% diameter stenosis.
Follow-up	6.2 months-angiographic follow-up. 11-month clinical follow-up.
Regimen	Lesions randomized to cutting balloon (conventional balloon catheter 10-15 mm in length with 3 or 4 micro beads) angioplasty, rotational atherectomy, additional stenting, and percutaneous transluminal coronary angioplasty.
Add'l Tx	Heparin, nitroglycerin, aspirin, ticlopidine.

Results	The stenting group had higher acute lumen gain (2.12±0.7 mm); the cutting balloon angioplasty group had similar gain to the rotational atherectomy group and angioplasty group (1.70±0.6 vs 1.79±0.5 mm vs 1.56±0.7 mm, respectively; p=NS). At angiographic follow-up the lumen loss was lower for cutting balloon angioplasty (0.63±0.6 mm) vs rotational atherectomy (1.30±0.8 mm) and stenting (1.36±0.8 mm); p<0.0001. Cutting balloon angioplasty resulted in a lower recurrent restenosis rate (20%) vs 36% and 41% with rotational atherectomy and stenting (p<0.05). At a mean of 11 months of clinical follow-up, death, Q-wave MI, CABG or repeat angioplasty occurred in 17.5% of cutting balloon angioplasty patients, 35.4% of rotational atherectomy patients, 37.9% of stent patients, and 43.2% of angioplasty patients (p=0.01). Death or MI rates did not differ among groups. There was a lower target lesion revascularization rate at long-term follow-up in the cutting balloon group (15.8%) vs rotational atherectomy (31.9%), stenting (35.5%) or angioplasty group (37.8%; p=0.03).
Concl.	Cutting balloon angioplasty was safe and efficient therapy for in-stent restenosis. Immediate results were similar to rotational atherectomy with better long-term angiographic and clinical outcomes.

5b

Cutting Balloon Global Randomized Trial

Title	Cutting balloon angioplasty for the prevention of restenosis: results of the cutting balloon global randomized trial.
Authors	Mauri L, Bonan R, Weiner BH, et al.
Reference	Am J Cardiol 2002;90:1079-1083.
Disease	Coronary artery disease, percutaneous intervention.
Purpose	To determine the immediate and long-term effects of cutting balloon (CB) angioplasty vs standard percutaneous transluminal coronary angioplasty on occlusive coronary artery disease.
Design	Multicenter, randomized.
Patients	1238 patients, age 25-75 years, who had evidence of myocardial ischemia due to a de novo stenosis that was <20 mm long in a native coronary artery ≥2 mm in diameter. Main exclusion criteria included history of angioplasty at the associated lesion, contraindication to emergency coronary artery bypass surgery, resting angina or Q-wave myocardial infarction in the past 48 hours, and congestive heart failure. Patients were also excluded if they were found at angiography to have total occlusion, thrombus, severe calcification, ulceration, vessel angle >45 °, and American College of Cardiology/American Heart Association class C lesions.
Follow-up	9 months.
Regimen	Patients were randomized to either CB or PTCA. In the CB group, a balloon-to-artery diameter ratio was restricted to between 0.9-1.1. At each lesion, a single inflation of the CB was performed with a final pressure of 4-8 atm for ≤90 seconds. Any residual stenosis >40% was treated with subsequent dilations with a normal angioplasty balloon. In the PTCA group, the number of inflations, the final pressure, and duration of pressure were left to the operator's decision.
Add'l Tx	All patients received aspirin and IV heparin prior to angioplasty.

Results	The primary end point was the binary angiographic resteno-

Results   The primary end point was the binary angiographic restenosis rate, which was defined as the percent with >50% diameter
stenosis at 6 months of follow-up. The primary adverse cardiac
event end point was the composite of death, Q-wave MI, emergency bypass surgery, and target lesion revascularization. 617
patients were in the CB group, and 621 in the PTCA group.
Baseline characteristics between the groups were similar. The
immediate procedural success rate was similar between the 2
groups (CB=92.9%, PTCA=94.7%). However, the CB procedures left a smaller minimal lumen diameter (2.05±0.52 mm vs
2.13±0.53 mm; p=0.01) and a larger residual percent diameter
stenosis (29%±14% vs 27%±13%; p=0.01) than PTCA. The
primary end point was similar between the 2 groups (restenosis,
CB=31.4% vs PTCA=30.4%; p=0.75). The minimal lumen
diameter and percentage of diameter stenosis were likewise
similar. The rate of major adverse cardiac events was similar in
both treatment groups at 30 days (CB=3.7% vs PTCA=2.7%;
p=0.34), and was also similar at 270 days (CB=13.6% vs
PTCA=15.1%; p=0.47). Patients who received CB had a higher likelihood of remaining free of target vessel revascularization
through 270 days (CB=88.5% vs PTCA=84.6%; p=0.04).
The CB group had a greater frequency of MI (4.7% vs 2.4%
for PTCA; p=0.03) and mortality (1.3% vs 0.3% for PTCA;
p=0.06) at the 9-month follow-up. There were 5 coronary per-
forations in the CB group, and 0 in the PTCA group.

Concl.   Cutting balloon angioplasty had similar efficacy vs conventional
balloon angioplasty in immediate and long-term angiographic
outcomes. Long-term clinical outcomes favored conventional
balloon angioplasty.

5b

Direct Coronary Stenting vs Predilatation Followed by Stent Placement

Title	Direct coronary stenting vs predilatation followed by stent placement.
Authors	Brueck M, Scheinert D, Wortmann A, et al.
Reference	Am J Cardiol 2002;90:1187-1192.
Disease	Coronary artery disease, percutaneous intervention.
Purpose	To compare the outcome of direct stenting vs usual stenting preceded by balloon dilatation.
Design	Randomized, prospective.
Patients	335 patients, who had at least 1 native coronary artery lesion noted on coronary angiography to have a diameter reduction of ≥60% in ≥1 projections and ≤95% in all projections; length of lesion ≤30 mm judged capable of being treated with 1 or 2 stents, and no significant stenosis ≥60% proximal to the lesion. Exclusion criteria included: unprotected left main diameter stenosis >50%, totally occluded target vessel, presence of a lesion that was highly calcified, excessively tortuous vessel, bifurcation or ostial stenosis, presence of thrombus, saphenous vein graft, in-stent restenosis, other pretreatment besides balloon angioplasty, and ejection fraction <30%.
Follow-up	6 months.
Regimen	Patients were randomized to either direct stenting or usual stenting following balloon dilatation. Before the procedure, all patients received a bolus of 10,000 U heparin. Usage of glycoprotein IIb/IIIa inhibitor was optional. All patients received 225 mg clopidogrel after the procedure or the day before, followed by 75 mg clopidogrel and 300 mg aspirin daily for 4 weeks. After this point, all patients received 100 mg qd.

Results	The primary study outcome was the procedural success, which was defined by normal perfusion of the distant vessel (Thrombolysis in Myocardial Infarction [TIMI] grade 3 flow), final stenosis diameter of ≤20%, and absence of major complications during the procedure and hospital period (death, MI, or target lesion revascularization). The secondary study outcomes were duration and cost of the procedure, radiation exposure, amount of contrast used, and events during follow-up, which included death, Q-wave infarction, and repeat intervention of the target lesion. 171 patients were assigned to the direct stenting group, and 164 patients to the predilatation followed by stenting group. The rate of procedural success was 98% in both groups. The numbers of in-hospital death, Q-wave MI, and acute stent thrombosis were nearly identical in both groups. The duration of the procedure was significantly shorter in the direct stent group (42.1±18.7 minutes vs 51.5±23.8 minutes; p=0.004), and time of exposure to radiation was significantly lower in the direct stent group (10.3±7.7 minutes vs 12.5±6.4 minutes; p=0.002). The amount of contrast dye used was significantly reduced in the direct stenting group (163±69 mL vs 197±84 mL; p<0.0001). During the 6-month follow-up, there was 1 death, which was in the direct stenting group. There were 8 Q-wave MIs in the direct stent group and 9 in the predilatation group (p=0.93). There was significantly less need for target vessel revascularization in the direct stent group (18% vs 28%; p=0.03), and significantly decreased composite of death/MI/revascularization (19% vs 30%; p=0.045). The rate of angiography restenosis was significantly reduced in the direct stent group (20% vs 31%; p=0.048). Angiography at follow-up showed significantly less late loss (p=0.01) and significantly increased net gain (p=0.04) in the direct stent group. There was less percent diameter stenosis with direct stenting (32.3%±28.9% with direct stenting vs 38.9±27.2% with predilatation; p=0.03). The MLD at follow-up was larger in the direct stent group (2.01±0.87 vs 1.82±0.96 mm; p=0.07).
Concl.	Direct stenting is safe and feasible, and results in a lower rate of angiographic restenosis as well as death, MI, and target vessel revascularization vs stenting preceded by balloon dilatation.

5b

5. Interventional Cardiology — b. Percutaneous Transluminal Coronary
Angioplasty vs Stenting vs Other Percutaneous Devices, IVUS-Guided Stenting

425

MultiLink Long Stents for Long Coronary Lesions

Title	Six-month angiographic and 12-month clinical follow-up of multiLink long (25 mm to 35 mm) stents for long coronary narrowing in patients with angina pectoris.
Authors	Ormiston JA, Webster MWI, Ruygrak PN, et al.
Reference	Am J Cardiol 2002;90:222-228.
Disease	Coronary artery disease.
Purpose	To determine the angiographic and clinical outcome of patients who receive stents for long coronary lesions.
Design	Prospective, multicenter registry.
Patients	120 patients who had stable or unstable angina or silent ischemia and an ejection fraction ≥40%. Patients had a single de novo stenosis greater than 20 mm long, in a native vessel ≥3 mm in diameter, which was amenable to a MultiLink stent 25-35 mm in length. Exclusion criteria included myocardial infarction in the previous 7 days and ejection fraction <30%. Lesion exclusion criteria were: previous intervention at the target site, diameter <3 mm, evidence of intracoronary thrombus, vessel blood supply from a venous or arterial surgically revascularized graft, significant calcification, aorto-ostial site, or presence of a side branch ≥2.5 mm in diameter that would be covered by the stent.
Follow-up	1 year.
Regimen	Stents were placed according to usual clinical practice. 1 long MultiLink (25-35 mm long) stent was required, and additional MultiLink stents could be used to cover the target area as needed. Residual stenosis of less than 20% was recommended. All patients received ≥100 mg/d of aspirin before the procedure, which was continued indefinitely. Ticlopidine 250-500 mg was given periprocedurally followed by 250 mg bid for 2 weeks thereafter.

Results   The clinical characteristics of the 120 patients were as fol-
           lows: mean age 59, 68% men, 46% were hypertensive, 59%
           had dyslipidemia, 11% had diabetes, 37% had a previous MI,
           16% were current smokers, 62% had stable angina, and 38%
           had unstable angina. 77% were on a β-blocker, 49% were
           on a calcium channel-blocker, 53% were on nitrates, 96%
           were on aspirin, 50% were on cholesterol-lowering drugs, and
           24% were on an ACE inhibitor. The average length of the
           stent placed was 35.8±14.6 mm, and the average lesion length
           was 30.1±13.5 mm. The minimum luminal diameter before
           stenting was 0.81±0.36 mm, after stenting 2.49±0.45 mm,
           and 1.64±0.61 mm at 6 months. The reference diameter was
           3.12±0.56 mm before stenting, 3.05±0.45 mm after stenting,
           and 2.90±0.55 mm at 6 months. Angiographic follow-up at
           6 months was available in 112 patients (93%). The percent
           stenosis was 74%±11% before stenting, 18%±8 % after stent-
           ing and 44%±19% at 6 months. The mean acute gain was
           1.68±0.48 mm, late loss 0.85±0.59 mm, and late loss index
           was 0.52±0.35. At 6 months, the rate of restenosis (≥50% loss
           of diameter) was 32%, and restenosis ≥70% occurred in 8%
           of patients. The rate of restenosis for lesions <35 mm (26%)
           was less than the rate for lesions ≥35 mm in length (44%),
           p=0.02. 12% of patients underwent or were scheduled for a
           repeat revascularization of the target vessel at 12 months.

Concl.   Stenting of long lesions was associated with a low rate of reste-
           nosis and a satisfactory clinical outcome.

A Randomized, Controlled Trial of the Use of Pulmonary-Artery Catheters in High-Risk Surgical Patients

Title	A randomized, controlled trial of the use of pulmonary-artery catheters in high-risk surgical patients.
Authors	Sandham JD, Hull RD, Brant RF, et al.
Reference	N Engl J Med 2003;348:5-14.
Disease	High-risk patients scheduled for urgent or elective major surgery followed in an intensive care unit environment.
Purpose	To compare treatment guided by use of a pulmonary artery catheter vs standard treatment (without the use of a pulmonary artery catheter) in a group of elderly surgical patients in the intensive care unit (ICU) considered to be high-risk.
Design	Multicenter, randomized, controlled.
Patients	1994 patients, 997 each in the catheter group and the standard group. Patients were ≥60 years and had American Society of Anesthesiologists (ASA) class III or IV risk, who were to undergo elective or urgent major abdominal, thoracic, vascular, or hip fracture surgery.
Follow-up	12 months.

Regimen   Patients in the standard care group underwent treatment without placement of a pulmonary-artery catheter. The measurement of the central venous pressure was permitted. Patients in the catheter group had a pulmonary artery catheter placed before surgery, and treatment was given according to prespecified goals and treatment priorities that were defined by consensus before study start. Treatment goals in order of priority were: oxygen delivery index of 550-600 mL/min/m^2 of body surface area; cardiac index of 3.5-4.5 L/min/mm^2, mean arterial wedge pressure of 70 mm Hg, pulmonary capillary wedge pressure of 18 mm Hg, heart rate <120 bpm; and hematocrit >27%. Therapy given in order to achieve these goals in the order of priority included: fluid loading, inotropic therapy, vasodilator therapy, vasopressors for hypotension, and blood transfusion for hematocrit <27%. Thromboprophylaxis was recommended to all patients using low-dose SC heparin, before and after surgery. The postoperative stay in the ICU was a minimum requirement of 24 hours.

5b

Results	The primary end point was inhospital mortality. The secondary end points were 6-month mortality, 12-month mortality, and inhospital morbidity. Morbidities included: MI, LV failure, arrhythmia, pneumonia, pulmonary embolism, renal insufficiency, liver insufficiency, and sepsis. The characteristics of patients in the 2 groups were similar at baseline. Inhospital mortality was similar between the 2 groups: (standard care vs catheter group: 7.7% vs 7.8%; p=0.93). 6-month survival was also similar between the 2 groups (standard care vs catheter group: 88.1% vs 87.4%), as was 12-month survival: (standard care vs catheter group: 83.9% vs 83.0%). The difference in survival at 6 months was -0.7 percentage points (95% CI= -3.6 to 2.2) and at 12 months was -0.9 percentage points (95% CI=-4.3 to 2.4). After adjustment for age, history of angina, type of surgery, preoperative ASA risk class, Goldman index, and hemoglobin level, the adjusted risk ratio for death in the catheter group was 1.0 (95% CI=0.7-1.3). The incidence of pulmonary embolism was higher in the catheter group (0 pulmonary embolisms in standard group vs 8 in catheter group; p=0.004). The incidence of MI, CHF, supraventricular tachycardia, ventricular tachycardia, hepatic insufficiency, sepsis from the central venous catheter or pulmonary artery catheter, and pneumonia were similar between the two groups. 15 patients in the catheter group had an adverse effect from the use of the catheter. Patients in the catheter group were more likely to have received inotropic agents (48.9% vs 32.8%, p<0.001), vasodilators (8.5% vs 3.9%, p<0.001), antihypertensive medication (25.5% vs 16.9%, p<0.001), packed red blood cells (56.6% vs 47.0%, p<0.001), and colloid (54.8% vs 47.7%, p=0.002). Central venous pressure was similar between the two groups.
Concl.	There was no evidence of benefit from treatment directed by a pulmonary artery catheter vs standard care in a group of high-risk elderly surgical patients.

ABACAS

Adjunctive Balloon Angioplasty After Coronary Atherectomy Study

Title	Effects of adjunctive balloon angioplasty after intravascular ultrasound guided optimal directional coronary atherectomy. The results of ABACAS.
Authors	Suzuki T, Hosokawa H, Katoh O, et al.
Reference	J Am Coll Cardiol 1999;34:1028-1035.
Disease	Coronary artery disease.
Purpose	To determine the effect of adjunctive PTCA after directional coronary atherectomy vs stand alone atherectomy and to assess the outcome of intravascular ultrasound guided, aggressive atherectomy.
Design	Prospective, randomized, multicenter.
Patients	225 patients who had intravascular ultrasound guided directional coronary artherectomy. Optimal debulking was achieved in 214 patients who were than randomized to no further therapy or PTCA.
Follow-up	12 months.
Regimen	Directional coronary atherectomy with a Simpson Coronary AtheroCath and guidance with intravascular ultrasound to obtain angiographic criteria of <30% or adequate debulking (estimated plaque area <50%). Patients randomized to adjunctive PTCA or no further therapy.
Add'l Tx	IV nitroglycerin during procedure.

5b

5. Interventional Cardiology — b. Percutaneous Transluminal Coronary Angioplasty vs Stenting vs Other Percutaneous Devices, IVUS-Guided Stenting

431

Results	Primary end point was angiographic restenosis rate at 6 months (>50% stenosis by angiography). Quantitative coronary angiography and quantitative coronary ultrasound also assessed. Secondary end point was clinical event rate (death, MI, target vessel revascularizaton) at 6 months. Acute post-procedure analysis revealed an improved minimum luminal diameter (2.88±0.48) in the adjunctive PTCA group vs the no further therapy group (2.6±0.51 mm; p=0.006). The adjunctive PTCA group had less residual stenosis (10.8% vs 15%; p=0.009). Acute quantitative ultrasound also showed a larger minimum luminal diameter (3.26±0.48 mm) in the adjunctive PTCA group vs the no further therapy group (3.04±0.5 mm; p<0.001). The adjunctive PTCA group also had a lower residual plaque mass (42.6%) vs the no therapy group (45.6%; p<0.001) on the ultrasound. However, at 6 months minimal luminal diameter was 33.4±19.9 mm in the adjunctive PTCA group vs 32.3±15.9 in the no further therapy group (p=NS); and restenosis rates were 23.6% for adjunctive PTCA vs 19.6% for the no further therapy group (p=NS). Cumulative clinical event rate at 6 months was 20.6% in the adjunctive PTCA group and 17.1% in the no further therapy group (p=NS). At 12 months there also was no difference between groups.
Concl.	Adjunctive PTCA following aggressive directional atherectomy improved acute quantitative coronary angiographic and intravascular ultrasound outcomes. The benefit was not maintained at 6 months. Adjunctive PTCA also did not improve clinical outcomes over aggressive ultrasound guided directional atherectomy alone.

ADVANCE

Additional Value of NIR Stents for Treatment of Long Coronary Lesions

Title	A randomized comparison of the value of additional stenting after optimal balloon angioplasty for long coronary lesions.
Authors	Serruys PW, Foley DP, Suttorp M-J, et al.
Reference	J Am Coll Cardiol 2002;39:393-399.
Disease	Coronary artery disease.
Purpose	To determine if there were benefits to additional stent implantation following optimal balloon angioplasty in long coronary artery lesions.
Design	Randomized, multicenter.
Patients	437 patients with stable or unstable angina, reversible ischemia due to single and native coronary lesion 20-50 mm in length.
Follow-up	9 months.
Regimen	Following baseline angiography with quantitative coronary angiography, target lesion balloon angioplasty was performed to achieve a diameter stenosis of <30%. When optimal result was achieved patients were randomized to no further therapy vs additional stenting. Bail-out stenting reserved for cases where repeated stenosis <50% or dissections, or reduction in TIMI flow.
Add'l Tx	Ticlopidine or clopidogrel given to all patients within 12 hours before intervention and for 1 month. Heparin given for the procedure. Aspirin given for the procedure and then indefinitely.

5. Interventional Cardiology — b. Percutaneous Transluminal Coronary
Angioplasty vs Stenting vs Other Percutaneous Devices, IVUS-Guided Stenting

433

Results | Of 437 patients, 149 (34%) underwent bail-out stenting. Bail-out stenting was associated with more periprocedural myocardial infarction (MI) (3-fold increase). 288 patients were randomized to additional stenting (n=145) or to no stenting (n=143). Primary end point was major adverse cardiac events (MACE) during 9 months of follow-up, defined as: cardiac death, MI, coronary artery bypass graft surgery (CABG), or repeat percutaneous transluminal coronary angioplasty (PTCA) that is target vessel revascularization. Besides initial angiography, follow-up angiograms performed in randomized patients at about 6 months. Angiographic success rate was 95.1% in control and 95.9% in additional stenting group. Procedural success defined by angiography and the absence of MACE during hospitalization, was 90% for the control group and 93% in the additional stent group. Additional stenting led to decreased angiographic restenosis (27% vs 42%; p=0.022), and greater gain (mm) in coronary diameter (1.47±0.47 mm vs 0.92±0.39 mm) compared to controls. Freedom from MACE was the same in both groups at 93% in the control group and 97% in the additional stent group at 31 days by intention-to-treat. At 300 days, MACE was 77% in both groups.

Concl. | Provisional stenting for long coronary lesions resulted in lower angiographic restenosis rate but no improvement in MACE at 9 months vs angioplasty without additional stenting. Bail-out stenting for long coronary lesions occurred in about one third of patients and was associated with an increase in periprocedural MIs.

ARTIST

Angioplasty vs Rotational Atherectomy for the Treatment of Diffuse In-Stent Restenosis Trial

Title	Rotational atherectomy does not reduce recurrent in-stent restenosis.
Authors	vom Dahl J, Dietz U, Haager PK, et al.
Reference	Circulation 2002;105:583-588.
Disease	Coronary artery disease.
Purpose	To compare rotational atherectomy followed by percutaneous transluminal coronary angioplasty (PTCA) with PTCA alone in patients with diffuse in-stent restenosis.
Design	Multicenter, randomized.
Patients	298 patients with in-stent restenosis, angina, or target vessel-related ischemia. In-stent restenosis of >70% and length of in-stent restenosis of 10-50 mm.
Follow-up	6 months.
Regimen	Rotational atherectomy (burr: artery [stent] ratio of ≥0.7, 160,000 rpm then 140,000 rpm later in the study; followed by adjunctive low pressure PTCA; vs PTCA.
Add'l Tx	Heparin, aspirin, ticlopidine.

5b

Results	146 patients received PTCA and 152 patients received rotational atherectomy. Initial procedural success rates defined as residual stenosis <30% was achieved in 89% of angioplasty and 88% of rotational atherectomy group. However, at 6-month angiography the net gain in minimal luminal diameter was 0.67 mm for PTCA and 0.45 mm for rotational atherectomy (p=0.0019). Restenosis ≥50% rates were 51% in the angioplasty group and 65% in the rotational atherectomy group (p=0.039). Mean percent diameter stenosis was 55.7% for angioplasty and 63.6% for rotational atherectomy (p=0.005). In an intravascular ultrasound subgroup there was less over-expansion during PTCA after rotational atherectomy. Event-free survival (absence of death, myocardial infarction, or clinically driven target lesion revascularization) was 91.3% in the angioplasty group vs 79.6% in the atherectomy group (p=0.0052).
Concl.	PTCA resulted in better long-term outcome than rotational atherectomy followed by adjunctive low pressure PTCA, for patients with in-stent restenosis.

ARTIST (Substudy)

Angioplasty vs Rotational Atherectomy for the Treatment of Diffuse In-Stent Restenosis Trial

Title	Angiographic analysis of the angioplasty vs rotational atherectomy for the treatment of diffuse in-stent restenosis trial (ARTIST).
Authors	Dietz U, Rupprecht HJ, de Belder MA, et al.
Reference	Am J Cardiol 2002;90:843-847.
Disease	Coronary artery disease, restenosis, percutaneous coronary intervention.
Purpose	To compare the acute and long-term outcomes of balloon angioplasty and rotational ablation for diffuse in-stent restenosis.
Design	Randomized, open label, multicenter.
Patients	298 patients with stable angina and/or evidence of effort-induced myocardial ischemia 2-12 months after 10-50 mm stent implantation with angiographic evidence of ≥70% in-stent restenosis. Patients with <2.5 mm in diameter stents and not fully expanded stents or those with planned multi-lesion interventions were excluded.
Follow-up	6 months.
Regimen	Patients were randomized to balloon angioplasty (PTCA) (n=146) or percutaneous transluminal rotational ablation (PTCR) (n=152).
Add'l Tx	All patients received aspirin 100 mg/d for 6 months and ticlopidine or clopidogrel for ≥2 weeks.

5b

5. Interventional Cardiology — b. Percutaneous Transluminal Coronary
Angioplasty vs Stenting vs Other Percutaneous Devices, IVUS-Guided Stenting

437

Results	Clinical and angiographic success were achieved in 86% and 95.2% of the patients in the PTCA group, respectively, and in 84% and 94.7% of the patients in the PTCR group, respectively (p=NS). More patients were crossed over from PTCR to PTCA (8/152) than from PTCA to PTCR (1/146; p=0.037). Immediately after procedure the diameter stenosis was reduced from 80%±12% to 29%±10% in the PTCA group and from 80±11% to 28±12% in the PTCR group. The minimal lumen diameter (MLD) increased from 0.55±0.3 mm to 1.9±0.3 mm in the PTCA group and from 0.54±0.3 mm to 1.9±0.4 mm in the PTCR group. Spasm (17.7% vs 8.6%; p=0.001) and intermittent slow flow (5.3% vs 0%; p=0.007) occurred more often with PTCR than with PTCA. A total of 123 patients in the PTCA group and 131 patients in the PTCR group underwent repeat coronary angiography at 6 months. After 6 months, the percent diameter stenosis was 56±20% in the PTCA group and 64±22% in the PTCR group (p=0.005). MLD was 1.2±0.6 mm and 1.0±0.6 mm, respectively (p=0.008). The restenosis rate was 51.2% with PTCA and 64.9% with PTCR (p=0.027). Late vessel occlusion occurred more often with PTCR (7.6% vs 1.6%; p=0.03). Procedural factors did not influence long-term outcome. In the PTCR group there was an inverse correlation between the vessel diameter size and restenosis rate.
Concl.	The immediate angiographic and clinical results of PTCA and PTCR of diffuse in-stent restenosis were comparable. However, PTCR resulted in more restenosis than PTCA.

ASCENT

ACS MultiLink Stent Clinical Equivalence in De Novo Lesions Trial

Title	Final results of a randomized trial comparing the MULTI-LINK stent with the Palmaz-Schatz stent for narrowings in native coronary arteries.
Authors	Baim DS, Cutlip DE, Midei M, et al.
Reference	Am J Cardiol 2001;87:157-162.
Disease	Coronary artery disease, stent, percutaneous coronary intervention.
Purpose	To show equivalence of the results of the MULTI-LINK stent (Guidant, Santa Clara, CA) and the Palmaz-Schatz stent (Cordis, Johnson & Johnson Interventional Systems, Miami, FL) in single de novo native coronary artery lesions.
Design	Randomized, open-label, multicenter.
Patients	1040 patients, >18 years old, with angina pectoris or objective evidence of myocardial ischemia, with a <20 mm de novo 50%-99% diameter stenotic lesion in a native coronary artery with a reference artery diameter of 3.0-3.75 mm. Patients who underwent pretreatment with nonballoon device, those with a need to stent across a large side branch, recent myocardial infarction, a neurologic event within the last 6 months, bleeding disorder, or intolerance to aspirin or ticlopidine were excluded.
Follow-up	9-month clinical follow-up. A subset of 538 patients was also scheduled for repeated angiography at 9 months.
Regimen	Randomization to MULTI-LINK stent or Palmaz-Schatz stent.
Add'l Tx	All patients received aspirin, started before PCI and intravenous heparin during PCI (target activated clotting time >275 sec). After stenting, all patients received aspirin 325 mg/d and ticlopidine 250 mg bid for 4 weeks.

5b

Results	Device success was 97.9% with the MULTI-LINK and 96.5% with the Palmaz-Schatz stent. Failure to place the stent occurred in 2.5% vs 4.2% of the patients, respectively (p=0.12). In 1.2% of the MULTI-LINK and 3.1% of the Palmaz-Schatz group, the randomized stent was not delivered. Procedural success was 95.7% with the MULTI-LINK and 93.9% with the Palmaz-Schatz stents. Postprocedural in-stent residual stenosis was 8±11% in the MULTI-LINK vs 10±12% in the Palmaz-Schatz group (p=0.04). Major adverse events occurred within 30 days in 5.0% vs 6.5%, respectively (p>0.20). Zero patients in the MULTI-LINK group vs 6 in the Palmaz-Schatz group died within 30 days (incidence 0% vs 1.1%; p=0.03). At 9 months, 7.7% of the patients in the MULTI-LINK vs 9.8% in the Palmaz-Schatz underwent target lesion revascularization. Target vessel failure occurred in 15.1% vs 16.7%, respectively (p<0.001 by test for equivalency). Angiographic restenosis at 9 months occurred in 16.0% of the MULTI-LINK group vs 22.1% in the Palmaz-Schatz group (p=0.31).
Concl.	The deliverability, acute and 9-month clinical and angiographic results of the MULTI-LINK stent were equivalent or better than the results of the Palmaz-Schatz stent.

BENESTENT-I (5-Year Follow-Up)

Belgium Netherlands Stent

Title	Continued benefit of coronary stenting versus balloon angioplasty: 5-year clinical follow-up of BENESTENT-I trial.
Authors	Kiemeneij F, Serruys PW, Macaya C, et al.
Reference	a. N Engl J Med 1994;331:489-495. b. J Am Coll Cardiol 1996;27:255-261. c. J Am Coll Cardiol 2001;37:1598-1600.
Disease	Coronary artery disease.
Purpose	To determine whether early favorable results in BENESTENT-I randomized trial of Palmaz-Schatz stent vs balloon angioplasty in patients with stable angina was maintained at 5 years.
Design	Randomized, multicenter.
Patients	516 patients with stable angina, single de novo lesion <15 mm in length suitable for a stent and coronary artery >3 mm in diameter.
Follow-up	5 years.
Regimen	Randomized to either Palmaz-Schatz stent (n=259) implant or balloon angioplasty (n=257).
Add'l Tx	Heparin, oral anticoagulation for 3 months in-stent group. Balloon group received heparin, calcium antagonists, aspirin, dipyridamole.

Results	Primary clinical end points included death, cerebrovascular accident, Q-wave MI, non-Q-wave MI, CABG or second percutaneous coronary intervention of previously treated lesion. At 5 years data were available from 511 patients. Of 256 patients randomized to stenting, 168 (65.6%) were free of major adverse cardiac and cerebrovascular events vs 153 of 256 (59.8%) patients randomized to PTCA (p=0.20). In-stent group vs PTCA group 5-year incidence of mortality was 5.9% vs 3.1%, respectively; 5-year incidence of cerebrovascular accident was 0.8% vs 1.2%, Q-wave MI was 7.8% vs 3.9%; non-Q-wave MI was 1.6 vs 2.3%; CABG 11.7% vs 9.8%; (p=NS for all). 17.2% of patients in the stent group underwent target lesion revascularization with second percutaneous coronary intervention vs 27.3% in the PTCA group (p=0.008). Anginal class and use of cardiac medicines was similar between groups at 5 years. Use of nitrates was lower in the stent group.
Concl.	Original 10% absolute difference in target lesion revascularization was maintained long-term by stenting.

BESMART

Bestent in Small Arteries

Title	Stent placement compared with balloon angioplasty for small coronary arteries.
Authors	Koning R, Eltchaninoff H, Commeau P, et al.
Reference	Circulation 2001;104:1604-1608.
Disease	Coronary artery disease.
Purpose	To determine whether stenting in small coronary artery vessels might lead to better clinical results and lower restenosis rates.
Design	Prospective, randomized, multicenter.
Patients	381 symptomatic coronary artery patients with de novo focal lesions in a small coronary segment (<3 mm). The angiographic lesion had to be ≥50% stenosis.
Follow-up	6-month angiographic follow-up.
Regimen	Patients were randomly assigned to either stent placement (n=192) or balloon angioplasty (n=189). The Bestent small for 2.5-3.0 mm diameter vessels were used in all cases with balloon predilation.
Add'l Tx	Heparin, aspirin. In stent patients, ticlopidine for 1 month.

5. Interventional Cardiology — b. Percutaneous Transluminal Coronary
Angioplasty vs Stenting vs Other Percutaneous Devices, IVUS-Guided Stenting

443

Results	Primary end point was restenosis rate ≥50% measured by quantitative coronary angiography. Initial angiographic procedural success rate was 97.9% in the stent group and 93.9% in the angioplasty group (p=NS). Rate for in-hospital major adverse cardiac events was similar in the 2 groups. There were no in-hospital deaths. There was 1 Q-wave MI in each group. At 6 months, restenosis occurred in 21% of lesions in stent patients vs 47% of the angioplasty patients (p=0.0001), for a risk reduction of 55%. Following the initial procedure there was a large acute gain with stent placement (1.35±0.45) vs 0.94±0.47 mm in the balloon group; p=0.0001. This resulted in a larger minimal lumen diameter in the stent group (2.06±0.42 mm) vs the balloon group (1.70±0.46 mm; p=0.0001). There was a reduction in repeat target lesion revascularization in the stent group (13%) vs the balloon group (25%; p=0.0006). There were no significant differences in death or MI at 6 months between groups.
Concl.	Elective stent deployment in small coronary arteries with focal de novo lesions reduced restenosis rates and subsequent target vessel revascularization at 6 months.

BET

Benefit Evaluation of Direct Coronary Stenting

Title	Comparison of direct coronary stenting with and without balloon predilatation in patients with stable angina pectoris.
Authors	Carrié D, Khalife K, Citron B, et al.
Reference	Am J Cardiol 2001;87:693-698.
Disease	Coronary artery disease, percutaneous coronary intervention.
Purpose	To compare the feasibility and 6-month clinical outcome of primary coronary artery stenting without balloon predilatation and standard stenting with balloon predilatation.
Design	Randomized, open-label, single-center.
Patients	338 patients with stable angina, scheduled to undergo PCI of a single de novo lesion in a native coronary artery without contraindication to anticoagulant therapy or antiplatelet agents. Patients with unstable angina or myocardial infarction within the previous 2 days were excluded. Only patients with ≥70% diameter stenosis, a lesion length ≤15 mm and a reference vessel diameter of ≥2.5 mm were included. Patients with an ostial lesion, a bifurcational lesion, a highly calcified lesion, severe vessel tortuosity, thrombotic lesion, or a lesion in a previously grafted artery were not included.
Follow-up	8 month clinical follow-up.
Regimen	Randomization to direct (without balloon predilatation) (n=173) or conventional (with balloon predilatation) (n=165) coronary artery stenting (Tenax coronary stent, Biotronik Inc., Berlin, Germany).
Add'l Tx	All patients received aspirin 250 mg/d, started 24 hours before PCI, and intravenous heparin during procedure. Abciximab was administered at the discretion of the treating physician. After PCI, all patients received ticlopidine 500 mg/d for 1 month and aspirin 100-250 mg/d.

5b

5. Interventional Cardiology — b. Percutaneous Transluminal Coronary
Angioplasty vs Stenting vs Other Percutaneous Devices, IVUS-Guided Stenting

445

Results	355 stents were implanted in 338 patients. In 13.9% of the cases in the direct stenting group, the operator was unable to cross the lesion with the stent. Procedural success was achieved in 97.5% of the patients in the conventional stenting group vs 98.3% in the direct stenting group (p=NS). Residual stenosis after stent implantation was 13.04±8.3% in the direct stenting group and 11.54±7.4% in the conventional stenting group. Subacute closure occurred in 1 patient in each group. There was no in-hospital repeat revascularization in both groups. CK elevation >150 IU/mL occurred in 5 patients in the conventional stenting and 3 patients in the direct stenting group. The duration of the procedure was 10.34±6.30 minutes with the conventional stenting and 7.04±6.52 minutes for the direct stenting group (p<0.0001). The quantity of contrast media used was 156.7±87.3 mL vs 135.5±85.3 mL, respectively (p<0.3). The procedural cost was $1164.6±389.9 vs $956.4±352.2, respectively (p<0.0001). After 8 months of follow-up, 5.5% of the patients in the conventional stenting vs 3.5% in the direct stenting group underwent target vessel revascularization. Major adverse cardiac events (death, myocardial infarction or repeat target lesion revascularization) occurred in 11.4% vs 5.3% of the patients, respectively (p=NS). Multivariate analysis showed that major adverse cardiac events were unrelated to the technique of stenting, but to the stent length and diameter and to the complexity of the lesion (type C).
Concl.	Direct stenting without predilatation was safe and associated with shorter procedure length and lower costs, without increasing the rates of in-hospital and 8-month clinical adverse events.

BET

Benefit Evaluation of Direct Coronary Stenting

Title	Is direct coronary stenting the best strategy for long-term outcome? Results of a multicentric randomized BET study.
Authors	Elbaz MN, El Mokhtar E, Khalife K, et al.
Reference	Am Heart J 2002;144:e7.
Disease	Coronary artery disease, percutaneous coronary intervention.
Purpose	To compare the long-term outcome after direct coronary stenting and stenting after balloon predilatation.
Design	Randomized, open-label, multicenter.
Patients	338 patients scheduled to undergo percutaneous coronary intervention because of stable angina caused by a single de novo lesion in a coronary artery. Patients with contraindications to anticoagulation or antiplatelet therapy were excluded. Patients with unstable angina or recent (<2 days) myocardial infarction were excluded. Angiographic inclusion criteria were ≥70% diameter stenosis in a vessel with a reference diameter ≥2.5 mm, lesion length ≤15 mm, and ability to cover the lesion with 1 stent. Patients with ostial lesion, bifurcational lesion, a highly calcified lesion, severe vessel tortuosity, thrombus-containing lesion, or a lesion in a previously grafted artery were not included.
Follow-up	Mean 16.4±4.6 months (range 3.1-23.7 months).
Regimen	Randomized to direct stenting (n=173) or balloon predilatation followed by stenting (n=165).
Add'l Tx	All patients received aspirin 250 mg within 24 hours before PCI. All patients received IV heparin during procedure. Abciximab was administered when needed. All patients received ticlopidine 500 mg/d for 1 month. 100-250 mg/d aspirin was given to all patients.

5b

Results	In 13.9% of the patients assigned direct stenting, the stent could not cross the lesion. In all cases the stent was withdrawn and balloon predilatation was performed. Glycoprotein IIb/IIIa inhibitors were used in 2.4% and 0.5% of the predilatation and direct stenting groups, respectively. Minimal lumen diameter postprocedure was 2.84±0.44 mm in the predilatation group and 2.83±0.52 mm in the primary stenting group (p=NS). The percent diameter stenosis after PCI was comparable between the groups (11.54%±7.4% vs 13.04%±8.3%, respectively; p=NS). Clinical success was 97.5% with predilatation and 98.3% with direct stenting (p=NS). There was no significant difference in the rate of in-hospital MI, subacute thrombosis, or death between the groups. During follow-up, major adverse cardiac events occurred in 11.3% of the patients in the predilatation group vs 18.2% in the primary stenting group (p=NS). 5.2% of the patients in the predilatation group vs 7% in the primary stenting group underwent target lesion revascularization (p=NS). At 12 months, major adverse cardiac events occurred in 9.1% vs 10.8% of the patients, respectively (p=NS). Multivariate regression analysis showed that direct stenting had no significant effect on the risk of major adverse cardiac events.
Concl.	The long-term clinical outcomes after a strategy of direct stenting and stenting after conventional balloon predilatation were comparable.

CAPAS

Cutting Balloon Angioplasty vs Plain Old Balloon Angioplasty Randomized Study in Type B/C Lesions

Title	Final results of the CAPAS trial.
Authors	Izumi M, Tsuchikane E, Funamoto M, et al.
Reference	Am Heart J 2001;142:782-789.
Disease	Coronary artery disease, percutaneous coronary intervention (PCI).
Purpose	To compare cutting balloon angioplasty (CBA) with balloon angioplasty (PTCA) in small coronary arteries.
Design	Randomized, single-center, open-label.
Patients	232 patients (248 lesions) with American College of Cardiology/American Heart Association type B or C lesions in a <3.0 mm diameter target native coronary artery. Heavily calcified or angulated lesions were excluded. Unprotected left main lesions, bypass graft lesions, and culprit lesions of a recent (<1 month) acute myocardial infarction were not included.
Follow-up	Repeat angiography at 90 days. Clinical follow-up for 1 year.
Regimen	Randomization to CBA (n=120) or PTCA (n=128).
Add'l Tx	All patients received IV heparin (150 IU/kg) and intracoronary nitroglycerin (200-300 mg). After PCI, all patients received aspirin, ticlopidine, or cilostazol for >3 months.

5b

5. Interventional Cardiology — b. Percutaneous Transluminal Coronary
Angioplasty vs Stenting vs Other Percutaneous Devices, IVUS-Guided Stenting

449

Results	Residual stenosis >50% after PCI was detected in 1.7% of the lesions in the CBA and in 3.9% in the PTCA group (p=0.287). Stents were implanted in 5.8% and 8.6% of the lesions, respectively (p=0.402). In 6.7% of the lesions assigned to CBA there was delivery failure and crossover to PTCA. Final balloon size was comparable between the groups (2.64±0.42 mm and 2.61±0.35 mm; p=0.665). However, maximal inflation pressure was lower with CBA (6.4±1.4 ATM vs 8.8±2.7 ATM; p<0.0001). No perforations were noted in either group. Procedural success was 98.3% with CBA and 96.1% with PTCA. Residual diameter stenosis after PCI was 26.2%±11.7% with CBA and 28.9%±10.3% with PTCA (p=0.072). At 90 days, the percent diameter stenosis was 40.8%±19.2% and 47.5%±20.4%, respectively (p=0.011). Immediately after PCI the minimal lumen diameter was 1.65±0.39 mm with CBA and 1.63±0.45 mm with PTCA (p=0.663). At 90 days minimal lumen diameter was 1.31±0.48 mm and 1.18±0.58 mm, respectively (p=0.080). Restenosis was noted in 25.2% of the CBA treated lesions vs 41.5% in the PTCA treated lesions (p=0.009). In lesions with reference diameter of <2.25 mm, restenosis occurred in 24.2% in the CBA and in 49.2% in the PTCA group (p=0.003). In lesions with reference diameter ≥2.25 mm, there was no significant difference in restenosis between CBA (26.7%) and PTCA (33.3%; p=0.472). 1-year mortality was comparable (2.6% and 2.5%, respectively; p=0.986). None of the patients had Q-wave myocardial infarction or needed emergency CABG. 22.1% of the lesions in the CBA and 33.9% in the PTCA group underwent target lesion revascularization (p=0.049), and 24.8% vs 36.4%, respectively, underwent target vessel revascularization (p=0.050). Major adverse cardiac events occurred in 27.2% and 39.0% of the CBA and PTCA treated lesions (p=0.047).
Concl.	Cutting balloon angioplasty was superior to balloon angioplasty for revascularization of small coronary arteries.

COBRA

Comparison of Balloon Angioplasty vs Rotational Atherectomy

Title	A randomized comparison of balloon angioplasty vs rotational atherectomy in complex coronary lesions (COBRA study).
Authors	Dill T, Dietz U, Hamm CW, et al.
Reference	Eur Heart J 2000;21:1759-1766.
Disease	Coronary artery disease.
Purpose	To compare the short- and long-term effects of percutaneous transluminal coronary angioplasty and rotational atherectomy in patients with complex coronary artery lesions.
Design	Randomized, open-label, multicenter.
Patients	502 patients, 20-80 years old, with angiographically documented coronary artery disease and angina pectoris. The target coronary artery lesion should have to be with 70%-99% luminal area stenosis with minimal lumen diameter of ≤1 mm for a length of ≥5 mm. The lesion should be complex (calcified, ostial or bifrucational, eccentric, diffuse or within angulated segment). Patients with unstable angina, recent (<4 weeks) myocardial infarction, previous percutaneous coronary intervention of the target vessel within 2 months, left ventricular ejection fraction <30% were excluded.
Follow-up	Clinical follow-up and repeated angiography at 6 months.
Regimen	Randomization to rotablation (burr sizes 1.25-2.5 mm) or balloon angioplasty.
Add'l Tx	All patients received aspirin, nitroglycerin, nifedipine and heparin (15,000-20,000 units with a target activated clotting time of ≥350 seconds). The use of stents for bail out or unsatisfactory results was permitted.

5b

Results	250 patients were randomized to PTCA and 252 to rotablation. 5 patients did not undergo the randomized intervention. The procedure was complicated by spasm in 23.0% of the patients in the rotablation group vs only 2.8% in the angioplasty group (p=0.0001). Transient vessel occlusion occurred in 5.6% and 2.8% of the patients, respectively (p=0.29). Slow flow was observed in 6.4% and 2.0%, respectively (p=0.024). Stents were used in 14.9% of the patients in the angioplasty group vs 6.4% in the rotablation group (p=0.002). The procedural success rate was 78% in the angioplasty group vs 85% in the rotablation group (p=0.038). 4% of the patients were crossed over from angioplasty to rotablation and 10% from rotablation to angioplasty. Death occurred in 1.6% of the patients in the angioplasty group vs 0.4% in the rotablation group (p=0.18). There was no difference in the rates of Q-wave myocardial infarction (1.6% vs 2.4%) or emergency CABG (1.2% vs 2.4%) between the angioplasty and rotablation groups. At 6 months, target vessel revascularizations were done in 23% of the angioplasty group vs 21% of the rotablation group. 6.5% of the patients in the angioplasty group and 4.2% of the patients in the rotablation group underwent CABG. After 6 months 63.8% of the patients in the angioplasty group vs 59.4% in the rotablation group were free of angina (p=0.37). There was no difference between the groups with respect to exercise tolerance. There was no difference in acute gain and late lumen diameter loss between the groups. Restenosis occurred in 51.1% of the angioplasty group vs 48.9% in the rotablation group (p=0.333).
Concl.	There were no significant differences in short- and long-term clinical and angiographic results between standard angioplasty and rotablation for complex coronary artery lesions.

CRUISE

Can Routine Ultrasound Influence Stent Expansion?

Title	Final results of the Can Routine Ultrasound Influence Stent Expansion (CRUISE) study.
Authors	Fitzgerald PJ, Oshima A, Hayase M, et al.
Reference	Circulation 2000;102:523-530.
Disease	Coronary artery disease.
Purpose	To determine whether routine intravascular ultrasound guidance of stent implantation improves clinical outcome vs angiographic guidance alone.
Design	Multicenter; use of intravascular ultrasound (IVUS) assigned to certain centers as part of Stent Anti-Thrombotic Regimen Study (STARS).
Patients	525 patients undergoing stent implantation for symptomatic ischemic heart disease, new lesions or restenotic lesions of native coronaries, and planned stent implantation; up to 2 stents per patient.
Follow-up	9 months.
Regimen	9 centers prospectively assigned to stent deployment with use of ultrasound guidance; 7 centers assigned to angiographic guidance alone with documentary (blinded) IVUS at conclusion of procedure.
Add'l Tx	As per STARS trial, patients randomly assigned to aspirin alone, aspirin plus ticlopidine, or aspirin plus cumarin.

5b

5. Interventional Cardiology — b. Percutaneous Transluminal Coronary Angioplasty vs Stenting vs Other Percutaneous Devices, IVUS-Guided Stenting

453

Results	Primary end point was post procedural minimal stent dimensions determined by angiography and IVUS. Secondary end point was major cardiac events (death, Q-wave MI, target vessel revascularization) at 9 months. IVUS guided patients demonstrated a larger minimal lumen diameter than angiographic guidance alone (2.9±0.4 vs 2.7±0.5 mm; p<0.001) by quantitative coronary angiography and a larger minimal stent area by quantitative IVUS (7.78±1.72 vs 7.06±2.13 mm^2; p<0.001). Target vessel revascularization occurred less frequently with IVUS guidance (8.5%) vs angiographic guidance alone (15.3%; p<0.05). There was no difference in incidence of death or MI between groups.
Concl.	IVUS guidance of stent deployment resulted in more effective stent expansion compared with angiographic guidance alone.

DANSTENT

The Danish Multicenter Stent Study

Title	Low restenosis rate of the NIR coronary stent: results of the Danish multicenter stent study (DANSTENT)—a randomized trial comparing a first-generation stent with a second-generation stent.
Authors	Jorgensen E, Kelbaek H, Helqvist S, et al.
Reference	Am Heart J 2003;145:e5.
Disease	Coronary artery disease, stent, restenosis.
Purpose	To compare the outcomes after implantation of a first-generation Palmaz-Schatz stent and a second-generation stainless NIR stent.
Design	Randomized, open-label, multicenter.
Patients	424 patients scheduled for percutaneous coronary intervention because of stable or unstable angina or silent ischemia, and de novo coronary lesion in a native coronary artery that could be covered by a 15 mm-long stent in a coronary artery with a reference diameter of 2.5-4.5 mm. Patients with recent myocardial infarction, child-bearing potential, severe chronic disease, malignancy, renal insufficiency, intolerance to aspirin or ticlopidine, and patients with ostial, bifurcational, or heavily calcified lesions were excluded. In addition, patients with unprotected left main lesion and with thrombus-containing lesions were not included.
Follow-up	1-year clinical follow-up with repeat angiography at 6 months.
Regimen	After balloon angioplasty, patients were randomized to Palmaz-Schatz (n=210) or NIR stent (n=214) implantation.
Add'l Tx	All patients received aspirin ≥75 mg and ticlopidine 500 mg before stent implantation. Heparin was given during the procedure. Ticlopidine was given for 1 month.

5b

5. Interventional Cardiology — b. Percutaneous Transluminal Coronary
Angioplasty vs Stenting vs Other Percutaneous Devices, IVUS-Guided Stenting

455

Results	Crossover to other stent or balloon occurred in 0.4% of the patients in the NIR stent and in 3.4% in the Palmaz-Schatz (PS) stent group (p=0.02). The overall procedure success rate was 98% with the NIR stent and 99% with the PS stent (p=0.90). Minimal lumen diameter (MLD) immediately post-procedure was larger in the NIR stent group (2.97±0.64 mm vs 2.87±0.59 mm; p=0.004). 91% of the patients underwent repeat coronary angiography at 6 months. Follow-up angiography showed that MLD was 2.21±0.80 mm in the NIR stent group and 2.23±0.88 mm in the PS stent group (p=0.76). Accordingly, the late loss was significantly larger in the NIR stent group (0.65±0.69 mm vs 0.57±0.66 mm; p=0.02). There was no difference in percent diameter stenosis at follow-up between the NIR and PS stent group (25.2±19.0% vs 26.3±22.5%; p=0.87). Restenosis rate was comparable (9.9% vs 12.6%, respectively; p=0.35). Total mortality was 1.9% in the NIR stent group and 0.5% in the PS stent group (p=0.37). MI occurred in 4.2% and 2.9% of the patients, respectively (p=0.60). Target lesion revascularization was done in 11.7% and 9.5% of the patients, respectively (p=0.47). Any major adverse cardiac events occurred in 15.9% and 11.9% of the NIR and PS stent groups, respectively (p=0.24). Multivariate regression analysis did not show that the type of stent affected restenosis rate.
Concl.	The angiographic and clinical outcomes after NIR stent implantation were comparable to those of first-generation PS stent implantation.

DEBATE II

Doppler End Points Balloon Angioplasty Trial Europe II

Title	Randomized comparison of primary stenting and provisional balloon angioplasty guided by velocity measurement.
Authors	Serruys PW, de Bruyne B, Carlier S, et al.
Reference	Circulation 2000;102:2930-2937.
Disease	Coronary artery disease.
Purpose	To determine whether elective treatment should be by stenting or whether limited stent use should be reserved for patients with a suboptimal result after angioplasty (provisional angioplasty). Determine costs of these approaches. To determine whether optimal balloon angioplasty obtains additional benefit from stenting.
Design	Randomized, multicenter.
Patients	CAD patients scheduled for single-vessel angioplasty. 97 patients received primary stenting; 523 patients received balloon angioplasty guided by Doppler flow velocity and angiography.
Follow-up	1 year.
Regimen	Patients initially randomized to primary stenting vs percutaneous transluminal coronary angioplasty guided by Doppler flow velocity and angiography. Patients in latter group further randomized after optimization of PTCA to either additional stenting or termination of procedure. Optimal PTCA defined as flow reserve >2.5 and diameter stenosis <36%.

5b

Results	Optimal PTCA results were achieved in 35% of cases. (Average diameter stenosis [DS] was 22% and coronary flow reserve [CFR] 3.1). In suboptimal group DS was 23% and CFR was 2.0. Adding stenting to patients with optimal PTCA yielded a DS of 8% and CFR 3.3%. In patients with suboptimal PTCA, stenting resulted in DS of 7% and CFR 2.4%. Efficacy end point was composite of major adverse cardiac events within 12 months, including death, nonfatal MI, percutaneous or surgical target lesion revascularization. Event-free survival at 1 year was 86.6% for primary stenting and 85.6% for provisional angioplasty. Costs were higher for provisional angioplasty. After second randomization in optimized PTCA group to additional stenting or termination of procedure, stenting was more effective after optimal PTCA than termination of procedure with a 1-year event-free survival rate of 84.1% in stenting vs 93.5% of optimized PTCA alone, p=0.066.
Concl.	At 1-year follow-up provisional angioplasty was costlier and without clinical benefit compared to primary stenting. Benefits of stenting are not limited to patients with suboptimal PTCA.

DEBATE II (Substudy)

Doppler End Points Balloon Angioplasty Trial Europe II

Title	Coronary hemodynamics of stent implantation after suboptimal and optimal balloon angioplasty.
Authors	Voskuil M, van Liebergen RAM, Albertal M, et al.
Reference	J Am Coll Cardiol 2002;39:1513-1517.
Disease	Coronary artery disease.
Purpose	To evaluate the hemodynamic alterations following stent implantation in patients who had suboptimal or optimal Doppler flow-guided balloon angioplasty.
Design	Substudy of multicenter DEBATE II.
Patients	523 patients with coronary disease with angina or documented ischemia due to single coronary stenosis who underwent guided balloon angioplasty (with angiography and Doppler flow velocity measurements) with hemodynamic analysis before and after stenting.
Follow-up	12 months.
Regimen	620 patients in DEBATE II initially randomized to guided percutaneous transluminal coronary angioplasty (PTCA) (n=523) or direct stenting (n=97). PTCA was considered optimal when diameter stenosis was ≤35% and coronary flow reserve was >2.5 and suboptimal if these criteria were not met. Bail-out stenting due to this approach occurred in 129 patients, the remaining 379 patients underwent a second randomization to stenting or completion of PTCA. Coronary flow reserve assessed with intracoronary adenosine.

5b

Results	End point was major adverse cardiac events (MACE) defined as death, nonfatal MI, or need for target lesion revascularization. Of the 379 patients, 184 (49%) appeared to have an optimal PTCA result. 195 (51%) did not meet these criteria. Baseline coronary flow velocity increased in the suboptimal group (after additional balloon angioplasty) from 15±8 to 22±11 cm/sec; while it remained unchanged in the optimal group (14±8 to 16±10 cm/sec; p<0.01). Diameter stenosis improved following guided PTCA from 70%±11% in the suboptimal group and 68%±11% in the optimal groups to 23%±10% and 22%±8%, respectively. Percent diameter stenosis further improved after stenting in the suboptimal group and optimal groups to 7%±8% and 8%±8%, respectively. Following stenting, baseline flow velocity remained elevated (22±11 cm/sec) in the suboptimal group, but a trend toward being lower in the optimal group (17±7 cm/sec; p=NS). Hyperemic blood flow velocity increased after stenting in both groups (49±26 cm/sec in suboptimal and 52±24cm/sec in optimal groups). Coronary flow reserve further improved following stenting in both suboptimal (2.36±0.7) and optimal groups (3.30±0.7). Total MACE was decreased from 16% to 6.5% (p=0.08) with stenting in the optimal group and from 27% to 11% with stenting in the suboptimal group (p=0.007).
Concl.	Stenting improved coronary flow reserve and residual stenosis in patients with or without suboptimal Doppler-guided PTCA. Stenting resulted in better clinical outcomes.

DESTINI

Doppler End Point Stenting International Investigation

Title	Randomized comparison of elective stent implantation and coronary balloon angioplasty guided by online quantitative angiography and intracoronary Doppler.
Authors	DiMario C, Moses JW, Anderson TJ, et al.
Reference	Circulation 2000;102:2938-2944.
Disease	Coronary artery disease.
Purpose	To compare long-term outcomes of coronary stenting in all lesions (elective stenting) or only in lesions with inadequate (angiographic and physiologic results assessed by quantitative coronary angiography and Doppler coronary flow velocity reserve) results following guided percutaneous transluminal coronary angioplasty.
Design	Randomized, multicenter.
Patients	735 patients with CAD who had lesions suitable for stent implantation.
Follow-up	1 year.
Regimen	Patients randomized to elective stenting (n=370) or guided PTCA (n=365). Optimal PTCA with residual stenosis ≤35% and coronary flow reserve assessed by Doppler guide wire >2.0, and absence of threatened dissection was achieved in 166 (43%) lesions. Remaining 218 lesions underwent provisional stenting.
Add'l Tx	Aspirin; and ticlopidine (in-stent patients).

5b

Results	Primary end point was development of ≥1 lesion-related major adverse cardiac event (death, MI, repeat target lesion revascularization) at 12 months. End point achieved in 17.8% in elective stenting group vs 18.9% in guided PTCA group (20.1% for optimal PTCA result and 18.0% for provisional stenting [p=NS]). Repeat target lesion revascularization at 12 months was 14.9% for elective stenting and 15.6% for guided PTCA (17.6% for optimal PTCA vs 14.1% for provisional stenting; p=NS). At end of procedure, residual diameter stenosis was lower in elective and provisional stent groups (9.3% and 10.2%) compared to optimal PTCA patients (24.8%; p<0.00001).
Concl.	Clinical outcomes were comparable between elective stenting and balloon angioplasty guided by online quantitative angiography and Doppler-determined coronary flow reserve with provisional stenting for patients with suboptimal PTCA results.

DIRECT

Comparison of Direct Stenting vs Stenting with Predilation for the Treatment of Selected Coronary Narrowings

Title	Comparison of direct stenting vs stenting with predilation for the treatment of selected coronary narrowings.
Authors	Brito FS, Caixeta AM, Perin MA, et al.
Reference	Am J Cardiol 2002;89:115-120.
Disease	Coronary artery disease, percutaneous coronary intervention (PCI).
Purpose	To compare the safety and efficacy of direct coronary stenting and stenting after conventional balloon predilation.
Design	Randomized, open-label, multicenter.
Patients	411 patients with angina pectoris or documented myocardial ischemia and coronary lesions suitable for direct stenting (without predilation) (de novo or restenotic lesions in native coronary arteries or vein grafts, ≥2.7 mm in diameter, and lesion length ≤35 mm). Patients with multivessel disease were included. Patients within 48 hours of acute myocardial infarction or patients with severe coronary calcifications, tortuosity, unprotected left main disease, total occlusion, bifurcational lesion, or left ventricular ejection fraction <30% were excluded.
Follow-up	6 months.
Regimen	Patients were randomized to predilation before stenting (using balloon diameter 0.5-mm lower than the vessel reference diameter and/or low-pressure inflation) (201 patients, 209 lesions) or to direct stenting without predilation (210 patients, 216 lesions). If crossing the lesion with the stent was impossible, another attempt was made after balloon dilation. Stent type and deployment pressure were at the discretion of the operator.

5b

Add'l Tx	All patients received heparin before the procedure with target activated clotting time of 250-350 seconds. All patients received aspirin ≥200 mg/d and ticlopidine 250-500 mg/d for 2-4 weeks. The use of glycoprotein IIb/IIIa antagonists was permitted.
Results	Stent deployment was successful in all lesions in the predilation group vs in 97.2% of the lesions in the direct stenting group. In the other 6 cases, the lesion could not be crossed with the stent. In all 6 cases, the stent was withdrawn, the lesion was dilated with balloon, and the same stent was implanted. In the direct stenting group, positioning of the stent was considered a "laborious" task by the operator in 39.3% of the patients with ≥90% diameter stenosis and in none with <90% diameter stenosis. Post-stenting dissection was found in 5.6% of the lesions in the direct stenting group vs 7.7% of the lesions in the predilation group (p=0.38). Distal embolization occurred in 0.9% and 1.0% of the lesions, respectively (p=1.00), and no-reflow in 1.9% and 1.4%, respectively (p=0.96). Final angiographic success was 100% in the direct stenting group and 98.6% in the predilation group (p=0.12). Stent maximal deployment pressure was 16.0±2.5 ATM in the direct stenting vs 15.6±3.0 ATM in the predilation group (p=0.14). The number of stents used per lesion was comparable. Residual diameter stenosis, acute gain (mm) and stent/artery ratio was comparable between the groups. Procedure time was 22.7±15.0 minutes in the direct stenting group vs 25.6±18.2 minutes in the predilation group (p=0.073). Fluoroscopy time was comparable (7.2±5.9 minutes vs 7.8±5.1 minutes, respectively; p=0.26). Contrast volume used was 127±53 vs 135±51 mL (p=0.11). In noncomplex (types A/B1) and <90% diameter stenosis lesions, direct stenting was associated with significant reduction in procedure time, fluoroscopy time, and contrast media used. The average balloon per lesion used was 0.15 and 1.09, respectively (p<0.001). In-hospital major adverse cardiac events (MACE) occurred in 3.8% of the patients in the direct stenting vs 3.5% in the predilation group (p=0.86). At 1 month, MACE were noted in 4.8% vs 3.5%, respectively (p=0.68). 6-month mortality was 1.4% and 2.5%, respectively (p=0.50). At 6 months, myocardial infarction occurred in 5.3% of the patients in the direct stenting and 5.0% in the predilation group (p=0.90).

At 6 months, 8.2% and 10.5% of the patients in the direct stenting and predilation groups underwent target vessel revascularization (p=0.42). Overall, 6-month survival free of MACE was 87.5% in the direct stenting vs 85.5% in the predilation group (p=0.0002).

Concl.	Direct stenting is equivalent or even superior to the standard strategy of balloon predilation before stenting in terms of 6-month clinical outcomes when performed on selected coronary lesions without significant calcification or tortuosity. In non-complex lesions and <90% diameter stenosis lesions direct stenting was associated with significant reduction in procedure time, fluoroscopy time, and contrast media used.

5b

5. Interventional Cardiology — b. Percutaneous Transluminal Coronary
Angioplasty vs Stenting vs Other Percutaneous Devices, IVUS-Guided Stenting

465

FROST

French Randomized Optimal Stenting Trial

Title	The French randomized optimal stenting trial: A prospective evaluation of provisional stenting guided by coronary velocity reserve and quantitative coronary angiography.
Authors	Lafont A, Dubois-Rande JL, Steg PG, et al.
Reference	J Am Coll Cardiol 2000; 36:404-409.
Disease	Coronary artery disease.
Purpose	To prospectively compare systematic stenting vs provisional stenting (stents placed if there is unsatisfactory immediate result of balloon angioplasty or as a bail-out procedure, in coronary patients).
Design	Prospective, randomized.
Patients	251 patients undergoing elective angioplasty.
Follow-up	6 month angiographic follow-up.
Regimen	Systematic stenting or provisional stenting (if postangioplasty coronary velocity reserve <2.2 and/or residual stenosis ≥35%, or as bail-out).
Add'l Tx	Aspirin, heparin; ticlopidine in stent patients.
Results	Primary end point was final minimal lumen diameter at 6 months. Stenting was performed in 48.4% of patients in the provisional group and all of the patients in the systematic group. Minimal lumen diameter did not differ between groups at 6 months (1.90±0.79 mm vs 1.99±0.79 mm; p=0.39) nor did the rate of binary restenosis (27.1% vs 21.4%; p=0.37). Among patients that developed restenosis, 40.6% in the provisional group and 100% in the systematic group, had in-stent restenosis. The incidence of major adverse cardiac events (death, acute myocardial infarction, target lesion revascularization) did not differ between groups.
Concl.	Systematic stenting did not provide an advantage over provisional stenting.

ISAR-SMART

Intracoronary Stenting or Angioplasty for Restenosis Reduction in Small Arteries

Title	A randomized trial comparing stenting with balloon angioplasty in small vessels in patients with symptomatic coronary artery disease.
Authors	Kastrati A, Schömig A, Dirschinger J, et al.
Reference	Circulation 2000;102:2593-2598.
Disease	Coronary artery disease.
Purpose	To determine whether stenting compared to percutaneous transluminal coronary angioplasty of small coronary arteries (2 to 2.8 mm in size) reduces restenosis.
Design	Randomized, multicenter.
Patients	404 patients with angina or exercise-induced ischemia with ≥70% diameter stenosis by angiography of a native coronary vessel between 2.0-2.8 mm in size.
Follow-up	6-month angiographic follow-up; 7-month clinical follow-up.
Regimen	204 patients randomized to stent and 200 randomized to PTCA.
Add'l Tx	Heparin, abciximab, ticlopidine, aspirin.

5b

Results	Primary end point was angiographic restenosis (diameter stenosis ≥50%). Secondary end points were adverse clinical events including death, myocardial infarction, stroke, and target vessel revascularization. Restenosis occurred in 35.7% of patients in the stenting group and 37.4% in the PTCA group (p=0.74). Compared with PTCA, stenting had an initial better acute result, but with greater late lumen loss. Net lumen gain was 0.76±0.78 mm in the stent group and 0.76±0.63 mm in the PTCA group (p=NS). Infarct-free survival rate at 7 months was 96.6% for stent group and 97.0% for PTCA group (p=0.80). Target vessel revascularization rate was 20.1% in-stent patients and 16.5% in PTCA patients (p=0.35). 30-day death rates were low in both groups (0.5%). At end of follow-up period, 77% of stent group and 81% of PTCA group survived event-free (p=0.22).
Concl.	In coronary patients with small coronary vessels, stenting and PTCA were equally favorable.

ISAR-SMART Trial (Substudy)

Intracoronary Stenting or Angioplasty for Restenosis Reduction in Small Arteries

Title	Comparative analysis of stent placement vs balloon angioplasty in small coronary arteries with long narrowings (ISAR-SMART) Trial.
Authors	Hausleiter J, Kastrati A, Mehilli J, et al.
Reference	Am J Cardiol 2002;89:58-60.
Disease	Coronary artery disease.
Purpose	To determine whether patients with both small coronary arteries and long lesions benefited from stenting vs percutaneous transluminal coronary angioplasty (PTCA) in the ISAR-SMART study.
Design	Randomized, multicenter, subgroup analysis.
Patients	98 patients as part of the ISAR-SMART trial with coronary arteries between 2.0-2.8 mm in diameter and with a lesion length of ≥15 mm.
Follow-up	6 month (angiographic); 12 month (clinical).
Regimen	Stent placement vs PTCA to achieve a final diameter stenosis <30% with TIMI flow grade of 3.
Add'l Tx	As per ISAR-SMART.

5b

Results	Primary end point was angiographic restenosis (diameter stenosis ≥50%) at 6 month follow-up. 3.7% of patients randomized to stenting crossed over to PTCA; 27.3% of patients randomized to PTCA crossed over to stenting. At the end of the procedure acute lumen gain was greater in the stent group (1.8±0.49) vs the PTCA group (1.55±0.61; p=0.012). Angiographic follow-up data were available in 79.6% of the subgroup. Restenosis occurred in 35.6% of stented patients vs 60.6% for the PTCA group (p=0.028). Minimal lumen diameter was 1.37±0.67 mm in the stent group vs 0.90±0.59 mm in the PTCA group (p=0.002). Net gain was 0.90±0.74 mm in the stent group vs 0.53±0.61 in the PTCA group (p=0.022). Adverse events (death, nonfatal MI, CABG, repeat PTCA) at 1 year follow-up occurred in 20% of stent patients and 21% of PTCA patients.
Concl.	Stent placement resulted in a reduced incidence of restenosis compared to PTCA in patients with small coronary arteries who had long lesions.

ISAR-STEREO-2

Intracoronary Stenting and Angiographic Results: Strut Thickness Effect on Restenosis Outcome Trial

Title	Intracoronary stenting and angiographic results: strut thickness effect on restenosis outcome trial.
Authors	Pache J, Kastrati A, Mehilli J, et al.
Reference	J Am Coll Cardiol 2003;41:1283-1288.
Disease	Coronary artery disease, percutaneous intervention.
Purpose	To assess the influence of strut thickness on restenosis in comparing 2 stents with differing designs.
Design	Randomized, multicenter.
Patients	611 patients (n=309 in thin-strut, n=302 in thick strut) with symptomatic coronary artery disease and coronary artery lesions in native vessels.
Follow-up	6 months.
Regimen	Patients were randomized to receive either the thin-strut stent (ACS RX Multi-Link, strut thickness 50 mm, strut width 100 mm, and interconnected ring design) or the thick-strut stent (BX Velocity, strut thickness 140 mm, strut width 130 mm, and a closed cell design). All patients received heparin and aspirin during the intervention. Patients considered to be high-risk received a bolus of abciximab followed by a 12-hour IV infusion and heparin dosage reduced by 50%. The procedure was deemed successful if there was a residual stenosis <30% and a Thrombolysis in Myocardial Infarction flow grade ≥2. After the procedure, all patients received aspirin 100 mg bid indefinitely and clopidogrel 75 mg/d for at least 4 weeks.

5b

Results   The primary study end point was the incidence of angiographic restenosis at the 6-month follow-up. Secondary end points were the incidence of target-vessel revascularization and the combined rate of death and MI. The baseline characteristics of the 2 groups were similar. There were no differences in the early lumen gain and final diameter stenosis between the 2 groups. Follow-up angiography was carried out in 77% of the eligible patients in the thin-strut group and 80% in the thick-strut group. The primary end point, the incidence of angiographic restenosis, occurred in 17.9% of those in the thin-strut group and 31.4% in the thick-strut group, (relative risk [RR] 0.57; 95% CI=0.39-0.84; p<0.001). At follow-up, the minimal lumen diameter (MLD) was significantly greater in the thin-strut group (p<0.001); the diameter stenosis and late lumen loss were significantly smaller (p<0.001). At 1 year, the incidence of target vessel revascularization was 12.3% in the thin-strut group and 21.9% in the thick-strut group (RR 0.56; 95% CI=0.38-0.84; p=0.002). Also at 1 year, 4.9% of patients in the thin-strut group died or had an MI, vs 6.3% in the thick-strut group (RR 0.77; 95% CI=0.39-1.52; p=0.46).

Concl.   In 2 stents with differing designs, stents with thinner struts were associated with significantly improved angiographic characteristics and decreased rates of clinical restenosis vs thick-strut stents.

LARS

Laser Angioplasty of Restenosed Stents

Title	Laser angioplasty of restenosed coronary stents. Results of a multicenter surveillance trial.
Authors	Köster R, Hamm CW, Seabra-Gomes R, et al.
Reference	J Am Coll Cardiol 1999;34:25-32.
Disease	Coronary artery disease. Restenosis or occluded stents.
Purpose	Determine the feasibility, safety, and efficacy of excimer laser angioplasty, with saline flush and adjunctive balloon angioplasty for in-stent restenosis.
Design	Prospective, nonrandomized, multicenter, surveillance trial.
Patients	440 patients with restenosis or occlusions in 527 coronary artery stents.
Follow-up	In-hospital.
Regimen	Xenon chloride excimer laser unit used to debulk as much tissue in the in-stent restenosis as possible.
Add'l Tx	Aspirin, heparin, IV nitroglycerin; abciximab if necessary.
Results	Laser angioplasty success was defined as ≤50% residual stenosis or successful pass with a 2.0 mm or an eccentric 1.7 mm laser catheter. Success was attained in 92% of patients. Adjunctive PTCA was carried out in 99% of patients. Procedural success was defined as laser angioplasty success followed by ≤30% residual stenosis with or without PTCA and occurred in 91% of cases. Success was not dependent upon length of the lesion, size of vessel, or procedure in native vessels vs vein grafts. Death occurred in 1.6%, Q-wave infarct in 0.5%, and non-Q-wave infarct in 2.7% of patients. Laser treatment caused perforation of the coronary artery in 0.2% cases. Dissections occurred in 4.8% of patients following laser treatment and 9.3% after PTCA. Cardiac tamponade occurred in 0.5%.

5b

5. Interventional Cardiology — b. Percutaneous Transluminal Coronary
Angioplasty vs Stenting vs Other Percutaneous Devices, IVUS-Guided Stenting

473

Concl.   Excimer laser angioplasty with adjunctive PTCA was safe and effective for treating in-stent coronary artery restenoses and a randomized comparison to PTCA alone is justified.

Magic 5L

Magic 5L Wallstent Study

Title	The influence of stent length on clinical and angiographic outcome in patients undergoing elective stenting for native coronary artery lesions. Final results of the Magic 5L study.
Authors	Foley DP, Pieper M, Wijns W, et al.
Reference	Eur Heart J 2001;22:1585-1593.
Disease	Coronary artery disease, restenosis.
Purpose	To study whether stent length has influence on 6-month angiographic and clinical outcome in patients with ≤45 mm native coronary artery lesions, treated with the self-expandable Magic Wallstent.
Design	Multicenter.
Patients	276 patients (302 lesions), scheduled for percutaneous coronary intervention (PCI) of native coronary artery lesions ≤45 mm in length. Patients with intolerance to aspirin and/or ticlopidine, peptic ulcer disease, recent (<1 week) acute myocardial infarction, Q-wave myocardial infarction in the territory supplied by the culprit artery, large akinesia in the territory supplied by the culprit artery, left ventricular ejection fraction (LVEF) <30%, cardiogenic shock, left bundle branch block, left main coronary artery lesion, bifurcational lesions, lesions with angiographic evidence of a thrombus, heavily calcified coronary lesions, severe hepatic disease, and hematologic disorder were excluded.
Follow-up	9 months of clinical follow-up. Repeated angiography at 6 months.
Regimen	After successful balloon dilatation, patients underwent stenting with the Magic Wallstent. Stent length was either mini, extra-short, short, medium, or long. The recommendation was that stent length would be 4-8 mm longer than the lesion. Stent diameter was either 3.5, 4.0, 4.5, or 5.0 mm.

5. Interventional Cardiology — b. Percutaneous Transluminal Coronary
Angioplasty vs Stenting vs Other Percutaneous Devices, IVUS-Guided Stenting

475

Add'l Tx	All patients received aspirin 80-325 mg/d, started before the procedure, and continued throughout the study period. All patients received ticlopidine for ≥2 weeks. All patients received IV heparin during the procedure. Glycoprotein IIb/IIIa was permitted.
Results	Magic Wallstent was successfully implanted in 301 of the 302 lesions studied. In 98.6% of the patients the residual stenosis was <20%. Stent length was mini in 33 lesions, extra-short in 62 lesions, short in 72 lesions, medium in 52 lesions, and long in 45 lesions. A total of 38 lesions (12.6%) were treated with an additional stent. At 30 days, 6.2% of the patients had major adverse cardiac events (1.8% subacute occlusion). At 6 and 9 months 27.5% and 30.4% of the patients, respectively, had experienced major adverse cardiac events. Angiographic restenosis occurred in 37% of the cases. Restenosis rate was 25.9% with the mini, 25% with the extra-short, 22.6% with the short, 36.2% with the medium, and 67.5% with the long Wallstents. Multivariate analysis revealed stent length to be an independent predictor of restenosis and to be associated with increased risk for major adverse cardiac events.
Concl.	The longer Wallstents were associated with excessive restenosis rates, while the results with the shorter Magic Wallstents were comparable with short balloon-expandable stents.

NIRVANA

NIR Vascular Advanced North American Trial

Title	Final results of a randomized trial comparing the NIR stent to the Palmaz-Schatz stent for narrowings in native coronary arteries.
Authors	Baim DS, Cutlip DE, O'Shaughnessy CD, et al.
Reference	Am J Cardiol 2001;87:152-156.
Disease	Coronary artery disease, percutaneous coronary intervention.
Purpose	To compare the results of NIR and Palmaz-Schatz stents.
Design	Randomized, open-label, multicenter.
Patients	849 patients, >18 years old, with a focal ≤25 mm de novo 50%-99% diameter stenosis lesion in a native coronary artery, with a reference diameter of 3-4 mm. Patients with left main coronary artery stenosis, ostial lesions, the need to cover a large side branch by the stent, a recent myocardial infarction, left ventricular ejection fraction <25%, intolerance to aspirin or ticlopidine or bleeding were excluded.
Follow-up	Clinical follow-up for 9 months. A cohort of 302 consecutive patients were scheduled for repeated coronary angiography at 9 months.
Regimen	Randomization to Palmaz-Schatz stent or the NIR stent. Stents were deployed by 8-10 atm slow inflation of the delivery balloon, followed by ≥12 atm inflation of a high-pressure balloon inflation.
Add'l Tx	Intravascular ultrasound was used in 7.3% of the patients. All patients received aspirin before procedure and intravenous heparin during procedure (target activated clotting time >250 seconds). After stent implantation all patients received aspirin 325 mg/d and ticlopidine 250 mg bid for 30 days.

5b

5. Interventional Cardiology — b. Percutaneous Transluminal Coronary
Angioplasty vs Stenting vs Other Percutaneous Devices, IVUS-Guided Stenting

477

Results	Stent was delivered successfully in 100% and 98.8% of the cases in the NIR and Palmaz-Schatz groups. Device success (residual diameter stenosis <50% by using the assigned device only) was 99.5% with the NIR stent and 97.9% with the Palmaz-Schatz stent. Procedural success (device success, no myocardial infarction, emergency CABG or in-hospital death) was 95.4% and 94.3%, respectively. Postprocedural in-stent residual stenosis was significantly greater in the Palmaz-Schatz group (9±12% vs 7±11%; p=0.04). The incidence of major adverse events at 30 days was 4.3% in the NIR and 4.4% in the Palmaz-Schatz (p>0.20). Mortality at 9 months was 1.0% in the NIR and 0.9% in the Palmaz-Schatz groups. Acute myocardial infarction occurred in 4.8% and 4.2%, respectively. 9.6% and 11.6%, respectively, underwent target lesion revascularization, and 12.2% and 13.4%, respectively underwent target vessel revascularization. Target vessel failure was 16.0% with the NIR stent and 17.2% with the Palmaz-Schatz stent (p<0.001 by test for equivalency). Among the 71% of the 298 eligible patients for repeated coronary angiography at 9 months, restenosis occurred in 19.3% of the patients in the NIR group and 22.4% of the patients in the Palmaz-Schatz group (p=NS).
Concl.	The NIR stent was associated with slightly better acute angiographic results than the Palmaz-Schatz stent and with equivalent or better 9-month target vessel failure rate.

OPTICUS

Optimization with ICUS (Intracoronary Ultrasound) to Reduce Stent Restenosis

Title	Randomized comparison of coronary stent implantation under ultrasound or angiographic guidance to reduce stent restenosis.
Authors	Mudra H, di Mario C, de Jaegere P, et al.
Reference	Circulation 2001;104:1343-1349.
Disease	Coronary artery disease (CAD).
Purpose	To determine whether ultrasound guided stent implantation strategy improves long-term angiographic and clinical outcomes.
Design	Randomized, multicenter.
Patients	550 patients with symptomatic CAD stenosis or silent ischemia. Lesion length ≤25 mm to be covered with 1 or 2 stents in an artery with a diameter of ≤2.5 mm.
Follow-up	6 month angiographic; 6-, 12-month clinical evaluation.
Regimen	Patients were randomly assigned to ultrasound guided or angiographically guided implantation of the stents. By ultrasound and angiography, a <10% residual stenosis was the target.
Add'l Tx	IV heparin, aspirin. Ticlopidine for 4 weeks.

5b

Results   Primary end points were incidence of angiographic restenosis
           (>50% lumen diameter reduction), minimal lumen diameter,
           percent diameter stenosis at 6 months. Assigned treatment
           received in 252 ICUS patients and 269 angiographic-guided
           patients. At 6 months restenosis rate was 24.5% in the ultra-
           sound group and 22.8% in the angiographically guided group
           (p=0.68). There also was no difference in minimal lumen diam-
           eter at 1.95±0.72 mm vs 1.91±0.68 mm; p=0.52 in the ultra-
           sound vs angiographic groups, respectively. Percent diameter
           stenosis was 34.8%±20.6% vs 36.8%±19.6%; p=0.29, in the 2
           groups. At 12 months, there was no reduction in major adverse
           cardiac events (death, myocardial infarction, CABG, repeat
           PCI) in the ultrasound-guided group (relative risk [RR] 1.07;
           95% CI=0.75-1.52; p=0.71). Ultrasound guided deployment
           of stents was not associated with less repeat PCI (RR 1.04; 95%
           CI=0.64-1.67; p=0.87).

Concl.   The use of routine ultrasound guidance for coronary stenting
           was not supported by the results of this trial.

OPUS-1

Optimum Percutaneous Transluminal Coronary Angioplasty vs Routine Stenting-1

Title	Optimum percutaneous transluminal coronary angioplasty compared with routine stent strategy trial (OPUS-1): a randomized trial.
Authors	Weaver DW, Reisman MA, Griffin JJ, et al.
Reference	Lancet 2000;355:2199-2203.
Disease	Coronary artery disease.
Purpose	To compare the clinical outcomes and economic implications of patients treated with routine coronary stenting vs standard balloon angioplasty followed by stenting only in cases with suboptimal results.
Design	Randomized, open-label, multicenter.
Patients	479 patients, 21-81 years old, with stable or unstable angina, a positive functional test for ischemia or a recent myocardial infarction, with ≥70% stenosis in a single lesion of ≤20 mm of length in a native coronary artery with a reference diameter of ≥3.0 mm. Patients who needed to undergo revascularization of >1 coronary artery, >1 previous intervention at the target-vessel site, and contraindication to aspirin, severe illness with a limited life expectancy were excluded. Angiographic exclusion criteria were: a coronary lesion with ≥45° angulation, moderate to severe calcification, and ostial lesions.
Follow-up	6 months.
Regimen	Randomization to a strategy of routine stenting (stent, n=230) or a strategy of balloon angioplasty with provisional stenting (percutaneous transluminal coronary angioplasty, n=249).
Add'l Tx	The use of glycoprotein IIb/IIIa inhibitors and multiple stents were permitted. All patients received aspirin 325 mg/d and ticlopidine for 4 weeks.

5b

Results	The mean residual stenosis after PCI was 1±7% in the stent group and 9±14% in the PTCA group (p<0.001). 37% of the patients in the PTCA group received stents. The average number of stents used per patient was 1.17±0.5 in the stent group and 0.52±0.77 in the PTCA group (p<0.001). The mean length of the initial hospitalization was 2.5±0.9 days in the stent group and 2.6±2.2 days in the PTCA group (p=NS). Initial hospital costs were higher in the stent group ($9234) than in the PTCA group ($8434) (p<0.001). 6-month mortality was 0.4% in the stent group vs 1.2% in the PTCA group. MI occurred in 1.7% and 2.4%, respectively. 1.3% of the patients in the stent group vs 2.9% in the PTCA group underwent cardiac surgery and 3.0% vs 10.1% underwent target vessel revascularization (p<0.05). Overall, 5.2% of the patients in the stent group vs 14.9% of the patients in the PTCA group underwent revascularization or CABG (p<0.01). Events (death, MI, or revascularization) occurred in 6.1% of the patients in the stent group and 14.9% of the patients in the PTCA group (hazard ratio 2.53; 95% CI=1.38-4.71; p=0.003). Mean total costs at 6 months were $10,206 in the stent group and $10,490 in the PTCA group (p=NS). Functional status, frequency of angina, treatment satisfaction and overall Seattle angina questionnaire scores were comparable between the groups.
Concl.	Routine stent implantation was associated with better acute and 6-month clinical outcome at comparable cumulative costs than a strategy of PTCA with provisional stenting.

PARAGON Stent Study

Platelet IIb/IIIa Antagonism for the Reduction of Acute Coronary Syndrome Events in a Global Organization Network

Title	The PARAGON stent study: a randomized trial of a new martensitic nitinol stent vs the Palmaz-Schatz stent for treatment of complex native coronary arterial lesions.
Authors	Holmes DR, Lansky A, Kuntz R, et al.
Reference	Am J Cardiol 2000;86:1073-1079.
Disease	Coronary artery disease, stent.
Purpose	To compare the safety and efficacy of a new martensitic nitinol stent (with presumed improved flexibility and radiopacity, better side branch access, and no articulation artifact) with those of the conventional Palmaz-Schatz stent.
Design	Randomized, open-label, multicenter.
Patients	688 patients scheduled for percutaneous coronary intervention of a native coronary arterial de novo or restenotic lesion, with a reference diameter ≥3.0 mm and ≤4.0 mm, lesion length ≤25 mm and percent diameter stenosis ≥50 and <100. Patients with myocardial infarction of <48 hours, previous stenting of the target vessel, left ventricular ejection fraction <25%, angiographic evidence of intraluminal thrombus, moderate or severe calcification, diffuse target vessel disease, or excess tortuosity unsuitable for stent delivery were excluded.
Follow-up	6 months.
Regimen	Randomization to the PARAGON (n=349) or conventional Palmaz-Schatz (n=339) stent.
Add'l Tx	All patients received oral aspirin and ticlopidine for 2 weeks. All patients received intravenous heparin before and during the PCI with a target acitvated clotting time of 250-300 seconds.

Results	The reference vessel diameter was significantly larger in the Palmaz-Schatz group (3.05±0.51 mm) than in the PARAGON group (2.97±0.51; p=0.05), however, the lesion length was similar. 73% of the patients in the Palmaz-Schatz group required a single 15 mm stent and 83% of the patients in the PARAGON group needed a single stent. Device success was 99.1% in the PARAGON group vs 94.3% in the Palmaz-Schatz group (p<0.05). In 16 patients in the Palmaz-Schatz group there was a failure to deliver the stent, vs in only 1 patient in the PARAGON group. Stent thrombosis occurred in 2.0% of the PARAGON patients vs 0.3% in the Palmaz-Schatz patients (p=0.06). The composite end point of in-hospital death, myocardial infarction, target lesion revascularization and emergency CABG occurred in 8.3% in the PARAGON group vs 4.4% in the Palmaz-Schatz group (p=0.04). At 6 months, the composite end point of death, myocardial infarction related to the target vessel, and target vessel revascularization because of clinical indications, occurred in 20.3% in the PARAGON group vs 12.4% in the Palmaz-Schatz group (p=0.005). Myocardial infarctions occurred in 9.2% of the PARAGON group vs 4.7% in the Plamaz-Schatz group (p=0.025). Target lesion revascularization was needed in 12.0% of the PARAGON group vs 5.9% of the Palmaz-Schatz group (p=0.005). Follow-up angiography was performed in 79% of the PARAGON group and 71% of the Palmaz-Schatz group. In-stent restenosis occurred in 29.1% in the PARAGON group and 23.7% in the Palmaz-Schatz group (p=0.345).
Concl.	Both stents were safe and associated with infrequent adverse events. The PARAGON stent can be delivered with a higher success rates than the conventional Palmaz-Schatz stent. However, clinical events were more frequent with the PARAGON stent.

PREDICT

Predilatation vs Direct Stenting in Coronary Treatment

Title	Comparison of predilatation vs direct stenting in coronary treatment using the Medtronic AVE S670 coronary stent system (The PREDICT Trial).
Authors	Baim DS, Flatley M, Caputo R, et al.
Reference	Am J Cardiol 2001;88:1364-1369.
Disease	Coronary artery disease, percutaneous coronary intervention (PCI).
Purpose	To compare the strategy of balloon predilatation with that of direct stenting on restenosis after PCIs.
Design	Randomized, open-label, multicenter.
Patients	399 patients undergoing elective PCI with focal (≤15 mm) non-calcified, de novo native coronary lesions suitable for stenting with a single (9, 12, or 15 mm) stent, and without significant proximal or distal disease. The reference artery should have been 3.0-4.0 mm. Patients with recent myocardial infarction, evidence of lesion-associated thrombus, or left ventricular ejection fraction <30% were not included.
Follow-up	6 months clinical follow-up with repeated coronary angiography after 6 months. In addition, 62 patients (31 patients from each group) underwent intravascular ultrasound (IVUS) after stent implantation and at 6 months.
Regimen	All patients received Medtronic AVE S670 coronary stents (9, 12, or 15 mm long). Patients were randomized to conventional balloon predilatation before stenting (number of lesions=203), or to stenting without predilatation (number of lesions=201). If unable to cross the lesion with the stent, the stent was retrieved and the vessel was predilated with a balloon.
Add'l Tx	All patients received aspirin 325 mg/d, and either ticlopidine 250 mg bid or clopidogrel 75 mg/d for 2 weeks after PCI.

5b

5. Interventional Cardiology — b. Percutaneous Transluminal Coronary
Angioplasty vs Stenting vs Other Percutaneous Devices, IVUS-Guided Stenting

485

Results	The primary success rate of the procedure was 92.0% for direct stenting and 96.6% for predilatation. After additional balloon predilatation or rotablation, the procedure success rate was 99.5% and 99.0%, respectively. Immediately post-procedure the in-stent minimal lumen diameter was 2.92±0.43 mm in the direct stenting group and 2.98±0.42 mm in the predilatation group. The residual diameter stenosis was 5.9%±9.4% vs 4.5%±9.3%, respectively. Procedure time was 33.2±18.4 minutes with direct stenting and 35.9±16.5 minutes for predilatation. The fluoroscopy time was 9.2±7.5 minutes vs 10.4±8.1 minutes, and the contrast used was 154±86 mL vs 169±82 mL, respectively. The average number of balloons used was 0.56±0.79 in the direct stenting group vs 1.3±0.62 in the predilatation group (p=0.001). The average number of stents per lesion was comparable (1.20±0.54 vs 1.16±0.42, respectively). Major adverse cardiac events at 14 days occurred in 6.1% of the patients in the direct stenting group vs 7.5% in the predilatation group. Stent thrombosis occurred in 0.5% of the patients in each group. None of the patients died or had Q-wave MI. 7% vs 8% of the patients in the direct stenting and predilatation groups had non-Q-wave MI. At 180 days, major adverse cardiac events occurred in 19% of the patients in each group. Death occurred in 0.5% of the patients in the direct stenting vs 2% in the predilatation group. 12% of the patients in each group had target lesion revascularization. 7% and 8% had non-Q-wave MI, respectively. Follow-up angiography revealed in-stent restenosis in 20.4% of the lesions in the direct stenting vs 20.9% in the predilatation group. The loss index was comparable. The IVUS substudy showed that the acute postintervention minimal stent area was 7.1 mm^2 in the direct stenting vs 7.6 mm^2 in the predilatation group (p=NS). The 6-month minimal stent areas were comparable (8.3 vs 8.4 mm^2).
Concl.	Direct stenting was safe and highly successful. However, it was associated with only modest cost savings and no reduction in late restenosis compared with conventional approach of stenting after balloon predilation.

SAFE

Saphenous Vein Graft Angioplasty Free of Emboli

Title	Evaluation of a balloon occlusion and aspiration system for protection from distal embolization during stenting in saphenous vein grafts.
Authors	Grube E, Schofer J, Webb J et al.
Reference	Am J Cardiol 2002;89:941-945.
Disease	Coronary artery disease; saphenous vein graft degeneration.
Purpose	To evaluate feasibility, safety, efficacy of distal protection using PercuSurge GuardWire Occlusion and Aspiration System (PercuSurge, Inc., Sunnyvale, CA).
Design	Prospective, controlled, international, multicenter registry.
Patients	103 patients requiring stenting of 1 or 2 lesions in a single degenerated saphenous vein graft with evidence of symptomatic or inducible ischemia, and target lesion with diameter stenosis ≥50% and <100% and at least TIMI 1 flow.
Follow-up	30 days.
Regimen	All patients treated with the PercuSurge GuardWire Occlusion and Aspiration System. Prior to angioplasty, protection of distal circulation established with this distal balloon occlusion system, followed by stenting and aspiration of debris.
Add'l Tx	Aspirin, ticlopidine.

5b

Results	Primary end point was in-hospital rate of major adverse cardiac event, defined as: death, Q-wave or non-Q-wave MI, emergent CABG, or repeat PCI of target vessel. Average age of graft was 8.9 years. Duration of distal inflation of the balloon was 5.4 minutes. 5 patients had MIs defined as post procedural creatine kinase-MB >3 times normal. 97 (94%) patients were free of major adverse events at 30 days. Macroscopically visible red and/or yellow debris was extracted by the device in 91% of patients. By microscopy, fibrin and necrotic core were present in 100% of specimens, foams cells in 80%; and cholesterol clefts in 29%. Angiographic analysis in a core laboratory showed post-procedure TIMI 3 flow in 98.9% of grafts vs 83.5% prior to intervention. TIMI 0/1 was present in 4.1% at baseline and 1.1% after the procedure. None of the patients had angiographic evidence of no reflow or distal embolization. 47% of patients had angiographic thrombus at baseline vs 13.5% following the procedure.
Concl.	This study suggests that the guard wire distal balloon occlusion and aspiration device is safe and effective in capturing distal emboli and debris during percutaneous interventional procedures within degenerated saphenous vein grafts.

SCORES

Stent Comparative Restenosis

Title	Comparison of self-expanding and balloon-expandable stents for the reduction of restenosis.
Authors	Han RO, Schwartz RS, Kobayashi Y, et al.
Reference	Am J Cardiol 2001;88:253-259.
Disease	Coronary artery disease.
Purpose	To compare angiographic and clinical outcomes of the self-expanding stent with a balloon expandable stent in native coronary arteries.
Design	Prospective, randomized, multicenter.
Patients	1096 patients with new or restenotic coronary artery lesions with angina pectoris and/or objective evidence of myocardial ischemia (ECG at rest or during stress testing).
Follow-up	9 months.
Regimen	Patients randomized to self-expanding stent (n=545) or balloon expandable stent (n=551). Nitinol self-expanding stents expand over time in response to body temperature. The stent was available in diameters of 3.0, 3.5, and 4.0 mm and in lengths of 14, 20, and 31 mm. The stents expand to a diameter of 0.75 mm greater than labeled diameter if left at body temperature.
Add'l Tx	Aspirin. Ticlopidine for 1 month.

5b

Results	Primary end point was incidence of target vessel failure at 9 months defined as composite of acute procedural failure, death, MI, and/or target vessel revascularization. At 9 months there was no difference between the 2 stent groups in rates of death, Q-wave MI, non-Q-wave MI, CABG, repeat PTCA, or target vessel failure. Target vessel failure occurred in 19.3% of patients receiving the self-expanding stent and in 20.1% in the balloon expandable stent group (p=NS). At 1 month there also was no difference in incidence of major adverse cardiac events between groups. A subgroup of patients had follow-up angiography (n=250) at 6 months. Binary restenosis rates were 24.2% in the self-expanding and 18.7% in the balloon expandable groups (p=NS). Late loss and loss index did not differ between groups. Intravascular ultrasound performed in 62 patients suggested a lower incidence of edge tears in the self-expanding group (6% vs 23%; p=0.06). At 6 months of intravascular ultrasound follow-up, the minimum stent area of the self-expanding stents increased by 33% but no change occurred in the balloon-expandable group. However there was more intimal proliferation in the self-expandable stent group vs the balloon expandable group (3.1 ± 2.0 vs 1.7 ± 1.7 mm^2). Late lumen area loss was similar in the 2 groups.
Concl.	Self-expanding stents and balloon expandable stents had similar angiographic and clinical outcomes in native coronary artery lesions.

SISA

Stent in Small Arteries

Title	Stent placement to prevent restenosis after angioplasty in small coronary arteries.
Authors	Doucet S, Schalij MJ, Vrolix MC, et al.
Reference	Circulation 2001;104:2029-2033.
Disease	Coronary artery disease, angina.
Purpose	To determine whether stents reduce angiographic restenosis in small coronary arteries vs standard percutaneous transluminal coronary angioplasty (PTCA).
Design	Randomized, multicenter.
Patients	351 patients with angina or documented silent ischemia with reference vessel diameter ≤2.9 mm and ≥2.3 mm and lesion length ≤12 mm.
Follow-up	6 months.
Regimen	Patients were randomized to angioplasty alone (n=182) or stenting (n=169).
Add'l Tx	Heparin; aspirin; ticlopidine if a stent was implanted.
Results	Primary end point was angiographic restenosis (% diameter stenosis ≥50%) at follow-up angiogram (6 months). There was a trend toward fewer adverse in-hospital events with stenting (3%) vs PTCA (7.1%; p=0.076). 20.3% of patients in PTCA group crossed over to stenting; 2.4% of the stent group crossed over to angioplasty. Procedural success was 98.3% in the PTCA group and 98.2% in the stent group. 4.9% in the PTCA group had an in-hospital non-Q wave MI vs 1.8% in the stent group (p=0.142). 85.3% of patients had repeat angiography at 6 months. At 6 months angiographic restenosis occurred in 32.9% of the PTCA group vs 28% of the stent group (p=0.36). There was no difference in need for target revascularization between the PTCA group (20.3%) vs the stent group (17.8%; p=NS). Minimal lumen diameter at 6 months was 1.37±0.57 in the PTCA group vs 1.44±0.53 in the stent group (p=NS).

5b

5. Interventional Cardiology — b. Percutaneous Transluminal Coronary
Angioplasty vs Stenting vs Other Percutaneous Devices, IVUS-Guided Stenting

491

Concl.   There was no difference in restenosis rates at 6 months in small coronary arteries subjected to PTCA or stenting. There was a lower overall in-hospital complication rate with stenting compared to PTCA of the small vessels.

SISCA

Stenting in Small Coronary Arteries

Title	Stenting in small coronary arteries (SISCA) trial. A randomized comparison between balloon angioplasty and the heparin-coated Bestent.
Authors	Moer R, Myreng Y, Molstad P, et al.
Reference	J Am Coll Cardiol 2001;38:1598-1603.
Disease	Coronary artery disease, percutaneous coronary intervention (PCI).
Purpose	To compare clinical and angiographic outcome after elective stenting and balloon angioplasty of small coronary arteries (reference diameter of 2.1-3.0 mm).
Design	Randomized, open-label, multicenter.
Patients	145 patients, referred for angioplasty of de novo >50% diameter stenosis lesions in coronary arteries with a reference diameter of 2.1-3.0 mm. Patients with single and multivessel disease and with stable or unstable angina were included. Patients with functionally occluded arteries, vessels with multiple lesions, thrombus containing lesions, bifurcational lesions, vessels with patent grafts, and ongoing myocardial infarction were not included. Only 1 lesion in each patient was included in the study.
Follow-up	6-month clinical follow-up with repeated angiography (on day 179±35).
Regimen	Patients were randomized to PTCA alone (n=71) or PTCA + stent implantation (heparin coated [Hepamed] 15 mm long Bestent [Medtronic InStent, Minneapolis, MN]) (n=74).
Add'l Tx	All patients were pre-treated with aspirin. Heparin and glycoprotein IIb/IIIa inhibitors were administered according to local standards. All patients received ticlopidine or clopidogrel immediately after PCI. Aspirin ≥75 mg/d for ≥1 month and thienopyridine (ticlopidine or clopidogrel) for 1 month after PCI was given to all patients.

5. Interventional Cardiology — b. Percutaneous Transluminal Coronary Angioplasty vs Stenting vs Other Percutaneous Devices, IVUS-Guided Stenting

493

5b

Results	4.1% of the patients in the stent group and 14.1% in the PTCA group crossed over to the alternative treatment. Procedural success was 94.6% with stenting and 80.3% with PTCA (p=0.011). 6-month survival free of major adverse cardiac events was 90.5% in the stent group vs 76.1% in the PTCA group (p=0.016). 1 patient in the PTCA group and none in the stent group died during follow-up and 1 patient in each group had acute myocardial infarction. 1 patient in each group underwent target lesion revascularization during the first month, and 6 and 12 patients between the first to the 6th month (p=0.13). At 6 months, 9.6% of the patients in the stent group vs 23.2% in the PTCA group underwent repeat revascularization (p=0.041). Immediately after PCI minimal lumen diameter was 2.22±0.27 mm in the stent group and 1.79±0.36 mm in the PTCA group (p<0.001). At 6 months, minimal lumen diameter was 1.69±0.52 mm and 1.57±0.44 mm, respectively (p=0.096). Immediately after PCI the diameter stenosis was 11.3%±8.0% in the stent group and 25.3%±13.0% in the PTCA group (p=0.001). At 6 months, the diameter stenosis was 29.8%±18.1% and 35.1%±17.2%, respectively (p=0.025). The restenosis rate was 9.7% with stenting and 18.8% with PTCA (p=0.15).
Concl.	Elective implantation of heparin coated stents in small coronary arteries improved clinical outcomes as compared with PTCA alone. However, the differences in the angiographic results at 6 months between stenting and PTCA were not statistically significant.

START (Stent vs Atherectomy)

Stent vs Directional Coronary Atherectomy Randomized Trial

Title	Final Results of the Stent vs directional coronary atherectomy randomized trial (START).
Authors	Tsuchikane E, Sumitsuji S, Awata N, et al.
Reference	J Am Coll Cardiol 1999;34:1050-1057.
Disease	Coronary artery disease.
Purpose	To compare primary stenting with optimal directional coronary atherectomy (DCA).
Design	Randomized clinical study.
Patients	Patients with coronary artery disease who had suitable coronary lesions for both stenting and DCA, by angiography and intra-vascular ultrasound (IVUS).
Follow-up	6 month angiography; 1 year clinical outcome.
Regimen	Stenting (62 lesions) with high pressure adjunctive PTCA to achieve a minimal lumen cross sectional area of ≥ 7.5 mm^2 assessed by IVUS. In the DCA group (n=60 lesions) aggressive debulking using a Simpson Atherocath and increasing balloon pressures to 40 psi. Debulking was guided by IVUS with the goal of a residual percent plaque plus media cross sectional area of <50%. Low pressure adjunct balloon dilatation was performed.
Add'l Tx	Ticlopidine and aspirin for stenting. Aspirin in DCA group. Glycoprotein IIb/IIIa antagonists or anticoagulants were not used.

5b

Results	Serial quantitative angiography and IVUS performed at pre and post procedure and 6 months. Primary end point was restenosis (≥50% diameter stenosis at 6 months) defined by angiography. Initial procedural success (<50% residual diameter stenosis); minimal luminal diameter and percent diameter stenosis at baseline, postprocedure and 6 months were also assessed. Clinical end points also were determined. Initial procedural success was achieved in all patients in both groups. Postprocedural minimal luminal diameter was 2.79±0.39 mm in the stent group vs 2.90±0.38 mm in the DCA group. Postprocedural percent diameter stenosis was 14.8±10% in the stent and 12.9±8.1% in the DCA group (p=NS). Luminal cross sectional area was 8.1±2.2 mm^2 in the stent and 8.5±1.8 mm^2 in the DCA group. Postprocedural percent plaque plus media cross sectional areas was higher for stent arm vs DCA arm (58.6±5.9% vs 52.4±8.2%; p=0.0001). At 6 months the minimal lumen diameter was smaller (1.89±0.73 mm) in the stent group vs the DCA group (2.18±0.62 mm; p=0.023) and diameter stenosis was higher in the stent group (40.1±19.2%) vs the DCA group (32.1±16.9%; p=0.018). The primary end point of angiographic restenosis was lower in the DCA group (15.8%) vs the stent group (15.8%; p=0.032). Follow-up IVUS showed larger area in the DCA group (7.0 mm^2) vs stent group (5.3 mm^2; p=0.03) and more intimal proliferation in the stent group (3.1 mm^2) vs the DCA group (1.1 mm^2; p<0.0001). There was a trend toward lower 1 year target vessel failure in the DCA arm (18.3%) vs stent group (33.9%; p=0.056). Death occurred in 1 stent and zero DCA patients. Target lesion revascularization was 29% in the stent group and 15% in the DCA group (p=0.062).
Concl.	Aggressive DCA including IVUS directed debulking may provide better angiographic and clinical outcomes compared to primary stenting.

START (Stenting vs PTCA)

Stent Implantation and Balloon Angioplasty in the Treatment of De Novo Coronary Artery Lesions

Title	Randomized comparison of coronary stent implantation and balloon angioplasty in the treatment of de novo coronary artery lesions (START).
Authors	Betriu A, Masotti M, Serra A, et al.
Reference	J Am Coll Cardiol 1999;34:1498-1506.
Disease	Coronary artery disease.
Purpose	To determine whether stenting of de novo coronary artery lesions would decrease restenosis rates and lead to better long-term clinical outcomes compared to PTCA.
Design	Randomized, multicenter.
Patients	452 patients with either stable (n=129) or unstable angina (n=229), with angiographic evidence of a coronary stenosis of at least 70% and had not undergone previous dilation.
Follow-up	6 month repeat angiography. 4 year clinical follow-up.
Regimen	Stenting (n=229) vs angioplasty (n=223).
Add'l Tx	For stenting aspirin, dipyridamole, dextran, calcium blocker, heparin, warfarin. After first 100 stents, oral ticlopidine replaced dextran, dipyridamole, and warfarin.

5b

Results	84% of PTCA and 95% of stented patients achieved procedural success, defined as residual stenosis <50% in absence of death, acute MI, need for emergency CABG, or bail out stenting. Rate of vessel closure was 4% in the PTCA group and 2.6% in stent group. At 6 months, 397 patients underwent angiography. The stent group had demonstrated a greater increase in immediate minimal luminal diameter (2.02±0.6 mm) vs the PTCA group (1.43±0.6 mm; p<0.0001) and a greater increase in the 6 month minimal luminal diameter (1.98±0.7 mm vs 1.63±0.7 mm; p<0.001). Restenosis rates were 37% in the PTCA group and 22% in the stent group (RR 0.60; 95% CI=0.43-0.82; p=0.0013). In-hospital mortality was 1.3% in the PTCA group and 0.9% in the stenting group. At 4 years mortality rates were 2.4% and 2.7% in the stent vs angioplasty group; MI rates were 2.8% and 2.2% respectively (p=NS). The need for further revascularization procedures of the target lesions was reduced in the stent (12%) vs the PTCA group (25%; RR 0.49; CI=0.32-0.75; p=0.0006). Repeat procedures were most likely to be carried out within the first 6 months of the study.
Concl.	Stenting reduced restenosis rates and resulted in better minimal luminal diameters compared to PTCA. Stenting also decreased the need for repeat revascularization compared to PTCA.

STRATAS

Study to Determine Rotablator and Transluminal Angioplasty Strategy

Title	Results of the study to determine rotablator and transluminal angioplasty strategy (STRATAS).
Authors	Whitlow PL, Bass TA, Kipperman RM, et al.
Reference	Am J Cardiol 2001;87:699-705.
Disease	Coronary artery disease, percutaneous coronary intervention.
Purpose	To compare the results of aggressive rotablation (maximum burr/artery ratio >0.70) with or without balloon angioplasty (≤1 atmosphere [atm]) vs routine rotablation (maximum burr/artery ratio ≤0.70) followed by routine balloon angioplasty (≥4 atm).
Design	Randomized, open-label, multicenter.
Patients	497 patients undergoing rotational atherectomy for angina pectoris or a positive functional test. The arterial reference size had to be ≤3.25 mm. Patients with total occlusions, lesion length >20 mm, restenotic lesions with >2 prior PCIs, thrombotic lesions, lesions in vein grafts or arterial conduits, and acute myocardial infarction within the last 7 days were not included.
Follow-up	Follow-up angiography at 6-9 months.
Regimen	Randomization to a "routine" strategy of rotablation with a maximum burr/artery ratio ≤0.70, followed by routine balloon angioplasty (≥4 atm) (n=248) or to "aggressive" strategy of rotablation with a maximum burr/artery ratio of >0.70 (n=249). In the aggressive strategy, balloon dilatation was not routinely performed and if performed, the maximal pressure allowed was ≤1 atm.
Add'l Tx	Stents were used only in cases with extensive dissections, or persistent >50% stenosis. Nitroglycerin 4 mg, verapamil 5 mg, and heparin 2000 U/L were added to the rotablator flush solution in both groups.

5b

5. Interventional Cardiology — b. Percutaneous Transluminal Coronary
Angioplasty vs Stenting vs Other Percutaneous Devices, IVUS-Guided Stenting

499

Results	The number of burrs used was 1.9±0.8 in the routine strategy and 2.7±1.0 in the aggressive strategy (p=0.0001). Maximum burr size was 1.8±0.2 mm and 2.1±0.2 mm, respectively (p<0.0001). Maximum burr/artery ratio was 0.71±0.13 in the routine strategy and 0.82±0.14 in the aggressive strategy (p<0.0001). Maximal balloon pressure in patients without stenting was 5.8±2.4 atm vs 1.7±1.9 atm, respectively (p=0.0001). Minimal luminal diameter after procedure was comparable between the routine and aggressive strategies (1.97±0.50 mm and 1.95±0.54 mm). There was no difference in the acute gain (1.11 and 1.14 mm) or percent stenosis after procedure (26±14% vs 27±14%) between the groups. Stents were implanted in 8.8% of the patients in the aggressive strategy and in 6.5% of the patients in the routine strategy (p=NS). Angiographic success was 94.7% vs 95.5% in the aggressive vs routine strategy groups. Zero patients in the aggressive strategy vs 2.0% in the routine strategy underwent urgent or emergency bypass surgery (p=0.03). In-hospital mortality was 0.4% and 1.6%, respectively. Major complications (death, Q-wave myocardial infarction, or bypass surgery) occurred within 30 days in 2.0% vs 4.0% in the aggressive and routine strategies, respectively (p=0.20). TIMI flow <3 was noted in 15.7% and 7.7% of the patients, respectively (p=0.008). CK-MB elevation was noted in 31% vs 27% of the patients, and >5 times the upper limit of normal in 11% vs 7% of the patients, respectively. Patients who had a speed decrease of >5000 rpm from baseline for >5 seconds had more CK-MB elevation (42%) than patients without speed decrease (26%) (p=0.002). 2.0% of the patients in the aggressive strategy vs 3.2% in the routine strategy died after discharge. At 180 days, 22.3% vs 19.5% underwent repeat revascularization, respectively (p=0.18), and at 6-9 month clinical follow-up 23.5% vs 21.1% underwent target vessel revascularization (p=0.13). Target vessel failure (death, myocardial infarction, or repeated revascularization) was 24.9% in the aggressive strategy and 23.5% in the routine strategy (p=0.11). At follow-up angiography MLD was 1.16±0.7 mm in the aggressive strategy and 1.26±0.69 mm in the routine strategy group, and percent diameter stenosis was 56±24% and 53±24%, respectively. Restenosis (>50%) occurred in 58% vs 52% (p=NS). Operator technique reflected by an excessive speed decrease (>5000 rpm) from baseline was associated with CK-MB elevation and restenosis (OR 1.74; p=0.01).
Concl.	The aggressive strategy was comparable to the routine strategy of ≤0.70 maximum burr/artery ratio followed by routine balloon angioplasty. An excessive decrease in the speed of the rotablator was associated with CK-MB release and restenosis.

STRESS (Diabetic Substudy)

Stent Restenosis Study

Title	Coronary intervention in the diabetic patient. Improved outcome following stent implantation compared with balloon angioplasty.
Authors	Savage MP, Fischman DL, Schatz RA, et al.
Reference	Clin Cardiol 2002;25:213-217.
Disease	Coronary artery disease; diabetes.
Purpose	To determine whether stenting is better than percutaneous transluminal coronary angioplasty (PTCA) for reducing restenosis rates in the diabetic patient.
Design	Prospective, randomized, multicenter.
Patients	Of 594 patients randomized in STRESS, 92 (16%) were diabetic. Inclusion criteria as per STRESS.
Follow-up	Angiographic follow-up at 6 months; clinical follow-up at 1 year.
Regimen	Patients were randomized to elective placement of a Palmaz-Schatz stent or PTCA for treatment of new lesions in native coronary artery.
Add'l Tx	As per STRESS. Insulin, oral hypoglycemic agents.

5b

Results	45 patients assigned to PTCA and 47 to stenting. Primary outcome was restenosis determined angiographically at 1 year. Initial procedural success (<50% residual stenosis) achieved in 82% of PTCA patients and 100% of stented patients (p<0.01). Postprocedural lumen diameter was greater with stenting (2.34±0.44 mm) than with PTCA (1.87±0.52 mm; p<0.001). Stenting also resulted in greater luminal gain at 1.61±0.47 vs 1.06±0.46 mm; p<0.001. At 6-month follow-up angiography there was a larger net gain in stented patients (0.97) vs PTCA patients (0.52 mm; p<0.001) as well as a larger lumen (1.69±0.57 mm vs 1.38±0.60 mm; p=0.03). Minimal lumen diameter was 1.69 with stenting vs 1.38 mm with PTCA (p=0.03). Restenosis was present in 24% of stented patients vs 60% of PTCA patients (p=0.002). At 1 year there was no difference in death or MI rates between groups, but target vessel revascularization was performed in 13% of stent patients vs 31% of PTCA patients (p=0.029).
Concl.	Stenting was superior to PTCA in diabetic patients with de novo local coronary lesions. Stenting reduced restenosis rates and need for revascularization procedures.

SWIBAP

Stent Without Balloon Predilation

Title	Randomised comparison of coronary stenting with and without balloon predilatation in selected patients.
Authors	Le Breton H, Boschat J, Commeau P, et al.
Reference	Heart 2001;86:302-308.
Disease	Coronary artery disease, percutaneous coronary intervention (PCI).
Purpose	To assess the feasibility and safety of direct stenting in noncomplex coronary lesions.
Design	Randomized, open-label, multicenter.
Patients	396 patients, <76 years old, scheduled to undergo PCI with stent implantation of a single American College of Cardiology/ American Heart Association task force classification type A or B1 noncalcified de novo lesion in an artery of ≥3.0 mm diameter, and without contraindications to aspirin, ticlopidine, or clopidogrel. Patients with sharp angulation before or at the target lesion were not included. Patients with acute myocardial infarction or refractory unstable angina were excluded. Patients with lesions that could not be covered by a single 9-mm or 16-mm stent, bifurcation lesion, left main coronary artery lesion, and restenotic lesions were excluded. Patients could undergo multivessel PCI, but only 1 lesion could be randomized for the study.
Follow-up	30 days.
Regimen	Randomization to stenting without balloon predilation (SWIBAP) (n=197) or to predilation with balloon before stenting (PTCA-stent) (n=199). Crossover to balloon predilation was permitted when the stent could not be advanced. NIR stents (9 or 16 mm in length) were used in all patients.
Add'l Tx	All patients received aspirin 160 mg/d and ticlopidine 250 mg bid or clopidogrel 75 mg/d for 1 month after PCI. IV heparin 10,000 was given at the beginning of PCI.

5b

Results	SWIBAP was successful in 192/197 of the lesions (97.5%), and after balloon predilatation in the PTCA-stent group in 197/199 of the lesions (99%; p=0.283). In all 5 patients of the SWIBAP group in whom initial stent placement failed, stent was successfully deployed after balloon predilation. 4 patients in the PTCA-stent and none in the SWIBAP needed an additional stent for residual dissection. The final angiographic success was 100% in both groups. The mean duration of the procedure was longer in the PTCA-stent (27.96±15.23 minutes) than in the SWIBAP group (23.50±13.54 minutes; p=0.002). Fluoroscopic time was 6.67±3.65 and 6.04±4.13 minutes, respectively (p=NS). The average amount of contrast agent used was 135±65 mL in the SWIBAP and 157±62 mL in the PTCA-stent group (p<0.001). The minimal lumen diameter after stenting was comparable between the SWIBAP (2.82±0.43 mm) and the PTCA-stent (2.85±0.43 mm) groups (p=0.551). The residual diameter stenosis was also comparable (11.6%±7.2% vs 10.6%±8.0%, respectively; p=0.220). No major adverse cardiac event occurred in-hospital in both groups. There were 2 cases with non-Q-wave myocardial infarction in the SWIBAP group (1%). The primary success rate was 96.5% in the SWIBAP and 99% in the PTCA-stent group (p=NS). There were no cases of death, myocardial infarction, stent thrombosis, or need for target vessel revascularization in both groups during the 30-day follow-up.
Concl.	Direct stenting of selected and noncomplex de novo coronary lesions was feasible and safe. Direct stenting resulted in reduction in procedure time and contrast agent used.

TOSCA

Total Occlusion Study of Canada

Title	Primary stenting vs balloon angioplasty in occluded coronary arteries.
Authors	Buller CE, Dzavik V, Carere RG, et al.
Reference	Circulation 1999;100:236-242.
Disease	Coronary artery disease.
Purpose	To determine whether routine stenting improves late complete patency of recanalized total coronary artery occlusions.
Design	Randomized, controlled, multicenter.
Patients	Patients undergoing coronary interventions with a total coronary occlusion defined as high grade native coronary stenosis with TIMI grade 0 or 1 antegrade flow.
Follow-up	6 months.
Regimen	Percutaneous transluminal coronary angioplasty (PTCA) vs heparin coated 15 mm long PS-153 Palmaz-Schatz coronary stent.
Add'l Tx	Aspirin, ticlopidine, as per investigator.
Results	The primary end point was failure of sustained complete target vessel patency with TIMI flow of <3. Secondary end points included repeat revascularization, adverse cardiovascular events, and restenosis (>50% diameter stenosis on angiography). Primary stenting was associated with a 10.9% failed patency rate vs PTCA at 19.5%, p=0.025 resulting in a 44% decrease in failed patency at 6 months. Target vessel revascularization was 8.4% with stenting vs 15.4% with PTCA (p=0.03), reflecting at 45% decrease in revascularization rates. Incidence of adverse cardiovascular events (defined as any revascularization, myocardial infarction or death) was 23.3% in the stent group and 23.6% in the PTCA group; p=NS. By angiography, stenting was associated with a larger minimum lumen dimension at 6 months (1.48 mm) vs PTCA (1.23 mm; p<0.01) and decreased binary restenosis rate (55% vs 70%; p<0.01).

5b

Concl.   Primary stenting is superior to PTCA for nonacute total coronary occlusions.

TOTAL

Total Occlusion Trial with Angioplasty by Using Laser Guide Wire

Title	Total occlusion trial with angioplasty by using laser guide wire. The TOTAL trial.
Authors	Serruys PW, Hamburger JN, Koolen JJ, et al.
Reference	Eur Heart J 2000;21:1797-1805.
Disease	Coronary artery disease.
Purpose	To evaluate the efficacy and safety of crossing a chronic coronary total occlusion using a laser guide wire as compared to "conventional" mechanical guide wires.
Design	Randomized, open-label, multicenter.
Patients	303 patients with angina or ischemia and a TIMI 0 flow occlusion, detected by coronary angiography >4 weeks before randomization. Patients without clear visualization of the distal lumen via collaterals, ostial occlusion of the right cornary artery or the left main coronary artery, a nonvisible entry point of the target lesion, >1 anatomical curve expected within the missing arterial segment, or angiographic evidence of thrombus in the target lesion were excluded.
Follow-up	12 months.
Regimen	Randomization to a laser guide wire (n=144) or "conventional" mechanical guide wire (n=159).

5b

Results	The primary end point of reaching the true lumen distal to the occlusion within 30 minutes of fluoroscopic time was reached by 52.8% of the patients randomized to the laser guide wire vs 47.2% of the patients in the mechanical guide wire (p=0.33). The total amount of contrast dye used was 517±244 mL and 492±262 mL in the laser and mechanical guide wire groups (p=0.28). The total fluoroscopic time was comparable (42±26 minutes vs 41±26 minutes, respectively; p=0.84). The duration of hospital stay was longer in the laser guide wire group (4.6±3.7 days vs 4.0±4.9 days; p=0.03). Guidewire perforation was detected in 7.2% of the patients assigned to laser guide wire vs 8.8% of the patients assigned to mechanical guide wire. Serious adverse events following the initial guide wire attempt were detected in zero and 0.6% of the patients in the laser and mechanical guide wire, respectively. Clinical success rate of the percutaneous coronary intervention was achieved in 51% of the patients in the laser vs 60% of the patients in the mechanical guide wire group (p=0.12). Stents were used in 90% of the patients in the laser guide wire vs 78% of the patients in the mechanical guide wire group. At 6 months, restenosis occurred in 45.5% of the patients in the laser guide wire vs 38.3% of the patients in the mechanical guide wire group (p=0.38). Reocclusion occurred in 25.8% vs 16.1%, respectively (p=0.15). There was no significant difference in the angina and major adverse cardiac event-free survival between the groups (p=0.11).
Concl.	The laser guide wire was not more effective than conventional mechanical guide wires in crossing chronic total coronary occlusions. In both groups, the 1-year event-free survival was low (about 60%).

VeGAS 2

Vein Graft AngioJet Study 2

Title	A trial comparing rheolytic thrombectomy with intracoronary urokinase for coronary and vein graft thrombus (The Vein Graft AngioJet Study [VeGAS 2]).
Authors	Kuntz RE, Baim DS, Cohen DJ, et al.
Reference	Am J Cardiol 2002;89:326-330.
Disease	Coronary artery disease, percutaneous coronary intervention (PCI).
Purpose	To compare the clinical efficacy of rheolytic thrombectomy with AngioJet (Possis Medical, Minneapolis, MN) with intracoronary urokinase infusion for the treatment of thrombus-containing lesions in saphenous vein grafts and native coronary arteries.
Design	Randomized, open-label, multicenter.
Patients	349 patients undergoing PCI of a lesion with angiographically evident thrombus in a native coronary artery or vein graft. Patients who received thrombolytic therapy or had acute myocardial infarction within the preceding 24 hours were excluded. Patients with contraindications to aspirin or thrombolytic therapy were excluded. In addition, patients who needed PCI of more than 1 vessel and those with a target lesion in a <2.0 mm diameter vessel were not included.
Follow-up	30 days.
Regimen	Randomization to PCI with AngioJet or to urokinase (250,000 IU intracoronary bolus over 15-30 minutes followed by IV infusion 20,000 IU/h for 6-30 hours).
Add'l Tx	All patients received aspirin 325 mg/d, oral calcium channel blockers, IV nitroglycerin, and IV heparin (target activated clotting time ≥300 sec). Use of glycoprotein IIb/IIIa was permitted. Patients who underwent stent implantation received ticlopidine, clopidogrel, or warfarin at the discretion of the operator.

5b

5. Interventional Cardiology — b. Percutaneous Transluminal Coronary Angioplasty vs Stenting vs Other Percutaneous Devices, IVUS-Guided Stenting

509

Results	The treated vessel was vein graft in 53% of the patients in the AngioJet group and 54% in the urokinase group (p=0.914). The AngioJet was successfully delivered in 98% of the cases. Glycoprotein IIb/IIIa inhibitors were used in 14% of the patients in each group. Urokinase was infused for an average of 13.2±8.1 hours, and the mean dose was 1,112,780±968,750 IU. Stents were implanted in 73% of the patients in the AngioJet and 61% in the urokinase groups. The device success was 87% and 75% with the AngioJet and urokinase, respectively (p=0.005). The procedural success rate was 86% and 72%, respectively (p=0.002). Bradycardia occurred significantly more often in the AngioJet group (24% vs 2%). Hemolysis occurred in 73% and 38%, respectively. However, hemolysis did not lead to transfusions or renal failure. Major adverse cardiac events occurred in 16% of the patients in the AngioJet vs 33% in the urokinase group (p<0.001). Death occurred in 2% vs 3%, respectively (p=0.491); myocardial infarction in 14% vs 31% (p<0.001); and revascularization in 3% vs 4% (p=1.00). Vascular complications were noted in 4% of the AngioJet group vs 18% in the urokinase group (p<0.001). Bleeding complications occurred in 5% vs 12%, respectively (p<0.001). Residual diameter stenosis >50% was noted in 6% vs 15% of the AngioJet and urokinase groups (p=0.004). However, final TIMI grade flow 3 was comparable (89% and 83%, respectively; p=0.199).
Concl.	Rheolytic thrombectomy with AngioJet device was more effective and safer than urokinase infusion for treating thrombus-containing lesions in native coronary arteries and venous grafts.

WIDEST

Wiktor Stent in De Novo Stenosis

Title	Is provisional stenting the effective option? The WIDEST study (Wiktor stent in de novo stenosis).
Authors	Fluck DS, Chenu P, Mills P, et al.
Reference	Heart 2000;84:522-528.
Disease	Coronary artery disease, percutancous coronary.intervention.
Purpose	To compare the results of routine coronary stent implantation and routine balloon angioplasty with provisional stenting for suboptimal results.
Design	Randomized, multicenter.
Patients	300 patients with symptomatic CAD, scheduled for PCI in a single lesion. Patients with a recent myocardial infarction, after coronary artery bypass grafting or PCI to the target vessel or lesion, or those needing multivessel PCI were excluded. In addition, patients with a TIMI flow grade 0, thrombotic lesion, need for >1 stent, ostial lesion, left main stenosis, contraindications to aspirin or anticoagulation, and uncontrolled hypertension were not included.
Follow-up	12 months.
Regimen	Randomized to conventional balloon angioplasty (n=146) or to Wiktor GX stent implantation (n=154).
Add'l Tx	All patients received aspirin. Warfarin was recommended initially after stent implantation, but later was replaced by antiplatelet drugs. Abciximab was used in 1 patient only.

5b

Results   The procedure was successful in 96% of the patients. 2 patients in the balloon group did not undergo PCI. 30.1% of the patients in the balloon group needed stent implantation because of suboptimal results. 3 patients (1.9%) assigned to stent did not receive stents. 2 patients in the balloon group vs none in the stent group died at 30 days (p=NS). Death, MI, or further revascularization occurred in 6.8% of the patients in the balloon group vs 7.8% in the stent group at 30 days. Death or MI at 1 year occurred in 4.8% and 4.0% of the patients, respectively. Death, MI or revascularization at 1 year occurred in 19.2% of the patients in the balloon group vs 20.8% in the stent group. Acute and subacute vessel closure occurred in 2.1% of the patients in the balloon group vs 3.3% of the patients in the stent group. Hemorrhage requiring transfusion or surgical repair of the arterial access site occurred in 2.1% and 6.4% of the patients, respectively. At 30 days, 6.1% of the patients in the balloon group vs 5.8% in the stent group underwent repeat revascularization. At 1 year, 17.1% and 18.2% of the patients, respectively, underwent repeat revascularization. In 213 patients (69% of the balloon group and 73% of the stent group) follow-up angiography at 6 months was analyzed. Minimal lumen diameter was 0.96 mm in the balloon group and 1.01 mm in the stent group before PCI, and 2.27 mm and 2.68 mm, respectively, after PCI ($p<0.007$). At 6 months, minimal lumen diameter was 2.00 and 1.90, respectively ($p>0.05$). Restenosis occurred in 17.3% of the patients in the balloon group vs 21.6% in the stent group ($p>0.05$).

Concl.   The short-term and 1-year clinical outcomes and the 6-month angiographic results of conventional balloon angioplasty with provisional stenting and routine stenting were comparable.

Title	Early use of the pulmonary artery catheter and outcomes in patients with shock and acute respiratory distress syndrome. A randomized controlled trial.
Authors	Richard C, Warszawski J, Anguel N, et al.
Reference	JAMA 2003;290:2713-2720.
Disease	Patients with shock mainly of septic origin, acute respiratory distress syndromes, or both.
Purpose	To determine the outcome of early use of pulmonary artery catheters in patients with shock, mainly due to septic shock, acute respiratory distress syndrome, or both.
Design	Randomized, multicenter, controlled study.
Patients	676 patients with criteria for shock, adult respiratory distress syndrome, or both in 36 intensive care units in France.
Follow-up	28 days.
Regimen	Randomized to pulmonary artery catheter (n=335) or no catheter (n=341). Therapy was left to the discretion of the physician. The centers agreed upon optimizing circulating blood volume and vasoactive support, if necessary, to maintain mean arterial blood pressure of at least 60 mm Hg, and other standard therapies.

5b

Results	Primary end point was mortality at 28 days. Secondary end points included mortality at 14 and 90 days, duration of intensive care unit and hospital stay, and others. At day 28, there was no difference in mortality in the patients who received a pulmonary artery catheter (59.4%) vs those who did not (61.0%; relative risk [RR]=0.97; 95% CI=0.86-1.10; p=0.67). Also, there was no difference in mortality between those who did or did not receive the catheter at day 14 (49.9% vs 51.3%; RR=0.97; 95% CI=0.84-1.13; p=0.70) or at day 90 (70.7% vs 72.0%; RR=0.98; 95% CI=0.89-1.08; p=0.71). At day 28, mean number of days not in hospital with or without pulmonary artery catheter (0.9±3.6 vs 0.9±3.3) or free of intensive care unit (3.3±6.8 vs 3.3±6.9) or ventilator use were the same between groups. There was also no difference at day 14 between the 2 groups in number of days free of organ system failure, renal support, or vasoactive agents.
Concl.	The use of a pulmonary artery catheter in patients with shock, acute adult respiratory syndrome, or both did not improve morbidity or mortality.

5. Interventional Cardiology — b. Percutaneous Transluminal Coronary Angioplasty vs Stenting vs Other Percutaneous Devices, IVUS-Guided Stenting

Small Vessel Study

Title	Randomized comparison of balloon angioplasty vs silicon carbon-coated stent implantation for de novo lesions in small coronary arteries.
Authors	Hanekamp C, Koolen J, Bonnier H, et al.
Reference	Am J Cardiol 2004;93:1233-1237.
Disease	Coronary artery disease, percutaneous coronary intervention.
Purpose	To compare angiographic and clinical outcomes of percutaneous transluminal coronary angioplasty and stent implantation in de novo lesions in coronary arteries with a diameter less than 3.0 mm.
Design	Randomized, open-label, multicenter.
Patients	496 patients with de novo lesion of ≤15 mm in length, in a coronary artery with a reference diameter 2.0-3.0 mm. Patients with a lesion in an artery supplying akinetic area or segment with prior Q-wave infarction, primary or rescue percutaneous coronary intervention for an acute myocardial infarction, lesions involving a major side branch, arteries with additional lesions beside the "study" lesion requiring percutaneous coronary intervention, contraindications to aspirin or ticlopidine, and those receiving oral anticoagulation therapy were excluded.
Follow-up	6-month follow-up angiography. Clinical follow-up for 1 year.
Regimen	Randomization to conventional balloon angioplasty (percutaneous transluminal coronary angioplasty, n=246) or percutaneous transluminal coronary angioplasty with stent implantation (a silicon carbide-coated, stainless steel 2.5-3.0 mm in diameter and 15 mm in length; Tenax, Biotronik, GmbH, Berlin, Germany; n=250).

5b

5. Interventional Cardiology — b. Percutaneous Transluminal Coronary
Angioplasty vs Stenting vs Other Percutaneous Devices, IVUS-Guided Stenting

515

Add'l Tx	All patients received aspirin 75-150 mg/d and those who underwent stent implantation received also ticlopidine 250 mg/d for ≥15 days.
Results	In the stent-assigned group, stent was implanted in 236 patients (94.4%). In the PTCA-assigned group, 70 patients (29%) underwent stent implantation. Immediately postprocedure there was 24.9%±9.8% diameter stenosis in the PTCA group vs 20.8%±10.3% in the stent group (p=0.0001). The minimal lumen diameter was 1.77±0.35 mm vs 1.97±0.36 mm, respectively (p=0.0001). In the hospital, major adverse cardiac events occurred in 3.7% of the patients in the PTCA group and in 3.2% in the stent group. Follow-up angiography was performed in 355 patients (72%). At follow-up, the percent diameter stenosis was 39.1%±19.8% in the PTCA group and 37.0%±21.2%, respectively (p=NS), and the minimal lumen diameter was 1.41±0.49 mm and 1.46±0.53 mm, respectively (p=NS). Although the acute gain was larger in the stent group (1.08±0.46 mm vs 0.92±0.40 mm; p=0.001), the late loss was also larger in the stent group (0.51±0.56 mm vs 0.36±0.49 mm; p=0.005). >50% diameter restenosis was found in 25% of the patients in the PTCA group and in 21% of the patients in the stent group (p=NS). 1-year survival-free of major adverse cardiac events was comparable between the groups (p=0.35).
Concl.	When followed by half the recommended dose of ticlopidine, use of silicon carbon-coated stents did not improve angiographic and clinical outcomes as compared to PTCA for the treatment of de novo lesions in small coronary arteries.

AMIGO

Atherectomy Before Multi-Link Improves Lumen Gain and Clinical Outcomes

Title	Comparison of directional coronary atherectomy and stenting vs stenting alone for the treatment of de novo and restenotic coronary artery narrowing.
Authors	Stankovic G, Colombo A, Bersin R, et al.
Reference	Am J Cardiol 2004;93:953-958.
Disease	Coronary artery disease, percutaneous coronary intervention.
Purpose	To compare outcome following stenting alone with directional atherectomy before stenting in a variety of de novo and restenotic coronary lesions.
Design	Randomized, open-label, multicenter.
Patients	753 patients, ≥18 years old with a single ≥70% diameter lesion (either de novo or first-time, postangioplasty restenosis) in a native coronary artery, 2.75-3.75 mm in diameter and ≤32 mm in length. Pregnant women were excluded. Patients with recent (≤3 days) myocardial infarction, intolerance to heparin, aspirin, thienopyridines, or contrast media were excluded. In addition, patients with >40% left main stenosis, intention-to-treat multiple vessels within 30 days of the index intervention, severe vessel tortuosity, excessive coronary calcification, visible thrombus in the target lesion or left ventricular ejection fraction <35% were excluded.
Follow-up	12 months clinical follow-up. Repeat angiography at 8 months.
Regimen	Randomization to stenting alone (n=372), or to directional coronary atherectomy (n=381) followed by stenting. The stents that were used are the ACS Multi-link Coronary Stent System and the ACS Multi-link Duet Coronary Stent System (Guidant Corporation, Indianapolis, IN).

5b

5. Interventional Cardiology — b. Percutaneous Transluminal Coronary
Angioplasty vs Stenting vs Other Percutaneous Devices, IVUS-Guided Stenting

517

Add'l Tx	Decisions concerning abciximab use should have been made before randomization. All patients received aspirin 325 mg/d, and ticlopidine 250 mg bid or clopidogrel 75 mg/d for 4 weeks.
Results	In 20 patients (5.2%), directional coronary atherectomy (DCA) could not be performed and they were crossed over from the DCA to the stent-alone group. Dissections ≥type B were more frequent in the DCA group (20.7% vs 9.8%; p<0.0001). Procedural success rate was lower in the DCA group (91.5% vs 97.3%; p=0.00070. The rate of clinical success was also lower in the DCA group (89.9% vs 96.5%; p=0.0004). Baseline minimal lumen diameter was comparable between the groups (0.90±0.43 mm in the DCA and 0.87±0.41 mm in the stent group; p=0.438). Immediately postprocedure, minimal lumen diameter tended to be larger (2.67±0.56 mm vs 2.61±0.49 mm; p=0.054), and the diameter stenosis was significantly lower (14.8±12.6% vs 15.9±10.0%; p=0.018) in the DCA group, although there was no difference in the acute gain (1.77±0.61 mm vs 1.74±0.56 mm, respectively; p=0.443). 8-month follow-up angiography showed no difference in the minimal lumen diameter (1.90±0.74 mm vs 1.92±0.65 mm; p=0.868), diameter stenosis (37.7±22.1% vs 36.6±19.1%; p=0.925), late loss (0.79±0.76 mm vs 0.69±0.66 mm; p=0.283), or restenosis rate (26.7% vs 22.1%; p=0.237). The rates of clinical events were comparable between the groups. 1-year target vessel failure occurred in 23.9% of the patients in the DCA vs 21.5% in the stenting group (p=0.487). 1-year target vessel revascularization occurred in 19.7% vs 18.8%, respectively (p=0.782). 1-year mortality was 1.3% and 0.8%, respectively (p=0.725). Multivariate logistic regression analysis showed that the use of stents alone reduced restenosis vs suboptimal (OR 0.59; p=0.01) or optimal (OR 0.45; p=0.01) DCA before stenting.
Concl.	DCA before stenting failed to reduce angiographic restenosis or improve clinical outcome after coronary stenting of lesions in native coronary arteries.

ATLAS

Acolysis During Treatment of Lesions Affecting Saphenous Vein Bypass Grafts

Title	Treatment of saphenous vein bypass grafts with ultrasound thrombolysis: a randomized study (ATLAS).
Authors	Singh M, Rosenschein U, Ho KK, et al.
Reference	Circulation 2003;107:2331-2336.
Disease	Coronary artery disease, acute coronary syndrome, thrombus of saphenous vein grafts.
Purpose	To determine whether acolysis (therapeutic ultrasound) can break up thrombus and lead to better outcomes in patients undergoing percutaneous coronary intervention in saphenous vein grafts with thrombus vs patients receiving abciximab.
Design	Randomized, multicenter, controlled trial comparing acolysis to abciximab.
Patients	181 patients with prior coronary artery bypass graft surgery and lesions in a vein graft who presented with either acute coronary syndrome or angiographic or clinical evidence of a thrombus within the graft. Inclusion criteria included unstable angina, ischemic ST change on resting electrocardiogram, recent myocardial infarction with 24 hours before intended therapy, positive stress test, and others. Patients were undergoing percutaneous coronary intervention in their saphenous vein grafts.
Follow-up	30 days and 360 days.
Regimen	Patients were randomized to acolysis followed by percutaneous transluminal coronary angioplasty or stenting or to abciximab followed by balloon dilation and stent implantation.
Add'l Tx	Heparin, aspirin, ticlopidine.

5b

Results	Primary end point was frequency of successful procedures (final diameter stenosis of ≤30% by quantitative coronary angiography, TIMI 3 flow, and freedom from major cardiac events (composite of cardiac death, MI, emergency CABG surgery, repeat target lesion revascularization, disabling stroke). 87 of 92 (95%) patients in the acolysis group received ≥1 stents. 80 of 89 (90%) patients in the abciximab group received a stent. 63% of acolysis patients and 82% of abciximab patients achieved angiographic procedural success (p=0.008). At 30 days major adverse cardiac events occurred in 25% of patients in the acolysis group vs 12% in the abciximab group (p=0.036) primarily due to more non-Qwave MIs in the acolysis group (19.6%) vs the abciximab group (7.9%; p=0.03). There was a trend toward more Q-wave MIs in the acolysis group (5.4%) as compared to the abciximab group (2.2%; p=NS). The primary composite end point (postprocedural diameter stenosis ≤30%, TIMI 3 flow, and freedom from major adverse cardiac events) was achieved in 53.8% of the acolysis group vs 73.1% of the abciximab patients (p=0.014). At 360 days, cumulative frequency of major adverse cardiac events was 39.1% in acolysis group vs 22.5% in abciximab group (p=0.017). The authors postulated that acolysis may have fragmented the thrombus into smaller particles that embolized the microvasculature.
Concl.	The use of therapeutic ultrasound to treat vein graft thrombi in patients with acute coronary syndromes was detrimental compared to abciximab during PCI.

CADILLAC

Controlled Abciximab and Device Investigation to Lower Late Angioplasty Complications

Title	Outcomes of optimal or "stent-like" balloon angioplasty in acute myocardial infarction: the CADILLAC trial.
Authors	Cox DA, Stone GW, Grines CL, et al.
Reference	J Am Coll Cardiol 2003;42:971-977.
Disease	Acute myocardial infarction.
Purpose	To compare outcomes between patients with acute myocardial infarction undergoing percutaneous transluminal coronary angioplasty with an optimal, or "stent-like" result vs patients who undergo routine stent replacement.
Design	Large-scale, multicenter, prospective, randomized trial.
Patients	2082 patients with acute myocardial infarction.
Follow-up	1 year.
Regimen	Percutaneous transluminal coronary angioplasty alone, percutaneous transluminal coronary angioplasty + abciximab, stenting alone, or stenting + abciximab.

5b

Results	By core laboratory angiographic analysis, optimal PTCA was achieved in 40.7% of patients who had PTCA: 38.5% assigned to PTCA alone and 42.7% to PTCA + abciximab. Ischemic target-vessel revascularization (TVR) at 30 days was more common after optimal PTCA than routine stenting (5.1% vs 2.3%; p=0.007). The 1-year composite adverse event rate (death, reinfarction, disabling stroke, or TVR) was greater in patients with optimal PTCA than in those with routine stenting (21.9% vs 13.8%; p<0.001), largely due to increased rates of ischemic TVR (19.1% vs 9.1%; p<0.001). The rates of death, reinfarction, and disabling stroke were not significantly different between the groups. Angiographic restenosis was also more common with optimal PTCA than with routine stenting (36.2% vs 22.2; p=0.003). Abciximab as an adjunct to PTCA or stenting provided short-term clinical benefits, yielding a reduction in 30-day ischemic TVR and subacute vessel closure for both stent and PTCA patients; it did not affect long-term mortality or ischemic TVR.
Concl.	Recent studies in patients with acute MI undergoing stent implantation suggest that PTCA may no longer be a relevant treatment strategy for stent-eligible lesions. It is not known whether routine stent placement is superior or necessary when an optimal PTCA - a "stent-like" result - is achieved. The CADILLAC trial suggests that even if an optimal result is achieved after primary PTCA in patients with acute MI, early and late outcomes can be further improved with routine stent implantation.

FIRE

FilterWire EX Randomized Evaluation

Title	Randomized comparison of distal protection with a filter-based catheter and a balloon occlusion and aspiration system during percutaneous intervention of diseased saphenous vein aorto-coronary bypass grafts.
Authors	Stone GW, Rogers C, Hermiller J, et al.
Reference	Circulation 2003;108:548-553.
Disease	Coronary artery disease.
Purpose	To evaluate the safety and efficacy of distal microcirculatory protection with a novel filter-based catheter compared with the GuardWire (Medtronic, Minneapolis, MN) balloon occlusion and aspiration device during percutaneous coronary intervention of diseased saphenous vein grafts.
Design	Multicenter, prospective, randomized trial.
Patients	651 patients undergoing percutaneous coronary intervention of 682 saphenous vein graft lesions.
Follow-up	30 days.
Regimen	Distal protection during percutaneous coronary intervention with the filter-based FilterWire EX (Boston Scientific, Natick, MA) (n=332) or the GuardWire balloon occlusion and aspiration system (n=319).

5b

Results	Device success was 95.5% with the FilterWire EX and 97.2% with the GuardWire system. Postprocedural measures of epicardial flow and angiographic complications were similar between the 2 groups, although bailout glycoprotein IIb/IIIa inhibitors were required in 1.5% of cases with the GuardWire and in 0 cases with the FilterWire EX (p=0.03). A primary end point event (30-day composite of major adverse cardiac events: death, MI, target-vessel revascularization) occurred in 9.9% of FilterWire EX patients and 11.6% of GuardWire patients (95% CI=-6.4 to 3.1; p for superiority=0.53; p for noninferiority=0.0008). Most major adverse cardiac events were non-Q MIs. The extent of periprocedural myonecrosis was almost identical in the 2 groups.
Concl.	The FIRE study is the first to examine the comparative efficacy of distal microcirculatory protection with 2 competitive technologies. Distal protection with the 2 systems resulted in similar rates of major adverse cardiac events at 30 days. Periprocedural adverse outcomes occur in about 10% of patients. Complementary device-based innovations and pharmacologic regimens are needed to improve the safety of PCI in these high-risk patients.

RESCUT

Restenosis Cutting Balloon Evaluation Trial

Title	Cutting balloon versus conventional balloon angioplasty for the treatment of in-stent restenosis. Results of the Restenosis Cutting Balloon Evaluation Trial (RESCUT).
Authors	Albiero R, Silber S, DiMario C, et al.
Reference	J Am Coll Cardiol 2004;43:943-949.
Disease	Coronary artery disease.
Purpose	To compare cutting balloon angioplasty with conventional balloon angioplasty for treatment of in-stent restenosis.
Design	Multicenter, randomized, prospective trial.
Patients	428 patients with all types of in-stent restenosis (focal, multifocal, diffuse, proliferative).
Follow-up	7 months.
Regimen	Cutting balloon angioplasty (n=214) or percutaneous transluminal coronary angioplasty (n=214).

5. Interventional Cardiology — b. Percutaneous Transluminal Coronary
Angioplasty vs Stenting vs Other Percutaneous Devices, IVUS-Guided Stenting

525

Results   Most of the in-stent restenosis (ISR) lesions in both groups were <20 mm long. The number of balloons used to treat ISR was lower with cutting balloon angioplasty (CBA): 1 balloon was used in 82.3% of CBA cases and in 75% of PTCA procedures (p=0.03). Balloon slippage was less common with CBA (6.5% vs 25% with PTCA; p<0.01). Additional stenting was somewhat less common with CBA (3.9% vs 8% with PTCA; p=0.07). At 7-month angiographic follow-up, the binary restenosis rate was similar between the groups (29.8% with CBA vs 31.4% with PTCA). The pattern of recurrent restenosis was similar, as were clinical events at 7 months.

Concl.   CBA did not reduce the rate of recurrent ISR and major cardiac events over conventional PTCA; however, CBA had some procedural advantages: it required fewer balloons, less additional stenting, and had a lower incidence of balloon slippage. The question of long-term superiority of CBA over conventional PTCA for treatment of ISR will be addressed by the ongoing REDUCE II.

RIBS

Restenosis Intra-Stent: Balloon Angioplasty vs Elective Stenting

Title	A randomized comparison of repeat stenting with balloon angioplasty in patients with in-stent restenosis.
Authors	Alfonso F, Zueco J, Cequier A, et al.
Reference	J Am Coll Cardiol 2003;42:796-805.
Disease	Coronary artery disease.
Purpose	To compare repeat stenting with balloon angioplasty in patients with in-stent restenosis.
Design	Multicenter, randomized trial.
Patients	450 patients with in-stent restenosis.
Follow-up	1 year.
Regimen	Elective stent implantation (n=224) or conventional balloon angioplasty (n=226).
Results	The procedural success rate was similar in the 2 groups, 98% with stenting and 95% with balloon angioplasty. However, in-hospital complications were more common with angioplasty (4.9% vs 1.3%; p=0.039). Stenting produced a larger minimal lumen diameter (MLD) (2.77±0.4 vs 2.25±0.5 mm; p<0.001) after the procedure. At follow-up (6 months), MLD remained larger with stenting when the in-lesion site was considered (1.69±0.8 vs 1.54±0.7 mm, p=0.046); however, the binary restenosis rate was similar in the 2 groups, 38% with stenting and 39% with angioplasty. With 100% follow-up, the 1-year event-free survival was similar, 77% with stenting and 71% angioplasty (p=0.19); however, in the prespecified subgroup of patients with large vessels (≥3 mm), the restenosis rate (27% vs 49%; p=0.007) and event-free survival (84% vs 62%; p=0.002) were better after repeat stenting.

5. Interventional Cardiology — b. Percutaneous Transluminal Coronary
Angioplasty vs Stenting vs Other Percutaneous Devices, IVUS-Guided Stenting

527

Concl.   Repeat coronary stenting yielded better initial angiographic results but did not decrease the restenosis rate or improve clinical outcome compared with balloon angioplasty; however, in patients with large vessels, coronary stenting improved the long-term clinical and angiographic outcome.

X-TRACT

X-SIZER for Treatment of Thrombus and Atherosclerosis in Coronary Interventions Trial

Title	Prospective, randomized evaluation of thrombectomy prior to percutaneous intervention in diseased saphenous vein grafts and thrombus-containing coronary arteries.
Authors	Stone GW, Cox DA, Babb J, et al.
Reference	J Am Coll Cardiol 2003;42:2007-2013.
Disease	Coronary artery disease.
Purpose	To determine whether routine thrombectomy before stent implantation in diseased saphenous vein grafts and thrombus-containing native coronary arteries reduces periprocedural myonecrosis and subsequently enhances event-free survival.
Design	Large-scale, multicenter, prospective, randomized trial.
Patients	797 patients with 839 diseased saphenous vein grafts or thrombus-containing native coronary arteries.
Follow-up	1 year.
Regimen	Stent implantation with or without prior thrombectomy with the X-SIZER (ev3 Inc., Plymouth, MN) device.
Results	In patients who underwent thrombectomy with the X-SIZER, a mean of 1.1±0.1 catheters per case were used. Glycoprotein IIb/IIIa inhibitors were used prophylactically in three fourths of patients in both groups, and stents were implanted in almost all patients. The rate of periprocedural MI was similar in the 2 groups, 15.8% in patients undergoing thrombectomy and 16.6% in control patients; however, the rate of "large" MI (development of new pathologic Q-waves or creatine kinase-MB elevation >8 × upper limits of normal) was less with thrombectomy, 5.5% vs 9.6% (multivariate risk ratio 0.35; 95% CI=0.18-0.66; p=0.002). The rate of major adverse cardiac events (cardiac death, MI, repeat target vessel revascularization) was also similar: at 30 days, 16.8% in patients with thrombectomy and 17.1% in control patients, and at 1 year, 31.3% and 28.2%.

5b

Concl.   Thrombectomy with the X-SIZER device before stent implantation in high-risk diseased saphenous vein grafts (SVGs) and thrombus-containing native coronary arteries may reduce the extent, but not the occurrence, of cardiac events. Thrombectomy did not improve early or late event-free survival. In contrast, both balloon occlusion/aspiration and filter-based distal protection devices during SVG intervention have been shown to reduce the incidence of small and large MIs and are the preferred therapy for eligible SVG lesions. More studies are needed to determine whether removing thrombus before percutaneous intervention improves event-free survival.

5. Interventional Cardiology
c. Medical Therapy, Including Antiplatelet Therapy, for Prevention of Complications and Restenosis with Angiography and Percutaneous Coronary Intervention

5. Interventional Cardiology — c. Medical Therapy, Including Antiplatelet Therapy, for Prevention of Complications and Restenosis with Angiography and PCI

531

Clopidogrel as Adjunctive Antiplatelet Therapy During Coronary Stenting

Title	Clopidogrel as adjunctive antiplatelet therapy during coronary stenting.
Authors	Mishkel GJ, Aguirre FV, Ligon RW, et al.
Reference	J Am Coll Cardiol 1999;34:1884-1890.
Disease	Coronary artery disease.
Purpose	To determine procedural and 30-day clinical outcomes in patients receiving ticlopidine vs clopidogrel during coronary artery stenting.
Design	Prospective, single-center analysis.
Patients	875 consecutive patients undergoing stenting who received aspirin plus either clopidogrel or ticlopidine.
Follow-up	30 days.
Regimen	All patients received oral aspirin (325 mg) before the procedure and then daily. Therapy with oral ticlopidine (250 mg twice daily) or oral clopidogrel (75 mg once daily) was begun the night before or the day of the procedure and continued for 2-4 weeks after the procedure.
Add'l Tx	Heparin; glycoprotein IIb/IIIa antagonists and intracoronary nitroglycerin could be used.

Results	End points included procedural success (all lesions dilated and stented with angiographic residual stenosis of <10%). The presence of acute (≤24 hrs) and subacute (>24 hrs and ≤1 month) stent thrombosis noted. Major adverse cardiac events were also assessed. 514 patients received clopidogrel and 316 received ticlopidine. Procedural success occurred in 99.6% of patients on clopidogrel and 99.4% of patients on ticlopidine. Subacute stent thrombosis occurred in 1 clopidogrel and 1 ticlopidine patient. Combined rates of death, nonfatal myocardial infarction, and need for target revascularization were 2.1% in the clopidogrel patients and 1.4% in the ticlopidine patients. Death occurred in 0.9% of clopidogrel and 0.6% of ticlopidine patients. Bleeding complications occurred in 5.4% of clopidogrel and 4.4% of ticlopidine patients (p=0.35). There was no difference in hemorrhagic stroke, need for transfusion, or need for vascular access surgical repair between the 2 groups.
Concl.	Aspirin plus clopidogrel was as effective as aspirin plus ticlopidine in terms of the incidence of thrombotic complications and major adverse cardiovascular events in a broad spectrum of coronary artery disease patients undergoing stenting.

5c

Clopidogrel vs Ticlopidine After Intracoronary Stent Placement

Title	Clopidogrel vs ticlopidine after intracoronary stent placement.
Authors	Berger PB, Bell MR, Rihal CS, et al.
Reference	J Am Coll Cardiol 1999;34:1891-1894.
Disease	Coronary artery disease.
Purpose	To compare efficacy and safety of ticlopidine with clopidogrel in intracoronary stent patients.
Design	Comparison of events in 500 consecutive coronary stent patients who received aspirin plus clopidogrel to 827 consecutive stent patients who received aspirin plus ticlopidine. Single-center study.
Patients	1327 coronary artery disease patients receiving stents.
Follow-up	30 days.
Regimen	All patients received aspirin. Clopidogrel was given as a 300 mg load in the catheterization lab before stent implantation and then 75 mg/d for 14 days. Ticlopidine was given as 500 mg load before stent implantation and 250 mg that evening and 250 mg twice daily for 14 days.
Add'l Tx	Heparin; abciximab, enoxaparin could be given at the discretion of the cardiologist.

Results	Despite the fact that at baseline clopidogrel patients had more adverse clinical characteristics (older, more severe angina, more diabetes and hypertension, and lower LV ejection fraction), the frequency of death, nonfatal MI, stent thrombosis, and repeat angioplasty or bypass surgery was slightly, although not statistically significantly lower than patients treated with ticlopidine. The composite of death, MI, stent thrombosis, repeat revascularization was 0.8% in clopidogrel patients vs 1.6% in the ticlopidine group (p=NS). Death occurred in 0.4% vs 1.1% of clopidogrel vs ticlopidine patients, respectively. Nonfatal MI occurred in 0% vs 0.5%; stent thrombosis in 0.2% vs 0.7%, and repeat revascularization in 0.4% vs 0.5% of clopidogrel vs ticlopidine patients, respectively. Thrombotic thrombocytopenic purpura and neutropenia were not observed in any patient.
Concl.	Clopidogrel can safely be substituted for ticlopidine in coronary artery disease patients receiving stents.

5c

Title	Minimal heparinization in coronary angioplasty. How much heparin is really warranted?
Authors	Kaluski E, Krakover R, Cotter G, et al.
Reference	Am J Cardiol 2000;85:953-956.
Disease	Coronary artery disease, PTCA.
Purpose	To assess outcomes of nonemergency PCI, performed with a single low dose of heparin (2500 U).
Design	A cohort, single-center.
Patients	300 patients undergoing nonemergency PCI.
Follow-up	6 months.
Regimen	All patients received a bolus of 2500 U of unfractionated heparin before insertion of the guiding catheter. Additional heparin was at the discretion of the operator. Femoral arterial sheaths were removed within 2 hours of PCI.
Add'l Tx	All patients received aspirin 250 mg/d and patients with stents received ticlopidine 250 mg bid for 30 days. IV platelet glycoprotein IIb/IIIa were permitted. Coumadin or hirudin were prohibited for 12 hours after PCI.

Results	Angiographic success was obtained in 96% of the patients, clinical success in 93.3% of the patients. Mean activated clotting time 5 minutes after heparin administration was 185±19 seconds. In 61% of the patients stents were deployed. 16% of the patients received IV glycoprotein IIb/IIIa inhibitors. Mean post PCI sheath dwelling time was 45±58 minutes. 77.6% of the patients stayed in the hospital <24 hours. 2 patients (0.66%) had cardiac arrest and died during hospitalization. None of the patients needed emergency CABG or had a stroke. 1 patient had a Q-wave myocardial infarction due to acute target vessel occlusion 6 hours after PTCA and stenting. 6 patients (2%) had abrupt coronary artery occlusion within 14 days of PTCA. No bleeding or vascular complications were detected. At 6 months (184 patients) 4 patients died (2.1%) and 1 patient had Q-wave myocardial infarction. 9.7% of the patients had repeated target vessel revascularization.
Concl.	Very low dose heparin administration is safe in patients undergoing nonemergency PCI and may be associated with lower bleeding complications, hospitalization length, and probably costs.

5c

Title	Decreased rate of coronary restenosis after lowering of plasma homocysteine levels.
Authors	Schnyder G, Roffi M, Pin R, et al.
Reference	N Engl J Med 2001;345:1593-1600.
Disease	Coronary artery disease, percutaneous coronary intervention (PCI).
Purpose	To study whether a combination of folic acid, vitamin B_{12} and pyridoxine will reduce restenosis after PCI.
Design	Randomized, double-blind, placebo-controlled, multicenter.
Patients	205 patients who had undergone successful PCI of ≥1 coronary stenosis of ≥50% diameter stenosis. Patients with unstable angina, myocardial infarction within 2 weeks, significant left main coronary artery disease, PCI of a bypassed vessel with a patent graft, or renal dysfunction were excluded.
Follow-up	Clinical follow-up with repeated coronary angiography at 6 months.
Regimen	Randomization to placebo (n=100) or a combination of folic acid 1 mg, vitamin B_{12} 400 mg, and pyridoxine 10 mg per day (n=105).
Add'l Tx	Multivitamins were prohibited. PCI was performed using standard techniques. The use of heparin, aspirin, ticlopidine, clopidogrel, glycoprotein IIb/IIIa inhibitors, and stents were at the discretion of the operator.

Results	28 patients did not complete the protocol. 196 patients (95.6%) had clinical follow-up for 6 months and 177 (86.3%) underwent follow-up angiography at 6 months. Homocysteine levels at follow-up were lower in the active treatment group (7.2±2.4 vs 9.5±3.6 mmol/L; p<0.001). At follow-up minimal lumen diameter was larger for the active treatment group (1.72±0.76 vs 1.45±0.88 mm; p=0.02). The average diameter stenosis was 39.9%±20.3% in the active treatment vs 48.2%±28.3% in the placebo group (p=0.01). The late loss of luminal diameter was 0.61±0.74 and 0.82±0.76, respectively (p=0.03). Homocysteine levels at follow-up correlated with late loss of lumen diameter (r=0.27; p<0.001). The correlation was stronger for lesions treated with PTCA without stenting (r=0.48; p<0.001). For stented lesions there was no such correlation (r=0.07; p=0.44). Restenosis occurred in 19.6% of the patients in the active treatment group vs 37.6% in the placebo group (relative risk [RR] 0.52; 95% CI=0.32-0.86; p=0.01). Restenosis occurred in 15.7% of the lesions in the active treatment group vs 34.5% in the control group (RR 0.46; 95% CI=0.28-0.73; p=0.002). In the 101 lesions treated with PTCA without stenting, restenosis occurred in 10.3% of the lesions in the active treatment vs 41.9% in the placebo group (RR 0.25; 95% CI=0.11-0.57; p<0.001). In the 130 stented lesions, restenosis occurred in 20.6% vs 29.9%, respectively (RR 0.69; 95% CI=0.38-1.27; p=0.32). Multivariate analysis showed that only active treatment (p=0.007) and prior restenosis (p=0.011) were independently associated with restenosis. Major adverse cardiac events occurred in 12.7% of the patients in the active treatment group vs 24.5% in the placebo group (p=0.055). The active treatment reduced the rate of target-lesion revascularization (10.8% vs 22.3%; p=0.047). Cardiac death was 1.0% and 2.1%, respectively (p=0.95), and nonfatal myocardial infarction occurred in 4.9% and 7.4% of the patients, respectively (p=0.66).
Concl.	The combination of folic acid, vitamin B12, and pyridoxine reduced the levels of homocysteine and decreased the rate of restenosis, especially after PTCA without stenting. The combination therapy reduced the need for target-lesion revascularization after PCI. This inexpensive treatment, which is associated with minimal side effects, should be considered for patients undergoing PCI.

5c

The Swiss Heart Study

Title	Effect of homocysteine-lowering therapy with folic acid, vitamin B12, and vitamin B6 on clinical outcome after percutaneous coronary intervention. The Swiss Heart Study: a randomized controlled trial.
Authors	Schnyder G, Roffi M, Flammer Y, et al.
Reference	JAMA 2002;288:973-979.
Disease	Coronary artery disease, percutaneous coronary interventions.
Purpose	To assess whether homocysteine-lowering therapy will affect clinical outcomes after PCI.
Design	Randomized, double-blind, placebo-controlled, 1 center.
Patients	553 patients who had undergone successful angioplasty of ≥1 significant coronary stenosis. Patients with unstable angina, recent (<2 weeks) myocardial infarction, renal failure, and those taking vitamin supplements were not included.
Follow-up	1 year. A subgroup of 205 patients underwent follow-up angiography at 6 months.
Regimen	Randomization to placebo (n=281) or to homocysteine-lowering therapy (n=272) (folic acid 1 mg/d, vitamin B_{12} 400 μg/d, and vitamin B_6 10 mg/d). Treatment was continued for 6 months.
Add'l Tx	Open-label multivitamin supplements were prohibited during the study period.

Results	70 patients (110 lesions) were lost to follow-up. 54% and 53% of the patients in the folate+B12+B6 and placebo groups underwent stent implantation (p=0.78) and 11% in each group received IV glycoprotein IIb/IIIa inhibitors (p=0.97). All analyses were performed with the intention-to-treat principles. After an average follow-up of 11±3 months, 14.0% of the patients in the folate+B12+B6 therapy and 19.9% of the placebo-assigned patients underwent repeat revascularization (Adjusted hazard ratio [HR] 0.69; 95% CI= 0.51-0.98; p=0.04). 9.9% of the patients in the folate+B12+B6 vs 16.0% in the placebo group underwent target lesion revascularization (Adjusted HR 0.61; 95% CI= 0.41-0.95; p=0.02). Nonfatal MI occurred in 2.6% vs 4.3% of the patients in the active treatment and placebo group, respectively (p=0.17). Total mortality was 1.5% vs 2.8%, respectively (p=0.17). The primary end point of death, MI and need for repeat revascularization occurred in 15.4% of the active-treatment-assigned patients vs 22.8% in the placebo-assigned patients (Adjusted HR 0.66; 95% CI= 0.47-0.94; p=0.01). The benefit of folate+B12+B6 was most apparent in patients in the highest cholesterol tertile (relative risk [RR] 0.44; 95% CI=0.21-0.92; p=0.04) for patients with total cholesterol >228 mg/dL) than in the middle tertile (RR 0.55; 95% CI=0.25-1.23; p=0.20 for patients with cholesterol 189-228 mg/dL), or the lowest tertile (RR 0.72; 95% CI=0.33-1.55; p=0.53 for patients with cholesterol <189 mg/dL). A similar trend was fond for LDL-cholesterol levels. Adjustment for statin use did not significantly change these associations.
Concl.	6 month homocysteine-lowering therapy with folic acid, vitamin B12 and vitamin B6 reduced the incidence of major adverse events after successful PCI.

5c

ATLAST

Randomized, Placebo-Controlled Trial of Enoxaparin After High-Risk Coronary Stenting

Title	A randomized, placebo-controlled trial of enoxaparin after high-risk coronary stenting: the ATLAST trial.
Authors	Batchelor WB, Mahaffey KW, Berger PB, et al.
Reference	J Am Coll Cardiol 2001;38:1608-1613.
Disease	Coronary artery disease, percutaneous coronary intervention (PCI).
Purpose	To evaluate the efficacy and safety of 14-day treatment with enoxaparin in patients at high risk for stent thrombosis after stent implantation.
Design	Randomized, double-blind, placebo-controlled, multicenter.
Patients	1102 patients who had undergone coronary stent implantation and were considered to be at increased risk of stent thrombosis because of presence of intracoronary thrombus, urgent stenting, or suboptimal stent results. Patients with recent (<48 hours) myocardial infarction, abrupt closure, threatened abrupt closure before stenting, left ventricular ejection fraction <35%, fresh total occlusion (<7 d), stenting of degenerated venous graft of <4 mm in diameter, placement of a 2.5 mm stent in a vessel with a reference diameter of ≤2.5 mm, implantation of stents in bifurcation lesion, diffuse distal disease, or persistent dissection at the stent margin were considered candidates for the study. Patients with indications or contraindications to anticoagulation, blood pressure ≥180/110 mm Hg, anemia, thrombocytopenia, dipyridamole, or glycoprotein IIb/IIIa inhibitor therapy within the preceding 72 hours, thrombolytic therapy in the preceding 6 hours, planned coronary artery bypass grafting or additional PCI within 30 days, groin hematoma, intolerance to aspirin, ticlopidine or heparin, or serious noncardiac illness were excluded.
Follow-up	30 days.

Regimen	After removal of the arterial sheath, patients were randomized to enoxaparin (40 mg bid for patients <65 kg, and 60 mg bid for patients >65 kg) (n=553) or matching placebo (n=549) for 14 days.
Add'l Tx	All patients received unfractionated heparin before PCI. All patients received aspirin (325 mg/d for ≥6 m) and ticlopidine (250 mg bid for 14 d). A loading dose of aspirin (650 mg) and ticlopidine (500 mg) was given to those not already taking these agents. All patients underwent stent implantation. Glycoprotein IIb/IIIa inhibitors were prohibited.
Results	The trial was terminated prematurely because of low event rates and difficulties in recruiting patients. The primary composite end point of death, myocardial infarction, or urgent revascularization at 30 days occurred in 1.8% of the patients in the enoxaparin group vs 2.7% in the placebo group (OR 0.66; 95% CI=0.29-1.5; p=0.30). 14-day mortality was 0.4% and 0.5% in the enoxaparin and placebo groups, respectively (p=0.69), and 30-day mortality was 0.5% in each group (p=1.0). Reinfarction occurred in 0.2% in the enoxaparin patients vs 1.3% in the placebo group at 14 days (p=0.038) and in 0.4% vs 1.6%, respectively at 30 days (p=0.037). Death or reinfarction at 14 days occurred in 0.5% in the enoxaparin and 1.8% in the placebo group (p=0.049). Death or reinfarction at 30 days occurred in 0.9% in the enoxaparin and 2.2% in the placebo group (OR 0.41; 95% CI=0.14-1.2; p=0.084). 1.1% of the patients in the enoxaparin group vs 1.8% in the placebo group underwent urgent revascularization within 30 days (p=0.33). Overall bleeding was more common in the enoxaparin group (28% vs 6.7%; p<0.001). However, the difference in major bleeding was not statistically significant (3.3% vs 1.6%; p=0.08). Thrombocytopenia was detected in 0.4% of the patients in the placebo group but in none of the patients in the enoxaparin group (p=0.48). Adverse events were reported in 9.2% in the enoxaparin and 9.4% in the placebo group (p=0.97). 24% of the patients in the enoxaparin group vs 13% in the placebo group prematurely discontinued their study medication.

Concl.   Overall, with the use of aspirin and ticlopidine, the clinical outcome of patients traditionally considered at high risk of stent thrombosis is favorable. A 14-day course of subcutaneous enoxaparin may reduce the risk of reinfarction after high-risk coronary stenting and therefore, might be considered for carefully selected patients. The significance of enoxaparin in patients receiving glycoprotein IIb/IIIa inhibitors is unknown.

BAAS

Balloon Angioplasty and Anticoagulation Study

Title	a. Effects of coumarins started before coronary angioplasty on acute complications and long-term follow-up: a randomized trial. b. A randomized trial assessing the effect of coumarins started before coronary angioplasty on restenosis: results of a 6-month angiographic substudy of BAAS.
Authors	ten Berg JM, Kelder JC, Suttorp MJ, et al.
Reference	a. Circulation 2000;102:386-391. b. Am Heart J 2003;145:58-65.
Disease	Coronary artery disease, percutaneous coronary intervention.
Purpose	To evaluate the effects of pretreatment with coumarins on 6-month outcome of patients undergoing percutaneous coronary intervention.
Design	Randomized, open-label, multicenter.
Patients	1058 consecutive patients with symptomatic coronary artery disease scheduled for percutaneous coronary intervention. Patients with current treatment with anticoagulants or contraindications to anticoagulants or aspirin were not included. Patients with acute myocardial infarction and a bypass graft lesion were excluded.
Follow-up	1-year clinical follow-up. Repeat angiography at 6 months in half of the patients.
Regimen	Randomization to aspirin alone (n=530) or to open-label coumarin in addition to aspirin (n=528). Study treatment was started ≥7 days before PCI in stable patients and ≥1 day before intervention in patients with unstable angina. The target INR was 2.1-4.8. Coumarins were continued for ≥6 months.
Add'l Tx	Half of the patients were randomized to angiographic follow-up. All patients received aspirin 300 mg before intervention and 100 mg/d thereafter. All patients received IV heparin during procedure. Patients that underwent stent implantation received ticlopidine for 4 weeks.

5c

Results	Among patients who underwent repeat angiography, 261 patients were assigned aspirin and 270 aspirin plus coumarins. The mean INR was 2.7±1.2 at the start of angioplasty and 3.1±0.5 during follow-up. Stents were placed in 33% of the patients in the aspirin group and in 34% of the patients in the coumarins group. None of the patients received glycoprotein IIb/IIIa inhibitors. The primary clinical end point was death, MI, target lesion revascularization (TLR), and stroke. This occurred in 24.5% of patients in the aspirin group and in 16.7% in the coumarins group (p=0.03). MI occurred in 3.8% vs 2.2% in the aspirin and coumarins group, respectively (relative risk [RR] 0.58; 95% CI=0.21-1.57). TLR was done in 23.0% vs 15.6% of patients, respectively (RR 0.68; 95% CI=0.47-0.97). Recurrent angina was noted more often in the aspirin group (p=0.003). At 30 days 1.5% of the patients reaching the target INR had an event vs 11.7% in the suboptimal group (p=0.001). Follow-up angiography was performed in 96% of the aspirin group and 91% of the coumarins group. The minimal lumen diameter (MLD) at 6 months was 1.75±0.67 mm in the aspirin group and 1.77±0.67 mm in the coumarins group (p=0.72). There was no difference in percent diameter stenosis between the groups (39.1±19.8% vs 38.9±19.0%, respectively; p=0.71). Multivariate analysis revealed that 6 month restenosis was predicted by the MLD before and immediately after angioplasty and by the presence of diabetes mellitus. Coumarin therapy was not an independent predictor of restenosis. However, optimal anticoagulation was an independent predictor of restenosis. MLD was 0.21 mm (95% CI=0.05-0.37 mm) larger in those with optimal anticoagulation vs those with suboptimal anticoagulation. The group with optimal anticoagulation had a follow-up MLD that was 0.12 mm (95% CI=0.04-0.28 mm) larger than that in the aspirin-alone group.
Concl.	Coumarins did not improve the angiographic outcome 6 months after balloon angioplasty, although optimal anticoagulation was effective. Treatment with coumarins as aspirin reduced clinical outcomes 1 year after angioplasty vs treatment with aspirin alone.

CAPARES

Coronary Angioplasty Amlodipine Restenosis Study

Title	Restenosis and clinical outcome in patients treated with amlodipine after angioplasty: Results from the coronary angioplasty amlodipine restenosis study (CAPARES).
Authors	Jorgensen B, Simonsen S, Endresen K, et al.
Reference	J Am Coll Cardiol 2000:35:592-599.
Disease	Coronary artery disease, coronary angioplasty.
Purpose	To assess the effect of amlodipine, a calcium channel blocker, on restenosis and clinical outcome after PTCA.
Design	Randomized, double-blind, placebo-controlled, multicenter.
Patients	635 patients, with stable angina, scheduled for elective PTCA of ≥1 major native coronary artery. Patients with totally occluded arteries and those with small (<2 mm) reference lumen diameter were excluded.
Follow-up	4 months.
Regimen	Patients were randomized to placebo (n=317) or amlodipine (n=318), started 2 weeks before scheduled PTCA. The initial amlodipine dose was 5 mg/d and the dose was increased to 10 mg/d. Patients randomized to placebo received 20 mg of nifedipine twice before PTCA and once after the procedure.
Add'l Tx	All patients received aspirin. Lipid lowering agents, ACE inhibitors, diuretics, and β-blockers were permitted. Nonstudy calcium channel blockers were prohibited. Stents were implanted only in bail out situation or in cases with unsatisfactory post PTCA results. All patients received 10,000 U heparin before PTCA.

5c

Results	10 patients in the amlodipine group and 7 in the placebo group stopped study medications. PTCA was performed in 585 patients (92.1%), and stents were implanted in 91 patients (15.6%). 236 patients of the amlodipine group and 215 patients of the placebo group underwent follow-up angiography at a median time of 132 and 131 days, respectively, after the initial PTCA. The minimal lumen diameter was comparable between the amlodipine and the placebo group both before angioplasty (0.92±0.35 mm vs 0.92±0.40 mm; p=0.95), immediately after PTCA (1.82±0.37 mm vs 1.79±0.34 mm; p=0.40), and at follow-up (1.52±0.57 mm vs 1.50±0.59 mm; p=0.71). The mean loss in minimal luminal diameter at follow-up was 0.30±0.45 mm in the amlodipine group vs 0.29±0.49 mm in the placebo group (p=0.84). Similarly, percent diameter stenosis at follow-up was comparable (41.3±17.5% in the amlodipine group vs 42.9±19.3% in the placebo group; p=0.34). Restenosis occurred in 29.7% in the amlodipine group vs 29.9% in the placebo group (p=0.97). In contrast to the angiographic results, fewer patients in the amlodipine group needed repeated PTCA (3.1% vs 7.3%; relative risk [RR] 0.45; 95% CI=0.22-0.91; p=0.02). Mortality was 0.3% in the amlodipine group vs 0.6% in the placebo group (p=0.62), whereas myocardial infarction occurred in 2.5% vs 3.5%, respectively (p=0.49). The composite end point of death, myocardial infarction or repeated revascularization occurred in 9.4% vs 14.5% in the amlodipine and placebo group, respectively (RR 0.65; 95% CI=0.43-0.99; p=0.049).
Concl.	Amlodipine, started 2 weeks before elective PTCA and continued for 4 months after the procedure, did not prevent restenosis or late loss in minimal lumen diameter after 4 months. However, amlodipine was associated with a reduction in the rate of the composite end point of death, myocardial infarction, and repeated revascularization, mainly due to a reduction in the need for repeated PTCA.

CART-1

Canadian Antioxidant Restenosis Trial

Title	Effects of AGI-1067 and probucol after percutaneous coronary interventions.
Authors	Tardif J-C, Grégoire J, Schwartz L, et al.
Reference	Circulation 2003;107:552-558.
Disease	Coronary artery disease, percutaneous intervention, restenosis.
Purpose	To determine whether AGI-1067, an antioxidant, reduces stenosis as evaluated by intravascular ultrasound when given before and after percutaneous intervention.
Design	Multicenter, double-blind, placebo-controlled, randomized.
Patients	305 patients. Patients were eligible if they were to undergo percutaneous intervention with or without stenting on at least 1 native coronary artery and had at least 1 target lesion with ≥50% luminal narrowing. Exclusion criteria were numerous and included: myocardial infarction within 7 days, left main stenosis >50%, ejection fraction <30%, percutaneous intervention for another lesion within 6 months, and others.
Follow-up	6 months.
Regimen	Starting 14 days before percutaneous intervention, patients were randomized to receive either AGI-1067 at 70 mg, 140 mg, or 280 mg once a day, probucol 500 mg bid, or placebo. After the intervention, patients were maintained on their study medications for 4 more weeks. Aspirin 325 mg/d was given during the entire study. Patients who received stents also received clopidogrel 75 mg/d for 30 days after the intervention.

Results	The primary end point of the study was the minimal lumen area (LA) at follow-up as assessed by intravascular ultrasound. The 305 patients were distributed equally between the 5 groups. Stents were placed in 85.1% of patients, and glycoprotein IIa/IIIb inhibitors were used in 75 patients (approximately equal numbers in each group). The LA at the target lesion was similar among the groups before the intervention. At follow-up, the LA for placebo was 2.66±1.58 mm^2; 3.69±2.69 mm^2 for probucol, 2.75±1.76 mm^2 for AGI-1067 70 mg, 3.17±2.26 mm^2 for AGI-1067 140 mg, and 3.36± 2.12 mm^2 for AGI-1067 280 mg (p=0.046 for AGI-1067 280 mg vs placebo, and p=0.01 for probucol vs placebo). There was a dose-response relationship among the groups taking AGI-1067 (p=0.02). The rates of restenosis were 37.5% in the placebo group, 25.5% in the probucol group, and 26% in the 3 AGI-1067 groups (p=0.85 for AGI-1067 vs probucol; p=0.09 for AGI-1067 vs placebo, and p=0.24 for probucol vs placebo). When only compliant patients were analyzed, the rates of restenosis were 37.7%, 25.9%, and 23.6% in the placebo, probucol, and AGI-1067 groups, respectively (p=0.03 for AGI-1067 vs placebo). At baseline, the lumen volumes of the reference segments were similar in all study groups. The average change in lumen volume at follow-up was -5.3 mm^3 in the placebo group, -0.2 mm^3 in the probucol group, -2.4 mm^3 in the AGI-1067 70 mg group, +3.5 mm^3 in the 140 mg group, and +1.8 mm^3 in the 280 mg group (p=0.05 for the AGI-1067 140 mg group vs placebo; p=0.077 for a dose-response relationship). There were no deaths during the study. There were 11 MIs, (2 in the placebo group, 3 in the probucol group, and 1, 3, and 2 in the AGI-1067 groups). The rates of revascularization of the target lesion were 18.3% in placebo, 18.0% in probucol, and 16.9%, 14.1%, and 13.1% in the 3 AGI-1067 groups. An increased QTc interval was seen at least once in the study in 4.8% of placebo patients, 17.4% of the probucol patients, and 4.8%, 2.4%, and 2.5% of the patients in the AGI-1067 groups. Diarrhea occurred in 4.9% of placebo patients, 15.0% of probucol patients, and 8.5%, 7.8%, and 18.0% of patients in the AGI-1067 groups. Gastrointestinal side effects were generally self-limited.
Concl.	AGI-1067 and probucol are effective in reducing restenosis after percutaneous intervention. AGI-1067 did not cause prolongation of the QTc interval and improved the lumen volume of the reference segments.

CLASSICS

Clopidogrel Aspirin Stent International Cooperative Study

Title	Double-blind study of the safety of clopidogrel with and without a loading dose in combination with aspirin compared with ticlopidine in combination with aspirin after coronary stenting.
Authors	Bertrand ME, Rupprecht HJ, Urban P, et al.
Reference	Circulation 2000;102:624-629.
Disease	Coronary artery disease.
Purpose	To compare the safety of clopidogrel, with or without a loading dose, in combination with aspirin vs ticlopidine plus aspirin in patients who had received a coronary stent.
Design	Randomized, controlled, double-blind, parallel-group, multi-center.
Patients	1020 patients who had undergone successful placement of a coronary stent.
Follow-up	28 days.
Regimen	28 days of therapy with 1) a loading dose of 300 mg of clopidogrel and 325 mg/d aspirin on day 1 followed by 75 mg/d clopidogrel and 325 mg/d aspirin (days 2-28); 2) 75 mg/d clopidogrel and 325 mg/d aspirin (days 1-28); and 3) 250 mg bid ticlopidine and 325 mg/d aspirin (days 1-6).
Add'l Tx	Heparin during procedure; it was discontinued at end of procedure and 4 hours before sheath removal.

5c

Results   Primary end point was incidence of 1) major peripheral or bleeding complications, which included false aneurysms, need for surgical repair due to complication at puncture site, ≥2 units of blood transfusion, intracranial or retroperitoneal bleeding, overt hemorrhage; 2) neutropenia; 3) thrombocytopenia with a platelet count <100 x 109/L; and 4) early discontinuation of study due to noncardiac adverse event. Primary end point was reached in 9.1% of ticlopidine patients and 4.6% of patients in combined clopidogrel group (relative risk [RR]=0.5; 95% CI=0.31 to 0.81; p=0.005). Rates of major cardiovascular events, including cardiac death, MI, and need for target lesion revascularization, were low and comparable groups at 0.9% with ticlopidine, 1.5% with 75 mg/d clopidogrel, and 1.2% with the loading dose of clopidogrel p=NS.

Concl.   The safety and tolerability of clopidogrel plus aspirin was superior to ticlopidine plus aspirin. Both drugs were equally efficacious with regard to cardiac events in this population.

COURT

Contrast Media Utilization in High-Risk PTCA

Title	Randomized trial of contrast media utilization in high risk PTCA (The COURT Trial).
Authors	Davidson, CJ, Laskey WK, Hermiller JB, et al.
Reference	Circulation 2000;101:2172-2177.
Disease	Coronary artery disease.
Purpose	To compare the isosmolar nonionic dimer iodixanol with the low osmolar ionic agent ioxaglate in patients undergoing PTCA.
Design	Prospective, multicenter, randomized trial.
Patients	865 high risk coronary artery disease patients undergoing coronary artery intervention. High risk defined as angina at rest within the previous 2 hours, evolving MI within 72 hours, including patients who failed thrombolysis, post MI ischemia within 2 weeks of a MI.
Follow-up	In-hospital, 30 days.
Regimen	Patients randomly assigned to iodixanol (n=405) or ioxaglate (n=410).
Add'l Tx	Aspirin, ticlopidine if stents used. Abciximab and heparin could be used.
Results	Primary composite end point of in-hospital major adverse clinical events (emergency recatheterization or repeat PTCA, abrupt closure of target vessel, stroke, systemic thromboembolic event, periprocedural nonfatal MI, unplanned CABG, or cardiac death). This composite end point occurred in 5.4% of those receiving iodixanol vs 9.5% in those patients receiving ioxaglate (p=0.027). Angiographic success was achieved in 92.2% of patients receiving iodixanol vs 13.2% of patients receiving ioxaglate (p=0.07). Events from hospital discharge to 30 days did not differ between groups. A multivariate analysis showed that significant predictors for in-hospital major adverse clinical events were ioxaglate and treatment of de novo coronary artery lesions.

5c

Concl.   Although the incidence of in-hospital clinical events was low in both groups, it was lower in the patients receiving nonionic contrast (iodixanol) vs ionic contrast (ioxaglate) in high risk patients undergoing PTCA.

CREDO

Clopidogrel for the Reduction of Events During Observation

Title	Early and sustained dual oral antiplatelet therapy following percutaneous coronary intervention: a randomized controlled trial.
Authors	Steinhubl SR, Berger PB, Mann JT III, et al.
Reference	JAMA 2002;288:2411-2420.
Disease	Coronary artery disease, percutaneous intervention.
Purpose	To determine whether there is benefit from long-term continuation of clopidogrel after percutaneous intervention and if there is benefit of a preprocedure loading dose of clopidogrel.
Design	Randomized, double-blind, placebo-controlled, multicenter.
Patients	2116 patients, ≥21 years old, who had symptomatic coronary artery disease along with evidence of ischemia (ie, angina, positive stress test, electrocardiographic changes) and had been referred for PCI or were considered to have a high likelihood of undergoing PCI with stent placement (with or without balloon angioplasty) or another device for revascularization. Exclusion criteria included: greater than 50% stenosis of the left main coronary artery, coronary intervention failure in the prior 2 weeks, persistent ST elevation in the day prior to study entry, administration of GP IIb/IIIa inhibitor in the prior 7 days, clopidogrel in the prior 10 days, or thrombolytics in the prior 24 hours, and other criteria.
Follow-up	1 year.

5c

Regimen	3-24 hours before PCI, patients were given either a 300 mg loading dose of clopidogrel (pretreatment group) or matched placebo (no pretreatment group). All study participants received 325 mg aspirin. After the PCI procedure, all patients immediately received 75 mg/d of clopidogrel and 325 mg/d of aspirin through the 28th day after the procedure. After 28 days, patients in the pretreatment group continued to receive 75 mg/d of clopidogrel and the no pretreatment group received placebo for the remainder of the study. All patients continued to receive aspirin (dosed 81-325 mg/d per the investigator's discretion). At the time of randomization, 20% of patients were allowed to receive a GP IIb/IIIa inhibitor (usually abciximab) during the PCI. Bail-out GP IIb/IIIa use was permitted for all patients as deemed necessary by the performing physician.
Results	The primary study end point was the 1-year composite of death, MI, and stroke within the intent-to-treat population. The primary 28-day outcome was the composite of death, MI, or urgent target vessel revascularization within the per-protocol population. Other analyzed outcomes were each of the components of the composites, differences in outcome for administration of clopidogrel <6 hours or >6 hours before PCI, and incidence of target vessel revascularization or any revascularization at 1 year. Secondary outcomes were incidence of major bleeding events, and early stoppage of study medications at 28 days and 1 year. Major bleeding was defined as intracranial bleeding or bleeding with a decrease in hemoglobin of more than 5 g/dL. The intent-to-treat population consisted of 2116 patients. The per-protocol population consisted of the 1815 patients who underwent PCI (900 in the pretreatment/clopidogrel group, 915 in the no-pretreatment/placebo group). At 28 days, patients who received pretreatment with a loading dose of clopidogrel had a nonsignificant 18.5% relative reduction in the composite of death, MI, or urgent target vessel revascularization (6.8% pretreated vs 8.3% not pretreated; 95% CI=-14.2%-41.8%; p=0.23). MI, death, and revascularization each occurred less frequently in patients who received pretreatment (death: 0 vs 4; MI: 52 vs 60; urgent vessel revascularization: 9 vs 12; total; 61 vs 76). Similar results were obtained when analyzing the intent-to-treat population (6.2% vs 7.8%, relative risk reduction=20.9%; p=0.15). Patients who received clopidogrel more than 6 hours prior to the PCI had a 38.5% reduction in the composite end point; this was nearly statistically significant (95%

CI=-1.6% to 62.9%; p=0.051). In the per-protocol population, 45% received GP IIb/IIIa antagonists. Patients who received clopidogrel pretreatment but not GP IIa/IIIb antagonist had a similar primary outcome vs those who received neither (p=0.81). However, patients who received both had a trend toward benefit, with a 30% relative reduction in events (7.3% vs 10.3%; p=0.12). Clopidogrel treatment did not increase the risk of bleeding at 28 days. Approximately 60% of patients in each group completed the 1-year course of study medication. At 1 year, patients who were on long-term clopidogrel had a 26.9% relative risk reduction (RRR) of the composite end point vs those on placebo (95% CI=3.9%-44.4%; p=0.02, absolute reduction=3%), with similar results in the intent-to-treat population (RRR 19.7%; 95% CI=-13.3% to 43.1%; p=0.21). There was a trend for a similar benefit for each of the components, but these were not significant. Rates of revascularization were similar between the 2 groups (21.3% vs 21.0%). Patients in the clopidogrel group had a trend toward a higher incidence of major bleeding (8.8% vs 6.7%; p=0.07).

| Concl. | No significant benefit from pretreatment with clopidogrel was seen at 28 days after PCI. However, there was a trend toward benefit if pretreatment was started more than 6 hours prior to the procedure. 12-month treatment with clopidogrel after PCI resulted in a significantly decreased risk of adverse events at 1 year vs placebo. Clopidogrel use was associated with a nonsignificant increase in bleeding events. |

5c

EPISTENT

Evaluation of Platelet IIb/IIIa Inhibition in Stenting

Title	Randomized placebo-controlled and balloon angioplasty controlled trial to assess safety of coronary stenting with use of platelet glycoprotein-IIb/ IIIa blockade.
Authors	The EPISTENT Investigators.
Reference	Lancet 1998;352:87-92.
Disease	Coronary artery disease.
Purpose	To compare outcomes of stent + placebo; to stent + abciximab; to PTCA + abciximab.
Design	Randomized, controlled, multicenter.
Patients	2399 patients with coronary artery disease and ≥60% coronary artery stenosis eligible for PTCA or stenting. Patients with unprotected left main stenosis, bleeding diathesis, intracranial tumor, stroke within the preceding 2 years, uncontrolled hypertension, recent surgery or PTCA within 3 months, and those who received oral anticoagulants were excluded.
Follow-up	30 days.
Regimen	Randomization to sent + placebo (n=809); stent+abciximab (n=794), or PTCA + abciximab (n=796). Abciximab or identical placebo was administered as a bolus 0.25 mg/kg up to 1 hour before intervention, followed by an infusion of 0.125 µg/kg/min for 12 hours. Patients assigned to abciximab received heparin 70 U/kg as a bolus with repeated boluses to maintain activated clotting time ≥200 s. Patients assigned to placebo received heparin 100 U/kg as a bolus followed by additional boluses to maintain activated clotting time ≥300 s.
Add'l Tx	Aspirin 325 mg/d. Ticlopidine 250 mg bid before the start of the study agent.

Results	>98.5% of patients in each group received the study medications. 91.5% of the patients completed 12 hours of infusion. Abrupt closure occurred in 0.7% of the stent+placebo group vs 0% in the stent+abciximab and 0.5% in the PTCA+abciximab group (p=0.060). Side-branch closure occurred in 4.5%, 2.4%, and 1.7%, respectively (p=0.02). 19.3% of the patients assigned to PTCA+abciximab received stents because of suboptimal results. The primary end point (30-day mortality, myocardial infarction or severe myocardial ischemia requiring revascularization) occurred in 10.8% of the stent+placebo group, 5.3% of the stent+abciximab group (hazard ratio 0.48; 95% CI=0.33 to 0.69; p<0.001), and 6.9% of the PTCA+abciximab group (hazard ratio 0.63; 95% CI=0.45 to 0.88; p=0.007). 30-day mortality was 0.6% in the stent+placebo group, 0.3% in the stent+abciximab group, and 0.8% in the PTCA+abciximab group. Myocardial infarction occurred in 9.6%, 4.5%, and 5.3%, respectively. Death or large myocardial infarction occurred in 7.8%, 3.0% (p<0.001), and 4.7% (p=0.010), respectively. Major bleeding occurred in 2.2% of the stent+placebo, 1.5% of the stent+abciximab, and 1.4% of the PTCA+abciximab. Subgroup analysis revealed that abciximab was beneficial in patients younger and older than 65 years, patients with and without diabetes, and in patients with either unstable angina or stable angina pectoris. Women had better results with PTCA+abciximab (5.1% event rate) than with stent+abciximab (8.6% event rate). This may be explained by the smaller diameter of the coronary arteries in women.
Concl.	GP IIb/IIIa blockade with abciximab significantly improved outcome of percutaneous coronary artery interventions. PTCA+abciximab was better and safer than stenting without abciximab administration.

EPISTENT (6-Month Outcome)

Evaluation of Platelet IIb/IIIa Inhibition in Stenting

Title	Complementary clinical benefits of coronary artery stenting and blockade of platelet glycoprotein IIb/IIIa receptors.
Authors	Lincoff AM, Califf RM, Moliterno DJ, et al.
Reference	N Engl J Med 1999;341:319-327.
Disease	Coronary artery disease.
Purpose	To determine the efficacy of abciximab and stent implantation in improving cardiac outcomes.
Design	Randomized, multicenter, blinding to abciximab vs placebo.
Patients	2399 patients undergoing elective or urgent percutaneous coronary revascularization.
Follow-up	6 months.
Regimen	Patients were randomized to stenting plus placebo, stenting plus abciximab, and balloon angioplasty plus abciximab. Abciximab was given as a 0.25 mg per kg body weight bolus 10-60 minutes before balloon inflation, and then 0.125 µg/kg/min up to 10 µg per minute infusion for 12 hours.
Add'l Tx	Aspirin, ticlopidine to all patients receiving stents. Low dose, weight adjusted heparin in abciximab patients; standard, weight adjusted heparin in placebo group.

Results	The primary end points were composite of death or myocardial infarction at 6 months and repeated revascularization of the target vessel. In the stent plus placebo group, 11.4% reached the end point of death or myocardial infarction; vs 5.6% in stent plus abciximab group (hazard ratio, 0.47; 95% CI=0.33-0.68; p<0.001); vs 7.8% in balloon angioplasty plus abciximab (hazard zone 0.67; 95% CI=0.49-0.92; p=0.01). Hazard ratio for stenting plus abciximab vs angioplasty plus abciximab was 0.7 (95% CI=0.48-1.04; p=0.07). 10.6%, 8.7%, and 15.4% required repeat revascularization in the stent plus placebo, stent plus abciximab, and angioplasty plus abciximab group, respectively (p=0.22 stent plus abciximab vs stent plus placebo; p=0.005 for angioplasty plus abciximab vs stent plus placebo, and p<0.001 for stent plus abciximab vs angioplasty plus abciximab group). In diabetes, rates of repeated revascularization after stenting were lower among patients receiving abciximab vs placebo; in patients without diabetes abciximab had no effect on need for repeated revascularization. Angiographic substudy showed better early angiographic outcomes with stenting and a trend toward greater minimal luminal diameters at 6 months with a lower loss index in stented patients who received abciximab vs placebo.
Concl.	Abciximab plus stenting have long-term complementary beneficial effects.

5c

EPISTENT (Diabetic Substudy)

Evaluation of Platelet IIb/IIIa Inhibition in Stenting

Title	Optimizing the percutaneous interventional outcomes for patients with diabetes mellitus. Results of the EPISTENT Diabetic Substudy.
Authors	Marso SP, Lincoff AM, Ellis SG, et al.
Reference	Circulation 1999; 100:2477-2484.
Disease	Coronary artery disease, diabetes.
Purpose	To determine whether abciximab plus stenting is better than stenting alone or PTCA-abciximab in diabetic patients who were part of the EPISTENT Trial.
Design	As per EPISTENT.
Patients	491 diabetic patients in the EPISTENT study. Patients eligible to undergo stenting or PTCA with an epicardial coronary stenosis ≥60%.
Follow-up	6 months-1 year.
Regimen	As per EPISTENT. 173 diabetic patients randomized to stent-placebo; 162 to stent-abciximab; 156 to balloon angioplasty-abciximab.
Add'l Tx	Diabetes was managed with insulin, oral hypoglycemics, diet, or combination of these treatments.

Results	Main composite end point was 6 month rate of death, MI, or target vessel revascularization. This end point was achieved in 25.2% of stent-placebo diabetic patients, 23.4% of balloon-abciximab diabetic patients, and 13.0% of stent-abciximab diabetic patients (p=0.005). 6 month death or MI rates were reduced by abciximab whether patients received balloon angioplasty (7.8%) or stenting (6.2%) vs stent-placebo (12.7%; p=0.029). The 6 months target vessel revascularization rate was lowest for stent-abciximab (8.1%) compared to stent-placebo (16.6%) and balloon-abciximab (18.4%). By angiographic follow-up stent-abciximab demonstrated a significant increase in angiographic net gain and a decrease in the late loss index compared to stent-placebo. 1-Year mortality rates were 4.1% for stent-placebo diabetic patients, vs 1.2% for stent-abciximab diabetic patients (p=0.11).
Concl.	The composite end point of 6 month death, myocardial infarction, and target vessel revascularization in diabetics was lowest when abciximab was combined with stenting vs placebo plus stenting or PTCA plus abciximab.

ERASER

The Evaluation of ReoPro and Stenting to Eliminate Restenosis

Title	Acute platelet inhibition with abciximab does not reduce in-stent restenosis (ERASER Study).
Authors	The ERASER Investigators.
Reference	Circulation 1999;100:799-806.
Disease	Coronary artery disease, restenosis.
Purpose	To determine whether IV abciximab would decrease neointimal hyperplasia following intracoronary stenting.
Design	Double-blind, placebo-controlled, randomized, multicenter.
Patients	215 patients with a de novo target coronary artery stenosis of ≥50% referred for intracoronary stent implantation.
Follow-up	6 months.
Regimen	Intravascular ultrasound (IVUS) was used to guide optimal stenting. Patients undergoing stenting were randomized to 1 of 3 groups: 1) placebo bolus plus placebo infusion; 2) abciximab 0.25 mg/kg bolus plus 12 hours of 0.125 µg/kg/min (up to 10 µg/min) infusion; or 3) abciximab 0.25 mg/kg bolus plus 2 consecutive 12 hour 0.125 µg/kg/min (up to 10 µg/min) infusions.
Add'l Tx	Aspirin, heparin, ticlopidine, nitroglycerin.

Results	Primary end point was percent in-stent volume obstruction of the target lesion, measured at 6 months with IVUS. Secondary end points were target lesion mean and minimum lumen diameter (MLD), late loss and loss index by quantitative coronary angiography at 6 months, and composite end point of death, myocardial infarction, and target lesion revascularization. Tissue volume as percentage of stent volume was similar in the placebo, 12 hour, and 24 hour abciximab groups at 25±15%, 27±15%, and 29±14%, respectively (p=NS). Dichotomous restenosis rates assessed by late quantitative coronary angiography were 11.6%, 18.9%, and 19.4%, respectively (p=NS). Late loss index assessed by coronary angiography were 0.33, 0.52, and 0.47, respectively (p=NS). The composite end point of death, myocardial infarction, or target lesion revascularization at 6 months was similar among groups at 25.4% in placebo and 21.4% of the combined abciximab groups (p=NS).
Concl.	Platelet inhibition with abciximab did not decrease the rate of in-stent restenosis.

5c

ESPRIT

Enhanced Suppression of the Platelet IIb/IIIa Receptor with Integrilin Therapy

Title	a. Novel dosing regimen of eptifibatide in planned coronary stent implantation (ESPRIT): a randomized, placebo-controlled trial. b. Platelet glycoprotein IIb/IIIa integrin blockade with eptifibatide in coronary stent intervention. The ESPRIT trial: a randomized controlled trial.
Authors	a. The ESPRIT investigators. b. O'Shea JC, Hafley GE, Greenberg S, et al.
Reference	a. Lancet 2000;356:2037-2044. b. JAMA 2001;285:2468-2473.
Disease	Coronary artery disease, elective stent implantation.
Purpose	To assess the efficacy and safety of high-dose eptifibatide in elective coronary stent implantation.
Design	Randomized, double-blind, placebo-controlled, multicenter.
Patients	2064 patients with CAD scheduled to undergo percutaneous coronary intervention with stent implantation in a native coronary artery. Patients with a recent (<24 hours) myocardial infarction, urgent referral for PCI, PCI within the previous 90 days, previous stent implantation at the target lesion, treatment with thienopyridines or GP IIb/IIIa inhibitors within the previous 30 days, stroke or transient ischemic attack within 30 days, previous history of stroke or bleeding diathesis, major surgery within the previous 6 months, thrombocytopenia, uncontrolled hypertension or renal failure were excluded.
Follow-up	a. 30 days. b. 6 months.

Regimen	Randomization to receive either placebo or eptifibatide. Eptifibatide was given as 2 boluses of 180 µg/kg 10 minutes apart, and an infusion of 2.0 µg/kg/min for 18-24 hours.
Add'l Tx	All patients received aspirin and a thienopyridine (clopidogrel or ticlopidine) on the day of PCI. All types of stents were permitted. All patients received heparin (an initial bolus of 60 units/kg [maximum 6000 units] to a target activated clotting time of 200-300 seconds.)

5c

5. Interventional Cardiology — c. Medical Therapy, Including Antiplatelet Therapy,   567
for Prevention of Complications and Restenosis with Angiography and PCI

Results	a. The trial was terminated early by the data and safety monitoring board for efficacy. 1040 patients received eptifibatide and 1024 received placebo. 1025 patients in the eptifibatide group and 1015 patients in the placebo group underwent PCI (986 and 997, respectively, underwent stent implantation). The primary end point of death, MI, urgent target vessel revascularization, and thrombotic bailout GP IIb/IIIa inhibitor administration within the first 48 hr after enrollment was reached in 10.5% of the placebo vs 6.6% in the eptifibatide group (RR of 0.63; 95% CI=0.47 to 0.84; p=0.0015). Death occurred in 0.1% in the eptifibatide group vs 0.2% in the placebo group (p=0.55). Acute MI occurred in 5.4% in the eptifibatide group vs 9.0% in the placebo group (RR 0.60; 95% CI=0.44 to 0.83; p=0.0015). Death or acute MI occurred in 5.5% and 9.2%, respectively (RR 0.60; 95% CI=0.44 to 0.82; p=0.0013), and death/MI or urgent target vessel revascularization within 48 hr occurred in 6.0% and 9.3%, respectively (RR 0.65; 95% CI=0.47 to 0.87; p=0.0045). 1.0% vs 2.1% of the patients, respectively, needed bailout GP IIb/IIIA inhibitor infusion during the first 48 hr after randomization (p=0.029). Death, MI, and urgent target vessel revascularization at 30 days occurred in 6.8% in the eptifibatide group vs 10.5% in the placebo group (RR 0.65; 95% CI=0.49 to 0.87; p=0.0034). Major bleeding occurred in 1.3% in the eptifibatide group vs only 0.4% in the placebo group (p=0.027). Severe (<20×109/L) thrombocytopenia occurred in 0.2% in the eptifibatide group vs none in the placebo group.
	b. At 6 months, the primary end point of death or MI occurred in 7.5% of the patients in the eptifibatide group vs in 11.5% in the placebo group (hazard ratio [HR] 0.63; 95% CI=0.47-0.84; p=0.002). Death, MI, or target vessel revascularization occurred in 14.2% and 18.3%, respectively (HR 0.75; 95% CI=0.60-0.93; p=0.008). Mortality was 0.8% in the eptifibatide group and 1.4% in the placebo group (HR 0.56; 95% CI=0.24-1.34; p=0.19). 8.6% of the patients in the eptifibatide vs 9.4% in the placebo group underwent target vessel revascularization (HR 0.91; 95% CI=0.68-1.22; p=0.51). Most of the beneficial effect of eptifibatide was apparent within 48 hr after initiation of therapy and was maintained during the 6-month follow-up period.
Concl.	a. Routine administration of eptifibatide reduced ischemic complications after elective coronary stent implantation.
	b. The beneficial effect of eptifibatide therapy during coronary stenting on the combined end point of death and MI was maintained during the 6-month follow-up.

ESPRIT (Substudy)

Enhanced Suppression of the Platelet IIb/IIIa Receptor with Integrilin Therapy

Title	Effect of glycoprotein IIb/IIIa receptor inhibition on angiographic complications during percutaneous coronary intervention in the ESPRIT trial.
Authors	Blankenship JC, Tasissa G, O'Shea JC, et al.
Reference	J Am Coll Cardiol 2001;38:653-658.
Disease	Coronary artery disease, percutaneous coronary intervention (PCI).
Purpose	To investigate whether eptifibatide decreases the rate of angiographic complications during elective PCI and to assess the relationship of angiographic complications to elevations of creatine kinase-MB (CK-MB) enzyme levels following PCI.
Design	Retrospective subanalysis of a randomized, double-blind, placebo-controlled, multicenter trial.
Patients	2064 patients who participated in the ESPRIT trial and underwent nonurgent PCI with stent implantation.
Follow-up	Angiographic complications and CK-MB levels.
Regimen	Randomized to placebo or eptifibatide.

5c

Results	In 180 patients post-intervention CK-MB levels were unavailable and in 221 patients baseline CK or CK-MB was elevated. The eptifibatide group had a nonsignificant trend toward fewer angiographic complications (10.1% vs 12.2%; p=0.13). Major dissection occurred in 3.9% vs 3.6% of the patients in the eptifibatide and placebo groups, respectively (p=0.78), and abrupt closure in 1.0% and 1.1%, respectively (p=0.80). Eptifibatide did not reduce the rates of no-reflow (1.4% vs 1.2%; p=0.29), thrombus formation (0.9% vs 1.6%; p=0.15), residual thrombus (0.5% vs 1.0%; p=0.18), side branch closure (3.4% vs 4.9%; p=0.08), distal embolization (1.0% vs 0.5%; p=0.21), and TIMI grade flow <3 (1.8% vs 2.5%; p=0.71). Among patients with normal baseline CK and CK-MB levels and without angiographic complications, CK-MB elevations >3 times normal following PCI were detected in 4% of the patients in the eptifibatide group vs 7% in the placebo group (p=0.003). However, among the patients with normal baseline CK and CK-MB with angiographic complications, >3 times normal CK-MB elevations occurred in 21% vs 22% (p=0.91).
Concl.	Eptifibatide did not reduced angiographic complications in patients undergoing nonurgent PCI with stent implantation. However, among patients without angiographic complications, eptifibatide reduced the incidence of CK-MB leaks.

ESPRIT (Substudy)

Enhanced Suppression of the Platelet IIb/IIIa Receptor with Integrilin Therapy

Title	Long-term efficacy of platelet glycoprotein IIb/IIIa integrin blockade with eptifibatide in coronary stent intervention.
Authors	O'Shea JC, Buller CE, Cantor WJ, et al.
Reference	JAMA 2002;287:618-621.
Disease	Coronary artery disease, percutaneous coronary intervention (PCI).
Purpose	To assess the long-term effects of eptifibatide after elective coronary stent implantation.
Design	Subanalysis of a randomized, double-blind, placebo-controlled, multicenter trial.
Patients	2064 patients who participated in the ESPRIT trial and underwent nonurgent PCI with stent implantation.
Follow-up	1 year.
Regimen	Randomized to placebo or eptifibatide.
Add'l Tx	Treatment with clopidogrel or ticlopidine was allowed on the day of the procedure, but not before.
Results	1-year follow-up was available for 988 of 1040 patients (95.0%) assigned to eptifibatide and 976 of 1024 patients (95.3%) assigned to placebo. Death or myocardial infarction occurred in 12.4% of the patients in the placebo group vs only 8.0% in the eptifibatide group (hazard ratio [HR] 0.63; 95% CI=0.48-0.83; p=0.001). Death, myocardial infarction, or target vessel revascularization occurred in 22.1% and 17.5%, respectively (HR 0.76; 95% CI=0.63-0.93; p=0.007). Mortality was 2.0% and 1.4%, respectively (HR 0.69; 95% CI=0.35-1.36; p=0.28). Eptifibatide tended to reduce target vessel revascularization in both the diabetic patients (HR 0.90; 95% CI=0.57-1.41; p=0.65) and nondiabetic patients (HR 0.89; 95% CI=0.66-1.20; p=0.43).

5c

Concl.	Eptifibatide was associated with an improved 1-year outcome in patients undergoing nonurgent PCI with stent implantation.

ESPRIT

Esapent for Prevention of Restenosis Italian Study

Title	Prevention of postcoronary angioplasty restenosis by omega-3 fatty acids: main results of the ESPRIT study.
Authors	Schneider TL, Hopp HW, Vlaho D, et al.
Reference	Am Heart J 2003;145:e5.
Disease	Coronary artery disease, percutaneous coronary intervention.
Purpose	To study whether long-term (≥4 weeks) administration of omega-3 fatty acid before percutaneous transluminal coronary angioplasty reduces restenosis rates at 6 months after angioplasty.
Design	Randomized, double-blind, placebo-controlled, multicenter.
Patients	339 patients, 18-75 years old, scheduled for angioplasty for ≥1 de novo coronary artery with ≥70% diameter stenosis. Patients with recent myocardial infarction, unstable angina, left main culprit lesion, saphenous vein graft culprit lesion, excessive bleeding risk, thrombocytopenia, uncontrolled hypertension, contraindications of omega-3 fatty acid, need for anticoagulation therapy, liver or renal disease, limited life expectancy, or drug or alcohol abuse were excluded.
Follow-up	6 months clinical follow-up with repeat angiography.
Regimen	Randomization to placebo (olive oil with vitamin E) or omega-3 fatty acid with vitamin E capsules. Treatment was given for 1 month before angioplasty at a dose of 6 capsules/d and during follow-up at a dose of 3 capsules/d.

5c

Add'l Tx	All patients received 100-500 mg/d aspirin or indobufen beginning ≥48 hours before angioplasty. All patients received nitrates and IV heparin during the procedure.
Results	52 patients were disqualified before or at the time of angioplasty. 257 patients (89%) with 280 lesions were included in the final analysis (125 in the omega-3 group and 132 in the placebo group). Restenosis (>50% diameter stenosis at follow-up angiography) occurred in 29.4% of the lesions in the omega-3 group vs in 39.6% of the lesions in the placebo group (p=0.04). >50% loss of the short-term gain immediately after PTCA occurred in 31.6% and 35.4% of the lesions, respectively (p=NS). Periprocedural complication rates were comparable between the groups. Periprocedural bleeding occurred in 2.1% of the patients in the omega-3 and in 1.0% of the patients in the placebo group (p=NS). MI occurred in 0.7% and 0% of the patients, respectively. Recurrent angina occurred in 0% and 2.8%, respectively. 6-month clinical end points (death, MI, revascularization) occurred in 9.5% of the patients in the omega-3 and in 8.5% in the placebo group (p=NS). Significant angina during follow-up was noted in 9.6% and 15.1% of the patients, respectively (p=NS).
Concl.	Long-term pretreatment with omega-3 fatty acids before coronary angioplasty resulted in a small reduction in the restenosis rate. However, the effect on clinical adverse events was not significant.

EXCITE

Evaluation of Oral Xemilofiban in Controlling Thrombotic Events

Title	Long-term treatment with a platelet glycoprotein receptor antagonist after percutaneous coronary revascularization.
Authors	O'Neill WW, Serruys P, Knudtson M, et al.
Reference	N Engl M Med 2000;342:1316-1324.
Disease	Coronary artery disease.
Purpose	To determine whether long-term oral glycoprotein IIb/IIIa receptor antagonist, xemilofiban, would reduce death, MI, and need for urgent revascularization.
Design	Double-blind, randomized, placebo-controlled, multicenter.
Patients	7232 patients with angiographic evidence of clinically significant CAD in need of percutaneous transluminal coronary revascularization.
Follow-up	182 days.
Regimen	Single oral dose of 20 mg xemilofiban prior to percutaneous intervention and maintenance of 20 mg 3 times daily after procedure; 20 mg before and maintenance of 10 mg 3 times daily after; or placebo given before and after.
Add'l Tx	Ticlopidine in stent patient on placebo or placebo ticlopidine in xemilofiban patients; all patients received aspirin.

Results	1 primary end point was death, nonfatal myocardial infarction, or urgent revascularization at 182 days. The other primary end point was death or nonfatal myocardial infarction at 182 days. At 182 days, death, nonfatal myocardial infarction, or urgent revascularization occurred in 324 (13.5%) placebo patients, 332 (13.9%) who received 10 mg of xemilofiban, and 306 (12.7%) who received 20 mg of xemilofiban (p=NS among groups). Death or nonfatal myocardial infarction developed in 215 (8.9%) patients in the placebo group, 220 (9.2%) in the 10 mg xemilofiban group, and 199 (8.2%) in the 20 mg xemilofiban group. There were no significant differences among the 3 groups. The percent of patients who withdrew for bleeding was 6.1% and 11.6% at the 10 mg and 20 mg dose of xemilofiban vs 1.5% in the placebo group (p<0.001 vs treatment groups). Myocardial infarcts occurring within 1 day after randomization were lower in the 10 and 20 mg xemilofiban groups (4.1% and 4.0%, respectively) compared to placebo (5.5%; p=0.02).
Concl.	The glycoprotein IIb/IIIa antagonist xemilofiban given prior to percutaneous coronary intervention and then for up to 6 months did not decrease the incidence of death, myocardial infarction, or urgent revascularization.

IMPACT-II (Substudy)

Integrilin to Minimize Platelet Aggregation and Coronary Thrombosis-II

Title	Effect of eptifibatide on angiographic complications during percutaneous coronary intervention in the IMPACT-II trial.
Authors	Blankenship JC, Sigmon KN, Pieper KS, et al.
Reference	a. Lancet 1997;349:1422-1428. b. Am J Cardiol 2001;88:969-975.
Disease	Coronary artery disease.
Purpose	To determine whether the small-molecule glycoprotein IIb/IIIa receptor inhibitor reduces elevation of creatine kinase (CK)-MB isoenzyme release during coronary intervention.
Design	As per IMPACT-II.
Patients	4010 patients with coronary artery disease scheduled for elective, urgent, or emergency coronary intervention with a Food and Drug Administration approved device, although stents were discouraged except for abrupt closure.
Follow-up	In this analysis, up to 30 days.
Regimen	Patients randomized to 1 of 3 treatments: 135 mg/kg bolus of eptifibatide plus 0.5 mg/kg/min infusion for 20-24 hours (135/0.5 regimen); 135 mg/kg bolus plus 0.75 mg/kg/min infusion for 20-24 hours (135/0.75 regimen) or placebo bolus and placebo infusion.
Add'l Tx	Aspirin, heparin.

Results	CK and CK-MB drawn at 6, 12, and 20 hours after initial bolus. Angiographic complications (major dissection, distal embolization, residual thrombus, abrupt closure, residual stenosis >50%, side branch occlusion, TIMI flow grade <3) occurred in 31.5% of the eptifibatide (135/0.5 regimen) vs 37.7% of placebo patients (p<0.001) and in 34.5% of the 135/0.75 regimen vs 37.7% of placebo patients (p=0.096). Patients with angiographic complications had higher CK-MB and CK elevations (33% and 18%, respectively) than those without such complications (19% and 9.0%, respectively; p<0.001 for both). Eptifibatide treatment was associated with a trend toward a lower incidence of CK-MB elevations in patients with in-laboratory angiographic complications (29% in the 135/0.75 regimen; 33% in the 135/0.5 regimen, vs 37% in the placebo group). Similar trends were seen with CK. In patients without angiographic complications, there was also a trend toward lower incidence of CK-MB elevations with therapy (17% and 18% in the eptifibatide arms vs 21% with placebo).
Concl.	Eptifibatide reduced angiographic complications and reduced the incidence of elevated CK-MB in patients with and without angiographic complications.

IMPRESS

Immunosuppressive Therapy for the Prevention of Restenosis After Coronary Artery Stent Implantation

Title	Immunosuppressive therapy for the prevention of restenosis after coronary artery stent implantation.
Authors	Versaci F, Gaspardone A, Tomai F, et al.
Reference	J Am Coll Cardiol 2002;40:1935-1942.
Disease	Coronary artery disease, percutaneous intervention.
Purpose	To determine the effects of prednisone on restenosis rate after stent implantation in patients who had maintained high levels of C-reactive protein (CRP) after implantation.
Design	Double-blind, randomized, placebo-controlled.
Patients	83 patients, who had characteristic angina pectoris, document-ed myocardial ischemia, or both; single-vessel or multivessel disease, who underwent successful implantation of 1 stent of length <19 mm. Patients were to have a CRP £0.5 mg/dL before the procedure and >0.5 mg/dL 72 hours after the implantation. Exclusion criteria were numerous and included: diabetes treated with medical therapy, unstable angina, myocardial infarction in the previous 6 weeks, left ventricular ejection fraction <40%, New York Heart Association functional class >II, steroid therapy in the past 30 days, and others.
Follow-up	12 months.
Regimen	Patients were randomized to start either prednisone or placebo 72 hours after the procedure. Prednisone was given orally in the following manner: 1 mg/kg in the first 10 days, 0.5 mg/kg for day 11 to day 30, 0.25 mg/kg for day 31-45.

5c

Add'l Tx	All patients received aspirin 325 mg/d and ticlopidine 250 mg bid, starting 3 days before stent implantation. After the sheath was inserted, a bolus of 100 U/kg of heparin was given and additional doses given to maintain an activated clotting time >300 seconds. Patients were continued indefinitely on aspirin 325 mg/d; ticlopidine 250 mg bid for 4 weeks, and pantoprazole 40 mg/d for 45 days.

Results	The clinical end point was the 12-month event-free survival rate, with events being defined as death, MI, or recurring symptoms requiring revascularization. The angiographic end points were restenosis rate (≥50% in-stent stenosis at follow-up angiography) and late loss (minimal lumen diameter [MLD] after the procedure minus the MLD at 6-month follow-up). A clinical primary end point occurred in 3/41 in the prednisone group vs 15/42 in the placebo group (relative risk reduction [RRR] 0.18; 95% CI=0.05-0.61; p=0.0063). The rate of event-free survival was significantly higher in patients in the prednisone group (p<0.0016). Additional revascularization occurred in 3/41 in the prednisone group vs 14/42 in the placebo group (p=0.001). Predictors of the primary end point were presentation with stable angina (RRR 0.26; 95% CI=0.08-0.80; p=0.018), TIMI flow grade 3 after stenting (RRR 0.23; 95% CI=0.07-0.80; p=0.02), and β-blocker therapy (RRR 0.17; 95% CI=0.04-0.76; p=0.02). The rates of restenosis were 7% and 33% in the prednisone and placebo groups, respectively (p=0.001). Late loss at follow-up was significantly less in the prednisone group (0.39±0.6 mm vs 0.85±0.6 mm; p=0.001) as was MLD (2.36±0.7 mm vs 1.88±0.7 mm; p=0.003).

Concl.	In patients who have persistently elevated CRP levels after successful stent implantation, therapy with prednisone significantly reduces rates of clinical events and angiographic restenosis.

IMPRESS

Intramural Infusion of Low-Molecular-Weight Heparin to Prevent Restenosis After Stent Implantation

Title	Local delivery of nadoparin for the prevention of neointimal hyperplasia following stent implantation: results of the IMPRESS trial. A multicenter, randomized, clinical, angiographic and intravascular ultrasound study.
Authors	Meneveau N, Schiele F, Grollier G, et al.
Reference	Eur Heart J 2000;21:1767-1775.
Disease	Coronary artery disease.
Purpose	To evaluate whether intramural delivery of nadoparin, a low-molecular-weight heparin, would prevent in-stent restenosis.
Design	Prospective, randomized, open-label, multicenter.
Patients	250 patients, 20-75 years old, with coronary artery disease who were scheduled for percutaneous coronary intervention of de novo type A or type B native coronary artery lesions, <15 mm length and ≥3.0 mm diameter. Restenotic lesions, patients with acute myocardial infarction or unstable angina within the last 7 days, left main coronary stenosis, suboptimal stent deployment, chronic total occlusion or ostial lesions were excluded. Patients were eligible for randomization only after complete coverage of the target lesion using 15 mm Palmaz-Schatz stents.
Follow-up	Clinical follow-up and repeated angiography at 6 months.
Regimen	After successful stent implantation, patients were randomized to local delivery of 2 mL solution of 5000 IU anti-Xa nadoparin with a Crescendo catheter or no nadoparin delivery.
Add'l Tx	All patients underwent balloon angioplasty followed by stent implantation. All patients received oral aspirin and intravenous unfractionated heparin 10,000 IU with a target activated clotting time of >300 seconds.

Results	Local delivery of nadoparin was successful in 124 of 125 patients randomized to nadoparin (99.2%). Nadoparin delivery was not associated with an increase in coronary artery dissection, in-stent thrombosis, acute closure, side branch occlusion, or distal embolisation. Acute myocardial infarction occurred in 0.8% in the control group (1 patient) vs zero in the nadoparin group. None of the patients died or needed emergency CABG. In both groups, 1.6% of the patients needed re-PCI. Only 1 patient in the nadoparin group had a bleeding complication at the vascular access site. 15% of the patients in the control group vs 13% in the nadoparin group needed >2 days hospitalization after the procedure (p=0.72). The late lumen loss at 6 months was comparable between the control (0.84±0.62 mm) and the nadoparin (0.88±0.63 mm) groups (p=0.56). >50% diameter restenosis occurred in 20% of the patients in the control group vs 24% in the nadoparin group. 70 patients underwent intravascular ultrasound study. The average area of neointimal tissue within the stent was 2.86±0.64 mm^2 in the control vs 2.90±0.53 mm^2 in the nadoparin group (p=0.57). At 6 months, event-free survival was 88.8% in the control group vs 89.6% in the nadoparin group.
Concl.	Intramural delivery of nadoparin after intracoronary stent implantation did not reduce intimal hyperplasia or in-stent restenosis and did not reduce the rate of major adverse clinical events over 6 months of follow-up.

ISAR

Intracoronary Stenting and Antithrombotic Regimen

Title	Sustained benefit over four years from an initial combined antiplatelet regimen after coronary stent placement in the ISAR trial.
Authors	Schühlen H, Kastrati A, Pache J, et al.
Reference	Am J Cardiol 2001;87:397-400.
Disease	Coronary artery disease.
Purpose	To determine long-term outcome of patients who received aspirin and ticlopidine vs aspirin and phenprocoumon for 4 weeks after stenting.
Design	Randomized.
Patients	517 patients who underwent successful Palmaz-Schatz stenting of the coronary artery.
Follow-up	4 years.
Regimen	257 patients randomized to aspirin and ticlopidine; 260 to aspirin and phenprocoumon to achieve target international normalized ratio of 3.5-4.5. Ticlopidine and phenprocoumon given for 4 weeks.
Add'l Tx	At beginning of stenting procedure all patients received aspirin and heparin and received heparin for 12 hours.
Results	Ticlopidine patients had fewer adverse cardiac events (1.6% vs 6.2%; p=0.007), nonfatal MIs (0.8% vs 3.5%; p=0.034) and target vessel revascularization procedures (1.2% vs 5.4%; p=0.007) compared to phenprocoumon patients, at 30 days. After 4 years, rates for any adverse cardiac events in the ticlopidine group was 22.6% vs 28.5% for phenprocoumon (p=0.078), 0.9% and 5.8% for nonfatal MI (p=0.003) and 18.3% vs 22.7% for target vessel revascularization (p=0.21) for ticlopidine vs phenprocoumon, respectively. Absolute difference in event rates was maintained after 4 years at 5.9%. Event rates beyond 30 days were

5c

not significantly different and event rates beyond 1 year were low (5.2% vs 3.6%; p=0.50) and also not significantly different.

| Concl. | The initial absolute benefit of combined antiplatelet therapy during the first 4 weeks of therapy was well maintained throughout the 4 years. |

ISAR-3

Intracoronary Stenting and Antithrombotic Regimen-3

Title	Treatment of Chlamydia pneumoniae infection with roxithromycin and effect on neointima proliferation after coronary stent placement (ISAR-3): a randomised, double-blind, placebo-controlled trial.
Authors	Neumann FJ, Kastrati A, Miethke T, et al.
Reference	Lancet 2001;357:2085-2089.
Disease	Coronary artery disease, restenosis.
Purpose	To evaluate whether roxithromycin, a macrolide antibiotic with antichlamydial activity, will reduce the rate of restenosis after coronary stenting.
Design	Randomized, double-blind, placebo-controlled, multicenter.
Patients	1010 patients after successful coronary stenting. Patients with contraindications to roxithromycin and those with indications for antibiotic therapy were excluded.
Follow-up	1 year of clinical follow-up. Repeat angiography after 6 months.
Regimen	Within 2 hours after stenting, patients were randomized to roxithromycin 300 mg/d or placebo for 4 weeks.
Add'l Tx	All patients received aspirin 100 mg/d during the study period and ticlopidine 250 mg bid for 4 weeks. The use of glycoprotein IIb/IIIa inhibitors was left to the discretion of the operator.

5c

Results	1239 lesions were treated. 65% of the patients had IgG antibodies against Chlamydia pneumoniae. 90% of the patients in the roxithromycin and 91% in the placebo group completed a full 4-week course of study medication (p=0.60). 83% of the patients in the roxithromycin and 86% of the patients in the placebo group underwent repeat angiography after 6 months. Minimal lumen diameter immediately after stenting was comparable between the roxithromycin (2.99±0.51 mm) and the placebo (2.99±0.51 mm) groups. Percent residual diameter stenosis was 5.7%±7.2% and 5.8%±8.2%, respectively. After 6 months, restenosis (≥50% diameter stenosis) was found in 31% of the patients in the roxithromycin group vs 29% in the placebo group (RR 1.08; 95% CI=0.92-1.26; p=0.43). ≥70% diameter restenosis was found in 19% vs 17%, respectively (p=0.54). 19% of the patients in the roxithromycin vs 17% in the placebo group underwent target vessel revascularization (p=0.3). Minimal lumen diameter at 6 months was 1.78±0.95 mm in the roxithromycin group vs 1.81±0.98 mm in the placebo group (p=0.58). Late loss was 1.20±0.84 mm and 1.17±0.85 mm, respectively (p=0.57), and net gain was 1.20±0.93 mm and 1.19±1.00 mm, respectively (p=0.93). 1-year mortality was 3.2% in the roxithromycin and 2.6% in the placebo group (RR 1.23; 95% CI=0.75-2.00; p=0.58). Nonfatal MI occurred in 4.0% and 3.5%, respectively (RR 1.18; 95% CI=0.76-1.83; p=0.61). There was a significant interaction between treatment effect and Chlamydia pneumoniae antibody titre (p=0.038 for restenosis; p=0.006 for revascularization). Among patients with negative titre, the OR for restenosis (>50%) was 1.46 (95% CI=0.98-2.18), for restenosis (>70%) 1.75 (95% CI=1.08-2.85), and for target vessel revascularization 1.87 (95% CI=1.17-2.98). In contrast, among patients with 1/512 titre, the OR for restenosis (>50%) was 0.65 (95% CI=0.33-1.30), for restenosis (>70%) 0.43 (95% CI=0.20-0.95), and for target vessel revascularization 0.49 (95% CI=0.23-1.03). The adjusted OR for restenosis at a titre of 1/512 was 0.44 (95% CI=0.19-1.06) and for revascularization 0.32 (95% CI=0.13-0.81).
Concl.	Roxithromycin did not prevent restenosis after coronary stenting in a non-selected population. In patients with high titres of antibodies against Chlamydia pneumoniae, roxithromycin reduced the rate of restenosis (>70%).

ITALICS

Randomized Investigation by the Thoraxcenter of Antisense DNA Using Local Delivery and IVUS After Coronary Stenting Trial

Title	Local intracoronary administration of antisense oligonucleotide against c-myc for the prevention of in-stent restenosis.
Authors	Kutryk MJB, Foley DB, van den Brand M, et al.
Reference	J Am Coll Cardiol 2002;39:281-287.
Disease	Coronary artery disease, restenosis.
Purpose	To determine whether antisense oligodeoxynucleotides against proto-oncogene c-myc could inhibit restenosis when delivered locally following coronary stenting.
Design	Randomized, control.
Patients	85 patients with coronary disease, single symptomatic on ischemia-provoking de novo or restenotic native lesion suitable for stenting.
Follow-up	6 months.
Regimen	After successful balloon predilation; implantation of self-expanding stent. Delivery of saline or antisense oligonucleotides using a local delivery catheter consisting of an inner support balloon and outer delivery balloon. A total of 10 mg of antisense oligonucleotides was delivered to the stented segment.
Add'l Tx	Aspirin, heparin.

5c

Results   Primary end point was percent in-stent volume obstruction measured by intravascular ultrasound (IVUS) at 6-month follow-up catheterization. In-stent volume obstruction was 44±16% in the placebo group and 46±14% in the antisense oligonucleotide group (p=NS). Minimal luminal diameter (mm) increased from 0.84±0.36 to 2.70±0.37 after stenting in the placebo group. Minimal luminal diameter (mm) increased from 0.90±0.45 to 2.80±0.37 after stenting in the treated group (p=NS between treatment groups). By 6 months, minimum luminal diameter decreased to 1.50±0.61 mm in the placebo group and 1.50±0.53 in the treated group (p=NS). Angiographic restenosis rates were similar between groups at 38.5% in the placebo group and 34.2% in the antisense oligonucleotide group. There were no differences in clinical outcome. The percentage of patients free of major adverse cardiac events at 210 days was 72% in the placebo group and 71% in the treated group.

Concl.   Local intracoronary delivery of antisense oligonucleotide against c-myc did not prevent in-stent restenosis of the coronary arteries.

NICOLE

Nisoldipine in Coronary Artery Disease in Leuven

Title	Usefulness of nisoldipine for prevention of restenosis after percutaneous transluminal coronary angioplasty (results of the NICOLE study).
Authors	Dens JA, Desmet WJ, Coussement P, et al.
Reference	Am J Cardiol 2001;87:28-33.
Disease	Coronary artery disease, restenosis, percutaneous coronary intervention.
Purpose	To evaluate the efficacy of slow-release nisoldipine to prevent restenosis after coronary angioplasty.
Design	Randomized, double-blind, single-center.
Patients	826 patients, <75 years old, who underwent a successful single- or multi-vessel balloon angioplasty without stenting. Patients who underwent primary or rescue percutaneous transluminal coronary angioplasty for acute myocardial infarction, patients with familial hypercholesterolemia, patients with prior coronary artery bypass graft surgery, and patients with renal failure or severe hepatic disease were excluded.
Follow-up	Clinical follow-up and repeated angiography at 6 months and 3 years.
Regimen	The next morning after successful PTCA, patients were randomized to nisoldipine coat-core 20 mg/d or placebo. If well tolerated, the dose was doubled after 14 days.
Add'l Tx	Other calcium channel antagonists were prohibited. Rifampicine, cimetidine, and quinidine were not permitted.

5c

Results	This paper reports on the results of 6 month follow-up. Only 772 patients were included in the intention-to-treat analysis, and 646 patients were valid for per-protocol analysis. Minimal lumen diameter at 6 months was 1.34±0.69 mm in the nisoldipine (n=415) and 1.33±0.64 mm in the placebo group (n=439). Percent diameter stenosis at 6 months was 50.2±22.2% in the nisoldipine and 50.1±21.9% in the placebo group. The restenosis rate per lesion (≥50% diameter stenosis), for the per-protocol population, was 45% in the nisoldipine and 50% in the placebo group (p=NS). The restenosis rate per patient was 49% and 55%, respectively (p=NS). During the first 6 months of follow-up 2 patients in the nisoldipine and 1 in the placebo group died, and 2 and 5 patients, respectively, had a nonfatal acute myocardial infarction. 18% of the patients in the nisoldipine group vs 26% of the patients in the placebo group underwent ≥1 unscheduled coronary angiography (p=0.006), mainly because of lower incidence of recurrent angina in the nisoldipine group (12% vs 21%; p=0.004). Less patients in the nisoldipine group underwent CABG (1 vs 10 patients; p=0.012) and repeat target lesion PTCA (31 vs 59 patients; p=0.017). At 6 month follow-up angiography, an additional number of patients underwent revascularization (mainly for pure angiographic indications). Finally, 32% of the nisoldipine and 41% of the placebo group underwent repeat revascularization (p=0.057). More patients in the nisoldipine group were angina free at 4 months (88% vs 83%).
Concl.	Nisoldipine did not prevent restenosis after PTCA, but reduced the number of repeat revascularization procedure, probably because of its antianginal effects.

PARIS

Effect of ACE Inhibitors on Angiographic Restenosis From PARIS Investigators

Title	Effect of ACE inhibitors on angiographic restenosis after coronary stenting (PARIS): a randomized, double-blind, placebo-controlled trial.
Authors	Meurice T, Bauters C, Hermant X, et al.
Reference	Lancet 2001;357:1321-1324.
Disease	Coronary artery disease, restenosis, percutaneous coronary intervention.
Purpose	To evaluate whether high-dose quinapril, an angiotensin-converting enzyme inhibitor, will reduce neo-intimal proliferation and prevent restenosis after intracoronary stent implantation in patients carrying the DD genotype.
Design	Randomized, double-blind, placebo-controlled, single-center.
Patients	91 patients, <75 years old, with a DD genotype for the angiotensin-I converting enzyme deletion allele, who underwent successful NIR stent implantation. Patients with acute myocardial infarction within 48 hours before PCI, systolic blood pressure <120 mm Hg, renal or hepatic impairment, a history of bleeding, a contraindication to aspirin or ticlopidine, an angioplasty of a vein graft, and a need for ACE inhibitor treatment were excluded.
Follow-up	Clinical follow-up for 6 months. Repeated angiography at 6 months.
Regimen	The ACE genotype was established within 12-24 h after coronary stenting. Patients with the DD genotype were randomized to quinapril 40 mg/d (n=46) for 6 months or placebo (n=45). Trial medication was started within 48 hours of stenting.
Add'l Tx	Patients received aspirin 75-300 mg/d for 6 months and ticlopidine 500 mg/d for 1 month.

5c

Results	Zero patients died. Nonfatal myocardial infarction occurred in 1 patient in the quinapril group. 3 patients from the quinapril vs zero in the placebo underwent CABG. 10 patients from the quinapril group and 7 from the placebo group needed repeat PCI. 24% of the patients in the quinapril vs 16% in the placebo group had ≥1 clinical event. Minimal lumen diameter was 2.93±0.46 mm and 2.81±0.50 mm in the quinapril and placebo group after stenting (p=0.276) and 1.82±0.76 mm and 2.06±0.79 mm at 6 month follow-up (p=0.184). Mean percent stenosis at follow-up was 41±23% in the quinapril and 33±21% in the placebo group (p=0.091). Late loss in diameter was 1.11±0.70 mm and 0.76±0.60 mm, respectively (p=0.018). The restenosis rate was 37% in the quinapril group and 24% in the placebo group (p=0.229).
Concl.	In patients with DD genotype undergoing intracoronary stent implantation, therapy with the ACE inhibitor quinapril did not prevent restenosis. Quinapril was associated with an exaggerated restenosis process compared with placebo.

POLONIA Study

Polish-American Local Lovenox NIR Assessment Study

Title	Local delivery of enoxaparin to decrease restenosis after stenting: results of initial multicenter trial. POLONIA Study.
Authors	Kiesz RS, Buszman P, Martin JL, et al.
Reference	Circulation 2001;103:26-31.
Disease	Coronary artery disease.
Purpose	To determine whether intramural delivery of enoxaparin (low-molecular-weight heparin, potent factor Xa and thrombin inhibitor) prior to stenting of de novo lesions decreases restenosis.
Design	Prospective, randomized, multicenter.
Patients	100 symptomatic patients with documented myocardial ischemia and 1-vessel disease who were undergoing stenting with NIR stent.
Follow-up	6-month angiographic follow-up.
Regimen	Local administration of enoxaparin (10 mg) during predilation using a balloon with microporous holes and reduced systemic heparinization or stenting with standard systemic heparinization.
Add'l Tx	All patients received NIR stent, aspirin, ticlopidine.
Results	Primary end point was late luminal loss at 6 months and secondary end points were major adverse cardiac events (death, MI, emergency CABG, repeat balloon angioplasty); restenosis at 6 months. 6-month late luminal loss was decreased to 0.76±0.42 mm in local enoxaparin group vs 1.07±0.49 mm in standard stent group (p<0.001). Restenosis occurred in 10% of patients in enoxaparin group vs 24% in standard stent group (p<0.05). Target lesion revascularization was needed in 8% in the enoxaparin group vs 22% in systemic heparinization group (p<0.05) at 6 months. There were no other differences in clinical outcomes between the 2 groups.

5c

Concl.   Local drug delivery with enoxaparin significantly reduced late
          luminal loss and restenosis after stent implantation of de novo
          coronary lesions vs stenting alone.

PRESTO

Prevention of Restenosis with Tranilast and Its Outcomes

Title	Results of Prevention of Restenosis with Tranilast and Its Outcomes (PRESTO) Trial.
Authors	Holmes DR, Savage M, LaBlanche J-M, et al.
Reference	Circulation 2002;106:1243-1250.
Disease	Coronary artery disease; need for percutaneous coronary intervention.
Purpose	Tranilast is a drug that inhibits release and production of cytokines and mediators from inflammatory cells and interferes with proliferation and migration of vascular medial smooth muscle cells. The purpose of the study was to determine whether usage of tranilast after PCI reduces the risk of major adverse cardiovascular events and affects quantitative measures of restenosis.
Design	Double-blind, randomized, placebo-controlled, multicenter.
Patients	11,484 patients, >18 years old, who underwent successful PCI. Successful PCI was defined as at least 1 stenosed vessel improved to <50% residual stenosis without a major adverse cardiovascular event (MACE: death or myocardial infarction or ischemia-driven target vessel revascularization) before starting study medication. Patients using oral anticoagulants, phenytoin or investigational drugs, and patients with non-Q-wave MI within 48 hours before enrollment; PCI in the previous 3 months; chronic liver disease; renal impairment; gout; anemia; severe concomitant disease; or a history of contrast media-induced nephrotoxicity were excluded. 2 prespecified randomly selected subsets of patients were assigned to be evaluated with either angiography (n=2018) or intravascular ultrasound (n=1107).
Follow-up	9 months.

5c

Regimen	Randomization to 1 of 5 treatment groups: 1) 3 months placebo bid (n=2298); 2) 3 months tranilast 300 mg bid (n=2300); 3) 3 months tranilast 450 mg bid (n=2300); 4) 1 month tranilast 300 mg bid and then placebo bid for 2 months (n=2306); or 5) 1 month tranilast 450 mg bid and then placebo bid for 2 months (n=2280) (from Am Heart J 2000;139:23-31).
Results	The primary end point of the study was the first MACE (all-cause death, MI, and ischemia-driven vessel revascularization) within 9 months. The secondary end points were each of these components. Other studied outcomes were minimal lumen diameter determined by quantitative coronary angiography and plaque volume by intravascular ultrasound. The frequency of the first incidence of MACE in the treatment groups was similar (15.4%-16.0%) and was no different than placebo (15.7%). The hazard ratio for the treatment groups compared to placebo ranged from 0.98-1.02, with p=0.77-0.81. Most of the MACEs were ischemia-driven revascularizations; the incidence of death and MI across groups was low: 1%-1.8%. Analyses by subgroups of sex, age, ethnicity, comorbidities, and nature of coronary lesions revealed no differences between tranilast and placebo for any subgroup. There was no trend observed in favor of tranilast for death or revascularization. There was a trend toward favor for tranilast 450 mg bid compared to placebo in follow-up MIs (hazard ratio 0.62; 95% CI=0.38-1.03; p=0.061); and an analysis using only patients who had taken at least 84 days of tranilast revealed a significant difference in favor of tranilast for follow-up MIS (hazard ratio 0.44; 95% CI=0.23-0.85; p=0.012). There were no statistically significant differences in any of the angiographic variables between the placebo group and the tranilast groups at follow-up. Similarly, there were no differences in any of the intracoronary ultrasound measurements between the groups at follow-up. The most common adverse events in the treatment groups were hyperbilirubinemia, hepatic (transaminase) enzyme elevations, hepatic function abnormal (defined as at least 1 hepatic laboratory test >3 times the upper limit of normal [ULN] and either alkaline phosphatase or total bilirubin ≥ULN), increased serum creatinine and anemia. All abnormalities were related to both the dose and duration of tranilast treatment, and reversed after discontinuation of study medication.

Concl.   Tranilast was not more effective than placebo in reducing the risk of MACEs in patients who underwent PCI. Tranilast did not improve angiographic or ultrasound parameters of restenosis. Usage of tranilast was associated with reversible hepatic and renal laboratory abnormalities.

PRICE

Prairie ReoPro vs Integrilin Cost Evaluation

Title	Comparative 30-day economic and clinical outcomes of platelet glycoprotein IIb/IIIa inhibitor use during elective pecutaneous coronary intervention: Prairie reoPro vs integrilin cost evaluation (PRICE) trial.
Authors	The PRICE Investigators.
Reference	Am Heart J 2001;141:402-409.
Disease	Coronary artery disease.
Purpose	To compare the economics, pharmacodynamics and clinical results of abciximab and eptifibatide treatment during elective percutaneous coronary interventions.
Design	Randomized, double-blind, placebo-controlled, 2-center.
Patients	320 patients, >21 years old, undergoing elective percutaneous coronary intervention. Patients with a recent (<48 hours) acute myocardial infarction, unstable angina, degenerated venous graft lesions, type C lesions, major trauma or surgery within the last 6 weeks, thrombocytopenia, renal failure, abciximab or eptifibatide therapy within the last 7 days and those planned for staged PCI procedures were excluded.
Follow-up	30 days.
Regimen	Patients were randomized to abciximab (a bolus of 0.25 mg/kg, followed by 0.125 µg/kg/min infusion for 12 hours) or to eptifibatide (a bolus of 180 µg/kg, followed by 2.0 µg/kg/min for 18-24 hours).
Add'l Tx	All patients received aspirin 325 mg at least 2 hours before PCI and daily thereafter. All patients received clopidogril for 2-4 weeks and intravenous heparin (70 U/kg) before the procedure. Patients underwent coronary angioplasty or stent implantation.

Results	163 patients received abciximab and 157 received eptifibatide. Coronary stents were implanted in 91% of the patients. In-hospital ischemic complications (death, myocardial infarction and urgent repeated revascularization) occurred in 4.9% of the abciximab-treated patients and in 5.1% of the eptifibatide-treated patients (p=0.84). There was no difference in the rate of occurrence or enzymatic size of non-Q-wave myocardial infarction between the groups. 30-day ischemic complications occurred in 5.6% and 6.3% of the patients, respectively (p=0.95). Serious in-hospital bleeding complications occurred in 3.1% and 1.9% of the abciximab and eptifibatide groups, respectively (p=0.75). Blood transfusions were administered in 3.1% and 1.3% of the patients, respectively (p=0.47). The median and 95% CI in-hospital total cost were $8268 ($7715-$8666) for the abciximab and $7207 ($6588, $7729) for the eptifibatide group (p=0.009). The median and 95% CI total costs at 30 days were $8336 ($8223-$9276) for the abciximab and $7207 ($6588-$7229) for the eptifibatide groups (p=0.009). The difference was largely related to the higher price of abciximab. The degree of platelet inhibition remained stable in the eptifibatide group, whereas in the abciximab group there was marked late variability in the degree of platelet inhibition. 29% of the abciximab-treated patients vs only 4% of the eptifibatide-treated patients had <80% platelet inhibition within 30 minutes before the cessation of the study drug.
Concl.	In patients undergoing elective PCI, eptifibatide was associated with more stable and durable platelet inhibition, similar clinical outcome and safety, and lower in-hospital and 30-day costs, compared with abciximab.

TARGET

Do Tirofiban and ReoPro Give Similar Efficacy Trial

Title	Comparison of two platelet glycoprotein IIb/IIIa inhibitors, tirofiban and abciximab, for the prevention of ischemic events with percutaneous coronary revascularization.
Authors	Topol EJ, Moliterno DJ, Herrmann HC, et al.
Reference	N Engl J Med 2001;344:1888-1894.
Disease	Coronary artery disease, percutaneous coronary intervention.
Purpose	To compare the safety and efficacy of 2 GP IIb/IIIa inhibitors, tirofiban and abciximab in patients undergoing PCI.
Design	Randomized, double-blind, double-dummy, multicenter.
Patients	5308 patients scheduled for coronary stenting with >70% diameter stenosis coronary lesion (either de novo or restenotic lesions, either in a native coronary artery or in a bypass graft). Patients with cardiogenic shock or an ST elevation acute myocardial infarction were excluded. In addition, patients with serum creatinine ≥2.5 mg/dL, high risk for bleeding or ongoing bleeding, or a platelet count <120,000 platelet/mm^3 were not included.
Follow-up	30 days.
Regimen	Patients were randomized to tirofiban (10 µg/kg bolus, followed by 0.15 µg/kg/min for 18-24 hours) (n=2647) or abciximab (0.25 mg/kg bolus, followed by 0.125 µg/kg/min for 12 hours) (n=2661).
Add'l Tx	All patients received aspirin 250-500 mg and a loading dose of clopidogrel 300 mg before PCI. All patients received heparin 70 U/kg at the beginning of PCI with a target activated clotting time of 250 secends. Aspirin 75-325 mg/d and clopidogrel 75 mg/d were continued for 30 days.

Results	2398 patients in the tirofiban group and 2411 in the abciximab group actually received the study medication. 95% of the patients in both groups underwent stenting. The primary end point of death, nonfatal MI or urgent target vessel revascularization within 30 days occurred in 7.6% of the patients in the tirofiban group vs in 6.0% of the patients in the abciximab group (hazard ratio [HR] 1.26; 1-sided 95% CI=1.51, demonstrating lack of equivalence, 2-sided 95% CI=1.01-1.57; p=0.038). Nonfatal MI (creatine kinase MB ≥X3 the upper limit of the normal range or new abnormal Q-waves) occurred in 6.9% of the patients in the tirofiban group vs 5.4% in the abciximab group (HR 1.27; p=0.04). 30-day mortality was 0.5% in the tirofiban group and 0.4% in the abciximab group (HR 1.21; p=0.66). Death or nonfatal MI occurred in 7.2% and 5.7% of the patients in the tirofiban and abciximab group, respectively (HR 1.26; p=0.04). Urgent target vessel revascularization occurred in 0.8% and 0.7%, respectively (HR 1.26; p=0.49). Abciximab was better than tirofiban in patients <65 and ≥65 years old, both in women and men, in patients with and without diabetes mellitus, in patients who received or did not receive a loading dose of clopidogrel before PCI, and in patients undergoing PCIs for an acute coronary syndrome. Among patients undergoing PCI for other indications, tirofiban was better (4.5% vs 5.6%, HR 0.82; 95% CI=0.54-1.24). Major bleeding occurred in 0.9% in the tirofiban group vs 0.7% in the abciximab group (p=NS), and minor bleeding in 2.8% vs 4.3%, respectively (p<0.001). Thrombocytopenia (<100,000/mm^3) was detected in 0.5% and 2.4%, respectively (p<0.001), and severe thrombocytopenia (<50,000/mm^3) in 0.1% and 0.9%, respectively (p<0.001).
Concl.	Abciximab was more effective than tirofiban in preventing nonfatal MI and the composite end point of death or MI; or death, MI and urgent target vessel revascularization.

TARGET

Do Tirofiban and ReoPro Give Similar Efficacy Outcome Trial

Title	Outcomes at 6 months for the direct comparison of tirofiban and abciximab during percutaneous coronary revascularization with stent placement: the TARGET follow-up study.
Authors	Moliterno DJ, Yakubov SJ, DiBattiste PM, et al.
Reference	Lancet 2002;360:355-360.
Disease	Coronary artery disease.
Purpose	To compare 6 month clinical outcome after percutaneous coronary intervention with stent implantation in patients randomized to tirofiban or abciximab in the TARGET trial.
Design	Randomized, double-blind, double-dummy, multicenter.
Patients	4809 patients undergoing PCI (see above).
Follow-up	6 months.
Regimen	See above.
Add'l Tx	See above.

Results	Follow-up data was available for 97% of the patients. At 6 months, the primary end point of the study (death, MI, and target vessel revascularization) occurred in 14.8% in the tirofiban group vs 14.3% in the abciximab group (hazard ratio [HR] 1.04; 95% CI=0.90Đ1.21; p=0.591). Death occurred in 1.1% of the patients in the tirofiban and 1.0% in the abciximab group (p=0.893). 8% of the patients in the tirofiban group vs 6.6% in the abciximab group had acute MI (HR 1.21; 95% CI=0.98Đ1.50; p=0.074). The rates of target vessel revascularization were 8.1% and 8.6%, respectively (HR 0.93; 95% CI=0.77Đ1.14; p=0.495). At 6 months the primary end point occurred in 18.0% of the tirofiban and abciximab patients who had acute coronary syndromes at enrollment (HR 1.19; 95% CI=0.99Đ1.42), and in 10.3% and 13.4% among those without acute coronary syndrome on enrollment (HR 0.77; 95% CI=0.58Đ1.01). However, among patients who had acute coronary syndrome, the composite end point of death or MI occurred less often in the abciximab group (10.4% vs 8.2%; p=0.028). In contrast, among patients without acute coronary syndrome, target vessel revascularization rate was lower in the tirofiban group (5.8% vs 8.4%; p=0.040). There was no statistically significant difference between tirofiban and abciximab in patients with and without diabetes mellitus.
Concl.	Over all, 6-month clinical outcome tirofiban and abciximab was comparable between tirofiban and abciximab in patients undergoing PCI with stent implantation, although abciximab reduced the composite end point of death or MI in patients with acute coronary syndrome on enrollment and tirofiban reduced the rate of target vessel revascularization in patients without acute coronary syndrome.

TARGET (Subanalysis)

Do Tirofiban and ReoPro Give Similar Efficacy Outcomes Trial

Title	Impact of clinical syndrome acuity on the differential response to 2 glycoprotein IIb/IIIa inhibitors in patients undergoing coronary stenting. The TARGET trial.
Authors	Stone GW, Moliterno DJ, Bertrand M, et al.
Reference	Circulation 2002;105:2347-2354.
Disease	Coronary artery disease; acute coronary syndromes.
Purpose	To compare the impact of clinical syndrome acuity on differential response of abciximab vs tirofiban in patients having stent implantation.
Design	Randomized, double-blind, double-dummy design.
Patients	4809 patients of any age undergoing percutaneous coronary intervention (PCI). Could have unstable angina, non-ST elevation MI, recent non-acute ST elevation MI, or stable angina; ischemia that was asymptomatic.
Follow-up	6-24 hours; 30 days; 6 months.
Regimen	Patients randomized to either tirofiban (10 mg/kg IV bolus followed by infusion of 0.15 mg/kg per minute for 18-24 hours) or abciximab (0.25 mg/kg bolus followed by infusion 0.125 mg/kg per minute to a maximum of 10 mg/min for 12 hours).
Add'l Tx	Aspirin, clopidogrel.

Results	3025 (63%) of the patients had an acute coronary syndrome; 1784 had stable coronary syndromes. There were fewer periprocedural infarctions in patients receiving abciximab vs tirofiban. In those patients with acute coronary syndromes abciximab lowered rates of MI at 30 days (5.8% vs 8.5%; p=0.004). MI rate also was lower in the abciximab group (7.2%) vs tirofiban (9.8%; p=0.013) at 6 months. Mortality rate at 6 months was the same in both groups at 1.39%. Target vessel revascularization was 9.4% with abciximab vs 9.9% with tirofiban (p=NS). In those patients with stable coronary artery disease tirofiban and abciximab had similar periprocedural MI rates. The 30-day MI rate was 4.9% with abciximab vs 4.2% with tirofiban and at 6 months 5.8% vs 5.1%, respectively. At 6 months target revascularization was 8.4% with abciximab vs 5.8% with tirofiban (p=0.04). There was an overall trend toward enhanced 6 month event-free survival with tirofiban (89.7% vs 86.6%; p=0.056), in patients without acute coronary syndrome. In acute coronary syndrome patients minor bleeding occurred in 4.0% of abciximab vs 2.4% of tirofiban patients (p=0.01). Thrombocytopenia (<100,000 platelets/mm^3) was more common with abciximab (3.6%) vs tirofiban (0.8%; p<0.001) in acute coronary syndromes. Thrombocytopenia also was more common in patients with abciximab (3.2%) vs tirofiban (0.3%; p<0.001) in stable coronary syndrome patients.
Concl.	Abciximab resulted in less periprocedural infarction than tirofiban in patients with acute coronary syndromes. Patients with stable coronary syndromes had equivalent or better outcomes with tirofiban vs abciximab and fewer adverse hematologic and hemorrhagic events.

5c

TARGET

Do Tirofiban and ReoPro Give Similar Efficacy Outcome Trial

Title	Triple antiplatelet therapy during percutaneous coronary intervention is associated with improved outcomes including one-year survival: results from the Do Tirofiban and ReoPro Give Similar Efficacy Outcome Trial (TARGET).
Authors	Chan AW, Moliterno DJ, Berger PB, et al.
Reference	J Am Coll Cardiol 2003;42:1188-1195.
Disease	Coronary artery disease.
Purpose	To examine whether clopidogrel treatment initiated before coronary stenting improves clinical outcomes among patients receiving aspirin and a glycoprotein IIb/IIIa inhibitor.
Design	Multicenter, randomized, double-blind, double-dummy trial.
Patients	4809 patients undergoing percutaneous coronary intervention with stent placement.
Follow-up	1 year.
Regimen	Tirofiban or abciximab with percutaneous coronary intervention; 300 mg of clopidogrel before (93.1% of patients) or immediately after the procedure. Aspirin.

Results	The 30-day primary composite end point (death, MI, urgent target-vessel revascularization) was lower among clopidogrel-pretreated patients (6.6% vs 10.4%; p=0.009), primarily because of a reduced rate of MI (6% vs 9.5%; p=0.012). The benefit of clopidogrel pretreatment was sustained at 6 months (composite end point 14.6% vs 19.8%, hazard ratio (HR)=0.71; p=0.010), primarily because of a reduced rate of death and MI (7.8% vs 13%; p=0.001). At 1 year, clopidogrel pretreatment was associated with a lower mortality rate (1.7% vs 3.6%; p=0.011). Clopidogrel pretreatment was an independent predictor for death or MI at 30 days (HR=0.63; p=0.012) and at 6 months (HR=0.61; p=0.003) and survival at 1 year (HR=0.53; p=0.044). Clopidogrel pretreatment did not cause an excess of 30-day bleeding events. Outcome was not affected by the type of IIb/IIIa inhibitor.
Concl.	Among patients undergoing PCI with stent placement and receiving adjunctive aspirin and a GP IIb/IIIa inhibitor, clopidogrel was associated with a superior clinical outcome, which was evident within 24-48 hours after the procedure and was sustained at 6 months. The mortality benefit extended to 1 year.

TOPSTAR

Troponin in Planned PTCA/Stent Implantation with or Without Administration of the Glycoprotein IIb/IIIa Receptor Antagonist Tirofiban

Title	Effect of additional temporary glycoprotein IIb/IIIa receptor inhibition on troponin release in elective percutaneous coronary interventions after pretreatment with aspirin and clopidogrel.
Authors	Bonz AW, Lengenfelder B, Strotmann J, et al.
Reference	J Am Coll Cardiol 2002;40:662-668.
Disease	Percutaneous intervention, coronary artery disease.
Purpose	To determine the timing and incidence of troponin release after elective, nonacute percutaneous interventions in patients that received aspirin and clopidogrel, and the impact of peri- and post-procedural administration of additional GP IIb/IIIa inhibitor on postprocedural troponin release.
Design	Double-blind, randomized, prospective, single-center.
Patients	96 patients (age 18-81) with a history of stable angina and a target lesion ≥70% appropriate for PCI. Patients with an acute coronary syndrome, subacute or acute MI were excluded. Other exclusion criteria were: unstable angina, stenosis in venous or arterial bypass grafts, renal insufficiency, recent peptic ulcers or history of bleeding, thrombocytopenia or thrombolytic therapy within the past 24 hours, stroke in the previous 2 years, severe hypertension, malignancy, and previous or planned treatment with a GP IIb/IIIa agent.
Follow-up	9 months.

Regimen	Patients were randomized to receive either tirofiban or placebo during and after the PCI. All patients were administered a loading dose of clopidogrel 375 mg and aspirin 500 mg at least 1 day prior to the PCI. During the PCI, the guide wire was passed beyond the target stenosis, and either tirofiban or placebo was administered, followed by stent placement or balloon inflation. A bolus of the glycoprotein IIb/IIIa inhibitor tirofiban (10 mg/kg or placebo) was given, followed by continuous infusion (0.15 mg/kg/min tirofiban or placebo), continued for 18 hours.
Add'l Tx	All patients received unfractionated heparin in a dosage of 5000 U to 10,000 U during the procedure with an activated clotting time target of 250 seconds.
Results	50 patients were randomized into the tirofiban group, and 46 into the placebo group. The primary end point was the appearance of troponin T (TnT) after PCI. Incidence of death, MI, and target vessel revascularization were the secondary end points. A trend toward lower troponin levels in the tirofiban group vs placebo was found at all measured postprocedural time intervals: 12 hours (40% with positive TnT in the tirofiban group, 63% in placebo; $p<0.05$), 24 hours (48% vs 69%; $p<0.05$) and 48 hours (58% vs 74%; p=NS). There was a continuous increase in TnT levels during the entire follow-up period in both groups. At 30-day follow-up there were no secondary events in the tirofiban group, while there was 1 event (MI) in the placebo group, a nonsignificant difference. At 9-month follow-up, there was 1 readmission in the treatment group and 5 readmissions in the placebo group; this difference was significant ($p<0.05$).
Concl.	Release of troponin T occurs in a majority of patients already on aspirin and clopidogrel following PCI. Tirofiban decreases the release of troponin T and is possibly beneficial in reducing subsequent readmission, MI and revascularization.

TRAPIST

Trapidil for Prevention of In-Stent Stenosis

Title	The TRAPIST Study. A multicentre randomized placebo-controlled clinical trial of trapidil for prevention of restenosis after coronary stenting, measured by 3-D intravascular ultrasound.
Authors	Serruys PW, Foley DP, Pieper M, et al.
Reference	Eur Heart J 2001;22:1938-1947.
Disease	Coronary artery disease, restenosis.
Purpose	To evaluate the safety and efficacy of trapidil, a phosphodiesterase inhibitor, in preventing restenosis after coronary stenting.
Design	Randomized, placebo-controlled, multicenter.
Patients	312 patients with coronary artery disease, scheduled to undergo single Wallstent implantation in a de novo ≤40 mm in length coronary artery lesion in a vessel 3-6 mm in diameter. Patients with estimated life expectancy of <1 year, myocardial infarction within 7 days, left bundle branch block, side branch >2.0 mm, left main stenosis, thrombotic coronary lesion, active peptic disease, stroke within 6 months, bleeding disorder and treatment with ketanserin, oral anticoagulants, ticlopidine, pentoxyphilline, calcium channel blockers and molsidomine were excluded.
Follow-up	All patients underwent intravascular ultrasound at the end of procedure and at 6 months. Clinical follow-up for 7 months.
Regimen	Randomization to trapidil 600 mg/d or placebo. Study medication was administered ≥1 hours before percutaneous transluminal coronary angioplasty (PTCA) and continued for 6 months.
Add'l Tx	All patients received ticlopidine 500-100 mg 12-48 hours before PTCA. Oral ticlopidine 500 mg/d was continued for 1 month. All patients received aspirin 75-500 mg/d. All patients received IV heparin 10,000 units at the beginning of PTCA. All patients underwent Magic Wallstent implantation.

Results	303 patients (155 placebo and 148 trapidil) underwent successful Wallstent implantation. 90% of the patients in the placebo group and 88% in the trapidil group underwent repeat angiography at 26±2 weeks. At follow-up, in-stent neointimal volume was 108.6±95.6 mm^3 in the trapidil group and 93.3±79.1 mm^3 in the placebo group (p=0.16). The percent obstruction volume was 38%±18% and 36%±21%, respectively (p=0.32). The minimal lumen diameter at follow-up was 1.63±0.61 mm and 1.74±0.69 mm in the trapidil and placebo group, respectively (p=0.17). Restenosis occurred in 31% vs 24% of the patients in the trapidil and placebo group, respectively (p=0.24). Major adverse cardiac events occurred in 22% and 20% of the patients, respectively (p=0.71).
Concl.	Oral trapidil was not effective in reducing in-stent hyperplasia or restenosis and did not affect clinical outcome after successful Wallstent implantation.

5c

TREAT

Tranilast Restenosis Following Angioplasty Trial

Title	Impact of tranilast on restenosis after coronary angioplasty: Tranilast restenosis following angioplasty trial (TREAT).
Authors	Tamai H, Katoh O, Suzuki S, et al.
Reference	Am Heart J 1999;138:968-975.
Disease	Coronary artery disease, PCI, restenosis.
Purpose	To assess whether tranilast, an antiallergic drug that suppresses the release of platelet derived growth factor and other cytokines, will prevent restenosis after percutaneous balloon angioplasty.
Design	Randomized, double-blind, placebo-controlled, multicenter.
Patients	255 patients, ≤75 years old, with angina pectoris or old myocardial infarction, >50% diameter stenosis in de novo native type A coronary artery lesions with TIMI flow grade 2-3. Before enrollment patients had to undergo successful PTCA.
Follow-up	Follow-up angiography at 3 months. Clinical follow-up for 12 months.
Regimen	Randomization to tranilast 600 mg/d (86 patients, 100 lesions), tranilast 300 mg/d (84 patients, 94 lesions), or placebo (85 patients, 95 lesions) for 3 months after successful PTCA.
Add'l Tx	All patients received IV 10,000 IU heparin just before PTCA. It is unclear whether aspirin was mandatory, whether stents, other devices, and IV glycoprotein IIb/IIIa were permitted.

Results	The per-protocol population included 59 patients (68 lesions) in the tranilast 600 mg/d, 64 patients (71 lesions) in the tranilast 300 mg/d, and 65 patients (71 lesions) in the placebo group. ≥50% diameter stenosis occurred in 17.6% of the tranilast 600 mg/d (p=0.005 vs placebo), 38.6% in the tranilast 300 mg/d and 39.4% in the placebo group. ≥50% loss of the initial gain was found in 14.7%, 35.2%, and 46.5% of the patients, respectively (p=0.000065 for tranilast 600 mg vs placebo). Multivariable model showed that tranilast (odds ratio 0.275; 95% CI=0.116-0.612; p=0.002) and female gender (odds ratio 0.352; 95% CI=0.119-0.991; p=0.042) were independent predictors of restenosis. 23.1% of the patients in the placebo group, 32.8% in the tranilast 300 mg/d and 15.3% in the tranilast 600 mg/d underwent revascularization within the first year (p=NS). The overall incidence of side effects per patient was 7.2% for the placebo group, 16.3% for the tranilast 300 mg/d and 9.5% for the tranilast 600 mg/d.
Concl.	Oral administration of tranilast 600 mg/d for 3 months was safe and effective in reducing restenosis rate after percutaneous transluminal coronary angioplasty.

5c

TREAT-2

Tranilast Restenosis Following Angioplasty Trial-2

Title	The impact of tranilast on restenosis after coronary angioplasty: the second tranilast restenosis following angioplasty trial (TREAT-2).
Authors	Tamai H, Katoh K, Yamaguchi T, et al.
Reference	Am Heart J 2002;143:506-513.
Disease	Coronary artery disease, percutaneous coronary intervention (PCI).
Purpose	To evaluate whether tranilast reduces restenosis after percutaneous transluminal coronary angioplasty (PTCA) for de novo as well as restenotic lesions.
Design	Randomized, double-blind, placebo-controlled, multicenter.
Patients	297 patients (329 lesions), ≥20 years old, with angina or old myocardial infarction, and ≥50% diameter stenotic de novo or restenotic lesions in native coronary arteries with TIMI flow grade 2 or 3 who underwent successful PTCA. Patients with left main coronary artery disease, severe congestive heart failure, liver insufficiency, renal failure, pulmonary disease, hematologic insufficiency, and women of childbearing potential were excluded. Lesions with long dissection after PTCA, thrombus containing lesions, and culprit lesions for acute myocardial infarction (within 14 days before randomization) were not included. Total occlusions, bifurcational lesions, ≥20 mm long lesions, and heavily calcified lesions were excluded.
Follow-up	Follow-up angiography after 3 months. Clinical follow-up for 1 year.
Regimen	Patients were randomized to placebo (146 patients, 167 lesions) or tranilast (N-[3,4-dimethoxycinamoyl] anthranilic acid) 600 mg/d (151 patients, 162 lesions), started on the day after PTCA and continued for 3 months.
Add'l Tx	All patients received heparin 10,000 IU before PTCA.

Results   288 patients (319 lesions) were included in the intention-to-treat analysis. The per-protocol analysis included 216 patients (239 lesions). 23.6% of the lesions were restenotic lesions in the placebo group and 33.9% in the tranilast group (p=0.086). On baseline, lesions were longer in the placebo group (6.3±3.5 mm) than in the tranilast group (5.8±3.5 mm; p=0.033). The percent diameter stenosis at baseline was lower in the placebo group (70.8%±11.0% vs 74.0%±11.9%; p=0.018). However, immediately after PTCA it was comparable (28.4%±11.9% vs 30.5%±11.9%, respectively; p=0.214). At follow-up, the percent diameter stenosis was significantly greater in the placebo group (47.7%±20.0% vs 42.3%±20.7%; p=0.025). Restenosis occurred in 44.1% in the placebo group and 18.8% in the tranilast group (p=0.0005). Restenosis in de novo lesions was 41.2% vs 18.9%, respectively (p=0.003). Restenosis in restenotic lesions was 53.3% vs 18.4%, respectively (p=0.004). Tranilast was equally effective in lesions with reference diameter ≥2.5 mm (33.8% vs 11.1%; p=0.001) and <2.5 mm (56.9% vs 30.8%; p=0.019). Minimal lumen diameter was significantly larger in the placebo group before PTCA (0.78±0.34 mm vs 0.69±0.35 mm; p=0.02). Immediately after PTCA minimal lumen diameter was comparable (p=0.840). However, at follow-up, minimal lumen diameter was significantly smaller in the placebo (1.39±0.64 mm) than in the tranilast group (1.55±0.66 mm; p=0.033). Multivariate analysis showed that tranilast treatment was independently associated with a reduction in restenosis rate (OR 0.412; 95% CI=0.198-0.831; p=0.0149). None of the patients in both groups died. Myocardial infarction occurred in 1% of the patients in the placebo group vs 2.1% in the tranilast group (p=0.608). Target vessel revascularization was performed in 31.4% and 28.7% of the patients, respectively (p=0.756). 28.7% of the lesions in the placebo group vs 27.0% in the tranilast group needed revascularization (p=0.879). The overall incidence of side effects was 9.2% in the placebo vs 18.5% in the tranilast group (p=0.034). The most common side effects of tranilast were elevation of liver transaminases, abdominal discomfort, nausea, diarrhea, skin rash, itching, and frequent urination.

Concl.   Oral administration of tranilast for 3 months reduced the rates of angiographic restenosis after balloon angioplasty of both de novo and restenotic lesions in native coronary arteries. In this study tranilast did not reduce the incidence of clinical events during the 1-year clinical follow-up. However, the drug is associated with side effects.

VIP

Visipaque in Percutaneous Transluminal Coronary Angioplasty

Title	Influence of a nonionic, iso-osmolar contrast medium (Iodixanol) vs an ionic, low osmolar contrast medium (Ioxaglate) on major adverse cardiac events in patients undergoing percutaneous transluminal coronary angioplasty (PTCA). A multicenter, randomized, double-blind study.
Authors	Bertrand ME, Esplugas E, Piessens J, et al.
Reference	Circulation 2000;101:131-136.
Disease	Coronary artery disease.
Purpose	To determine the influence of both nonionic and ionic contrast media on major adverse cardiac events (MACE) in coronary artery disease patients undergoing PTCA.
Design	Randomized, parallel group, double-blind, multicenter.
Patients	1141 patients undergoing PTCA. They had to have stable or unstable angina or silent ischemia. Recent MIs not included.
Follow-up	2 day, 1 month.
Regimen	697 received iodixanol (nonionic) and 714 received ioxaglate (ionic) contrast medium.
Add'l Tx	Heparin and aspirin, ticlopidine to patients with stents.

Results	Primary end point was a composite of MACE which included: death, stroke, myocardial infarction, coronary artery bypass grafting, and repeat PTCA at 2 days. MACE were similar in the iodixanol (4.7%) and ioxaglate group (3.9%; p=0.45). Between 2 days and 1 month follow-up there was again no difference in MACE between the 2 groups. The frequency of adverse events during the 2 day follow-up were similar in the iodixanol (27.5%) and ioxaglate group (27.6%). Hypersensitivity reactions were less common in the iodixanol (nonionic) group at 0.7% vs the ioxaglate (ionic) group at 2.5% (p<0.007). Contrast related adverse events were less common in the iodixanol group (1.0%) vs the ioxaglate group (3.5%; p<0.002). Rash, urticaria, or pruritis occurred in 5 iodixanol vs 12 ioxaglate patients. 1 patient in the ioxaglate group developed anaphylactic shock.
Concl.	While there was no overall difference in major adverse cardiac events between the use of iodixanol vs ioxaglate, hypersensitivity reactions and adverse drug reactions were less frequent with the use of the nonionic contrast agent, iodixanol.

5c

ISAR-REACT

Intracoronary Stenting and Antithrombotic Regimen-Rapid Early Action for Coronary Treatment

Title	A clinical trial of abciximab in elective percutaneous coronary intervention after pretreatment with clopidogrel.
Authors	Kastrata A, Mehilli J, Schühlen H, et al.
Reference	N Engl J Med 2004;350:232-238.
Disease	Coronary artery disease.
Purpose	To determine whether the glycoprotein IIb/IIIa inhibitor abciximab is beneficial in patients undergoing elective percutaneous coronary intervention after pretreatment with clopidogrel.
Design	Randomized, double-blind, placebo-controlled trial.
Patients	2159 patients with coronary artery disease who underwent elective percutaneous coronary intervention. Patients with acute myocardial infarction or unstable angina were not included.
Follow-up	30 days.
Regimen	Abciximab (0.25-mg/kg bolus followed by infusion of 0.125 µg/kg/min, maximum 10 µg/min for 12 hours) or placebo.
Add'l Tx	Patients received 600 mg clopidogrel at least 2 hours prior to percutaneous coronary intervention as well as 325-500 mg aspirin.
Results	The primary end point was the composite of death, MI, and urgent target-vessel revascularization within 30 days. The incidence of the primary end point was 4% in the abciximab group and 4% in the placebo group (relative risk 1.05; 95% CI=0.69-1.59; p=0.82). The rate of adverse events (mostly MIs) was 4% in both the abciximab group and in the placebo group (p=0.91). 1% of patients in the abciximab group and 1% in the placebo group had major bleeding complications. 10 patients in the abciximab group and none in the placebo group had profound thrombocytopenia (p=0.002).

Concl.   In low- to intermediate-risk patients undergoing PCI after pre-
          treatment with clopidogrel, abciximab shows no clinically mea-
          surable benefit within the first 30 days.

KAT

Kuopio Angiogenesis Trial

Title	Safety and feasibility of catheter-based local intracoronary vascular endothelial growth factor gene transfer in the prevention of postangioplasty and in-stent restenosis and in the treatment of chronic myocardial ischemia: phase II results of the Kuopio Angiogenesis Trial (KAT).
Authors	Hedman M, Hartikainen J, Syvanne M, et al.
Reference	Circulation 2003;107:2677-2683.
Disease	Coronary artery disease.
Purpose	To examine the safety and feasibility of vascular endothelial growth factor (VEGF) gene transfer in the prevention of postangioplasty and in-stent restenosis and in the treatment of myocardial ischemia.
Design	Multicenter, randomized, placebo-controlled, double-blind, phase II study.
Patients	103 patients with coronary artery disease.
Follow-up	6 months.
Regimen	Percutaneous transluminal coronary angioplasty, usually with stenting, followed by gene transfer with a perfusion-infusion catheter: VEGF adenovirus (VEGF-Adv, n=37), VEGF plasmid liposome (VEGF-P/L, n=28); or followed by Ringers lactate (control, n=38).
Results	Gene transfer to coronary arteries was well tolerated. The overall clinical restenosis rate was 6%. Coronary angiography revealed that minimal lumen diameter and percent diameter stenosis did not differ significantly between the study groups. Myocardial perfusion improved significantly in the VEGF-Adv-treated patients after 6 months. Some patients in this group showed a transient inflammatory response, but there were no increases in the incidence of serious adverse events. No increases were noted in serum VEGF levels in the treated groups, and no transgene was detected in serum or urine 2 days after gene transfer.

Concl.   Intracoronary gene transfer can be performed safely. Clinical restenosis rate and minimal lumen diameter did not differ at 6 months. Myocardial perfusion increased in the VEGF-Adv-treated patients. KAT is the first randomized, double-blind, placebo-controlled trial of local intracoronary VEGF gene transfer for treatment of CAD and prevention of restenosis after coronary angioplasty.

5c

5. Interventional Cardiology — c. Medical Therapy, Including Antiplatelet Therapy,   621
for Prevention of Complications and Restenosis with Angiography and PCI

LIPS

Lescol Intervention Prevention Study

Title	Fluvastatin for prevention of cardiac events following successful first percutaneous coronary intervention: a randomized controlled trial.
Authors	Serruys PW, de Feyter P, Macaya C, et al.
Reference	JAMA 2002;287:3215-3222.
Disease	Hyperlipidemia, coronary artery disease.
Purpose	To assess if the lipid-lowering agent fluvastatin reduces major adverse cardiac events in patients who have undergone percutaneous coronary intervention.
Design	Randomized, double-blind, placebo-controlled, multicenter.
Patients	1667 patients with stable or unstable angina or silent ischemia after percutaneous coronary intervention with baseline total cholesterol of 135-270 mg/dL and fasting triglycerides <400 mg/dL.
Follow-up	3.9 years.
Regimen	Fluvastatin 80 mg/d (n=844) vs placebo (n=833) at hospital discharge for 3-4 years. Median time between percutaneous coronary intervention and first dose of fluvastatin was 2.0 days.

Results	Primary clinical composite end point was occurrence of MACE (any death, unless noncardiac cause could be established), non-fatal MI, reintervention procedure. 181 (21.4%) in the flu-vastatin group vs 222 (26.7%) in the placebo group had at least one MACE (relative risk [RR] 0.78; 95% CI=0.64-0.95; p=0.01). Benefit was independent of baseline cholesterol levels. MACE-free survival time was longer in the fluvastatin group than placebo group (p=0.01). Kaplan-Meier curves for fluvas-tatin and placebo groups began to separate at about 1.5 years and continued to diverge throughout the course of the study. 13 (1.5%) patients in the fluvastatin group and 24 (2.9%) in the placebo group died from cardiac causes (p=0.07). Risk of MACE was lower in the subgroup of patients with multivessel disease (23% vs 33.9%; RR 0.66; 95% CI=0.48-0.91; p=0.01) in the fluvastatin vs placebo group. The risk of MACE was also reduced in diabetics (21.7% vs 37.8%; RR 0.53; 95% CI=0.29-0.97; p=0.04) in the fluvastatin vs placebo group. Fluvastatin reduced LDL cholesterol by 27% at 6 weeks vs placebo (median increase of 11%). There were no increases of creatine phosphokinase of 10 × upper limit of normal, nor were there cases of rhabdomyolysis.
Concl.	Fluvastatin given to patients undergoing first successful PCI and who had average cholesterol levels reduced MACE.

PRIMO-CABG

Pexelizumab for Reduction in Infarction and Mortality in Coronary Artery Bypass Graft Surgery

Title	Terminal complement blockade with pexelizumab during coronary artery bypass graft surgery requiring cardiopulmonary bypass. A randomized trial.
Authors	Verrier ED, Sherman SK, Taylor KM, et al.
Reference	JAMA 2004;291:2319-2327.
Disease	Coronary artery disease, coronary artery bypass graft.
Purpose	To evaluate whether pexelizumab, a C5 complement inhibitor, reduces perioperative myocardial infarction and clinical events in patients undergoing coronary artery bypass graft.
Design	Randomized, double-blind, placebo-controlled, multicenter.
Patients	3099 patients, ≥18 years old, requiring coronary artery bypass graft (with or without concurrent valve surgery). To be included, patients had to have ≥1 risk factors: 1) need for urgent revascularization (while staying in the hospital); 2) diabetes mellitus; 3) female gender; 4) prior coronary artery bypass graft; 5) history of stroke or transient ischemic attack or carotid endarterectomy; 6) history of congestive heart failure; 7) history of prior ≥2 myocardial infarctions; or 8) myocardial infarction 48 hours to 4 weeks before enrollment. Patients with myocardial infarction <48 hours before enrollment, surgery for aortic dissection, salvage intervention, cardiogenic shock, acute ventricular septal defect, acute papillary muscle rupture, uncontrolled diabetes, creatinine ≥3.0 mg/dL, liver disease, malignancy, hereditary complement deficiency, active infection, pregnancy, breastfeeding, or recent exposure to investigational agent were excluded.
Follow-up	Primary end point: events at 30 days. Follow-up for 180 days.
Regimen	Randomized to IV infusion of placebo (n=1546) or pexelizumab (2.0 mg/kg bolus followed by 0.05 mg/kg/h for 24 hours) (n=1553). The study drug was administered after induction of general anesthesia and more than 10 minutes before cardiopulmonary bypass.

Add'l Tx	All patients underwent coronary artery bypass graft with or without additional valvular surgery.
Results	1368 patients assigned placebo underwent CABG without valve surgery, 1359 patients were included in the analysis of primary end points. 1378 patients assigned pexelizumab underwent CABG without valve surgery, 1373 were included in the final analysis. Adverse events occurred at similar rates between the groups, except that pneumonia occurred more frequently in the pexelizumab group (2.4% vs 1.1%; p=0.009). On the other hand, septicemia was reduced by pexelizumab (1.9% vs 3.1%; p=0.03). 30-day mortality among patients undergoing CABG alone was 2.9% in the placebo and 2.3% in the pexelizumab group (19% risk reduction [RR]; p=0.36). MI in the first 30 days among the CABG-only patients occurred in 10.3% in the placebo group and 8.1% in the pexelizumab group (22% RR; p=0.04). The combined end point of 30-day mortality or MI in the CABG-only patients occurred in 11.8% of the patients in the placebo and in 9.8% in the pexelizumab group (18% RR; p=0.07). Among all patients (including those who underwent additional valve surgery) 30-day mortality or infarction occurred in 14.0% in the placebo group and 11.5% in the pexelizumab group (18% risk reduction; p=0.03), 30-day mortality was 3.4% and 2.5%, respectively (26% RR; p=0.15), and MI occurred in 12.0% and 9.8%, respectively (18% RR; p=0.04). At day 4, pexelizumab reduced the rate of death or MI in all patients (9.1% vs 11.9%; RR 24%; p=0.008) and in the CABG-only population (7.4% vs 10.0%; RR 26%; p=0.01). 6-month death or MI occurred less frequently in the pexelizumab group (relative RR 17%; absolute RR 2.6%; p=0.03).
Concl.	Pexelizumab reduced the risk of 30-day mortality and MI among the entire population; however, the primary end point of the study (30-day death or MI in the CABG only patients) was not significantly reduced by pexelizumab.

5c

REPLACE-1

Randomized Evaluation of PCI Linking Angiomax to Reduced Clinical Events

Title	Comparison of bivalirudin vs heparin during percutaneous coronary intervention (the Randomized Evaluation of PCI Linking Angiomax to Reduced Clinical Events [REPLACE]-1 trial).
Authors	Lincoff AM, Bittl JA, Kleiman NS, et al.
Reference	Am J Cardiol 2004;93:1092-1096.
Disease	Coronary artery disease, percutaneous coronary intervention.
Purpose	To compare the efficacy and safety of bivalirudin, a direct thrombin inhibitor, and unfractionated heparin during percutaneous coronary interventions.
Design	Pilot, randomized, open-label, multicenter.
Patients	1056 patients undergoing percutaneous coronary intervention with an approved device. Patients with an acute myocardial infarction or at high risk of bleeding were excluded. Patients who received unfractionated heparin in the preceding 6 hours and those who received low-molecular-weight heparin in the preceding 12 hours before randomization were not included. In addition, patients who received abciximab in the preceding 7 days or tirofiban or eptifibatide in the preceding 12 hours were not included.
Follow-up	Hospital discharge.
Regimen	Randomization to bivalirudin (bolus 0.75 mg/kg followed by 1.75 mg/kg/h for the duration of the procedure) or to unfractionated heparin (bolus 60-70 U/kg followed by additional doses to maintain activated clotting time 200-300).
Add'l Tx	All patients received aspirin. Clopidogrel from ≥30 days was added to those who received stents. The decision about the use of glycoprotein IIb/IIIa inhibitors was made prior to randomization.

Results	524 patients were randomized to heparin (72.5% received GP IIb/IIIa inhibitors) and 532 to bivalirudin (71.1% received GP IIb/IIIa inhibitors). The primary end point (death, MI, or repeat revascularization before hospital discharge) occurred in 6.9% of the patients in the heparin group and in 5.6% in the bivalirudin group (p=0.40). Death occurred in 0.6% and 0%, respectively, and MI in 5.2% and 4.9%, respectively. 2.3% of the patients in the heparin vs 1.5% in the bivalirudin group underwent revascularization. Major bleeding occurred in 2.7% and 2.1% of the patients, respectively (p=0.52). The combined end point of death, MI, repeat revascularization, and major bleeding occurred in 8.8% of the patients in the heparin group and in 7.1% in the bivalirudin group (relative risk reduction 19%, p=0.32). Thrombocytopenia (<100,000/μL or >25% decrease) occurred in 1.5% and 1.0% of the patients, respectively. All patients who had thrombocytopenia had received GP IIb/IIIa inhibitors. Among patients who received GP IIb/IIIa inhibitors, death, MI, or revascularization at 48 hours occurred in 7.2% of the 377 heparin-treated patients vs 6.1% of the 375 bivalirudin-treated patients. Among patients who did not receive GP IIb/IIIa inhibitors, death, MI, or revascularization at 48 hours occurred in 6.2% of the 147 heparin-treated patients vs 4.5% of the 157 bivalirudin-treated patients. Major bleeding occurred in 2.9% of the patients in each group among those who received GP IIb/IIIa inhibitors and in 2.0% and 0, respectively, among those who did not receive GP IIb/IIIa inhibitors.
Concl.	Bivalirudin was safe and was associated with a trend toward less ischemic and adverse bleeding events vs unfractionated heparin when given to patients undergoing PCI and treated with aspirin and clopidogrel, with and without GP IIb/IIIa inhibitors; however, none of the differences in outcome reached statistical significance.

5c

5. Interventional Cardiology
d. Irradiation for Preventing Restenosis After Percutaneous Coronary Intervention

3-Year Clinical and Angiographic Follow-Up After Intracoronary Radiation

Title	3 year clinical and angiographic follow-up after intracoronary radiation. Results of a randomized trial.
Authors	Teirstein PS, Massullo V, Jani S, et al.
Reference	Circulation 2000;101:360-365.
Disease	Coronary artery disease, restenosis.
Purpose	To determine angiographic and clinical outcome 3 years following treatment of restenosis with catheter based intracoronary radiation.
Design	Double-blind, randomized.
Patients	55 patients with previous restenosis following coronary angioplasty who either had a stent or were candidates for a stent.
Follow-up	3 years.
Regimen	Patients received a 0.76 mm ribbon with sealed sources of 192Ir (n=26) vs placebo (n=29) for 20-45 minutes.
Results	Target lesion revascularization was lower in the 192Ir group (15.4%) vs the placebo group (48.3%) by 3 years (p<0.01). Restenosis rates were lower in the group receiving intracoronary radiation (33%) vs placebo (64%; p<0.05). There was no difference in rates of death in the radiation group (11.5%) vs placebo group (10.3%) or rates of myocardial infarction (3.9% vs 10.3%, respectively). In patients with 3 year angiographic follow-up who did not undergo target lesion revascularization, mean minimal luminal diameter decreased between 6 months to 3 years (2.49 to 2.12 mm) in radiation treated patients, but was unchanged in the placebo patients.
Concl.	At 3 year follow-up intracoronary radiotherapy was associated with lower rates of target lesion revascularization and restenosis in patients who had undergone stenting for restenosis.

Gamma-1 Study

Title	Localized intracoronary gamma-radiation therapy to inhibit the recurrence of restenosis after stenting.
Authors	Leon MB, Teirstein PS, Moses JW, et al.
Reference	N Engl J Med 2001;344:250-256.
Disease	Coronary artery disease, post-stent restenoses.
Purpose	To determine the effect of intracoronary radiation therapy on in-stent restenosis.
Design	Randomized, double-blind, multicenter.
Patients	252 patients who developed in-stent coronary artery stenosis.
Follow-up	9 months.
Regimen	In stent lesion (>60% of luminal diameter) was treated by high pressure balloon dilation, rotational atherectomy or ablation with excimer laser, or both). After successful coronary intervention patients received indwelling intracoronary ribbon containing iridium-192 (n=131) or nonradioactive ribbon (n=121).
Add'l Tx	Aspirin, oral ticlopidine or clopidogrel, heparin, new stents in some cases.
Results	The primary end point was a composite of death, MI, and need for repeat revascularization of the target balloon; it occurred in 53 patients (43.8%) receiving placebo and 37 (28.2%) of patients receiving gamma radiation. The benefit was solely due to a decreased need for target revascularization. At 6 months, binary in-lesion restenosis was lower in radiation patients (32.4 vs 55.3%; p=0.01). Other measures of restenosis were lower in the radiation group. Late thrombosis (occurring 31-270 days after the index procedure) occurred more frequently in the radiation group (5.3%) than the placebo group (0.8%; p=0.07). This resulted in a trend toward more late MIs in patients receiving radiation (9.9% vs 4.1%; p=0.09). Late thrombosis did not

occur in patients receiving ticlopidine or clopidogrel, or within 1 month of stopping these drugs. It occurred only in patients that had received new stents at the time of radiation therapy.

| Concl. | Iridium-192 intracoronary therapy decreased clinical and angiographic restenosis but was associated with higher rates of late thrombosis and MI. |

Title	Effect of intracoronary γ-radiation therapy on in-stent restenosis. An intravascular ultrasound analysis from the Gamma-1 study.
Authors	Mintz GS, Weissman NJ, Teirstein PS, et al.
Reference	Circulation 2000;102:2915-2918.
Disease	Coronary artery disease.
Purpose	To evaluate the effect of γ-radiation on recurrent in-stent restenosis using serial volumetric intravascular ultrasound.
Design	Randomized, double-blind, multicenter, placebo-controlled trial.
Patients	70 patients with in-stent restenosis received primary catheter-based intervention followed by randomization to either Ir-192 vs placebo. 4 centers part of intravascular ultrasound analysis study. This study focuses on IVUS results.
Follow-up	8 months.
Regimen	Ir-192 vs placebo of the coronary artery. Sources inserted into noncentered, blind lumen catheter. Initial in-stent restenosis treated at operator's discretion with percutaneous transluminal coronary angioplasty, atheroblation, and/or additional stent implantation (>80% of lesions were restented). Dwell time of radioactive ribbon calculated to deliver 800 cGy to target farthest from radiation source, provided no more than 3000 cGy delivered to target closest to source. IVUS performed acutely and at 8 months.
Results	Decrease in stented segment lumen volume was -25±34 mm^3 in Ir-192 patients vs -48±42 mm^3 in placebo patients (p=0.0225). Increase in volume of intimal hyperplasia was 28±37 mm^3 in stented segment in Ir-192 patients vs 50±40 mm^3 in placebo patients (p=0.0352). Increase in mean area of intimal hyperplasia averaged over the length of the stented segment was 0.8±1.0 mm^2 in the Ir-192 group vs 1.6±1.2 mm^2 in placebo group (p=0.0065).

Concl.   γ-radiation prevented recurrent in-stent restenosis by inhibiting neointimal formation within the stent. There were no significant differences at the stent edge between groups.

Title	Endoluminal β-radiation therapy for the prevention of coronary restenosis after balloon angioplasty.
Authors	Verin V, Popowski Y, DeBruyne B, et al.
Reference	N Engl J Med 2001;344:243-249.
Disease	Coronary artery disease.
Purpose	To determine the lowest dose of β-radiation that can prevent restenosis following coronary angioplasty.
Design	Prospective, randomized, multicenter, dose-finding trial.
Patients	181 patients undergoing successful balloon angioplasty of previously untreated coronary stenosis.
Follow-up	6 month angiographic follow-up.
Regimen	Patients were randomized to receive 9 Gy, 12 Gy, 15 Gy, or 18 Gy of radiation following coronary angioplasty. Mean duration of radiation therapy varied from 1.8-3.2 minutes.
Add'l Tx	Beta irradiation was not performed if there was an urgent need for stent implantation or if glycoprotein IIb/IIIa receptor blockers had been given.

Results   Primary end point was minimal luminal diameter at 6 months
           assessed by quantitative coronary angiography. Secondary end
           points were incidence of serious cardiac events: death, MI,
           PTCA, in target vessel-additional intervention, CABG. 45
           patients received 9 Gy, 45-12 Gy, 46-15 Gy, and 45-18 Gy.
           PTCA was performed in 130 patients; stenting was required fol-
           lowing brachy therapy in 51 patients (either because of residual
           stenosis or dissection). There were no differences in the mean
           degree of stenoses between groups prior to angioplasty or mean
           degree of residual stenosis after the procedure. At 6 months a
           significant dose-dependent benefit of β radiation on minimal
           lumen diameter was present (p=0.006). Mean minimal luminal
           diameter was 1.67 mm, 1.76 mm, 1.83 mm, and 1.97 mm
           in the 9, 12, 15 and 18-Gy groups, respectively (p=0.06 for
           comparison of 9 Gy vs 18 Gy). Restenosis rates were 29%,
           21%, 16%, and 15% respectively. In the 130 patients that had
           angioplasty but did not require a stent, restenosis rates were
           28%, 17%, 16%, and 4%, respectively (p=0.02 for 9 Gy vs
           18 Gy) and there was a significant dose-dependent enlargement
           of the coronary lumen at 28%, 50%, 45% and 74% of patients
           (p<0.001 for 9 Gy vs 18 Gy). The incidence of serious cardiac
           events did not differ among dose groups.

Concl.   Intracoronary β-radiation produced a dose dependent decrease
           in rate of restenosis following PTCA. An 18 Gy dose induced
           luminal enlargement.

Title	Endovascular brachytherapy for prophylaxis of restenosis after femoropopliteal angioplasty. Results of a prospective randomized study.
Authors	Minar E, Pokrajac B, Maca T, et al.
Reference	Circulation 2000;102:2694-2699.
Disease	Peripheral vascular disease; atherosclerosis.
Purpose	To determine the effect of endovascular brachytherapy on restenosis after percutaneous transluminal angioplasty of the femoropopliteal region.
Design	Randomized.
Patients	113 patients with claudication or critical limb ischemia with rest pain, de novo lesion in the femoropopliteal region, a technical successful angioplasty procedure with residual stenosis of <30% and no further stent implantation.
Follow-up	12 months.
Regimen	Randomized to brachytherapy (n=57) or no brachytherapy (n=56). Dose of 12 Gy applied by an Ir-92 source.
Add'l Tx	Aspirin before procedure and long-term heparin during the procedure.
Results	Primary end point was patency at 6 months. Restenosis defined as angiographically verified stenosis of >50% narrowing of the luminal diameter. Overall recurrence rate at 6 months was 28.3% in the angioplasty plus brachytherapy group vs 53.7% of the angioplasty alone group (p<0.05). Cumulative patency rate at 12 months was 63.6% in the angioplasty plus brachytherapy group vs 35.3% in the angioplasty alone group (p<0.005). Ankle-brachial index at follow-up was 0.77 in the angioplasty and 0.88 in the angioplasty plus brachytherapy group, and after 3 months was 0.74 and 0.84.
Concl.	Endovascular brachytherapy was effective for prophylaxis of restenosis following femoropopliteal angioplasty.

Intravascular Gamma Radiation for In-Stent Restenosis in Saphenous Vein Bypass Grafts

Title	Intravascular gamma radiation for in-stent restenosis in saphenous vein bypass grafts.
Authors	Waksman R, Ajani AE, White RL, et al.
Reference	N Engl J Med 2002;346:1194-1199.
Disease	Coronary artery disease.
Purpose	To determine the effects of intravascular gamma radiation on in-stent restenosis of saphenous vein bypass grafts.
Design	Randomized, double-blind trial, multicenter.
Patients	120 patients with in-stent restenosis of saphenous vein grafts. Majority of patients had in-stent restenosis.
Follow-up	12 months.
Regimen	Patients had percutaneous transluminal coronary angioplasty (PTCA), atherectomy, additional stenting or a combination. If the intervention was successful, patients randomized to intravascular treatment with a ribbon containing iridium-192 vs nonradioactive seeds.
Add'l Tx	Aspirin, ticlopidine, or clopidogrel for 1 month.

Results	Primary end points were cardiac death, Q wave MI, repeat revascularization of the target vessel, and a composite of these end points at 12 months. Initial revascularization and radiation therapy were successful. Minimal luminal diameter at 6 months was 1.92±0.77 mm in the iridium-192 group vs 1.32±0.87 mm in the placebo group (p<0.001). Restenosis rate was 21% in the iridium-192 group vs 44% in the control group. There was an 80% reduction in late loss in the radiation group (0.23±0.75 mm) vs the placebo group (1.14±0.85 mm; p<0.001). There was no "edge-effect" type of restenosis in the radiation group, nor were aneurysms present in the iridium group. In a subgroup analysis, intravascular ultrasound revealed less intimal hyperplasia in the radiation group. Rate of major cardiac events was 32% in the radiation group vs 63% in the placebo group, at 12 months (p<0.001). 17% in the radiation group vs 57% in the placebo group required additional target revascularization.
Concl.	Gamma radiation therapy for in-stent restenosis of saphenous bypass grafts was effective in reducing cardiac events and preventing future restenosis.

PREVENT (Radiotherapy)

Proliferation Reduction with Vascular Energy Trial

Title	Inhibition of restenosis with β-emitting radiotherapy: report of the PREVENT.
Authors	Raizner AE, Oesterle SN, Waksman R, et al.
Reference	Circulation 2000;102:951-958.
Disease	Coronary artery disease.
Purpose	To demonstrate safety and performance of intracoronary radiation therapy using an automated source-delivery unit and a source centering mechanism in a broad spectrum of patients undergoing percutaneous coronary interventions.
Design	Prospective, randomized, sham-control, multicenter.
Patients	105 coronary artery disease patients with denovo (70%) or restenotic (30%) lesions being treated by stenting (61%) or balloon angioplasty (39%).
Follow-up	6 month angiography; 12 month clinical events.
Regimen	Patients randomized to 1 of 4 radiation treatments: 0, 16, 20, 24 Gy to 1 mm beyond the lumen surface.

Results	Primary clinical end point was in-hospital and 12 month major adverse clinical events (MACE); defined as composite of death, MI, target lesion revascularization for restenosis. There were additional angiographic end points. At 6 months target site late loss index was $11\pm36\%$ in radiotherapy patients vs $55\pm30\%$ in controls ($p<0.001$). Restenosis at the target site ($\geq50\%$) was 8% in radiotherapy patients vs 39% in control patients ($p=0.012$). Restenosis at the target plus adjacent segments was also less in the radiotherapy group (22% vs 50%; $p=0.018$). At 12 months, target lesion revascularization occurred in 6% of radiotherapy patients vs 24% of controls ($p<0.05$). 12-month MACE (death, MI, target lesion revascularization) occurred in 16% of radiotherapy patients and 24% of control patients ($p=NS$). Myocardial infarction occurred in 10% of radiotherapy and 4% of control patients. Death occurred in 1 radiotherapy patient and none of the controls. 7 MIs had occurred late (5-188 days) after the procedure in the radiotherapy group and were considered acute occlusive events. In some cases restenosis involving adjacent segments was observed.
Concl.	β-radiotherapy was safe and effective in inhibiting restenosis at the target site and decreasing the need for target revascularization. Late thrombotic events and edge narrowing were a problem in some patients.

WRIST

Washington Radiation for In-Stent Restenosis Trial

Title	Intracoronary γ-radiation therapy after angioplasty inhibits recurrence in patients with in-stent restenosis.
Authors	Waksman R, White L, Chan RC, et al.
Reference	Circulation 2000;101:2165-2171.
Disease	Coronary artery disease.
Purpose	To determine the effects of intracoronary γ-radiation on clinical and angiographic outcomes in patients with in-stent restenosis.
Design	Prospective, randomized, double- blind trial.
Patients	130 symptomatic patients with in-stent restenosis (≥50% diameter stenosis in the stent site) who underwent successful (<30% residual stenosis with no complications) with balloons, ablative devices, additional stents, or combinations of these techniques.
Follow-up	6 months, 12 months.
Regimen	Patients randomized to receive a nylon ribbon containing either placebo or seed trains of 192Ir at the lesion site.
Add'l Tx	Routine postangioplasty care; ticlopidine for 1 month.

Results	Primary clinical end point was cumulative composite of death, MI, repeat target lesion revascularization at 6 months. At 6 months angiographic end points were restenosis (diameter stenosis ≥50%), magnitude of late loss, and late loss index. Restenosis (binary angiographic) was 19% in the irradiated group vs 58% in the placebo group (p=0.001). The main angiographic pattern of restenosis in the radiation group occurred at the edges of the stent. Late luminal loss was lower in the radiated vs placebo patients. Late loss index was 0.16±0.73 mm in the radiated patients vs 0.70±0.46 in placebo patients (p=0.0001). At 6 months 29.2% of radiated patients had a major cardiac event (death, Q-wave MI, and target vessel revascularization) vs 67.6% in the placebo group (p<0.001). There was no difference in death at 6 months between radiated (4.6%) or nonradiated groups (6.2%) and no patients had Q-wave infarcts. Hence the major clinical difference was a reduction in target vessel revascularization in the radiation group (26.1%) vs the placebo group (67.6%; p<0.001). Target lesion revascularization also was lower in the radiation group (13.8%) vs the placebo group (63.1%) and the same pattern was observed at 12 months.
Concl.	Gamma radiation as adjunct therapy for patients with in-stent restenosis reduced angiographic evidence of restensois and reduced the need for target lesion and target vessel revascularization.

ECRIS

Endocoronary-Rhenium-Irradiation Study

Title	Intracoronary β-irradiation with a rhenium-188-filled balloon catheter: a randomized trial in patients with de novo and restenotic lesions.
Authors	Hoher M, Wohrle J, Wohlfrom M, et al.
Reference	Circulation 2003;107:3022-3027.
Disease	Coronary artery disease.
Purpose	To evaluate the efficacy of β-irradiation with a liquid rhenium-188-filled balloon in patients with de novo or restenotic lesions.
Design	Randomized, controlled trial.
Patients	225 patients (71% with de novo lesions) who had undergone successful percutaneous transluminal coronary intervention with or without stenting.
Follow-up	12 months.
Regimen	After percutaneous transluminal coronary intervention, 22.5 Gy intravascular β-irradiation in 0.5-mm tissue depth (n=113) or no additional intervention (n=112, control group).
Results	The groups were similar in terms of clinical and procedural data except that more patients in the control group underwent stenting (63% vs 45% in the irradiation group; p<0.02). At 6 months of follow-up, the rate of late loss was significantly lower in the irradiation group than in the control group, both of the target lesion (0.11±0.54 vs 0.69±0.81 mm; p<0.0001) and of the total segment (0.22±0.67 vs 0.70±0.82; p<0.0001). This was also evident in patients with de novo lesions and independent of stenting. Brachytherapy yielded lower rates of binary restenosis of the target lesion, 6.3% vs 27.5% (p<0.0001), and of the total segment, 12.6% vs 28.6% (p<0.007). The target-vessel revascularization rate was significantly lower with brachytherapy, 6.3% vs 19.8% (p=0.006).

Concl.   Intracoronary β-brachytherapy with a rhenium-188 liquid-filled balloon is safe and reduces restenosis and revascularization rates after coronary angioplasty. Whether this therapy will be as successful in patients with diabetes, small vessels, or bypass grafts is not yet clear.

5. Interventional Cardiology
e. Covered Stents and Drug-Eluting Stents

TENISS

The Tenax vs NIR Stent Study

Title	Comparison of a silicon carbide-coated stent vs a noncoated stent in human beings: the Tenax vs NIR stent study's long-term outcome.
Authors	Unverdorben M, Sippel B, Degenhardt R, et al.
Reference	Am Heart J 2003;145:e17.
Disease	Coronary artery disease, stent.
Purpose	To compare the long-term outcome after silicon carbide-coated (Tenax) stent and noncoated (NIR) stent.
Design	Randomized, open-label, 2 centers.
Patients	497 patients (mean age 63.4±9.8 years), scheduled for percutaneous coronary intervention for a single lesion in a vessel (either native artery or a bypass graft) with a reference diameter ≥2.8 mm, length <20 mm, and diameter stenosis ≥70% and ≤100%. Patients with contraindications to aspirin and ticlopidine, unprotected left main lesion, lesion within 2 mm of the left main artery, lesion covering a major side branch, recent myocardial infarction, multiple-lesion percutaneous coronary intervention, left ventricular ejection fraction <20%, TIA in the last year, and life expectancy <1 year were excluded.
Follow-up	81±12 weeks.
Regimen	Patients were randomized to the Tenax or NIR stent. The choice of stent diameter and length was done by the operator.
Add'l Tx	All patients received IV heparin and nitroglycerin. All patients received aspirin 100 mg/d and if not tolerated, ticlopidine 250 mg bid, started before the procedure and continued throughout the follow-up period. All patients received ticlopidine 250 mg bid for 4 weeks after PCI. Patients with visible thrombus received glycoprotein IIb/IIIa inhibitors.

Results   3 patients were excluded before PCI. Stent deployment fail-
           ure occurred in 6 patients (2.4%) in the Tenax group and in
           8 patients (3.3%) in the NIR group (p=0.6). 1 patient in the
           Tenax group and 7 in the NIR group needed ≥1 additional stent
           to cover the lesion (p=0.07). 450 patients were available for fol-
           low-up (233/250 [93.2%] in the Tenax group and 217/244
           [88.9%] in the NIR group). Major adverse cardiac events
           occurred in 12% of patients in the Tenax group and in 14.3%
           in the NIR group (p=0.50). Acute MI occurred more often in
           the NIR group (11 vs 3 patients; p<0.04 after 60 weeks). Target
           lesion revascularization was performed in 6.9% of patients
           in the Tenax group and in 5.1% in the NIR group (p=0.55).
           Mortality was 3% and 3.7%, respectively (p=0.88). Survival free
           from death, MI, repeat angina, and target lesion revasculariza-
           tion was comparable (72.1% vs 71.9%, respectively; p=0.95).
           365 patients underwent repeat coronary angiography. There was
           no difference in the percent diameter stenosis or restenosis rate
           between the groups.

Concl.   The Tenax and the NIR stents were equally effective with no
           differences in outcome between them.

Title	Short- and long-term clinical benefit of sirolimus-eluting stents compared to conventional bare stents for patients with acute myocardial infarction.
Authors	Lemos PA, Saia F, Hofma SH, et al.
Reference	J Am Coll Cardiol 2004;43:704-708.
Disease	Acute myocardial infarction.
Purpose	To investigate the clinical outcomes of patients with ST-segment elevation myocardial infarction treated with sirolimus-eluting stents or with conventional bare stents.
Design	Long-term evaluation; nonrandomized comparison to historic control group.
Patients	369 unselected patients with ST-segment elevation acute myocardial infarction.
Follow-up	300 days.
Regimen	Primary angioplasty performed with a sirolimus-eluting stents (n=186) or with a bare stent (n=183).
Results	Postprocedural vessel patency, enzymatic release, and incidence of short-term adverse events were similar with the sirolimus-eluting stents (SES) and bare stents (30-day rate of death, reinfarction, or repeat revascularization was 7.5% vs 10.4%, respectively). No patient with a SES had stent thrombosis vs 1.6% in patients with a bare stent, an NS difference. At 300 days, patients with SESs had a lower incidence of combined adverse events (9.4% vs 17%) (hazard ratio [HR] 0.52; 95% CI=0.30-0.92; p=0.02), mainly because of a lower risk of repeat intervention (1.1% vs 8.2%; HR 0.21; 95% CI=0.06-0.74; p=0.01).
Concl.	The rate of stent thrombosis was similar with the SES and bare stents at 30 days; the incidence of adverse events and repeat intervention at 300 days was significantly lower in patients receiving the SES stent. These favorable results require further confirmation in a randomized controlled trial.

Carbostent-Trial

Carbofilm-Coated Stent vs a Pure High-Grade Stainless Steel Stent

Title	Comparison of early and late results of a Carbofilm-coated stent vs a pure high-grade stainless steel stent (the Carbostent-Trial).
Authors	Sick PB, Gelbrich G, Kalnins U, et al.
Reference	Am J Cardiol 2004;93:1351-1356.
Disease	Coronary artery disease, percutaneous coronary intervention.
Purpose	To evaluate whether Carbofilm-coated stents reduce neointimal proliferation and restenosis.
Design	Randomized, open-label, multicenter.
Patients	420 patients, 18-80 years old, with stable or unstable angina.
Follow-up	Follow-up angiography at 6 months.
Regimen	Randomization to a stainless steel stent (Medtronic Vascular, Minneapolis, MN) (n=210) or to Carbofilm-coated Sirius stent (Sorin Biomedica Cardio, Via Crescentino, Italy) (n=210).
Add'l Tx	All patients received heparin 10,000 IU and aspirin 500 mg before angioplasty. All patients received ticlopidine or clopidogrel and aspirin 100-300 mg for 1 month.

Results	A total of 461 stents were implanted. Dissections were noted in 12.9% of the Carbofilm-coated stents and in 6.7% of the control stents (p=0.048). The angiographic success rate was 98.8%. 365 lesions (86.9%) were available for follow-up angiography analysis. Postprocedure diameter stenosis was 11.6±4.0 mm in the Carbofilm stent group and 11.4±4.4 mm in the control stent group (p=0.63). Postprocedure minimal lumen diameter was 2.87±0.37 mm and 2.87±0.34 mm, respectively (p=0.85). Follow-up minimal lumen diameter was 1.86±0.78 mm in the Carbofilm stent group and 1.95±0.70 mm in the control stent group (p=0.68). Follow-up diameter stenosis was 40.7%±22.9% and 38.0%±20.1%, respectively. Late luminal loss was comparable between the groups (1.00±0.72 mm and 0.93±0.62 mm, respectively; p=0.94). ≥50% diameter stenosis was found in 23.5% of the patients in the Carbofilm stent group and in only 15.9% of the patients in the control stent group (p=0.07). Death occurred in 0.5% and 0% of the patients, respectively (p=1.00), stent thrombosis in 2.0% vs 1.0% (p=0.68), MI in 3.9% vs 1.5% (p=0.22), and target vessel revascularization was needed in 17.6% vs 12.7% of the patients, respectively (p=0.21). MACE occurred in 20.1% of the patients in the Carbofilm stent and in 13.7% in the control stent group (p=0.11).
Concl.	Carbofilm-coated stents failed to reduce angiographic restenosis or decrease major adverse cardiac event rates vs bare stainless steel stents.

C-SIRIUS

The Canadian Study of the Sirolimus-Eluting Stent in the Treatment of Patients with Long De Novo Lesions in Small Native Coronary Arteries

Title	The Canadian study of the sirolimus-eluting stent in the treatment of patients with long de novo lesions in small native coronary arteries (C-SIRIUS).
Authors	Schampaert E, Cohen EA, Schlüter M, et al.
Reference	J Am Coll Cardiol 2004;43:1110-1115.
Disease	Coronary artery disease.
Purpose	To assess the safety and effectiveness of the sirolimus-eluting stent in treating single de novo long lesions in small native coronary arteries compared to an identical bare-metal stent.
Design	Multicenter, randomized, double-blind trial.
Patients	100 patients with documented angina pectoris or silent ischemia who had a single de novo lesion, 15-32 mm long and 50%-99% diameter stenosis in a native vessel.
Follow-up	8 months.
Regimen	Placement of a sirolimus-eluting stent (n=50) or identical bare-metal stent (n=50).
Results	The in-stent minimal lumen diameter at 8 months (primary end point) was 2.46 ± 0.37 mm in the sirolimus-eluting stent vs 1.49 ± 0.75 mm in the bare-metal stent, a 65% difference ($p<0.001$). Angiographic restenosis occurred in 1 of 44 patients with a sirolimus-eluting stent (SES) (2.3%) and in 23 of 44 patients with a bare-metal stent (52.3%) ($p<0.001$). At 270 days, there were 2 clinically driven target-lesion revascularizations in the SES group (4%) and 9 in the bare metal stent group (18%) ($p=0.05$). The Kaplan-Meier estimate of freedom from major adverse cardiac events at 270 days was 96% for SES patients and 81.7% for patients with a bare-metal stent ($p=0.029$).

Concl. Patients with long lesions in small vessels are at high risk for restenosis. The SES dramatically reduces the risk of restenosis at 8 months, yielding a very favorable clinical outcome at 9 months.

E-SIRIUS

Sirolimus-Eluting Stents for Long Lesions in Small Coronary Arteries

Title	Sirolimus-eluting stents for treatment of patients with long atherosclerotic lesions in small coronary arteries: double-blind, randomised controlled trial (E-SIRIUS).
Authors	Schofer J, Schluter M, Gershlick AH, et al.
Reference	Lancet 2003;362:1093-1099.
Disease	Coronary artery disease.
Purpose	To determine the risk of restenosis with use of sirolimus-eluting stents compared with bare-metal stents.
Design	International, multicenter, randomized trial.
Patients	352 patients with 1-vessel coronary artery disease (lesion diameter 2.5-3 mm and 15-32 mm long).
Follow-up	9 months.
Regimen	Patients randomly assigned to receive sirolimus-eluting (n=175) or bare-metal (n=177) stents.
Results	Implantation was successful in all patients receiving sirolimus-eluting stents and in 99.4% receiving bare-metal stents. Mean (±SE) diameter of treated coronary arteries was 2.55±0.37 mm and mean lesion length was 15±6 mm. Nearly half of patients required multiple stents. At 8 months, minimum lumen diameter was higher with sirolimus-eluting stents than with bare-metal stents (2.22 vs 1.33 mm, p<0.0001). The rate of binary restenosis was significantly reduced with sirolimus-eluting stents (5.9% vs 42.3% with bare-metal stents, p=0.0001). The rate of major adverse cardiac events (death, MI, CABG, target-lesion revascularization) was significantly lower at 9 months in patients receiving the sirolimus-eluting stents (8% vs 22.6%, p=0.0002); this was mainly due to a lesser need for target-lesion revascularization (4% vs 20.9%, p<0.0001).

Concl.   Sirolimus-eluting stents yielded an improved rate of event-free survival compared with bare-metal stents. The sirolimus-eluting stents were efficacious along the entire length of the lesions in these patients, who had high-risk clinical profiles for restenosis. More studies are needed to assess this drug-eluting stent's effectiveness over several years and in other high-risk subsets.

SIRIUS

Sirolimus-Eluting Balloon Expandable Stent in the Treatment of Patients with De Novo Native Coronary Artery Lesions

Title	Sirolimus-eluting stents vs standard stents in patients with stenosis in a native coronary artery.
Authors	Moses JW, Leon MB, Popma JJ, et al.
Reference	N Engl J Med 2003;349:1315-1323.
Disease	Coronary artery disease, angina pectoris.
Purpose	To determine the clinical usefulness of a sirolimus-eluting stent in patients with newly diagnosed lesions in a native coronary artery in which the coronary artery disease was deemed as complex because of diabetes (26% of patients), longer lesions (mean 14.4 mm), and smaller vessels (mean 2.80 mm).
Design	Randomized, double-blind, multicenter.
Patients	Patients with stable or unstable angina with signs of myocardial ischemia (n=1058). Patients had to have a single newly diagnosed target lesion in a native coronary artery with a stenosis of 51%-99%, measuring 15-30 mm in length assessed by angiography. Recent myocardial infarction (within 48 hours), an ejection fraction <25%, and other exclusions existed.
Follow-up	270 days.
Regimen	Patients were randomized to a sirolimus-eluting stent vs a standard stent.

Add'l Tx	Oral aspirin daily, oral clopidogrel for 3 months, IV heparin during the procedure. Use of IV glycoprotein IIb/IIIa inhibitors were at the physician's discretion.
Results	Primary end point was failure of the target vessel (composite of cardiac death, MI, repeated PCI, or CABG of the target vessel) within 270 days. The primary end point occurred in 21.0% of patients receiving the standard stent vs 8.6% receiving the sirolimuseluting stent (p<0.001). This improvement with the sirolimus stents was driven primarily by a decrease in need for revascularization of the target lesion (16.6% with standard stenting vs 4.1% with sirolimus stenting; p<0.001) and was observed in all subgroups. Follow-up angiographic data available in 85%86% of patients revealed minimal luminal diameter (mm) of the in-stent zone at 240 days of 1.69±0.79 mm in the standard stent group vs 2.50±0.58 in the sirolimus stent group (p<0.001). Percent stenosis of the in-stent zone at 240 days was 40.1%±25.3% in the standard stent group vs 10.4%±16.5% in the sirolimus stent group (p<0.001). The restenosis rate, defined as stenosis of 50% of the luminal diameter on the 240 day follow-up angiogram, was 35.4% in the standard stent group vs 3.2% (p<0.001) in the sirolimusstent group. Intravascular ultrasound study showed significant decrease in neointimal volumes within the in-stent zone in the sirolimus group (4.4 mm^3) vs the standard stent group (57.6 mm^3; p<0.001). There were no acute stent thromboses within 24 hours after the procedure. There was 1 case of subacute stent thrombosis (1-30 days after placement) in each group.
Concl.	Sirolimus-eluting stents decreased the rate of restenosis and adverse clinical events in patients with complex CAD vs patients receiving standard stents.

SIRIUS

Sirolimus-Eluting Balloon Expandable Stent in the Treatment of Patients with De Novo Native Coronary Artery Lesions

Title	Analysis of 1-year clinical outcomes in the SIRIUS trial: a randomized trial of a sirolimus-eluting stent vs a standard stent in patients at high risk for coronary restenosis.
Authors	Holmes DR, Leon MB, Moses JW, et al.
Reference	Circulation 2004;109:634-640.
Disease	Coronary artery disease.
Purpose	To evaluate whether the initial clinical improvement seen with sirolimus-eluting stents in previous smaller series is maintained out to 12 months and to study the potential treatment effect in patient subsets known to be at increased risk of restenosis.
Design	Retrospective evaluation of a double-blind, randomized trial.
Patients	1058 patients with de novo native coronary stenosis undergoing clinically indicated percutaneous coronary intervention.
Follow-up	1 year.
Regimen	Percutaneous coronary intervention with a sirolimus-eluting stent (n=533) or a control bare-metal stent (n=525).
Results	The procedural success rate was 97.4% with the sirolimus-eluting stent and 98.5% with the bare-metal stent. At 9 months, the rate of clinical restenosis (target-lesion revascularization) was 4.1% with the sirolimus-eluting stent vs 16.6% with the bare-metal stent (p<0.001). At 12 months, the rate of target-lesion revascularization continued to increase to 4.9% vs 20%. Rates of death and MI were similar in the 2 groups. In high-risk patient subsets, defined by vessel size, lesion length, and presence of diabetes, there was a 70%-80% reduction in clinical restenosis at 1 year with the sirolimus-eluting stent. 6 factors were found to be associated with target lesion revascularization: treatment group, total stent length, postprocedure in-stent minimum lumen diameter, history of diabetes, prior CABG surgery, and Canadian Cardiovascular Society class III or IV.

Concl.   The major finding of this analysis is that at 12 months, target lesion revascularization is dramatically reduced with the sirolimus-eluting stent. The reduction in clinical restenosis between the 2 stent groups was concordant among all patient and lesion subsets.

DELIVER

Angiographic Follow-Up of the DELIVER Trial

Title	Non-polymer-based paclitaxel-coated coronary stents for the treatment of patients with de novo coronary lesions. Angiographic follow-up of the DELIVER clinical trial.
Authors	Lansky AJ, Costa RA, Mintz GS, et al.
Reference	Circulation 2004;109:1948-1954.
Disease	Coronary artery disease.
Purpose	To report the angiographic outcomes of the non-polymer-based, paclitaxel-coated ACHIEVE stent (Cook Incorporated, Bloomington, IN) evaluated in the DELIVER clinical trial.
Design	Prospective, randomized, blinded, multicenter clinical evaluation.
Patients	1043 patients with focal de novo coronary lesions <25 mm long in 2.5- to 4-mm vessels.
Follow-up	9 months for primary clinical end point; 8 months for major secondary end point.
Regimen	Randomly assigned to receive the non-polymer-based paclitaxel-coated ACHIEVE stent (n=524) or the stainless steel Multi-Link PENTA stent (Guidant Corporation, Indianapolis, IN) (n=519).

Results	The prespecified primary end point was a 40% reduction in target-vessel failure at 9 months; the major secondary end point was a 50% reduction in binary restenosis at 8 months. Baseline clinical characteristics were similar in the 2 groups, although patients in the ACHIEVE group had more type C lesions. The procedural success rate was 99% for ACHIEVE and 99.8% for the Multi-Link (ML) PENTA stent. Stent late loss was 0.81 vs 0.98 mm (p=0.003), stent binary restenosis was 14.9% vs 20.6% (p=0.076), and target-vessel failure was 11.9% vs 14.5% (p=0.12) for the ACHIEVE and ML PENTA stents, respectively. In the multivariate model, independent predictors of binary restenosis included use of a 2.5-mm stent, diabetes that required treatment, glycoprotein IIb/IIIa inhibitor use, and prior MI. Among patients who received IIb/IIIa inhibitors, restenosis was 17.5% for the ACHIEVE stent and 23.9% for the ML PENTA stent (p=0.02); among patients who did not receive IIb/IIIa inhibitors, restenosis was 8.8% for ACHIEVE and 14.5% for ML PENTA (p=0.4).
Concl.	The ACHIEVE paclitaxel-coated stent system decreased neointimal proliferation vs the bare-metal stent; however, the reduction was insufficient to meet the end point of target-vessel failure and the secondary end point of binary restenosis.

DRASTIC

The Diamond Randomization Against Stainless Steel in Coronaries

Title	Comparison of diamond-like carbon-coated stents vs uncoated stainless steel stents in coronary artery disease.
Authors	Airoldi F, Colombo A, Tavano D, et al.
Reference	Am J Cardiol 2004;93:474-477.
Disease	Coronary artery disease, percutaneous coronary intervention.
Purpose	To compare angiographic and clinical outcomes of bare stainless steel stents and carbon-coated stents.
Design	Randomized, double-blind, multicenter.
Patients	347 patients with de novo or restenotic >50% diameter stenosis in native coronary arteries in vessels ≥2.5 mm in diameter. Patients with contraindications to aspirin or thienopyridines and those with an acute myocardial infarction in the preceding 72 hours were not included. Patients with in-stent restenosis, use of rotational or directional atherectomy, and unprotected left main lesions were excluded.
Follow-up	Repeat angiography at 6 months. 6-month clinical follow-up.
Regimen	Randomization to carbon-coated (CC) (n=172) or stainless-steel (SS) (n=175) stents. All stents were the Diamond Flex AS (Phytis Medical Devices, GmbH, Berlin, Germany).
Add'l Tx	All patients received ticlopidine 250 mg bid or clopidogrel 75 mg/d for 4 weeks and aspirin 100 mg/d indefinitely. The use of glycoprotein IIb/IIIa inhibitor was permitted.

Results	Procedural success was 95.9% with CC and 96.2% with SS stents (p=0.866). Q-wave MI during hospitalization occurred in 1 patient in the CC group and in 2 in the SS group (p=0.93). Non-Q-wave infarction occurred in 2.3% and 3.4% of the patients, respectively (p=0.523). None of the patients died during the index admission. 6-month rates of major adverse cardiac events were 30.5% in the CC and 32.7% in the SS group (p=0.675). Mortality was 1.8% and 2.2% (p=0.926). There was no difference in the rate of MI (3.4% vs 5.6%; p=0.392) or the need for target vessel revascularization (25.9% vs 26.1%; p=0.586) between the CC and SS groups. Immediately postprocedure, minimal lumen diameter was comparable between the CC (2.75±0.49 mm) and the SS (2.70±0.51 mm) groups (p=0.411), and residual diameter stenosis was 11%±10% and 12%±11%, respectively (p=0.100). After 6 months, minimal lumen diameter did not differ between the CC (1.72±0.85 mm) and the SS (1.62±0.81 mm) group (p=0.733). There was no difference in the average diameter stenosis (38%±25% vs 41%±26%; p=0.440) or late loss (1.02±0.78 mm vs 1.00±0.78 mm; p=0.837) between the CC and SS groups. ≥50% restenosis occurred in 31.8% of the patients in the CC group and in 35.9% in the SS group (p=0.448).
Concl.	Carbon-coated stents did not reduce angiographic restenosis or clinical end points compared to bare SS stents.

ELUTES

The European Evaluation of Paclitaxel-Eluting Stent

Title	Inhibition of restenosis with a paclitaxel-eluting, polymer-free coronary stent: the European Evaluation of Paclitaxel Eluting Stent (ELUTES) trial.
Authors	Gershlick A, De Scheerder I, Chevalier B, et al.
Reference	Circulation 2004;109:487-493.
Disease	Coronary artery disease.
Purpose	To investigate the safety and efficacy of the V-Flex Plus coronary stent coated with escalating doses of paclitaxel (0.2, 0.7, 1.4, and 2.7 $\mu g/mm^2$ stent surface area) applied directly to the abluminal surface of the stent in de novo lesions compared with bare-metal stent alone.
Design	Multicenter, randomized, controlled, and triple-blinded clinical study.
Patients	190 patients with single de novo type A or B1 lesions <15 mm long in a native coronary artery who were candidates for coronary surgery, if required.
Follow-up	12 months.
Regimen	Paclitaxel-eluting, polymer-free coronary stent with surface area of 0.2 (n=37), 0.7 (n=40), 1.4 (n=39), or 2.7 $\mu g/mm^2$ (n=37) stent surface area or bare stent (control, n=39).

5e

Results	By 6-month angiographic follow-up, 1 patient had died and 14 patients refused angiographic follow-up. The primary efficacy end point was angiographic percent diameter stenosis (%DS) at 6 months. At that point, the %DS was 33.9%±26.7% in control patients (n=34) and 14.2%±16.6% in patients receiving the 2.7µg/mm^2-density stent (n=31) (p=0.006). Late loss was 0.11±0.5 mm in paclitaxel-eluting stents (2.7) vs 0.73±0.73 mm in controls (p=0.002). Binary restenosis (≥50% at 6 months) decreased from 20.6% in controls to 3.2% in the 2.7 µg/mm^2 (p=0.056); there were no significant benefit from intermediate paclitaxel doses. Freedom from major adverse cardiac events in the highest dose group was 92%, 89%, and 86% at 1, 6, and 12 months, respectively (NS vs control). No treated group had late stent thrombosis despite only 3 months of clopidogrel treatment.
Concl.	The paclitaxel-eluting stent at a dose density of 2.7 µg/mm^2 reduced angiographic in-stent restenosis without short- or medium-term adverse effects. Paclitaxel in effective doses is safe. Future studies should examine long-term safety and efficacy of coated-stent technology.

RECOVERS

Randomized Evaluation of Polytetrafluoroethylene-Covered Stent in Saphenous Vein Grafts

Title	Randomized evaluation of polytetrafluoroethylene-covered stent in saphenous vein grafts: the Randomized Evaluation of polytetrafluoroethylene COVERed stent in Saphenous vein grafts (RECOVERS) trial.
Authors	Stankovic G, Colombo A, Presbitero P, et al.
Reference	Circulation 2003;108:37-42.
Disease	Coronary artery disease.
Purpose	To compare angiographic restenosis rates and early and late clinical outcome between a polytetrafluoroethylene-covered stent and a bare stent in patients undergoing saphenous vein graft intervention.
Design	Prospective, randomized, multicenter trial.
Patients	301 patients with saphenous vein graft lesions.
Follow-up	6 months.
Regimen	Saphenous vein graft treatment with the polytetrafluoroethylene-covered JoStent or the bare stainless-steel JoFlex stent (control group).
Results	Angiographic and procedural success rates were similar with the 2 stents: 97.4% (polytetrafluoroethylene [PTFE]) vs 97.9% (stainless steel) and 87.3% vs 93.8%, respectively. The primary end point was angiographic restenosis at 6 months; 242 patients (81%) with 257 lesions (80%) underwent repeat angiography at 6-month follow-up. The rate of angiographic restenosis was similar between the 2 groups, 24.2% (PTFE) vs 24.8% (stainless steel). Secondary end points were 30-day and 6-month MACE (death, MI, target lesion revascularization). The incidence of 30-day MACE was higher in the PTFE group (10.9% vs 4.1%; p=0.047). Although the rate of non-Q-wave MI at 6 months rate was higher in the PTFE group (12.8% vs 4.1%; p=0.013), the cumulative MACE rate was not significantly different (23.1% vs 15.9%).

Concl.   Restenosis rates and 6-month clinical outcomes did not differ significantly with use of a PTFE stent or a stainless-steel stent; however, patients with the PTFE stent had a higher incidence of nonfatal MI. The aggressive approach used to deploy and postdilate the PTFE stents may have contributed to the higher incidence of MI. The late occurrence of non-Q-wave MI in PTFE group (4 patients had angiographically documented total occlusions) is disturbing. Delayed re-endothelialization of the PTFE-covered stents predisposing to thrombotic occlusion can help to explain this finding.

RESEARCH

Rapamycin-Eluting Stent Evaluated at Rotterdam Cardiology Hospital Registry

Title	Early outcome after sirolimus-eluting stent implantation in patients with acute coronary syndromes: insights from the Rapamycin-Eluting Stent Evaluated At Rotterdam Cardiology Hospital (RESEARCH) registry.
Authors	Lemos PA, Lee CH, Degertekin M, et al.
Reference	J Am Coll Cardiol 2003;41:2093-2099.
Disease	Acute myocardial infarction, unstable angina.
Purpose	To evaluate the early outcomes of patients with acute coronary syndromes (acute myocardial infarction or unstable angina) treated with sirolimus-eluting stents.
Design	Single-center registry evaluation.
Patients	198 consecutive patients with acute coronary syndrome treated with sirolimus-eluting stents during the first 4 months of the RESEARCH registry and a control group of 301 consecutive patients treated with bare-metal stents (control patients) in the same time period.
Follow-up	30 days.
Regimen	Implantation of a sirolimus-eluting stent from April 16 to August 15, 2002.

Results   End points were major cardiac events (death, nonfatal MI, or repeat target lesion revascularization or target-vessel revascularization). Compared with control patients, patients treated with sirolimus-eluting stents had more primary angioplasty procedures (95% vs 77%), more bifurcation stenting (13% vs 5%), fewer previous MIs (28% vs 45%), and less use of glycoprotein IIb/IIIa inhibitors (27% vs 42%) (p<0.01 for all differences). The 30-day rate of major adverse cardiac events was similar (6.1% for patients with sirolimus-eluting stents and 6.6% for control patients). Most complications occurred in the first week. The rate of stent thrombosis was 0.5% in the registry patients and 1.7% in control patients, a nonsignificant difference. In multivariate analysis, sirolimus-eluting stent utilization did not influence the incidence of MACE (OR 1.0; 95% CI=0.4-2.2).

Concl.   Implantation of sirolimus-eluting stents in patients with acute coronary syndromes is safe as it is in patients with chronic stable disease. Early outcomes are comparable to those with bare-metal stents. Maintenance of the good short-term results is crucial to validate sirolimus-eluting stents as a useful strategy in the treatment of complex cases.

TAXUS II

Polymer-Controlled Paclitaxel-Eluting Stents

Title	Randomized study to assess the effectiveness of slow- and moderate-release polymer-based paclitaxel-eluting stents for coronary artery lesions.
Authors	Colombo A, Drzewiecki J, Banning A, et al.
Reference	Circulation 2003;108:788-794.
Disease	Coronary artery disease.
Purpose	To evaluate the safety and efficacy of 2 different release formulations of paclitaxel-eluting stent (TAXUS).
Design	Multicenter, randomized, double-blind trial.
Patients	536 patients with single de novo coronary lesions randomly assigned into 2 consecutive and independent cohorts: TAXUS-slow-release slow-release and TAXUS-moderate-release.
Follow-up	12 months.
Regimen	Cohort I: TAXUS-slow-release or control stents; cohort II: TAXUS moderate release or control stents. Control stents were uncoated stents.
Results	At 6 months, percent net volume obstruction with the stent measured by intravascular ultrasound (primary end point) was significantly lower with TAXUS stents (7.9% slow-release [SR] and 7.8% moderate-release [MR]) than for the respective controls 23.2% and 20.5%; p<0.0001 for both). There was a reduction in angiographic restenosis from 17.9% to 2.3% in the SR group (p<0.0001) and from 20.2% to 4.7% in the MR group (p=0.0002). The incidence of major adverse cardiac events at 12 months (a secondary end point) was significantly lower in the TAXUS-SR (10.9%) and TAXUS-MR (9.9%) groups than in the control groups (22% and 21.4%), primarily because of a significant reduction in repeat target-lesion revascularization in TAXUS-treated patients (64% reduction with TAXUS-SR and 76% reduction with TAXUS-MR).

Concl.   The paclitaxel-eluting stents reduced in-stent neointimal
          formation and restenosis and improved 12-month clinical
          outcome in patients with single de novo coronary lesions.
          Persistence of these benefits at 12 months indicates that the
          paclitaxel-eluting stents may inhibit, not just delay, restenosis.
          These beneficial effects must be balanced against concerns
          about vascular cytotoxicity and associated clinical correlates.
          The slow- and moderate-release formulations did not yield
          differences in ultrasound, angiographic, or clinical outcomes.
          The similar efficacy of the 2 formulations suggests that the
          dosing threshold to interrupt the restenotic cascade had been
          reached with the slow-release formulation. Whether the same
          threshold will apply for patients at higher risk (eg, diabetic)
          or with more complex lesions is not known.

TAXUS-IV

Paclitaxel-Eluting Coronary Stent Implantation

Title	A polymer-based, paclitaxel-eluting stent in patients with coronary artery disease.
Authors	Stone GW, Ellis SG, Cox DA, et al.
Reference	N Engl J Med 2004;350:221-231.
Disease	Coronary artery disease.
Purpose	To examine the safety and efficacy of a paclitaxel-eluting stent in reducing the risk of clinical and angiographic restenosis in a broad population of patients and lesions.
Design	Large-scale, prospective, double-blind, randomized, multi-center trial.
Patients	1314 patients with angina or provocable ischemia undergoing a percutaneous intervention, receiving a stent in a single, previously untreated coronary artery stenosis.
Follow-up	9 months.
Regimen	Bare-metal stent (n=652) or slow-release, polymer-based, paclitaxel-eluting stent (n=662).
Add'l Tx	Angiographic follow-up prespecified at 9 months in 732 patients. Before and after stenting patients received aspirin and clopidogrel.

Results	The 2 groups were well matched at baseline. Diabetes mellitus was present in 24.2%, mean reference-vessel diameter was 2.75 mm, and mean lesion length was 13.4 mm. A mean of 1.08 stents (21.8 mm long) were implanted per patient. At 9 months, the rate of ischemia-driven target-vessel revascularization was 12% with bare-metal stents and 4.7% with the paclitaxel-eluting stent (relative risk [RR] 0.39; 95% CI=0.26-0.59; $p<0.001$). Target-lesion revascularization was required in 3% of the patients receiving the paclitaxel-eluting stent vs 11.3% of those receiving the bare-metal stent (RR 0.27; 95% CI=0.16-0.43; $p<0.001$). The angiographic restenosis rate was 26.6% with the bare-metal stent and 7.9% with the paclitaxel-eluting stent (RR 0.30; 95% CI=0.19-0.46; $p<0.001$) The 9-month composite rates of death from cardiac causes or MI (4.7% in the paclitaxel vs 4.3% in the bare-metal stent group) and stent thrombosis (0.6% paclitaxel and 0.8% bare-metal) were similar in the 2 groups.
Concl.	The slow-release, polymer-based, paclitaxel-eluting stent is safe and markedly reduces the rates of clinical and angiographic restenosis at 9 months.

Sirolimus-Eluting Stents

Title	Sustained suppression of neointimal proliferation by sirolimus-eluting stents. One-year angiographic and intravascular ultrasound follow-up.
Authors	Sousa JE, Costa MA, Abizaid AC, et al.
Reference	Circulation 2001;104:2007-2011.
Disease	Coronary artery disease.
Purpose	To determine whether sirolimus-eluting stents result in sustained reduction in restenosis over 1 year.
Design	Nonrandomized, multicenter.
Patients	45 patients with de novo coronary artery disease. 32 had stable angina; 13 had unstable angina.
Follow-up	6-12 months.
Regimen	Treatment with single sirolimus-eluting Bx Velocity stent (fast or slow releasing). Stents implanted as per standard protocols, after balloon predilatation. Stents were 18 mm long and 3-3.5 mm in diameter.
Add'l Tx	Heparin, aspirin.
Results	Angiographic and volumetric intravascular ultrasounds were performed at 4 and 12 months or 6 months. 1-year in-stent minimum luminal diameter and percent diameter stenosis remained unchanged in all groups. In 3 groups of patients with fast or slow releasing sirolimus in either Brazil or The Netherlands, follow-up in lesion minimal lumen diameter was 2.28-2.48 mm. At 1 year no patient approached $\geq$50% diameter stenosis assessed by angiography or intravascular ultrasound. In addition no edge restenosis was detected. Neointimal hyperplasia assessed by intravascular ultrasound was absent at 6 months (2% obstruction volume) and 12 months (2%).

Concl.   Sirolimus-eluting Bx Velocity stents showed sustained suppression of neointimal proliferation and prevented restenosis up to 1 year after implantation into coronary artery lesions of patients with angina.

ASPECT

Asian Paclitaxel-Eluting Stent Clinical Trial

Title	A paclitaxel-eluting stent for the prevention of coronary restenosis.
Authors	Park S-J, Shim WH, Ho DS, et al.
Reference	N Engl J Med 2003;348:1537-1545.
Disease	Coronary artery disease, percutaneous intervention.
Purpose	To determine the ability of a paclitaxel-coated stent to prevent restenosis.
Design	Multicenter, randomized, controlled, triple-blind.
Patients	177 patients. Subjects were at least 18 years old and symptomatic. There were numerous exclusion criteria. These included ejection fraction less than 35%, MI in the prior 72 hours, other revascularization procedures in the prior 1 month, presence of coronary thrombus, total occlusion, lesion length greater than 15 mm, and others.
Follow-up	Mean 174 days.
Regimen	Angioplasty and stent placement were performed in the usual manner, with a stent-to-artery ratio of 1.1:1.0 and a residual stenosis <10%. Treatment with aspirin and clopidogrel or ticlopidine before the procedure was recommended. Heparin was given during the procedure. After the procedure, aspirin, ticlopidine, or clopidogrel was recommended for 1 month at 2 centers and 6 months at the other center. At 2 centers, cilostazol was given in place of ticlopidine or clopidogrel.

Results	The primary end point was the percentage stenosis at angiographic follow-up. Secondary angiographic end points were late loss, rate of restenosis, and the in-stent minimal lumen diameter. Secondary clinical end points were death, acute and subacute thrombosis, need for coronary bypass surgery or intervention to treat ischemia due to target lesion restenosis, and MI due to restenosis of the target lesion. 60 patients were randomized to the high-dose group, 58 to the low-dose group and 59 to the control group (uncoated stent). Baseline characteristics were similar between the groups. There was a dose-dependent reduction of the primary end point: the percent stenosis was 39%±27% in the control group, 23%±25% in the low-dose group, and 14%±21% in the high-dose group (p<0.001). There was dose-dependent reduction in late loss of luminal diameter: 1.04±0.83 mm in the control group, 0.57±0.71 mm in the low-dose group, and 0.29±0.72 in the high-dose group (p<0.001). The rate of restenosis, was 27% in the control group, 12% in the low-dose group, and 4% in the high-dose group (p<0.001). There was a dose-dependent improvement in the minimal lumen diameter (1.79±0.86 mm in the control group, 2.28±0.83 mm in the low-dose group, and 2.53±0.72 mm in the high-dose group; p<0.001). There was an increased number of adverse events associated with the use of cilostazol: 1 death and 4 subacute thromboses. Overall, 96% of patients in the aspirin with ticlopidine or clopidogrel group remained event-free, compared to 81% in the aspirin with cilostazol group (p=0.007).
Concl.	When used with conventional antiplatelet therapy, paclitaxel-eluting stents effectively prevent restenosis and neointimal hyperplasia compared to uncoated stents.

ASPECT (Substudy)

Asian Paclitaxel-Eluting Stent Clinical Trial

Title	Paclitaxel coating reduces in-stent intimal hyperplasia in human coronary arteries. A Serial Volumetric Intravascular Ultrasound Analysis From The Asian Paclitaxel-Eluting Stent Clinical Trial (ASPECT).
Authors	Hong MK, Mintz GS, Lee CW, et al.
Reference	Circulation 2003;107:517-520.
Disease	Coronary artery disease, percutaneous intervention.
Purpose	To determine the effect of a paclitaxel coating on in-stent intimal hyperplasia.
Design	3-center, triple-blind, randomized, placebo-controlled.
Patients	177 patients who had single de novo lesions.
Follow-up	6 months.
Regimen	Patients were randomized to receive placebo (bare metal stents) or 1 of 2 doses of the coated stent (low dose: 1.28 mg/mm^2 stent surface area and high dose: 3.10 mg/mm^2; overall dose 54-60 mg and 130-146 mg, respectively, depending on diameter of stent). Patients were given antiplatelet agents for 6 months. The intravascular ultrasound (IVUS) analysis was a substudy of the ASPECT trial. Ultrasound analysis was performed on 81 patients.

Results   The primary end point of the study was the intra-stent intimal hyperplasia (IH) accumulated at follow-up. At follow-up, there was a decrease in lumen volume and increase in volume of intimal hyperplasia (IH) in all groups ($p<0.0001$ for all comparisons). There was a reduction in IH accumulation with increasing doses of paclitaxel (31 ± 22 mm^3 in control, 18 ± 15 mm^3 in low-dose patients, and 13 ± 14 mm^3 in high-dose patients; $p<0.001$). There was less IH accumulation when the low- and high-dose patients were compared with placebo ($p=0.009$ and $p<0.001$, respectively), but not when low-dose patients were vs the high-dose patients ($p=0.2$). As the dosage increased, there were no significant changes in the measurements of the reference segments (i.e. proximal and distal reference segments).

Concl.   Compared to uncoated stents, paclitaxel-coated stents are effective in reducing neointimal tissue proliferation within the stent.

COAST

Heparin-Coated Stents in Small Coronary Arteries Trial

Title	Heparin-coated stent placement for the treatment of stenoses in small coronary arteries of symptomatic patients.
Authors	Haude M, Konorza TFM, Kalnins U, et al.
Reference	Circulation 2003; 107:1265-1270.
Disease	Coronary artery disease, percutaneous intervention.
Purpose	To evaluate the outcome of treatment of stenoses in small coronary arteries with heparin-coated stents compared with bare stents and angioplasty.
Design	Prospective, randomized, multicenter.
Patients	588 patients, who had stable or unstable angina, with stenoses in the native coronary arteries between 2.0 and 2.6 mm in diameter. Exclusion criteria included acute or evolving MI, severe heart failure (left ventricular ejection fraction <30%), or contraindication to aspirin, ticlopidine, or clopidogrel.
Follow-up	6 months.
Regimen	Angioplasty or stent implantation was performed in the usual manner. Patients were randomly assigned to balloon angioplasty, implantation of a bare stent, or implantation of a heparin-coated stent. Predilatation was strongly recommended in the stent groups. The target balloon-to-artery ratio was 1.1 and the target stent implantation pressure was 14 atm. Aspirin was prescribed, and 10,000 U of heparin were given before the procedure. Use of glycoprotein IIb/IIIa inhibitors was discouraged. Following the procedure, all patients received aspirin 100 mg/d; patients in the stent arms received 500 mg ticlopidine daily or a loading dose of 300 mg clopidogrel followed by 75 mg/d for 4 weeks.

Results	The primary study end point was the mean lumen diameter at the 6-month follow-up angiography. The secondary end points were procedural success rates and incidence of death, myocardial infarction, thrombotic events, angiographic restenosis (>50% diameter stenosis), target vessel revascularization, and event-free survival at the end of hospitalization, at 30 days, and at 250 days. 195 patients were in the angioplasty-only group, 196 in the bare stent group, and 197 in the heparin-coated stent group. At baseline, the groups were comparable. Approximately 20% of patients were diabetic, 80% had multivessel disease, and 25% had complex lesions. The primary study end point, mean lumen diameter (MLD), was significantly different between the groups at the 6-month follow-up: MLD was 1.34 ± 0.48 mm in the angioplasty group, 1.47 ± 0.48 in the bare stent group, and 1.45 ± 0.54 in the heparin-coated group ($p=0.049$ for difference of angioplasty group vs stent groups). There was no significant difference between the 2 stent groups for MLD. The percent diameter stenosis was significantly larger in the angioplasty-only group: $42\%\pm20\%$ in the angioplasty group, $36\%\pm20\%$ in the bare stent group, and $38\%\pm23\%$ in the heparin-coated group, ($p=0.038$ for difference of angioplasty group vs stent groups). Initial procedural success rates were significantly higher in the stent groups vs the angioplasty group: 97.9% in the bare stent group, 97.9% in the heparin-coated stent group, and 72.8% in the angioplasty group ($p<0.0001$). There were no significant differences in the number of postprocedural adverse major cardiac events (ie death, MI, thrombotic event, target vessel revascularization) between the 3 groups. 15.4% of those in the angioplasty-only group had any such event within 250 days vs 11.7% and 11.7% in the 2 stent groups ($p=NS$).
Concl.	Bare and heparin-coated stents offer significantly better angiographic results and were associated with a nonsignficant reduction in clinical events vs angioplasty-only treatment. There was no difference in outcome between bare and heparin-coated stents for treatment of stenotic small coronary arteries.

RAVEL

Randomized Study with the Sirolimus-Coated Bx Velocity Balloon-Expandable Stent in the Treatment of Patients with De Novo Native Coronary Artery Lesions

5e

Title	A randomized comparison of a sirolimus-eluting stent with a standard stent for coronary revascularization.
Authors	Morice M-C, Serruys PW, Sousa JE, et al.
Reference	N Engl J Med 2002;346:1773-1780.
Disease	Coronary artery disease.
Purpose	To determine whether a sirolimus (rapamycin) eluting stent would reduce in-stent coronary restenosis rates to a greater extent than a standard uncoated stent in patients with angina pectoris.
Design	Randomized, double-blind, multicenter.
Patients	238 patients with stable or unstable angina or silent ischemia. Single primary target lesion in native coronary artery 2.5-3.5 mm in diameter appropriate for stent therapy.
Follow-up	30 days; 6 and 12 months.
Regimen	Patients were randomized to sirolimus-eluting stent vs standard uncoated stent. Sirolimus was fixed to the stent at a dose of 140 mg of drug per square centimeter of metal surface. 80% of drug was released within 30 days after implantation.
Add'l Tx	Heparin, aspirin, clopidogrel, or ticlopidine.

Results   Primary end point was in-stent late luminal loss (difference between minimal luminal diameter directly after the procedure and on 6 month follow-up angiogram). Intravascular ultrasound (IVUS) performed in a subgroup of patients at 6-month visit. At 6 months mean minimal luminal diameter was greater in the sirolimus-stented group (2.42 ± 0.49) vs the standard stent 1.64 ± 0.59; $p<0.001$). Stenosis (percent of luminal diameter) was $14.7\%\pm7.0\%$ in the sirolimus vs $36.7\%\pm18.1\%$ ($p<0.01$) in the standard stent group. Mean late luminal loss was lower in the sirolimus group (-0.01 ± 0.33 mm) vs the standard stent group (0.80 ± 0.53 mm; $p<0.001$). Restenosis of 50% or more of the luminal diameter was present in none of the patients receiving sirolimus stent vs 26.6% of those that received the standard stent. IVUS showed that the sirolimus group had less neointimal hyperplasia (2 ± 5 mm^3) vs the standard stent group (37 ± 28 mm^3) and less volume obstruction as well. No stent thrombosis occurred. A composite of major cardiac events (death, myocardial infarction, CABG, revascularization of the target lesion or vessel) occurred in 5.8% of sirolimus stent group vs 28.8% of standard stent group (<0.001).

Concl.   Sirolimus-eluting stent prevented restenosis, neointimal proliferation and reduced clinical event rate compared to standard stents.

RAVEL

Randomized Study with the Sirolimus-Eluting Velocity Balloon-Expandable Stent in the Treatment of Patients with De Novo Native Coronary Artery Lesions

Title	Intravascular ultrasound findings in the multicenter, randomized, double-blind RAVEL (Randomized Study with the Sirolimus-Eluting Velocity Balloon-Expandable Stent in the Treatment of Patients with De Novo Native Coronary Artery Lesions) trial.
Authors	Serruys PW, Degertekin M, Tanabe K.
Reference	Circulation 2002;106:798-803.
Disease	Coronary artery disease.
Purpose	To elucidate the local morphologic effects of implantation of a sirolimus-eluting stent, as compared to a noneluting stent, by using intravascular ultrasound (IVUS).
Design	Randomized, double-blind, multicenter.
Patients	Criteria for eligibility were: diagnosis of stable or unstable angina pectoris or documented silent ischemia, along with a single de novo target lesion in a native coronary artery which was between 2.5 and 3.5 mm in diameter and could be covered with a 18-mm stent. Exclusion criteria were: an evolving myocardial infarction; an unprotected left main coronary artery stenosis ≥50%; an ostial target lesion; a calcified lesion that could not be dilated; a thrombus within the target lesion which was angiographically visible; left ventricular ejection fraction less than 30%; or aspirin, clopidogrel, or ticlopidine intolerance.
Follow-up	12 months.
Regimen	After predilatation, patients were randomized to receive either an uncoated metal Bx Velocity Balloon-Expandable Stent or a sirolimus-eluting Bx Velocity Balloon-Expandable Stent. Randomization was double blind. After stent implantation, postdilatation was performed as needed to achieve stenosis less than 20% with a TIMI grade 3 flow.

Add'l Tx	Heparin was given to all patients during the procedure to maintain an activated clotting time >250 seconds, and was discontinued within 12 hours after the procedure. Aspirin, 100 mg minimum, was given 12 hours prior to the procedure and continued afterward. Clopidogrel was given 48 hours before the procedure at a loading dose of 300 mg, and 75 mg qd for 8 weeks afterward. Other patients received ticlopidine 250 mg bid (in place of clopidogrel) starting 1 day before the procedure and then continued for 8 weeks afterward.
Results	238 patients were enrolled and randomized. Of these, 95 patients underwent IVUS evaluation at 6 months. The primary end point was angiographic in-stent late loss at 6 months, determined by angiography. The secondary end point of the study was a composite of major cardiac events, which included death (cardiac and noncardiac), MI, CABG, or revascularization of target lesion or vessel, measured at 30 days, 6 months, and 12 months after the initial procedure. The restenosis rate and late angiographic stent loss in the sirolimus stents were 0% and 0.06±0.30 mm, respectively, and 23.4% and 0.91±0.58 mm in the noneluting stents; p values between the groups were not given. Mean diameter of the stented coronary artery segment in the sirolimus group was similar at study start compared to the 6 month evaluation: 2.87±0.46 vs 2.87±0.49 mm; mean stented diameter in the uncoated group decreased from 2.90±0.42 to 2.17±0.48 (p<0.001). Total vessel volume and amount of plaque behind stent was similar in the 2 groups. However, there were significant differences in the amounts of neointimal hyperplasia (2±5 vs 37±28 mm^3, coated vs uncoated; p<0.001) and percent of volume obstruction (1%±3% vs 29%±20%; p<0.001). In the group of patients who underwent IVUS evaluation (95 patients), the event-free survival rate at 1-year follow-up in the sirolimus group was 98%, vs 72% for the uncoated group (p<0.001). These rates were similar to the rates for the entire randomized cohort (94% and 72%, respectively; p<0.0001).
Concl.	Sirolimus-eluting stents significantly decreased neointimal hyperplasia and increased event-free survival compared to uncoated stents.

RAVEL

Randomized, Double-Blind Study with the Sirolimus-Eluting Bx Velocity Balloon Expandable Stent in the Treatment of Patients with De Novo Native Coronary Artery Lesions. (Substudy)

Title	Fate of side branches after coronary arterial sirolimus-eluting stent implantation.
Authors	Tanabe K, Serruys PW, Degertekin M, et al.
Reference	Am J Cardiol 2002;90:937-941.
Disease	Coronary artery disease.
Purpose	To determine the outcome of side branches after implantation of a sirolimus-eluting stent vs an uncoated metal stent.
Design	Substudy of a randomized, double-blind trial.
Patients	238 patients in the RAVEL study. Patients had a single de novo lesion in a native coronary artery capable of being covered with one 18-mm stent. Exclusion criteria included a target lesion with a side branch >2.5 mm in diameter that would need side branch stenting.
Follow-up	6 months.
Regimen	Enrolled patients were randomized equally to receive either an uncoated metal Bx VELOCITY stent or sirolimus-eluting Bx VELOCITY stent. Lesions were treated according to standard interventional techniques, and direct stenting was not allowed. All patients received at least 100 mg aspirin daily for an indefinite period, as well as either clopidogrel (75 mg qd) or ticlopidine (250 mg bid) for 8 weeks. Side branches that were seen on angiography and thereafter covered with a stent were analyzed by 2 blinded observers. The TIMI grade flow was determined before and after the stenting. An occluded side branch was defined as TIMI flow grade 0, and spontaneous recanalization was defined as an increase in TIMI flow from grade 0 to at least 1.

Results   63 patients with 118 side branches received a coated stent; 65 patients with 124 side branches received an uncoated stent. The 2 groups were well matched at baseline with respect to age, coronary risk factors, and prior cardiac events and procedures. After the procedure, the reference lumen diameter was similar in the coated stent group vs the uncoated stent group: (2.63±0.53 mm vs 2.68±0.58 mm; p=0.62). The minimal lumen diameters were also similar between the 2 groups after the procedure (2.48±0.41 vs 2.42±0.46 mm; p=0.46). At 6 months, the minimal lumen diameter was significantly greater in the coated group (2.40±0.48 mm) vs the uncoated group (1.63±0.59 mm; p<0.001). Quantitative analysis by intravascular ultrasound revealed neointimal hyperplasia was significantly less in the coated group vs the uncoated group (1 ± 1 and 37 ± 26 mm^3, respectively; p<0.001) at follow-up. Post-procedure occlusion of side branches occurred in 10% in the coated group and 7% in the uncoated group (p=non-significant). At 6-month follow-up, 11/12 side branches had spontaneously recanalized in the coated group, and 6/9 had spontaneously recanalized in the uncoated group (p=0.15). At follow-up, the percentage of patients who had improvement in TIMI grade flow was similar between the 2 groups (coated group: 24/30, uncoated group: 13/19; p=0.36).

Concl.   The outcome of side branches after sirolimus-coated stent implantation is similar to the outcome after uncoated stent implantation. Coated stents did not adversely affect the spontaneous recanalization rate of occluded side branches.

RAVEL (Angiographic Findings)

Randomized Study with the Sirolimus-Eluting Bx Velocity Balloon-Expandable Stent

Title	Angiographic findings of the multicenter randomized study with the sirolimus-eluting Bx velocity balloon-expandable stent (RAVEL). Sirolimus-eluting stents inhibit restenosis irrespective of the vessel size.
Authors	Regan E, Serruys PW, Bode C, et al.
Reference	Circulation 2002;106:1949-1956.
Disease	Coronary artery disease; restenosis.
Purpose	To evaluate angiographic outcome vs vessel diameter in those coronary arteries treated with sirolimus-eluting stents.
Design	Randomized, double-blind, multicenter.
Patients	238 patients with a single de novo lesion of a coronary artery.
Follow-up	6 months.
Regimen	Patients randomized to 18 mm bare metal Bx VELOCITY stent (n=118) or sirolimus-eluting Bx VELOCITY stent (n=120). Quantitative coronary angiography performed at baseline and at 6-month follow-up.
Add'l Tx	Aspirin indefinitely. Clopidogrel or ticlopidine for 8 weeks.

Results	At 6 months, binary restenosis was 0.0% in the sirolimus-eluting stent group vs 26.6% in the bare metal stent group (p<0.001). At 6-month follow-up angiogram, the minimal luminal diameter was larger in the sirolimus stent group (2.42±0.49 mm) than in the bare metal stent group (1.64±0.59 mm; p<0.001). Also, late lumen loss was lower in the sirolimus stent group (-0.01±0.33 mm) than the bare metal stent group (0.80±0.53 mm; p<0.001). In sirolimus-eluting stent group, the minimal lumen diameter remained unchanged in 97% of lesions. Subgroups of patients were examined by terciles according to reference diameter (RD): (stratum 1, RD<2.36 mm; stratum II, RD 2.36-2.84 mm; stratum III, RD>2.84 mm). Restenosis was 0% in the sirolimus group in all strata; it was 35%, 26%, and 20% in stratum 1, 2, and 3, respectively, in the bare metal stent patients. In-stent late loss was less in the sirolimus-eluting vs bare metal stents for all strata.
Concl.	Sirolimus-eluting stents prevented restenosis independently of coronary artery vessel diameter.

5. Interventional Cardiology
f. Other Therapy Including Transmyocardial Laser Revascularization

Transmyocardial Revascularization with CO_2 Laser in Patients with Refractory Angina Pectoris. Clinical Results from the Norwegian Randomized Trial

Title	Transmyocardial revascularization with CO_2 laser in patients with refractory angina pectoris. Clinical results from the Norwegian randomized trial.
Authors	Aaberge L, Nordstrand K, Dragsund M, et al.
Reference	J Am Coll Cardiol 2000;35:1170-1177.
Disease	Coronary artery disease, angina pectoris.
Purpose	To determine the effects of CO_2 laser transmyocardial revascularization (TMR) plus maximal medical therapy vs maximal medical therapy alone on anginal symptoms, exercise performance, and maximal oxygen consumption.
Design	Open, randomized, prospective, single-center study.
Patients	100 patients with refractory angina pectoris (Class III or IV despite optimal medical therapy).
Follow-up	3 months and 12 months.
Regimen	800 W CO_2 laser, 30-50 J, pulse duration of 30-50 msec. Approximately 1 channel/cm^2 of myocardium, confirmed by transesophageal ultrasound probe (average of 48±7 channels).
Add'l Tx	Included β-blockers, calcium blockers, long acting nitrates, aspirin, warfarin, ACE inhibitors, statins, diuretics, and others as per physician.

Results	Primary end points were time to 1 mm ST segment depression on exercise testing and MVO_2 (maximal oxygen consumption). Secondary end points included time to chest pain, total exercise time and accumulated work. 63% of TMR patients experienced an improvement in 1 or more functional classes at 3 months; 71% at 12 months. While mean functional class in TMR patients was 3.3 at baseline, it decreased to 2.3 at 3 months and 2.0 at 1 year. In contrast, only 14% of patients on maximal medical therapy improved by 1 or more classes at 3 months and only 22% improved at 12 months. While baseline class in the maximal medical therapy group was 3.2, it remained 3.1 at both 3 and 12 months in contrast to TMR (p<0.01). TMR increased time to angina during exercise from baseline by 78 seconds after 3 months (p=NS) and 66 seconds (p<0.01) after 12 months, whereas maximal medical therapy failed to improve this parameter. TMR did not improve total exercise time or MVO_2. 1-Year mortality was 12% vs 8% in the TMR group vs maximal medical therapy group, respectively (p=NS). Postoperative mortality with TMR was 4%.
Concl.	TMR with CO_2 laser improved symptoms and time to chest pain during exercise in coronary artery disease patients with refractory angina, who were not candidates for CABG or PTCA. In this study, overall exercise capacity was not improved.

Norwegian Randomized Trial with Transmyocardial Revascularization

Title	Continued symptomatic improvement 3-5 years after transmyocardial revascularization with CO_2 laser.
Authors	Aaberge L, Rootwelt K, Blomhoff S, et al.
Reference	J Am Coll Cardiol 2002;39:1588-1593.
Disease	Coronary artery disease, angina pectoris.
Purpose	To determine late clinical outcome and left ventricular (LV) function in patients with refractory angina not eligible for routine revascularization, with CO_2 laser.
Design	Late follow-up of Norwegian, randomized study.
Patients	100 patients with refractory angina, New York Heart Association (NYHA) class III or IV or despite optimal medical therapy, not candidates for percutaneous transluminal coronary angioplasty (PTCA) or coronary artery bypass graft surgery (CABG).
Follow-up	43 months.
Regimen	Transmyocardial revascularization (TMR) achieved by 800 W CO_2 laser; average of 48 channels made during surgery (n=49) vs continued medical therapy (n=50).
Add'l Tx	Antianginal medicines at the discretion of treating physician.

Results	End points included angina, hospitalization for MI or unstable angina, heart failure, and LV ejection fraction (by multigated angiogram scanning). 24% of the medical treated group and 22% in the TMR group died before late follow-up (p=NS). Angina improvement by ≥2 NYHA functional classes occurred in 24% of the TMR group vs 3% of the medical group (p=0.001). Angina improvement by ≥1 NYHA functional classes occurred in 61% of the TMR group vs 24% of the medical treatment group (p=0.010). Hospitalization for unstable angina occurred in 53% of TMR patients vs 95% of the medical therapy group (p=0.047). Acute MI occurred in 8% of TMR patients vs 12% of medical patients (p=NS). Heart failure occurred in 19% of TMR patients vs 11% of medical therapy patients. antianginal medicine was only insignificantly reduced by TMR. There was greater use of diuretics and ACE inhibitors in the TMR group vs the medical group. There were no statistically significant differences in ejection fraction between groups.
Concl.	After 43 months, TMR with CO_2 laser was associated with less angina and hospitalization for unstable angina vs medical therapy only group; however, heart failure treatment was greater in the TMR group.

Percutaneous Transmyocardial Lasers in Chronic Total Occlusion

Title	A prospective, multicenter, randomized trial of percutaneous transmyocardial laser revascularization in patients with nonrecanalizable chronic total occlusions.
Authors	Stone GW, Teirstein PS, Robenstein R, et al.
Reference	J Am Coll Cardiol 2002;39:1581-1587.
Disease	Coronary artery disease.
Purpose	To assess safety and efficacy of percutaneous transmyocardial revascularization (PTMR) in patients with refractory angina due to 1 or more chronic total coronary occlusions.
Design	Prospective, single-blinded, randomized, multicenter.
Patients	141 patients with class III-IV angina and chronically occluded native coronary or coronaries in which a percutaneous coronary intervention had failed.
Follow-up	6 months.
Regimen	Patients randomized to PTMR plus maximal medical therapy (n=71) or maximal medical therapy only (n=70). PTMR achieved with holmium:YAG laser with fluoroscopic guidance. Blinding attempted with heavy sedation and dark goggles. Medium of 20 laser channels in PTMR group.
Add'l Tx	Antianginal medicine, maximized.

Results	Primary outcome was improvement in exercise duration from baseline to late follow-up (6 months). Median increase in exercise duration was 64 seconds in the PTMR group vs 52 seconds with maximal medical treatment alone (p=NS). Anginal class improved in both groups, by 2 or more classes in 49% of PTMR patients and 37% in maximal medical treatment alone group (p=0.33). 6-month death rates were 8.6% with PTMR vs 8.8% with maximal medical treatment (p=NS). Rate of MI was 4.3% in PTMR group vs 2.9% for maximal medical therapy (p=NS). Need for revascularization also was similar in the 2 groups (4.3% vs 5.9%). In-hospital complications tended to be more frequent in the PTMR group.
Concl.	PTMR was not superior to maximal medical therapy in patients with refractory angina and total coronary artery occlusion(s).

ATLANTIC

Angina Treatments—Lasers and Normal Therapies in Comparison

Title	Transmyocardial laser revascularization compared with continued medical therapy for treatment of refractory angina pectoris: A prospective randomised trial.
Authors	Burkhoff D, Schmidt S, Schulman SP, et al.
Reference	Lancet 1999;354:885-890.
Disease	Angina pectoris, coronary artery disease.
Purpose	To compare transmyocardial laser revascularization (TMR) with standard medical therapy in patients with medically refractory angina pectoris.
Design	Randomized, open-label, multicenter.
Patients	182 patients with Canadian Cardiovascular Society Angina (CCSA) Class III (38%) or IV (62%), despite maximum medical therapy, LVEF ≥30%, and reversible perfusion defects on dipyridamole thallium stress test. Patients with symptomatic heart failure, a history of significant ventricular arrhythmias, or who had cardiac transplantation were excluded. In addition, those patients who had been hospitalized for acute coronary syndromes or changes in antianginal medications were not included within 21 days of the last event or within 3 months for acute myocardial infarction.
Follow-up	12 months with repeated anginal class assessment, exercise test, dipyridamole thallium stress test, and angina questionnaire.
Regimen	Patients were randomized to TMR with continued medical therapy (n=92) or medical therapy alone (n=90). TMR was applied under general anesthesia through a limited muscle sparing left thoracotomy with a holmium:YAG laser (CardioGenesis Corp, Sunnyvale, CA, USA).

Results	5% of the TMR patients and 10% of the medical therapy patients died during the study. Unstable angina requiring hospitalization occurred in 37 patients of the TMR group vs 69 patients in the medical therapy group. Heart failure or left ventricular dysfunction occurred in 25 patients of the TMR group vs 10 patients in the medical therapy group, and myocardial infarction was noted in 14 and 8 patients of the TMR and medical therapy group, respectively. Exercise duration increased in the TMR group at all time points, with median improvement of >60 seconds. Over 50% of the medical therapy group had a decrease in their exercise time. At 12 months, total exercise time increased by a median of 65 seconds in the TMR group and decreased by 46 seconds in the medical therapy group (p<0.0001). Only 26% of the TMR patients had angina during the final exercise test, compared with 58% of the medical therapy group. After 12 months, CCSA score had decreased by ≥2 scores in 61% of the TMR group vs only 11% in the medical therapy group. Patients with more severe angina at baseline were more likely to have greater improvement with TMR. At 12 months 48% of the TMR group vs only 14% of the medical therapy group were in CCSA Class ≤2 (p<0.001). The quality of life index score increased significantly more in the TMR group than in the medical treatment group. However, the change in the percentage of myocardium with fixed and reversible perfusion defects at 3, 6, and 12 months was comparable between the TMR and medical therapy group. LVEF did not change in the medical therapy group from baseline to 3 months, whereas it decreased by 3% in the TMR group (p<0.0001).
Concl.	TMR was more effective than medical therapy alone in alleviating symptoms of angina and increasing exercise performance. However, it was not associated with improvement in myocardial perfusion, as assessed by dipyridamole thallium scan. TMR may provide benefits in patients with no other therapeutic options.

5f

PACIFIC

Potential Angina Class Improvement From Intramyocardial Channels

Title	Percutaneous transmyocardial laser revascularization for severe angina: the PACIFIC randomised trial.
Authors	Oesterle SN, Sanborn TA, Ali N, et al.
Reference	Lancet 2000;356:1705-1710.
Disease	Coronary artery disease, angina pectoris.
Purpose	To evaluate the efficacy and safety of percutaneous transmyocardial laser revascularization.
Design	Randomized, multicenter.
Patients	221 patients with refractory angina (Canadian Cardiovascular Society Angina Class III or IV) despite maximum medical therapy, left ventricular ejection fraction ≥30%, and reversible perfusion defects on thallium stress test. Patients with symptomatic heart failure, left ventricular wall thickness <8 mm, renal failure, aortic stenosis, severe peripheral vascular disease, significant ventricular arrhythmias, recent myocardial infarction and unstable angina were excluded.
Follow-up	1 year.
Regimen	Randomization to percutaneous transmyocardial laser revascularization or no PTMR. PTMR was performed using a 9F coaxial catheter system for positioning an optical fiber coupled to a holmium:YAG laser (Eclipse Surgical Technologies, Inc., Sunnyvale, CA).
Add'l Tx	Antianginal medical therapy.

Results	11 patients died (8 in the PTMR and 3 in the medical therapy group (p=0.21) and 19 withdrew from the study. 92 patients who underwent PTMR and 99 patients who were included in the medical therapy group completed the study. All patients assigned PTMR underwent the procedure. Patients received a median of 15 channels (range 8-35). During the 1 year follow-up 9 patients in the PTMR and 15 in the medical therapy underwent PTCA, CABG or PTMR. Exercise time at the end of follow-up increased by 89 seconds interquartile range (IQR) -15 to 183 seconds; median 14.4% increase) in the PTMR group vs by 12.5 seconds (IQR -67 to 125 seconds; median 5.5% increase) in the medical therapy group (p=0.008). When patients who underwent other revascularization procedures were excluded, the respective changes were 90.5 seconds (-18 to 188 seconds) vs 8.0 seconds (-81 to 123 seconds) (p=0.004). After 1 year, exercise duration had increased by >60 seconds in 54% of the PTMR group vs 39% of the medical therapy group (p=0.06). The Canadian Cardiovascular Society class had decreased by ≥2 classes in 45.7% in the PTMR group vs only 1.1% in the medical therapy group. On masked assessment, at the end of the 1 year follow-up, angina class was ≤2 in 34.1% of the PTMR group vs 13.0% in the medical therapy group (p=0.002). LVEF did not change from baseline to 3-month follow-up in either group.
Concl.	PTMR resulted in an increase in exercise time, low morbidity, improved quality of life, and lower anginal scores 1 year after treatment.

6. Hypertension

ALLHAT

Antihypertensive and Lipid-Lowering Treatment to Prevent Heart Attack Trial

Title	Major outcomes in high-risk hypertensive patients randomized to angiotensin-converting enzyme inhibitor or calcium channel blocker vs diuretic.
Authors	The ALLHAT Officers and Coordinators for the ALLHAT Collaborative Research Group.
Reference	JAMA 2002;288:2981-2997.
Disease	Hypertension.
Purpose	To determine the effect of treatment with calcium channel blocker or angiotensin-converting enzyme inhibitor vs diuretic on the incidence of coronary heart disease (CHD) and other cardiovascular disease (CVD) events.
Design	Randomized, double-blind, active-controlled, multicenter.
Patients	33,357 patients, age 55 and older, with stage 1 or stage 2 hypertension and at least 1 other coronary heart disease risk factor. Risk factors included: myocardial infarction or stroke >6 months prior; left ventricular hypertrophy shown on electrocardiography or echocardiography; type 2 diabetes, current smoking, high-density lipoprotein cholesterol <35 mg/dL, or history of other atherosclerotic CVD. Patients with a history of symptomatic heart failure and/or left ventricular ejection fraction <35% were excluded.
Follow-up	Mean 4.9 years.

Regimen	Patients were randomized to 1 of 3 groups: chlorthalidone (n=15,255; representing the diuretic group), amlodipine (n=9048; representing the calcium channel blocker group), or lisinopril (n=9054; representing the ACE inhibitor group). Patients continued taking their preexisting antihypertensive medications until they received randomized medication, at which point they stopped taking all other antihypertensive medications. Study medications were "step 1" drugs and were: chlorthalidone given in doses of 12.5, 12.5 (sham titration), and 25 mg/d; amlodipine given in 2.5, 5, and 10 mg/d; and lisinopril in 10, 20 and 40 mg/d. Doses of these step 1 medications were titrated and open-label agents added (step 2 and step 3) as necessary to achieve a target BP of <140/90 mm Hg. Step 2 medications included atenolol (25-100 mg/d), clonidine (0.1-0.3 mg twice a day), or reserpine (0.05-0.2 mg/d), all dosed at the discretion of the treating physician. The step 3 medication was hydralazine 25-100 mg twice a day as necessary in addition to step 1 and step 2 medications. Nonpharmacologic methods of reducing BP were also recommended to patients.
Results	The primary outcome was the composite of fatal CHD or non-fatal MI. The major secondary outcomes were all-cause mortality, fatal and nonfatal stroke, combined CHD (fatal CHD, nonfatal MI, coronary revascularization, angina with hospitalization), and combined CVD (combined CHD, stroke, other angina requiring treatment, all heart failure, and peripheral arterial disease). Coronary revascularization included CABG, percutaneous angioplasty, stent placement, and atherectomy. The other prespecified secondary outcomes were cancer, end-stage renal disease (dialysis, renal transplant, or death), and slope of the reciprocal of longitudinal serum creatinine measurements. The safety outcomes were angioedema and hospitalization for gastrointestinal bleeding (GI bleed). BP measurements at 5 years in the 3 groups were similar (for chlorthalidone, amlodipine, and lisinopril groups, BP= 133.9/75.4 mm Hg, 134.7/74.6 mm Hg, 135.9/75.4 mm Hg) although due to the large sample size the differences between chlorthalidone and both amlodipine and lisinopril were significant for reduction in systolic BP. The reduction in diastolic BP was significantly greater with amlodipine vs chlorathalidone.Amlodipine vs chlorthalidone: There was no significant difference in the primary outcome between amlodipine and chlorthalidone (relative risk [RR] 0.98; 95% CI=0.90-1.07; p=0.65). There were no significant differences between amlodipine and chlorthalidone in the secondary outcomes: all-cause

mortality (RR 0.96; 95% CI=0.89-1.02; p=0.20); combined CHD (RR 1.00; 95% CI=0.94-1.07; p=0.97); stroke (RR 0.93; 95% CI=0.82-1.06; p=0.28); combined CVD (RR 1.04; 95% CI=0.99-1.09; p=0.12); end-stage renal disease (RR 1.12; 95% CI=0.89-1.40; p=0.33); cancer (RR 1.01; 95% CI=0.92-1.11; p=0.77); hospitalization for GI bleeding (RR 0.92; 95% CI=0.82-1.03; p=0.15). There was a 38% higher risk of heart failure in the amlodipine group (RR 1.38; 95% CI=1.25-1.52; p<0.001) and a 35% higher risk of hospitalized or fatal heart failure (RR 1.35; 95% CI=1.21-1.50; p<0.001) compared with chlorthalidone. The effects of treatment were similar across all predefined subgroups and regardless of presence or absence of CHD. All-cause mortality and mortality due to all cardiovascular causes were similar in both groups. Lisinopril vs chlorthalidone: There was no significant difference in the primary outcome between lisinopril and chlorthalidone (RR 0.99; 95% CI=0.91-1.08; p=0.81). There was a 15% higher risk of stroke (RR 1.15; 95% CI=1.02-1.30; p=0.02) in the lisinopril group and a 10% higher risk of combined CVD (RR 1.10; 95% CI=1.05-1.16; p<0.001). The other secondary outcomes were similar between lisinopril and chlorthalidone: all-cause mortality (RR 1.00; 95% CI=0.94-1.08; p=0.90); combined CHD (RR 1.05; 95% CI=0.98-1.11; p=0.18); end-stage renal disease (RR 1.11; 95% CI=0.88-1.38; p=0.38); cancer (RR 1.02; 95% CI=0.93-1.12; p=0.67); hospitalization for GI bleeding (RR 1.11; 95% CI=0.99-1.24; p=0.07) or for most of the secondary outcomes. Also, patients in the lisinopril group had a 19% higher risk of heart failure (RR 1.19; 95% CI=1.07-1.31; p<0.001), and 10% higher risk of coronary revascularization (RR 1.10; 95% CI=1.00-1.21; p=0.05) compared with chlorthalidone. The effects of treatment were similar across the predefined subgroups of sex, diabetic status, and regardless of presence or absence of CHD. The mean systolic BP at follow-up was 2 mm Hg higher in the lisinopril group than the chlorthalidone group, 4 mm Hg higher in blacks, and 3 mm Hg higher in those over 65 years. Potassium levels at baseline were similar between patients in the 3 groups. At 4 years follow-up, potassium levels in patients on chlorthalidone were significantly lower than those in the amlodipine and lisinopril groups (4.1 vs 4.4 vs 4.5; p<0.001 for both amlodipine and lisinopril vs chlorthalidone). The number of patients who had potassium <3.5 mEq/L was significantly greater in the chlorthalidone group (8.5% vs 1.9% vs 0.8%; p<0.001 for both amlodipine and lisinopril vs chlorthalidone). Fasting glucose levels at baseline were similar between patients in the 3 groups. At 4 years follow-up, fasting glucose levels were significantly higher in the chlorthalidone group vs lisinopril (126.3 mg/dL vs 121.5 dL/mg; p=0.002) but not vs amlodipine (126.3 vs 123.7 dL/mg; p=0.20). The percentage of patients who had a fasting glucose ≥126 mg/dL was significantly greater in the chlorthalidone group vs lisinopril (32.7% vs 28.7%; p<0.001), but not vs amlodipine (32.7% vs 30.5%; p=0.11). The estimated glomerular filtration rate (GFR) was similar between patients in the 3 groups at baseline. At 4 years follow-up, GFR was significantly lower in the chlorthalidone group vs both amlodipine and lisinopril (70.0 mL/min per 1.73 m^2 vs 75.1 vs 70.7, respectively; p<0.001 and p=0.03). The slopes of the reciprocal of serum creatinine over the study period were very similar in the chlorthalidone and lisinopril groups (-0.018 and -0.019 dL/mg per year), but the decline in the slope of amlodipine (-0.012 dL/mg per year) was significantly less compared to the chlorthalidone slope (p<0.001). At 6 years, the rates of hospitalization for GI bleeding were 8.8%, 8.0%, and 9.6% in the chlorthalidone, amlodipine, and lisinopril groups, respectively. Angioedema occurred in 0.1%, <0.1%, and 0.4% of patients in the chlorthalidone, amlodipine, and lisinopril groups, respectively. The difference between the lisinopril and chlorthalidone groups was significant (p<0.001).

| Concl. | In patients with hypertension, amlodipine, lisinopril, and chlorthalidone all had similar effects on CAD death and nonfatal MI. All-cause mortality and cardiovascular mortality were similar among the 3 groups. Chlorthalidone was better than amlodipine in preventing overall heart failure and hospitalized or fatal cases of heart failure, and was similar to amlodipine in overall CVD prevention. Chlorthalidone was better than lisinopril in preventing stroke, combined CVD events, and heart failure. |

ALLHAT

Antihypertensive and Lipid-Lowering Treatment to Prevent Heart Attack Trial

Title	Major cardiovascular events in hypertensive patients randomized to doxazosin vs chlorthalidone.
Authors	The ALLHAT Officers and coordinators for the ALLHAT Collaborative Research Group.
Reference	JAMA 2000;283:1967-1975.
Disease	Hypertension.
Purpose	As part of the overall ALLHAT study which was to determine the incidence of fatal coronary heart disease and nonfatal MI in patients with hypertension randomized to 1 of 4 antihypertensives; this analysis compares the effect of the α-blocker doxazosin to the diuretic chlorthalidone.
Design	Randomized, double-blind, active controlled, multicenter.
Patients	24,335 patients with hypertension plus at least 1 other coronary disease risk factor who received the α-blocker doxazosin or diuretic chlorthalidone.
Follow-up	Median follow-up was 3.3 years.
Regimen	While the overall ALLHAT hypertensive protocol compares long-term outcome of chlorthalidone, doxazosin, amlodipine, and lisinopril, an independent data review committee recommended terminating the doxazosin arm based on comparison to chlorthalidone. Data here reflect outcomes from February 1994 to December 1999 and shows comparison of doxazosin (2-8 mg per day (n=9067) to chlorthalidone, 12.5-25 mg per day (n=15,268). Other limbs of the study are continuing.
Add'l Tx	There is also a lipid lowering protocol with pravastatin.

Results	365 patients in the doxazosin and 608 in chlorthalidone group achieved end point of fatal coronary heart disease or nonfatal MI and there was no difference between these 2 groups in this outcomes (RR 1.03; 95% CI=0.90-1.17; p=0.71). There was no difference in total mortality between groups (9.62%, 4 year rate for doxazosin vs 9.08% for chlorthalidone; RR 1.03; 95% CI=0.90-1.15; p=0.56). The secondary end point of combined cardiovascular disease (coronary heart disease death, nonfatal MI, stroke, revascularization, angina, congestive heart failure, and peripheral arterial disease) was higher in the doxazosin arm vs chlorthalidone arm (4 year rate of 25.45% vs 21.76%, respectively; RR 1.25; 95% CI=1.17-1.33; p<0.001); and stroke rate was higher in doxazosin vs chlorthalidone group (RR=1.19; 95% CI=1.0 -1.40; p=0.04). Considering other elements of combined cardiovascular disease outcome, congestive heart failure was higher in the doxazosin vs chlorthalidone group (4-year rates, 8.13% vs 4.45%; RR 2.04; 95% CI=1.79-2.32; p<0.001). RRs for angina and coronary revascularization also were higher at 1.16 (p<0.001) and 1.15 (p=0.05), respectively.
Concl.	Chlorthalidone and doxazosin resulted in comparable risks of coronary heart disease death and nonfatal MI, but chlorthalidone decreased the risk of combined cardiovascular events, notably congestive heart failure, compared to doxazosin, in high risk patients with hypertension.

Losartan and Low-Dose Hydrochlorothiazide in Essential Hypertension

Title	Losartan and low dose hydrochlorothiazide in patients with essential hypertension. A double-blind , placebo-controlled trial of concomitant administration compared with individual components.
Authors	MacKay JH, Arcuri KE, Goldberg AI, et al.
Reference	Arch Intern Med 1996;156:278-285.
Disease	Hypertension.
Purpose	To assess the effects of losartan + low dose hydrochlorothiazide as initial therapy in patients with essential hypertension.
Design	Randomized, double-blind, placebo-controlled, multicenter.
Patients	703 patients, ≥18 years old, with an untreated sitting diastolic blood pressure of 95-115 mm Hg. Patients with a significant hematological, renal, gastrointestinal, hepatic, immune, cerebrovascular or cardiovascular disorder were not included.
Follow-up	12 weeks of double-blind therapy phase.
Regimen	After 4 weeks of single blind, placebo run-in phase, patients were randomized to placebo (n=140), losartan (50 mg/d; n=139), hydrochlorothiazide (12.5 mg/d; n=142) and losartan (50 mg/d)+ hydrochlorothiazide (6.25 [n=144] or 12.5 mg/d [n=138]) for 12 weeks.

Results	18.6% of the placebo, 14.1% of the hydrochlorothiazide, 14.4% of the losartan, 10.4% of the losartan +6.25 mg hydrochlorothiazide, and 13.0% of the losartan +12.5 mg hydrochlorothiazide treated patients discontinued their study medication, mainly because of ineffective therapy. The combination of losartan +12.5 mg hydrochlorothiazide caused the largest reduction in systolic and diastolic blood pressure. The mean reduction in peak sitting diastolic blood pressure at 12 week was 5.4 ± 8.6 mm Hg with placebo, 7.4 ± 8.0 mm Hg with hydrochlorothiazide, 10.9 ± 9.5 mm Hg with losartan, 13.3 ± 13.2 mm Hg with losartan +6.25 mg hydrochlorothiazide, and 15.3 ± 8.9 mm Hg with losartan +12.5 mg hydrochlorothiazide ($p \leq 0.001$). After 12 weeks, 20.9%, 34.3%, 40.6%, 43.5%, and 57.8% of the patients treated with placebo, hydrochlorothiazide, losartan, losartan +6.25 mg hydrochlorothiazide and losartan +12.5 mg hydrochlorothiazide, respectively, had a sitting diastolic blood pressure <90 mm Hg.
Concl.	Combination therapy with losartan 50 mg/d and hydrochlorothiazide 12.5 mg/d resulted in greater reduction in trough sitting systolic and diastolic blood pressure. The combination was well tolerated and was not associated with increased adverse effects.

Comparison of ACE Inhibitors, Calcium Antagonists, β-Blockers, and Diuretic Agents on Reactive Hyperemia in Patients with Essential Hypertension: A Multicenter Study

Title	A comparison of ACE inhibitors, calcium antagonists, β-blockers, and diuretic agents on reactive hyperemia in patients with essential hypertension: A multicenter study.
Authors	Higashi Y, Sasaki S, Nakagawa K, et al.
Reference	J Am Coll Cardiol 2000;35:284-291.
Disease	Hypertension.
Purpose	To compare the effects of calcium antagonists, ACE inhibitors, β-blockers, diuretics, on endothelial function in patients with essential hypertension.
Design	Multicenter study evaluating forearm blood flow (measured using a strain gauge plethysmograph) and reactive hyperemia (induced by inflating a blood pressure cuff to 280 mm Hg for 5 minutes and then releasing the cuff) and flow after sublingual nitroglycerin in patients on various antihypertensives; normotensive control group for comparison.
Patients	296 Japanese patients with essential hypertension (>160/ >95 mm Hg). 47 normotensives as controls.
Follow-up	Acute study.
Regimen	Patients on monotherapy for at least 24 weeks with calcium blockers, ACE inhibitors, β-blockers, or diuretics were randomly recruited.

Add'l Tx	Nitroglycerin, Intraarterial infusion of NO synthase inhibitor NG-monomethyl-L-arginine (L-NMMA), indomethacin.
Results	Forearm reactive blood flow was lower in hypertensive patients compared to normotensive patients. Sublingual nitroglycerin induced an increase in forearm blood flow that was similar in normotensive and hypertensive individuals. All 4 antihypertensive agents were associated with equal systolic-diastolic blood pressures, and forearm vascular resistance. Maximal forearm blood flow response from reactive hyperemia was greatest with the ACE inhibitors ($p<0.05$) (40.5±5.2 mL/min per 100 mL tissue) vs calcium blockers (32.9±5.8), β-blockers (34.0±5.6), diuretics (32.1±5.9), or nothing (31.9±5.8 mL/min per 100 mL tissue). Changes in forearm blood flow after sublingual nitroglycerin were similar among all drug groups and untreated group. The nitric oxides synthase inhibitor, NG-monomethyl-L-arginine abolished the effect of ACE inhibitors on enhancing reactive hyperemia.
Concl.	ACE inhibitors augment reactive hyperemia, an index of endothelium dependent vasodilation, in hypertensive patients. An increase in NO may contribute to this effect by ACE inhibitors.

Long-Term Effects of Weight Loss and Dietary Sodium Reduction on Incidence of Hypertension

Title	Long-term effects of weight loss and dietary sodium reduction on incidence of hypertension.
Authors	He J, Whelton PK, Appel LJ, et al.
Reference	Hypertension 2000;35:544-549.
Disease	Hypertension.
Purpose	To determine if weight loss and sodium restriction could decrease the development of frank hypertension in a population with high-normal blood pressure.
Design	Randomized, multicenter.
Patients	208 participants, with high-normal blood pressure defined in this paper as diastolic blood pressure of 80-89 mm Hg and systolic blood pressure <160 mm Hg.
Follow-up	7 years.
Regimen	Structured weight loss program vs sodium restriction vs control, for 18 months.
Results	Body mass index was similar (overweight but not obese) in the weight loss group (29.0 body mass index) vs the control group (28.7) at baseline. Patients in the weight loss group lost 2.4 kg while those in the control group gained 1.1 kg. Sodium restriction was associated with a significant decrease in 24 hour urinary sodium excretion vs the control group. At 7 years among follow-up on 181 participants there was marked decrease in the incidence of frank hypertension in the weight loss group (19%) vs controls (41%) as well as the use of antihypertensive medicines (13% vs 29%). Sodium restriction led to a modest but not statistically significant decrease in the incidence of development of frank hypertension (22% vs 33% for controls). Use of antihypertensives also tended to be lower in the salt restricted participants (19% vs controls, 24%).
Concl.	Reduction in weight may forestall the development of frank hypertension.

Drug Classes in Black Hypertensives

Title	Efficacy of different drug classes used to initiate antihypertensive treatment in black subjects.
Authors	Sareli D, Radevski IV, Valtchanova ZP, et al.
Reference	Arch Intern Med 2001;161:965-971.
Disease	Hypertension.
Purpose	To test the recommendation that thiazides be used to initiate antihypertensive therapy in black patients.
Design	Randomized, open-label, single-center.
Patients	409 black men and women aged 18-70 with mean diastolic blood pressure between 90 and 114 mm Hg.
Follow-up	13 months.
Regimen	Randomized to nifedipine gastrointestinal therapeutic system 30 mg/d or 1 to 3 reference treatments starting with verapamil HCL sustained release 240 mg/d; hydrochlorothiazide 12.5 mg/d; or enalapril 10 mg/d. After first month, dose escalation and at 2 months additions of other drugs as per protocol.
Add'l Tx	Reserpine in patients whose blood pressure was uncontrolled while taking hydrochlorothiazide 25 mg/d.

Results   Target diastolic blood pressure was below 90 mm Hg. During the first 2 months on monotherapy decreases in daytime systolic/diastolic blood pressure was 22/14 mm Hg on nifedipine, 17/11 mm Hg on verapamil, 12/8 mm Hg on hydrochlorothiazide, and 5/3 mm Hg on enalapril. At 2 months blood pressure was better controlled with nifedipine (63%, p ≤0.03) vs verapamil (40%), hydrochlorothiazide (40%) or enalapril (21%). At 13 months into the study, more patients continued receiving monotherapy with nifedipine (61%) or verapamil (63%) than hydrochlorothiazide (26%) or enalapril (3%). Left ventricular mass was assessed by echocardiography and was reduced with no differences between groups.

Concl.   Calcium channel blockers were more effective than thiazides as initial treatment in black patients with hypertension.

A Comparison of Outcomes with Angiotensin-Converting-Enzyme Inhibitors and Diuretics for Hypertension in the Elderly

Title	A comparison of outcomes with angiotensin-converting-enzyme inhibitors and diuretics for hypertension in the elderly.
Authors	Wing LMH, Reid CM, Ryan P, et al.
Reference	N Engl J Med 2003;348:583-592.
Disease	Hypertension.
Purpose	To determine whether there is a differential outcome between treatment based on an ACE-inhibitor or treatment based on a diuretic in elderly hypertensive patients.
Design	Prospective, randomized, open-label.
Patients	6083 patients, aged 65-84 years, with an average systolic blood pressure of at least 160 mm Hg or average diastolic blood pressure of at least 90 mm Hg. Patients should not have had cardiovascular events in the past 6 months. Exclusion criteria were any life-threatening illness, contraindication to ACE inhibitor or diuretic, creatinine greater than 2.5 mg/dL, malignant hypertension, or dementia.
Follow-up	Median 4.1 years.
Regimen	The ACE inhibitor enalapril and the diuretic hydrochlorothiazide were recommended as the initial agents, but the choice was left to the discretion of the treating physician. Treatment guidelines were to reduce systolic BP by at least 20 mm Hg to less than 160 mm Hg, with reduction to 140 mm Hg if tolerated, and reduction of diastolic BP by at least 10 mm Hg to below 90 mm Hg and to 80 mm Hg if tolerated. In addition to the study medications, usage of β-blockers, calcium channel blockers, and α-blockers was recommended.

Results	The primary end point was all cardiovascular events, or all-cause death. 3044 patients were randomized to the ACE inhibitor group, and 3039 patients were randomized to the diuretic group. The mean systolic BP at baseline was 168±13 mm Hg, and mean diastolic BP was 91±8 mm Hg. At the end of the study, 58% of those assigned to the ACE inhibitor group and 62% of those in the diuretic group were still taking the assigned medication. 65% of patients in the ACE inhibitor group and 67% in the diuretic group were on monotherapy. Other medications being used were calcium channel blockers (approximately 23% in each group), β-blockers (10-13% in each group) and angiotensin receptor blockers (approximately 13% in each group). There were 695/3044 cardiovascular events or all-cause deaths in the ACE inhibitor group, and 736/3039 in the diuretic group (hazard ratio (HR) 0.89; 95% CI=0.79-1.00; p=0.05). There were 195 deaths in the ACE inhibitor group and 210 deaths in the diuretic group (HR=0.90; 95% CI=0.75-1.09; p=0.27). In male subjects, there was evidence of greater benefit from usage of ACE inhibitor, shown by a 17% reduction in the rates of all cardiovascular events and first cardiovascular events (HR for both 0.83; 95% CI=0.71-0.97; p=0.02). Also in males, there was a reduced risk of death associated with ACE inhibitor use (HR 0.83; 95% CI=0.66-1.06; p=0.14). Among female subjects, the HR for all and first cardiovascular events was 1.00 (p=0.98). The HR among females for death was 1.01 (95% CI=0.76-1.35; p=0.94). There was a significant reduction in the rate of first MIs in the ACE inhibitor group; (HR 0.68; 95% CI=0.47-0.98; p=0.04). The incidence of fatal stroke was higher in the ACE inhibitor group, (HR 1.91; 95% CI=10.4-3.5; p=0.04).
Concl.	Despite similar reductions in BP, treatment based on an ACE inhibitor appeared to lead to improved cardiovascular outcomes vs diuretics in elderly hypertensive patients, especially men.

6. Hypertension

AASK

African American Study of Kidney Disease and Hypertension

Title	Effect of ramipril vs amlodipine on renal outcomes in hypertensive nephrosclerosis. A randomized controlled trial.
Authors	Agodoa LY, Appel L, Bakris GL, et al.
Reference	JAMA 2001;285:2719-2728.
Disease	Hypertension.
Purpose	To compare the effects of amlodipine (a dihydropyridine calcium channel blocker), metoprolol (a β-blocker) and ramipril (an ACE inhibitor) on the progression of hypertensive renal disease in African American patients.
Design	Randomized, double-blind, 3 × 2 factorial, multicenter.
Patients	1094 African Americans, 18-70 years old, with hypertension (diastolic blood pressure ≥95 mm Hg) and glomerular filtration rate of 20-65 mL/min per 1.73 m^2 and no other causes of renal insufficiency except hypertension. Patients with diabetes mellitus, urinary protein/creatinine ratio >2.5, accelerated or malignant hypertension, secondary hypertension, serious systemic disease, congestive heart failure, contraindication or specific indication for 1 of the study drugs were excluded.
Follow-up	A median of 3 years.
Regimen	The study used a 3 × 2 factorial design. Patients were randomized to amlodipine 5-10 mg/d (n=217), ramipril 2.5-10 mg/d (n=436) and metoprolol 50-200 mg/d (n=441). In addition, patients were randomized to a goal of mean arterial pressure of 102-107 mm Hg or <92 mm Hg.
Add'l Tx	If the blood pressure goal was not achieved with the study drug, additional open-label antihypertensive drugs were added in the following order: furosemide, doxazosin, clonidine, hydralazine, and minoxidil.

Results   The Data and safety Monitoring Board terminated the amlodipine arm prematurely. The metoprolol and ramipril arms
continued. This paper concentrates on the comparison between
ramipril and amlodipine. Follow-up blood pressure results were
lower than the baseline values, without a significant difference
between the amlodipine and ramipril groups. After the 3-month
visit, the 2 groups were comparable in the number of antihypertensive drugs added or in the percentage of patients receiving
the highest dose of the study drug (57.4% in the ramipril vs
56.7% in the amlodipine group). After 32 months, 80.1% of
the patients in the ramipril group and 83.3% in the amlodipine group were still taking their study medications. During the
first 3 months of treatment GFR increased by 4.19 mL/min per
1.73 m^2/yr more in the amlodipine group than in the ramipril
group (p<0.001). However, the overall, mean GFR declined
by 2.07±0.21 mL/min per 1.73 m^2/year in the ramipril group
and by 3.22±0.33 mL/min per 1.73 m^2/year in the amlodipine group. The mean decline was 36% slower in the ramipril
group (p=0.002). Among patients with a urinary protein/cre-
atinine ratio of ≤0.22, mean GFR during the 3 years of follow-up declined by 1.02±0.25 mL/min per 1.73 m^2/year in the
ramipril and increased by 0.20±0.39 ml/min per 1.73 m^2/year
in the amlodipine group. Therefore, the decline in GFR was
1.22±0.44 mL/min per 1.73 m^2/year faster in the ramipril than
in the amlodipine group (p=0.006). In contrast, among patients
with urinary protein/creatinine ratio of >0.22, GFR declined
by 3.60±0.34 mL/min per 1.73 m^2/year in the ramipril and by
5.62±0.65 mL/min per 1.73 m^2/year in the amlodipine group.
Therefore, the total decline was 2.02±0.74 mL/min per 1.73
m^2/year (36%) slower in the ramipril than in the amlodipine
group (p=0.006). The total mean GFR decline was 0.97±0.47
mL/min per 1.73 m^2/year faster in the ramipril than in the
amlodipine group for patients with baseline GFR ≥40 mL/min
per 1.73 m^2. In contrast, among patients with baseline GFR <40
mL/min per 1.73 m^2, the GFR decline was 1.61±0.62 mL/min
per 1.73 m^2/year faster in the amlodipine than in the ramipril

group. Reduction in GFR by 50% or by 25 mL/min per 1.73 m^2 from baseline occurred in a rate of 0.028 events per person-year in the ramipril group vs 0.038 events per person-year in the amlodipine group (41% RR reduction; 95% CI=5%-63%; p=0.03). End-stage renal disease occurred at a rate of 0.030 and 0.043 events per person-year, respectively (44% RR reduction; 95% CI=13-65%; p=0.01). Death occurred at a rate of 0.011 and 0.016 events per patient-year in the ramipril and amlodipine groups, respectively (31% RR reduction; 95% CI=-41 to 66%; p=0.31). The combined end point of death, 50% reduction in GFR or reduction by 25 ml/min per 1.73 m^2 from baseline or end-stage renal disease occurred at a rate of 0.058 and 0.077 events per patient-year, respectively (38% RR reduction; 95% CI=13-56%; p=0.005). Proteinuria increased by 58% in the amlodipine group and decreased by 20% in the ramipril group (p<0.001).

| Concl. | Initial antihypertensive treatment with ramipril was associated with slower rate of progression of renal dysfunction than amlodipine in patients with mild-to-moderate chronic renal failure associated with hypertension. |

AASK

African American Study of Kidney Disease and Hypertension

Title	Effect of blood pressure lowering and antihypertensive drug class on progression of hypertensive kidney disease.
Authors	Wright JT, Bakris G, Greene T, et al.
Reference	JAMA 2002;288:2421-2431.
Disease	Hypertension.
Purpose	To compare the effects of 2 different levels of blood pressure control and 3 different antihypertensive medication classes on the decline of glomerular filtration rate in patients with hypertension.
Design	Randomized, double-blind, 3 x 2 factorial, multicenter.
Patients	1094 African Americans, aged 18-70 years, with renal disease cause by hypertension (glomerular filtration rate [GFR] 20-65 mL/min per 1.73 m^2), and no other cause of renal insufficiency. Exclusion criteria included diastolic blood pressure <95 mm Hg, diabetes mellitus, urinary protein to creatinine ratio >2.5, malignant hypertension in the past 6 months, secondary hypertension, chronic kidney disease not related to blood pressure, and congestive heart failure.
Follow-up	3-6.4 years.
Regimen	Patients were randomized to a goal mean arterial pressure of 102-107 mm Hg or to the lower goal of mean arterial pressure ≤92 mm Hg. Patients were also randomized to 1 of 3 antihypertensive medications (sustained release metoprolol 50-200 mg/d; ramipril 2.5-10 mg/d; amlodipine, 5-10 mg/d). Failure to achieve the BP goal with the randomized medications allowed adding open-label medications such as furosemide, doxazosin, clonidine, and hydralazine or minoxidil.

Results   The primary outcome was the rate of change in GFR (the GFR slope). The GFR slope was determined once during the first 3 months following randomization (acute slope) and again after 3 months (chronic slope). The chronic slope and the total slope from study start (both acute and chronic phases counted) were considered co-primary outcomes. The secondary outcome was a composite clinical outcome of any of the following: confirmed reduction of GFR by 50% or 25 mL/min per 1.73 m^2 from the average of the 2 baseline GFR measurements, end stage renal disease (dialysis or transplantation), or death. Another secondary outcome was the urinary protein excretion, measured as the ratio of urinary protein to creatinine from a 24-hour collection. Patient characteristics between the 2 BP groups and the 3 medications groups were similar. After study start, the BP decreased from 152/96 mm Hg to 128/78 mm Hg in the lower BP group and from 149/95 to 141/85 in the usual BP group. A difference of approximately 10 mm Hg in the mean arterial pressure was kept throughout the follow-up. Patients in the lower BP group were more likely to receive more antihypertensives, but there were no differences between the drug groups in the total number of antihypertensive medications or the percentage of patients receiving the highest dose of study drug. For the acute phase, the mean decline of GFR was 1.82 mL/min per 1.73 m^2/3 mo greater in the lower BP group compared to the usual BP group (p<0.001). The mean decline of GFR was not significantly different between the lower and usual BP groups during the chronic period (2.11 vs 2.32 mL/min per 1.73 m^2/yr; p=0.33) or the entire follow-up period (2.21 vs 1.95 mL/min per 1.73 m^2/yr; p=0.24). Ramipril vs Metoprolol. The mean decline of GFR was slower in the ramipril group compared to the metoprolol group in the acute phase (0.23 vs 1.73 mL/min per 1.73 m^2/3 mo; p=0.01) and the total follow-up period (1.81 vs 2.42 mL/min per 1.73 m^2/yr; p=0.007). The mean GFR slopes in the chronic period were not different; (1.87 vs 2.12 mL/min per 1.73 m^2/yr; p=0.26). Amlodipine vs Metoprolol. In the acute phase, GFR increased faster in the amlodipine and decreased in the metoprolol group (4.03 vs -1.73 mL/min per 1.73 m^2/3 mo; p<0.001). However, in the chronic period, GFR declined faster in the amlodipine group compared to the metoprolol group (3.22 vs 2.33 mL/min per 1.73 m^2/yr; p=0.02). GFR decline up to 3 years was significantly slower in the amlodipine group compared to the metoprolol group (1.60 vs 2.68 mL/min per 1.73 m^2/yr; p=0.004). Lower vs Usual BP. The numbers of events concerning the main composite clinical outcome were 173 and 167 in the low and usual BP groups, respectively. Adjustment for prespecified covariates found no significant differences between the groups in the risk of the composite outcome (relative risk reduction [RR] with low BP goal: 2%; 95% CI=−22% to 21%; p=0.85), or any of the outcomes by themselves. Ramipril vs Metoprolol. During the entire follow-up, 126 patients in the ramipril group and 155 patients in the metoprolol group had a main clinical outcome; this represented an RR of 22% (95% CI=1%-38%; p=0.04). Similar reductions of risk were seen for the individual components of the composite outcome, but were not statistically significant. Metoprolol vs Amlodipine. By the termination of the amlodipine arm at 2-years follow-up, 117 patients and 59 patients in the metoprolol and amlodipine groups had had a main clinical outcome; this represented a nonsignificant RR of 20% (95% CI=−10 to 41%; p=0.17). Compared to the amlodipine group, the metoprolol group had a significantly reduced risk of ESRD or death (p=0.003) and ESRD alone (p<0.001). Proteinuria (defined as the geometric mean of urinary protein to creatinine ratio) was increased by 58% in the amlodipine group and decreased by 14% in the metoprolol group at 6 months (p<0.001). Proteinuria was increased by 7% in the usual BP group and decreased by 17% in the lower BP group at 6 months. The percentage change in the geometric mean proteinuria at 4 years was significantly lower in the BP group compared to the usual BP group (p<0.001) and significantly higher in the amlodipine group compared to the other 2 drug groups (p<0.001). Proteinuria was slightly lower in the ramipril group compared to the metoprolol group at 4-years follow-up (p=0.06). There were no significant differences between the groups in all cause death, cardiovascular mortality, or first cardiovascular events.

| Concl. | The lower BP goal did not show any apparent additional benefit in retarding progression of hypertensive nephrosclerosis. Angiotensin-converting enzyme inhibitors were more effective in slowing decline of GFR compared to β-blockers or dihydropyridine calcium channel blockers. |

ABC Trial

Association of Black Cardiologists

Title	Evaluation of candesartan cilexetil in black patients with systemic hypertension: the ABC trial.
Authors	The Association of Black Cardiologists Candesartan Study Group.
Reference	Heart Disease 2000;2:392-399.
Disease	Hypertension.
Purpose	To address previous reports suggesting that drugs that block the renin-angiotensin-aldosterone system are not effective in black hypertensives.
Design	Randomized, double-blind, placebo-controlled, multicenter.
Patients	304 hypertensive black patients with a mean sitting diastolic blood pressure of 91 to 105 mm Hg.
Follow-up	≈19-20 weeks.
Regimen	1 week washout period if necessary; 4-5 week single-blind, placebo run-in phase; a 12-week double-blind treatment period; a 2-week follow-up period. Treatment was initiated with either candesartan cilexetil 16 mg or placebo once daily. At week 4 or 8 patients could be up-titrated to 32 mg once daily. Uncontrolled patients on candesartan 32 mg at week 8 had 12.5 mg hydrochlorothiazide added, as did placebo patients who remained uncontrolled. 156 patients randomized to candesartan; 148 to placebo.

Results	Primary measure was change in trough sitting diastolic blood pressure from end of placebo run-in period to end of double-blind period at week 8. Candesartan cilexetil 16 mg to 32 mg was more effective in reducing blood pressure (-5.1 mm Hg) than placebo (-2.7 mm Hg; p=0.024). At week 8 systolic blood pressure was also lower in the candesartan group (-6.4mm Hg) than the placebo group (-1.3 mm Hg; p=0.004). At 12 weeks, candesartan was more effective than placebo even with the addition of hydrochlorothiazide to 27% and 50% of patients in candesartan and placebo groups, respectively. At 12 weeks, candesartan reduced systolic/diastolic pressure by 9.3/7.5 mm Hg vs placebo at 5.7/5.2 mm Hg (p=0.062 for systolic and p=0.044 for diastolic). At 8 weeks, 40% of candesartan vs 21% of placebo had diastolic blood pressures that were controlled; at 12 weeks these numbers were 42% vs 33%. Adverse events and discontinuation rates were similar between the 2 groups.
Concl.	Candesartan cilexetil was effective in reducing blood pressure in a substantial proportion of black hypertensive patients; combination with hydrochlorothiazide further improved efficacy.

ARIC

Atherosclerosis Risk in Communities

Title	Hypertension and antihypertensive therapy as risk factors for type II diabetes mellitus.
Authors	Gress TW, Nieto J, Shahar E, et al.
Reference	N Engl J Med 2000;342:905-912.
Disease	Hypertension.
Purpose	To determine whether there was a relationship between antihypertensive medications and the development of type II diabetes mellitus.
Design	Prospective, multicenter, cohort study.
Patients	12,550 adults, 45-64 years of age without diabetes at the start of the study.
Follow-up	6 years.
Regimen	The categories for treatment of those with hypertension included ACE inhibitors, β-blockers, calcium channel antagonists, and thiazide diuretics.
Results	3804 patients had hypertension and 8746 did not have hypertension at baseline. 569 new cases of diabetes occurred in subjects with hypertension and 577 occurred in patients without hypertension. Thus there were 29.1 new cases of diabetes per 1000 person-years among patients with hypertension and 12.0 per 1000 person-years in patients without hypertension (RR 2.43; 95% CI=2.16-2.73). Much of the risk of developing diabetes was due to hypertension (rather than to antihypertensive drugs alone). For patients not taking antihypertensive medicines, the risk of diabetes was higher among patients with hypertension vs those without hypertension. After adjusting for a number of variables, subjects on thiazide diuretics, ACE inhibitors, or calcium channel blockers were not at greater risk for developing diabetes than untreated hypertensives. However development of diabetes was 28% more likely to occur in subjects on β-blockers vs those not taking medicines (relative hazard = 1.28; 95% CI=1.04-1.57).

Concl.   Type II diabetes is about 2.5 times as likely to develop in subjects with hypertension vs those that are normotensive. After taking into account the increased risk of diabetes among hypertensives, β-blockers but not thiazide diuretics, ACE inhibitors, or calcium blockers were associated with an increased risk of developing diabetes.

CANDLE

Candesartan vs Losartan Efficacy Comparison Study

Title	Comparative effects of candesartan cilexetil and losartan in patients with systemic hypertension.
Authors	Gradman A, Lewin A, Bowling BT, et al.
Reference	Heart Disease 1999;1:52-57.
Disease	Hypertension.
Purpose	To compare the efficacy of 2 angiotensin receptor blockers: candesartan cilexetil vs losartan in patients with hypertension.
Design	Multicenter, randomized, double-blind, parallel group, titration to effect.
Patients	332 patients with hypertension. Diastolic sitting blood pressure of 95-114 mm Hg as entry criteria.
Follow-up	8 weeks.
Regimen	Candesartan (16-32 mg) vs losartan (50-100 mg) daily.
Results	Candesartan was more effective than losartan in lowering blood pressure. Trough sitting diastolic blood pressure at 8 weeks was reduced by -11.0 mm Hg with candesartan vs -8.9 mm Hg with losartan. Responder rates (sitting diastolic blood pressure <90 mm Hg or reduction in blood pressure ≥10 mm Hg) were higher with candesartan (64%) vs losartan (54%). 1.9% of patients taking candesartan and 6.5% taking losartan discontinued the study prematurely because of lack of efficacy or adverse events.
Concl.	Candesartan was more effective than losartan in reducing blood pressure in this hypertensive cohort.

CASTLE

Candesartan and Amlodipine for Safety, Tolerability and Efficacy

Title	Comparative effects of candesartan cilexetil and amlodipine in patients with mild systemic hypertension.
Authors	Kloner RA, Weinberger M, MD, Pool JL, et al.
Reference	Am J Cardiol 2001;87:727-731.
Disease	Hypertension.
Purpose	To compare the efficacy and tolerability of amlodipine and candesartan in patients with mild hypertension.
Design	Randomized, double-blind, parallel-group, forced-titration, multicenter.
Patients	251 patients with mild hypertension (a mean sitting diastolic blood pressure of 90-99 mm Hg).
Follow-up	8 weeks.
Regimen	Randomization to candesartan cilexetil (16 mg/d) (n=123) or amlodipine (5 mg/d) (n=128). At week 4 visit, the drug dose was doubled.

Results	3.3% of the patients in the candesartan group and 9.4% of the patients in the amlodipine group discontinued treatment prematurely. Both drugs were equally effective in reducing blood pressure. At the end of the study trough, sitting systolic blood pressure was decreased by 15.2 mm Hg in the candesartan group and 15.4 mm Hg in the amlodipine group (p=0.88), and trough diastolic blood pressure by 10.2 mm Hg and 11.3 mm Hg, respectively (p=0.25). 79% of the patients receiving candesartan and 87% of the patients receiving amlodipine reached the goal of diastolic blood pressure <90 mm Hg. Peripheral edema was more common with amlodipine (22.1% vs 8.9%; p=0.005). However, only 1.6% of the patients in the amlodipine and zero in the candesartan group discontinued the study medication because of edema. ≥1 treatment adverse event occurred in 66.7% of the patients in the candesartan group vs 60.2% in the amlodipine group. Fatigue was reported by 1.6% of the patients in the amlodipine vs 8.9% of the patients in the candesartan group, headache by 7.0% and 6.5%, respectively, dizziness in 3.9% and 6.5%, respectively, diarrhea by 2.3% and 6.5%, respectively, and sinusitis by 0.8% and 5.7%, respectively. 4.7% of the patients in the amlodipine group vs 2.4% of the patients in the candesartan group discontinued the study because of adverse events.
Concl.	Amlodipine and candesartan cilexetil were equally effective in controlling blood pressure in patients with mild hypertension. Amlodipine was associated with a greater risk of developing peripheral edema; however, in most cases the edema was not severe enough to stop the medicine.

COOPERATE

Combination Treatment of Angiotensin-II Receptor Blocker and Angiotensin-Converting-Enzyme Inhibitor in Non-Diabetic Renal Disease

Title	Combination treatment of angiotensin-II receptor blocker and angiotensin-converting-enzyme inhibitor in non-diabetic renal disease (COOPERATE): a randomised controlled trial.
Authors	Nakao N, Yoshimura A, Morita H, et al.
Reference	Lancet 2003;361:117-124.
Disease	Non-diabetic renal disease.
Purpose	To compare the efficacy and safety of 3 regimens: an angiotensin-II receptor blocker, an angiotensin-converting enzyme inhibitor, and their combination on renal survival in patients with non-diabetic renal disease.
Design	Randomized, double-blind, single-center.
Patients	301 patients, 18-70 years old, with non-diabetic chronic renal disease (serum creatinine 133-398 μmol/L or GFR of 20-70 mL/min per 1.73 m^2). Patients with diabetes mellitus, overt heart failure, allergic reaction to the study medications, immediate need for renal replacement therapy, treatment-resistant edema, corticosteroid, NSAID, or immunosuppressive treatment were excluded. In addition, patients with >10 g/d proteinuria, hypoalbuminemia, renovascular hypertension, malignant hypertension, myocardial infarction or stroke in the preceding year, severe peripheral vascular disease, chronic hepatic disease, chronic lung disease, and obstructive uropathy were not included.
Follow-up	3 years.
Regimen	Patients entered a single-blind, 18-week, run-in phase of trandolapril therapy, then 3-week wash-out period. 263 patients were randomized to losartan 100 mg/d (n=89); trandolapril 3 mg/d (n=86), or their combination (n=88).

Add'l Tx	Nonstudy ACE inhibitors and angiotensin receptor blockers were prohibited. All patients received antihypertensive therapy to reduce BP to <130/80 mm Hg.
Results	9% of the patients reported adverse effects during the run-in phase. The primary end point of the study (doubling of serum creatinine or end-stage renal disease) was reached by 23%, 23%, and 11% of the patients in the trandolapril, losartan, and the combination group, respectively. The hazard ratio (HR) of the combination group vs trandolapril was 0.38 (95% CI=0.18-0.63; p=0.018), and vs losartan 0.40 (95% CI=0.17-0.69; p=0.016). Frequency of side effects with the combination therapy was comparable with the trandolapril and losartan groups.
Concl.	Combination therapy with losartan and trandolapril was safe and retarded progression of non-diabetic renal disease compared to single therapy with losartan or trandolapril.

DASH

Dietary Approaches to Stop Hypertension—
(Reduced Dietary Sodium Study)

Title	Effects on blood pressure of reduced dietary sodium and the dietary approaches to stop hypertension (DASH) diet.
Authors	Sacks FM, Svetkey LP, Vollmer WM, et al.
Reference	N Engl J Med 2001;344:3-10.
Disease	Hypertension.
Purpose	To determine whether reducing the level of sodium from average intake (150 mmol per day—equivalent to 3.5 g of sodium or 8.7 g of sodium chloride) to below 100 mmol per day would further lower blood pressure. To assess the effects of various levels of sodium reduction in patients on standard vs DASH diet.
Design	Multicenter, randomized.
Patients	412 participants with blood pressures exceeding 120/80 mm Hg including patients with Stage 1 hypertension—140-159 mm Hg/90-95 mm Hg.
Follow-up	Outcome at end of each 30-day period of dietary intervention.
Regimen	Participants randomized to 1 of 2 diets: 1) Control diet, typical of U.S. diet; and 2) DASH diet—emphasizing fruits, vegetables, lowfat dairy foods; includes whole grains, poultry, fish, nuts; smaller amounts of red meat, sweets, sugar-containing beverages than found in typical U.S. diet. Participants ate assigned diet at each of the 3 sodium levels for 30 days in random order and then crossed over. Participants received 1 of 3 sodium levels: High (target of 150 mmol per day and energy of 2100 Kcal, which reflects typical U.S. diet), Intermediate (target of 100 mmol per day, upper limit of current national recommendations) and Low (target of 50 mmol per day).

Results	Primary outcome was systolic blood pressure at end of 30-day period of dietary intervention and secondary outcome was diastolic blood pressure. Reduction in sodium intake from High to Intermediate decreased systolic blood pressure by 2.1 mm Hg ($p<0.001$) on control diet and 1.3 mm Hg ($p=0.03$) on DASH diet. Reduction in sodium intake from Intermediate to Low caused further reduction of 4.6 mm Hg on control diet ($p<0.001$) and 1.7 mm Hg on DASH diet ($p<0.001$). The effect of sodium reduction was observed in men, women, whites, blacks, in participants with and without hypertension. There were also reductions in diastolic blood pressure with sodium lowering. On control diet diastolic blood pressure fell significantly between high-sodium and low-sodium phase (-3.5 mm Hg; $p<0.001$); on the DASH diet it fell by -1.6 mm Hg; ($p<0.001$). The DASH diet was associated with a lower systolic blood pressure at any given sodium level, compared to the control diet. At high sodium level, the DASH diet had a mean systolic pressure that was 5.9 mm Hg lower than the control diet ($p<0.001$).
Concl.	Reducing sodium intake to levels below current recommendations of 100 mmol per day and DASH diet both lower blood pressure substantially, with greater effects in combination.

DRASTIC

Dutch Renal Artery Stenosis Intervention Cooperative Study

Title	The effect of balloon angioplasty on hypertension in atherosclerotic renal artery stenosis.
Authors	Van Jaarsveld BC, Krijnen P, Pieterman H, et al.
Reference	N Engl J Med 2000;342:1007-1014.
Disease	Hypertension, atherosclerotic renal artery stenosis.
Purpose	To determine the effect of balloon angioplasty vs antihypertensive therapy on hypertension associated with atherosclerotic renal artery stenosis in patients with mild or only mildly impaired renal function.
Design	Randomized, controlled, multicenter
Patients	106 patients with hypertension and angiographically documented atherosclerotic renal artery stenosis and serum creatinine of ≤2.3 mg/dL. Diastolic blood pressure had to be at least 95 mm Hg despite therapy with 2 antihypertensive drugs or an increase of at least 0.2 mg/dL in serum creatinine with an ACE inhibitor.
Follow-up	12 months.
Regimen	Antihypertensive drug therapy vs angioplasty. If after 3 months patients in the drug therapy group had a diastolic blood pressure that was 95 mm Hg or higher despite therapy with 3 or more drugs or if there was evidence of worsening renovascular disease, they underwent balloon angioplasty.
Add'l Tx	Aspirin in the angioplasty group.

Results	Primary outcome was systolic and diastolic blood pressure at 3 and 12 months. Other outcome measures included numbers and defined daily doses of drugs, the serum creatinine concentration as well as others. Baseline blood pressures were elevated to similar levels in the angioplasty group (179/104 mm Hg) and the drug-therapy group (180/103 mm Hg). At 3 months, blood pressure was 169±28/99±12 mm Hg in the angioplasty group (n=56), and 176±31/101±14 mm Hg in the drug group (n=50; p=NS). The number of defined daily doses of medicines in the angioplasty group was 2.1±1.3 vs the drug group at 3.2±1.5 (p<0.001). 22 patients in the drug-therapy group underwent angioplasty secondary to persistent hypertension despite therapy with 3 or more drugs or worsening renal function. At 12 months, by intention-to-treat analysis, there was no difference in systolic and diastolic blood pressure between the angioplasty group (160±26/93±13 mm Hg) vs the drug therapy group (163±25/96±10 mm Hg). The number of defined daily doses of medication was no longer significantly lower in the angioplasty vs drug therapy group at 12 months. However, at 12 months blood pressure control did improve in 38 of 56 patients in the angioplasty group (68%) vs 18 of 48 patients (38%) in the drug-therapy group (p=0.002). At 12 months there was no difference in serum creatinine or creatinine clearance between groups.
Concl.	Angioplasty has little advantage over antihypertensive drug therapy for the treatment of hypertension in patients with atherosclerotic renal artery stenosis.

IDNT

Irbesartan Diabetic Nephropathy Trial

Title	Renoprotective effect of the angiotensin-receptor antagonist irbesartan in patients with nephropathy due to type 2 diabetes.
Authors	Lewis EJ, Hunsicker LG, Clark WR, et al.
Reference	N Engl J Med 2001;345:851-860.
Disease	Hypertension, diabetic nephropathy.
Purpose	To determine whether the angiotensin II receptor blocker irbesartan slows the progression of nephropathy in patients with type 2 diabetes, independently of its blood pressure lowering effect.
Design	Randomized, double-blind, multicenter.
Patients	1715 hypertensive patients with nephropathy due to type 2 diabetes.
Follow-up	2.6 years.
Regimen	Patients were randomized to 1 of 3 regimens: irbesartan (75-300 mg per day), amlodipine (2.5-10 mg per day), or placebo.
Add'l Tx	Antihypertensive agents not including angiotensin-converting enzyme (ACE) inhibitors, angiotensin receptor blockers, or calcium channel blockers. Target blood pressure was systolic ≤135 mm Hg or 10 mm Hg lower than value at screening and diastolic blood pressure of 85 mm Hg or less.

Results   Mean arterial blood pressure was reduced in the losartan and amlodipine groups vs the placebo group by 3.3 mm Hg (p=0.001). Primary end point was the composite of doubling of base-line serum creatinine concentration, onset of end-stage renal disease (dialysis, renal transplant, serum creatinine concentration of at least 6.0 mg per deciliter), or death. Primary composite outcome occurred in 189 (32.6%) of irbesartan group; 233 (41.1%) of amlodipine group; and 222 (39.0%) of placebo group. Irbesartan resulted in a risk of achieving this primary composite end point that was 20% lower than in the placebo group (p=0.02) and 23% lower than in the amlodipine-treated patients (p=0.006). Doubling of serum creatinine occurred in 16.9%, 25.4%, and 23.7% of the irbesartan, amlodipine, and placebo groups respectively; the rate with irbesartan was 33% lower than placebo (p=0.003) and 37% lower than amlodipine (p<0.001). End-stage renal disease occurred in 14.2%, 18.3%, and 17.8%, respectively (23% lower RR with irbesartan than the other 2 groups; p=0.07). Benefits could not be explained by change in blood pressure. Rates of death or rates in composite cardiovascular events did not differ among groups. Patients on irbesartan had a 23% lower rate of hospitalization for CHF than placebo. Patients on amlodipine had a rate of nonfatal MI that was 41% lower than patients on placebo.

Concl.   The angiotensin II receptor blocker irbesartan decreased the progression of nephropathy in type 2 diabetic patients with hypertension. Its benefit could not be explained by lowering of blood pressure.

INSIGHT

International Nifedipine GITS Study: Intervention as a Goal in Hypertensive Treatment

Title	Morbidity and mortality in patients randomized to double-blind treatment with long-acting calcium channel blocker or diuretic in the International Nifedipine GITS study: Intervention as a Goal in Hypertensive Treatment (INSIGHT).
Authors	Brown, MJ, Palmer CR, Castaigne A, et al.
Reference	Lancet 2000;356:366-372.
Disease	Hypertension.
Purpose	To compare the effects of the once daily long acting calcium channel blocker, nifedipine GITS (gastrointestinal-transport system) with the diuretic combination co-amilozide (hydrochlorothiazide plus amiloride) on cardiovascular morbidity and mortality in high risk hypertensive patients.
Design	Prospective, randomized, double-blind, multicenter.
Patients	6321 patients, aged 55-80 years with blood pressure >150/95 mm Hg or >160 mm Hg systolic plus 1 additional cardiovascular risk factor beside hypertension.
Follow-up	>3 years.
Regimen	Nifedipine GITS (30 mg initially); or co-amilozide (hydrochlorothiazide 25 mg plus amiloride 2.5 mg, initially) with dose titration by dose doubling and if needed addition of atenolol or enalapril.

Results   Primary outcome was cardiovascular death, myocardial infarction, heart failure or stroke. 3/57 patients on nifedipine GITS completed 10,976 patient-years treatment; 3164 on co-amilozide completed 11,015 patient-years of treatment. 725 in the nifedipine group withdrew because of adverse events; 518 in the co-amilozide group withdrew because of adverse events. 255 patients in nifedipine group withdrew secondary to peripheral edema, but more patients on co-amilozide had metabolic disorders such as hypokalemia, hyponatremia, hyperglycemia, hyperuricemia, and renal impairment. Serious adverse events were more frequent in the co-amilozide group (880) vs the nifedipine group (796; p=0.02). Mean blood pressure fall was comparable between the 2 groups falling from 173/99 mm Hg to 138/82 mm Hg. The primary outcome did not differ between groups: 200 (6.3%) in the nifedipine group vs 182 (5.8%) in the co-amilozide group; with 18.2 events per 1000 patient-years in the nifedipine group vs 16.5 for co-amilozide; RR 1.10; 95% CI=0.91-1.34; p=0.35.

Concl.   Long acting, once daily nifedipine and co-amilozide had similar efficacy on blood pressure lowering and the primary outcomes of cardiovascular death, myocardial infarction, heart failure, or stroke.

IRMA II

Irbesartan in Patients with Type 2 Diabetes and Microalbuminuria Study II

Title	The effect of irbesartan on the development of diabetic nephropathy in patients with type 2 diabetes.
Authors	Parving H-H, Lehnert H, Bröchner-Mortensen J, et al.
Reference	N Engl J Med 2001;345:870-878.
Disease	Hypertension, diabetes, microalbuminuria.
Purpose	To determine whether irbesartan protects the kidneys in hypertensive patients with type 2 diabetes and microalbuminuria.
Design	Randomized, double-blind, placebo-controlled, multicenter.
Patients	590 hypertensive patients with type 2 diabetes and microalbuminuria (albumin excretion of 20-200 mg per minute) and serum creatinine of no greater than 1.5 mg per deciliter for men or 1.1 mg per deciliter for women.
Follow-up	2 years.
Regimen	Irbesartan 150 mg daily, irbesartan 300 mg once daily, or matching placebo.
Add'l Tx	Diuretics, β-blockers, calcium channel blockers other than dihydropyridines, and α-blockers.

Results	Primary outcome was time to onset of diabetic nephropathy (urinary albumin excretion rate in overnight specimen greater than 200 mg/min and at least 30% higher than on baseline for 2 consecutive visits). 10 of 194 patients (5.2%) in the 300 mg irbesartan group, 19/195 (9.7%) in the 150 mg irbesartan group vs 30/201 (14.9%) of the placebo patients reached the primary outcome (hazard ratio 0.30 [95% CI=0.14-0.61; p<0.001] for 300 mg irbesartan and 0.61 [95% CI=0.34-1.08; p=0.08] for 150 mg group vs placebo). Blood pressure during the study was 144/83 mm Hg, 143/83 mm Hg, and 141/83 mm Hg in the placebo, 150 mg, and 300 mg irbesartan group, respectively (p=0.004 systolic blood pressure in placebo vs combined irbesartan groups). Irbesartan reduced the level of urinary albumin excretion throughout the study (24% reduction in the 150 mg group and 38% reduction in the 300 mg group) vs 2% in the placebo group (p<0.001). High dose irbesartan restored normo-albuminuria. Serious adverse events were less frequent in the irbesartan group. Nonfatal cardiovascular events occurred in 4.5% of the irbesartan 300 mg group vs 8.7% in the placebo group (p=0.11).
Concl.	Irbesartan was renoprotective and prevented the development of diabetic nephropathy in hypertensive patients with diabetes and microalbuminuria.

LIFE

Losartan Intervention for End Point Reduction

Title	Cardiovascular morbidity and mortality in the Losartan Intervention For Endpoint reduction in hypertension study (LIFE): a randomised trial against atenolol
Authors	Dahlöf B, Devereux RB, Kjeldsen S, et al.
Reference	Lancet 2002;359:995-1003.
Disease	Hypertension.
Purpose	To compare the long-term effects of atenolol and losartan on cardiovascular mortality and morbidity in hypertensive patients with left ventricular hypertrophy (LVH).
Design	Randomized, double-blind, double-dummy, multicenter.
Patients	9193 patients, 55-80 years old, with hypertension and ECG signs of LVH. Patients with secondary hypertension; stroke, or myocardial infarction within the preceding 6 months; treatment with β-blockers or calcium channel blockers for angina pectoris; LV ejection fraction ≤40%; heart failure; or need for treatment with an angiotensin II receptor antagonist, angiotensin-converting enzyme inhibitors, hydrochlorothiazide, or blockers were excluded. Patients were enrolled only if after 1-2 weeks of placebo sitting blood pressure was 160-200/95-115 mm Hg.
Follow-up	≥4 years (mean 4.8±0.9 years).
Regimen	Randomization to losartan 50 mg (n=4605) or atenolol 50 mg (n=4588). Dose was increased to 100 mg/d and hydrochlorothiazide was added if blood pressure remained ≥140/90 mm Hg.
Add'l Tx	Other antihypertensive drugs were added if blood pressure remained ≥140/90 mm Hg despite 100 mg/d of losartan or atenolol and 25 mg/d hydrochlorothiazide.

Results 84% of the losartan group and 80% of the atenolol group remained on study drug throughout the study. Mean doses of losartan were 82±24 mg/d and atenolol 79±26 mg/d. Sitting systolic blood pressure at the end of follow-up was reduced by 30.2±18.5 mm Hg in the losartan group and by 29.1±19.2 mm Hg in the atenolol group (p=0.017). Sitting diastolic blood pressure was reduced by 16.6±10.1 mm Hg and 16.8±10.1 mm Hg, respectively (p=0.37). 49% of the patients in the losartan group and 46% in the atenolol group reached systolic blood pressure ≤140 mm Hg, and 89% of the patients in each group reached diastolic blood pressure ≤90 mm Hg. Cardiovascular mortality was 4% in the losartan group and 5% in the atenolol group (adjusted hazard ratio [HR] 0.89; 95% CI=0.73-1.07; p=0.206). Stroke occurred in 5% and 7%, respectively (HR 0.75; 95% CI=0.63-0.89; p=0.001). Myocardial infarction occurred in 4% and 4%, respectively (p=0.491). The primary end point of cardiovascular mortality, stroke, or myocardial infarction occurred in 11% of the patients in the losartan group and in 13% in the atenolol group (adjusted HR 0.87; 95% CI=0.77-0.98; p=0.021). Total mortality was 8% and 9%, respectively (p=0.128). Hospital admissions for angina pectoris (3% vs 3%; p=0.212) or heart failure (3% vs 4%; p=0.765) were comparable. There were no differences between the groups in the rates of revascularization (6% vs 6%; p=0.441) and resuscitated cardiac arrest (0.2% vs 0.1%; p=0.250). However, new-onset diabetes mellitus occurred less often in the losartan group (6%) than in the atenolol group (8%; p=0.001). Discontinuation as the result of adverse events, drug-related adverse events, and serious adverse events were more common in the atenolol group than in the losartan group. ECG scores of LVH (the Cornell voltage-duration product and the Sokolow-Lyon voltage) were reduced more in the losartan than atenolol group (p<0.0001 for both scores).

Concl. Losartan was more effective than atenolol in preventing the combined end point of cardiovascular death, stroke, and myocardial infarction. Losartan significantly reduced the rates of stroke compared to atenolol and tended to reduce cardiovascular mortality and total mortality.

LIFE

Losartan Intervention for End Point Reduction (Substudy)

Title	Effects of losartan on cardiovascular morbidity and mortality in patients with isolated systolic hypertension and left ventricular hypertrophy.
Authors	Kjeldsen SE, Dahlof B, Devereux RB, et al.
Reference	JAMA 2002;288:1491-1498.
Disease	Hypertension.
Purpose	To determine whether use of losartan is superior to atenolol in reducing CV morbidity and mortality in patients with isolated systolic hypertension and left ventricular hypertrophy.
Design	Substudy of a double-blind, randomized, prospective, multi-center.
Patients	1326 patients, age 55-80 (mean 70 years) who had systolic BP of 160-200 mm Hg and diastolic BP <90 mm Hg and ECG evidence of left ventricular hypertrophy (LVH).
Follow-up	Mean 4.7 years.
Regimen	As per LIFE.
Add'l Tx	As per LIFE.

Results   The primary study end point was a composite of cardiovascular death, stroke, and MI. Other measured outcomes were: angina pectoris, heart failure, resuscitated coronary or peripheral revascularization procedures, cardiac arrest, and new-onset diabetes mellitus. Mean BP reductions were similar in the 2 groups. Blood pressure <140/90 mm Hg was achieved for 44.4% in the losartan group and 42.9% in the atenolol group. The primary end point occurred at a rate of 25.1 events/patient-year in the losartan group vs 35.4/1000 patient-years in the atenolol group; this represented a 25% relative risk (RR) reduction and was statistically significant: (unadjusted RR 0.71; 95% CI=0.53-0.95, p=0.02). When the RR was adjusted for degree of LVH and baseline Framingham risk score, the risk reduction was no longer statistically significant (adjusted RR 0.75; 95% CI=0.56-1.01; p=0.06). Among the other measured outcomes there were significant reductions in CV mortality (adjusted RR 0.54; CI=0.34-0.87; p=0.01), stroke (adjusted RR 0.60; CI=0.38-0.92; p=0.02), total mortality (adjusted RR 0.72; CI=0.53-1.00; p=0.046) and new-onset diabetes (adjusted RR 0.62; CI=0.40-0.97; p=0.04) in the losartan group. The end point of MI between the 2 groups was not statistically significant (adjusted RR 0.89; CI=0.55-1.44; p=0.64). There was a trend toward benefit for losartan in the other measured outcomes (hospitalization for either angina or heart failure, and revascularization) but these were not statistically significant. Both agents reduced ECG evidence of LVH, but losartan did so to a greater degree.

Concl.   In patients with isolated systolic hypertension and ECG evidence of LVH, losartan-based anti-hypertensive therapy was more effective than atenolol-based therapy in reducing the incidence of stroke, CV death, and new-onset diabetes.

LIFE (Diabetes Mellitus Substudy)

Losartan Intervention for End Point Reduction

Title	Cardiovascular morbidity and mortality in patients with diabetes in the Losartan Intervention For Endpoint reduction in hypertension study (LIFE): a randomised trial against atenolol.
Authors	Lindholm LH, Ibsen H, Dahlöf B, et al.
Reference	Lancet 2002;359:1004-1010.
Disease	Hypertension, diabetes mellitus.
Purpose	To compare the long-term effects of atenolol and losartan on cardiovascular mortality and morbidity in hypertensive patients with left ventricular hypertrophy (LVH) and diabetes mellitus on enrollment for the study.
Design	Randomized, double-blind, double-dummy, multicenter.
Patients	1195 patients, 55-80 years old, with hypertension and ECG signs of LVH, and diabetes mellitus. For inclusion and exclusion criteria see the main LIFE study.
Follow-up	≥4 years (mean 4.7±1.1 years).
Regimen	Randomization to losartan 50 mg (n=586) or atenolol 50 mg (n=609). Dose was increased to 100 mg/d and hydrochlorothiazide was added if blood pressure remained ≥140/90 mm Hg.

Results   Cardiovascular mortality was 6% in the losartan group and 10% in the atenolol group (adjusted hazard ratio [HR] 0.63; 95% CI=0.42-0.95; p=0.028). Stroke occurred in 9% and 11% of the patients, respectively (0.79; 95% CI=0.55-1.14; p=0.204), and myocardial infarction in 7% and 8%, respectively (0.83; 95% CI=0.55-1.25; p=0.373). The composite end point of cardiovascular death, myocardial infarction, or stroke occurred in 18% of the patients in the losartan group vs 23% in the atenolol group (adjusted HR 0.76; 95% CI=0.58-0.98; p=0.031). Total mortality was 11% vs 17%, respectively (0.61; 95% CI=0.45-0.84; p=0.002). Hospital admissions for angina pectoris (5% vs 5%; p=0.828) and revascularization (11% vs 11%; p=0.533) were comparable. However, there were less hospital admissions for heart failure in the losartan group (5% vs 9%; p=0.019). At the end of the study more patients in the atenolol group (32%) than the losartan group (27%) stopped their study drug (p=0.076). The target systolic blood pressure of <140 mm Hg was reached by 38% of the patients in the losartan group vs 34% in the atenolol group. The target diastolic blood pressure of <90 mm Hg was reached by 85% of the patients in the losartan group vs 82% in the atenolol group. Albuminuria was noted in 7% vs 13%, respectively (p=0.002). Chest pain was reported by 12% vs 8% of patients, respectively (p=0.036).

Concl.   Losartan was more effective than atenolol in reducing total and cardiovascular mortality as well as the composite end point of cardiovascular morbidity and mortality, hospitalization for heart failure, and the risk of developing albuminuria in hypertensive patients with diabetes and ECG signs of LVH.

LIFE Substudy

Losartan Intervention for End Point Reduction in Hypertension

Title	Regression of electrocardiographic left ventricular hypertrophy by losartan vs atenolol. The Losartan Intervention for Endpoint Reduction in Hypertension (LIFE) study.
Authors	Chin PM, Devereux RB, Jern S, et al.
Reference	Circulation 2003;108:684-690.
Disease	Hypertension, left ventricular hypertrophy.
Purpose	To compare left ventricular hypertrophy regression in patients treated with losartan-based vs atenolol-based therapy.
Design	Prospective, double-blind, randomized.
Patients	Patients aged 55-80 years with untreated essential hypertension with a mean seated blood pressure of 160-200/95-115 mm Hg who did not have a myocardial infarction or stroke within 6 months and did not specifically require therapy with a β blocker, angiotensin-converting enzyme inhibitor, or angiotensin receptor blocker.
Follow-up	This study reports changes in electrocardiogram over 6 months up to 5 years.
Regimen	Blinded 50 mg losartan or 50 mg atenolol qd with a target blood pressure of ≤140/90 mm Hg. Hydrochlorothiazide 12.5 mg could be added, and doses of losartan or atenolol could be increased to 100 mg qd. Additional therapy as per LIFE protocol. Electrocardiograms were obtained at baseline, 6 months, and at 1-year intervals.

Results	Left ventricular hypertrophy (LVH) was assessed by Cornell product and Sokolow voltage criteria. At 6 months follow-up and adjusting for baseline, ECG LVH, pressures, and diuretic therapy, there was greater regression of LVH by both Cornell product -200 vs -69 mm · ms; p<0.001) and Sokolow-Lyon voltage criteria (-2.5 vs -0.7 mm; p<0.001) in the losartan vs the atenolol based therapy group. This greater regression in LVH in the losartan group persisted throughout the study with greater mean reductions of 140 to 164 mm · ms by the Cornell product and 1.7-2.2 mm greater reductions in Sokolow-Lyon voltage (p<0.001).
Concl.	Losartan resulted in greater ECG evidence of LVH regression than atenolol.

MARVAL

Microalbuminuria Reduction with Valsartan

Title	MARVAL: Microalbuminuria Reduction with Valsartan in patients with type 2 diabetes mellitus: a blood pressure independent effect.
Authors	Viberti G, Wheeldon NM; Micro Albuminuria Reduction With VALsartan (MARVAL) Study Investigators.
Reference	Circulation 2002;106:672-678.
Disease	Diabetes mellitus; hypertension.
Purpose	To determine the effect, independent of blood pressure, of valsartan on urine albumin excretion in type 2 diabetes patients who have microalbuminuria.
Design	Randomized, double-blind, active control, multicenter.
Patients	Patients were 35-75 years of age, with type 2 diabetes, and persistent microalbuminuria (median urine albumin excretion [UAER] of 3 timed overnight urine collections between 20-200 mg/min during the 5 weeks before study entry). Other inclusion criteria were normal serum creatinine level and BP at baseline <180/105 mm Hg. Patients were excluded if they had type 1 diabetes (onset <35 years of age and on insulin within the first year); use of angiotensin-converting enzyme inhibitors, angiotensin receptor blockers and calcium channel blockers within the 5 weeks before study entry; childbearing potential for women; heart failure in the prior 6 months necessitating use of an ACE inhibitor; history of myocardial infarction, percutaneous transluminal coronary angioplasty or cerebrovascular accident within the prior 3 months; severe diabetic neuropathy; history of hypertensive or hepatic encephalopathy; and hepatic disease.
Follow-up	24 weeks.

Regimen	5 weeks before study entry, patients on any calcium channel blockers, ACE inhibitors, or angiotensin receptor blockers were taken off those medications and switched to non-potassium-sparing diuretics for BP control during this run-in period. Other antihypertensive drugs were continued during this period. Hypertension was defined as BP ≥140/90 mm Hg and/or antihypertensive therapy at baseline. After the run-in period, all antihypertensive treatments were withdrawn, and patients were randomized to 80 mg/d valsartan (n=169) or 5 mg/d amlodipine (n=163) for 24 weeks. The target BP was 135/85 mm Hg. Doses of either medication could be doubled at week 4 if BP control was not adequate. Starting at week 8, 2.5 mg/d of bendrofluazide could be added and doxazosin from week 12 as necessary to control BP.
Results	The primary end point was the percent change of UAER from study start to week 24. The secondary end point was the proportion of patients who returned to normal albuminuria status (UAER <20 mg/min at last visit). The UAER at the end of the study was 56% of baseline on valsartan (95% CI=49.6%-63.0%), a 44% reduction. UAER at study finish on amlodipine was 92% of baseline (95% CI=81.7%-103.7%), an 8% reduction. The difference of effect on UAER between the 2 medications was significant ($p<0.001$; 95% CI=0.520-0.710). Similar treatment effects were seen regardless of whether patients were hypertensive or normotensive at baseline: change in UAER in hypertensive subgroup $p<0.001$; 95% CI=0.482-0.737; change in normotensive subgroup $p<0.001$; 95% CI=0.486-0.772. Reductions in BP were similar between the 2 groups; there was no time during the study when there was a significant difference in either the systolic or diastolic BP between the groups. The effect of treatment on UAER remained significant after adjustment for changes in BP, which indicated that valsartan lowered UAER independent of its BP-lowering effect. The proportion of patients who returned to normal albuminuria was greater in the valsartan group than the amlodipine group (29.9% vs 14.5%, difference 15.4%; 95% CI=5.6-25.8; $p<0.001$).
Concl.	Valsartan was more effective than amlodipine in decreasing urine albumin excretion and re-establishing normal albuminuric status in type 2 diabetics with microalbuminuria. These effects were independent of the decrease in BP.

NORDIL

Nordic Diltiazem Study

Title	Randomized trial of effects of calcium antagonists compared with diuretics and β-blockers on cardiovascular morbidity and mortality in hypertension. The Nordic Diltiazem Study.
Authors	Hansson L, Hedner T, Lund-Johansen P, et al.
Reference	Lancet 2000: 356:359-365.
Disease	Hypertension.
Purpose	To compare diltiazem with diuretics, β-blockers, or both on cardiovascular morbidity and mortality in middle-aged hypertensive patients.
Design	Prospective, randomized, open trial with blinded end point evaluation (PROBE).
Patients	10,881 patients aged 56-74 years with diastolic blood pressure of 100 mm Hg or more.
Follow-up	Mean of 4.5 years.
Regimen	Diltiazem (n=5410) given as 180-360 mg daily vs diuretics, β-blockers, or both (n=5471).
Add'l Tx	Additional antihypertensives could be added to lower diastolic blood pressure <90 mm Hg, including ACE inhibitor, diuretic, and/or α blocker.

Results   The primary combined end point was fatal and nonfatal stroke, fatal and nonfatal myocardial infarction, and other cardiovascular death. Mean blood pressure during the study was 154.9/88.6 mm Hg with diltiazem and 151.7/88.7 mm Hg with diuretic/β-blocker. Decrease in diastolic pressure was the same between groups (-18.7 mm Hg) and the decrease in systolic pressure was greater in the diuretic and β-blocker group (-23.3) vs the diltiazem group (-20.3; p<0.001). The primary end point occurred with equal frequency in both groups (403 patients in the diltiazem group; 16.6 events per 1000 patient-years; 400 patients in the diuretic and β-blocker group (16.2 events per 1000 patient-years; RR 1.00; 95% CI=0.87-1.15; p=0.97). The incidence of fatal plus nonfatal stroke was lower in the diltiazem group (159) vs the diuretic and β-blocker group (196); 6.4 vs 7.9 events per 1000 patient-years; RR 0.80; 95% CI=0.65-0.99; p=0.04. The incidence of fatal and nonfatal myocardial infarction did not differ significantly between groups (183 in diltiazem; 157 in diuretic and β-blocker group; 7.4 vs 6.3 events per 1000 patient-years; RR 1.16; 95% CI=0.94-1.44; p=0.17).

Concl.   Therapy based vs diltiazem vs diuretics, β-blockers, or both was effective in lowering blood pressure; both were equally effective in preventing the combined end point of stroke, myocardial infarction, cardiovascular death.

PROGRESS

Perindopril Protection Against Recurrent Stroke Study

Title	Randomised trial of a perindopril-based blood-pressure-lowering regimen among 6105 individuals with previous stroke or transient ischaemic attack.
Authors	PROGRESS Collaborative Group.
Reference	Lancet 2001;358:1033-1041.
Disease	Stroke.
Purpose	To study the efficacy and safety of blood pressure lowering with perindopril (an angiotensin-converting enzyme [ACE] inhibitor) and indapamide (a diuretic) in patients with a history of stroke or transient ischemic attack.
Design	Randomized, double-blind, placebo-controlled, multicenter.
Patients	6105 patients with a history of stroke or transient ischemic attack within the previous 5 years. Patients with definite indications (such as heart failure) or contraindications to ACE inhibitors were not included.
Follow-up	An average of 3.9 years.
Regimen	After 4-week run-in period with open-label perindopril 4 mg/d, patients were randomized to continue active treatment with perindopril (with or without the addition of indapamide) (n=3051) or to stop perindopril and start placebo (with or without placebo of indapamide) (n=3054).

Results	1770 patients received perindopril + indapamide, 1281 received perindopril alone, 1774 received double placebo, and 1280 received single placebo. 23% of the patients in the active treatment group and 21% in the placebo had prematurely discontinued study medications (p=0.02). Cough was noted in 2.2% and 0.4% of the patients in the active treatment and placebo groups, respectively, and hypotension in 2.1% and 0.9%, respectively. Blood pressure was reduced by 9.0/4.0 mm Hg in the active treatment group, compared with the placebo group. The blood pressure reduction was 12.3/5.0 mm Hg in those treated with perindopril + indapamide and 4.9/2.8 mm Hg in those treated with perindopril alone. Stroke occurred in 10% of the patients in the active treatment group and in 14% in the placebo group (relative risk reduction 28%; 95% CI=17%-38%; p<0.0001). Major vascular events occurred in 15% and 20%, respectively (RR reduction 26%; 95% CI=16%-34%). There were no differences between the groups in total mortality, cardiovascular mortality, or noncardiovascular mortality. 41% of the patients on active treatment vs 44% in the placebo group were hospitalized (RR reduction 9%; 95% CI=1%-15%). Stroke occurred in 14.4% of the patients receiving double placebo vs 8.5% of the patients receiving perindopril + indapamide (RR reduction 43%; 95% CI=30%-54%). Stroke occurred in 12.9% of the patients receiving single placebo and in 12.3% of the patients receiving perindopril alone (RR reduction 5%; 95% CI=-19% to 23%). Major vascular events occurred in 20.7% of the patients receiving double placebo vs 13.1% of the patients receiving perindopril + indapamide (40% RR reduction; 95% CI=29%-49%). Major vascular events occurred in 18.5% of the patients receiving single placebo vs 17.7% of the patients receiving perindopril alone (4% RR reduction; 95% CI=-15% to 20%). The standardized reductions in the risk of stroke and major vascular events were comparable in magnitude among hypertensive and nonhypertensive patients. The combination therapy was superior to perindopril alone in both hypertensive and nonhypertensive patients.
Concl.	The combination therapy of perindopril + indapamide reduced the risk of stroke and major vascular events in both hypertensive and nonhypertensive patients with a history of stroke or transient ischemic attack, whereas single therapy with perindopril 4 mg/d was not effective.

PROGRESS (Substudy)

Perindopril Protection Against Recurrent Stroke Study

Title	Effects of a perindopril-based blood pressure-lowering regimen on cardiac outcomes among patients with cerebrovascular disease.
Authors	PROGRESS Collaborative Group.
Reference	Eur Heart J 2003;24:475-484.
Disease	Coronary heart disease.
Purpose	To evaluate the effects of lowering blood pressure with perindopril on major cardiac events among patients with a history of stroke.
Design	Analysis of the PROGRESS study (see above).
Patients	6105 patients (see above).
Follow-up	An average of 3.9 years.
Regimen	See above.

Results   Major coronary events (nonfatal MI or coronary heart disease
           death) occurred in 3.8% of the patients assigned active treat-
           ment and in 5.0% of those assigned placebo (risk ratio [RR]
           26%; 95% CI=6%-42%; p=0.02). The effect tended to be
           greater among those treated with both perindopril and indap-
           amide (RR 35%; 95% CI= 12%-52%) than in those receiving
           perindopril alone (RR 7%; 95% CI=-37% to 38%). However,
           the difference was not statistically significant (p for homogene-
           ity 0.2). Coronary events (major coronary events, revasculariza-
           tion or admission for an acute coronary syndrome) occurred in
           7.6% of the patients in the active treatment group and in 9.5%
           in the placebo group (RR 21%; 95% CI=6%-33%; p=0.008).
           Heart failure was diagnosed in 3.7% of the patients in the active
           treatment group vs 4.9% in the placebo group (RR 26%; 95%
           CI=5%-42%; p=0.02). The effect was more apparent among
           those receiving both perindopril and indapamide (RR 34%;
           95% CI=7%-53%) than in those receiving only perindopril
           (RR 16%; 95% CI=-19% to 41%). However, the difference was
           not statistically significant (p for homogeneity 0.3). For each of
           the outcomes, there was no difference in the treatment effect
           in patients with or without hypertension at enrollment and in
           patients with and without a history of CAD.

Concl.   Blood pressure lowering with perindopril and indapamide
           reduced the risks of cardiac events, as well as the risk of stroke.

RENAAL

Reduction of End Points in NIDDM with Angiotensin II Antagonist Losartan

Title	Effects of losartan on renal and cardiovascular outcomes in patients with type 2 diabetes and nephropathy.
Authors	Brenner BM, Cooper ME, de Zeeuw D, et al.
Reference	N Engl J Med 2001;345:861-869.
Disease	Type 2 diabetes and nephropathy; hypertension.
Purpose	To determine whether the angiotensin II receptor antagonist losartan, with or without conventional antihypertensive therapy, would lengthen the time to doubling of serum creatinine concentration, end-stage renal disease (ESRD), or death.
Design	Double-blind, randomized, placebo-controlled, multicenter.
Patients	1513 patients with type 2 diabetes and nephropathy. 92%-95% of patients were on antihypertensive medicines.
Follow-up	3.4 years.
Regimen	Patients were randomized to losartan (50-100 mg once-a-day) vs placebo; both taken with patients on the following standard antihypertensive regimen: calcium blocker, diuretics, α-blockers, centrally acting agents. Patients who had been on angiotensin-converting enzyme inhibitors or angiotensin receptor blockers were switched to the above alternative agents. Target blood pressure was a systolic blood pressure less than 140 mm Hg and diastolic less than 90 mm Hg.

Results   Primary efficacy measure was time to composite end point of doubling of serum creatinine, ESRD, or both. Trough blood pressure at baseline was 152/82 mm Hg with losartan and 153/82 mm Hg with placebo. At 1 year it was 146/78 mm Hg in the losartan group vs 150/80 mm Hg in the placebo group. Primary composite end point occurred in 327 patients with losartan (43.5%) vs 359 with placebo (47.1%); losartan resulting in a 16% decrease in the primary composite end point (p=0.02). This benefit remained unchanged after adjusting for blood pressure. Losartan decreased the incidence of doubling of serum creatinine concentration by 25% (p=0.006) as well as ESRD by 28% (p=0.002) but did not alter death rate. There were no differences in the rates of most cardiovascular end points with the exception of first hospitalization for heart failure (11.9% in the losartan group vs 16.7% in the placebo group; p=0.005). There was a nonsignificant reduction in myocardial infarction rates (6.7% with losartan vs 8.9% in the placebo group; p=0.08). Losartan decreased proteinuria by 35% (p<0.001).

Concl.   Losartan preserved renal function in patients with type 2 diabetes and nephropathy and decreased first hospitalizations for heart failure.

SHEP (Subanalysis)

Systolic Hypertension in the Elderly Program

Title	Effect of treating isolated systolic hypertension on the risk of developing various types and subtypes of stroke. The Systolic Hypertension in the Elderly Program (SHEP).
Authors	a. SHEP Cooperative Research Group. b. Kostis JB, Davis BR, Cutler J, et al. c. Ofili EO, Cohen JD, St. Vrain J, et al. d. Curb JD, Pressel SL, Cutler JA, et al. e. Savage PL, Precsel SL< Curb JD, et al. f. Perry HM Jr, Davis BR, Price TR, et. al.
Reference	a. JAMA 1991;265:3255-3264. b. JAMA 1997;278:212-216. c. JAMA 1998; 279:778-780. d. JAMA 1996;276:1886-1892. e. Arch Intern Med 1998;158:741-751. f. JAMA 2000;284:465-471.
Disease	Isolated systolic hypertension.
Purpose	SHEP previously demonstrated that treating isolated systolic hypertension in the elderly decreased the incidence of stroke. The purpose of this analysis was to assess the effects of drug treatment on incidence of stroke by type, subtype, timing of strokes, case fatality rates, and stroke residual effects.
Design	As per SHEP. Determination of types of strokes included brain imaging, lumbar puncture, carotid duplex studies, and autopsy.
Patients	4736 men and women aged 60 or older with isolated hypertension at 16 clinical centers in the US.
Follow-up	4.5 years.
Regimen	Randomized to 12.5 mg/d of chlorthalidone (Step 1); either 25 mg/d of atenolol or 0.05 mg/d of reserpine (Step 2) could be added vs placebo.

Results	85 of active treatment group and 132 patients in the placebo group had ischemic strokes (adjusted RR 0.63; 95% CI=0.48-0.82); 9 of the active therapy group and 19 in the placebo group had hemorrhagic strokes (RR 0.46; 95% CI=0.21-1.02); 9 of active therapy group and 8 in placebo group had strokes of unknown type. The types of ischemic strokes were categorized as lacunar (23 in active treatment group vs 43 in placebo group; RR 0.59; 95% CI=0.32-0.88); embolic (9 vs 16); atheroclerotic (13 vs 13); and unknown (40 vs 60; RR 0.64; 95% CI=0.43-0.96). The timing of decrease in stroke depended on type with a treatment effect observed within 1 year for hemorrhagic strokes but 2 years required for ischemic strokes. Decrease in stroke incidence occurred for patients reaching the SHEP goal of 20 mm Hg decrease in systolic BP to less than 160 mm Hg, in those reaching a systolic BP below 160 mm Hg, and systolic BP decrease of 10 mm Hg. Participants in active treatment group tended to have fewer days of reduced activity and days in bed.
Concl.	Treatment of isolated systolic hypertension in the elderly decreased incidence of both hemorrhagic and ischemic (including lacunar) strokes.

STOP-Hypertension-2 (Update)

Swedish Trial in Old Patients with Hypertension-2

Title	Randomised trial of old and new antihypertensive drugs in elderly patients: Cardiovascular mortality and morbidity. The Swedish Trial in Old Patients with Hypertension-2 study.
Authors	Hansson L, Lindholm LH, Ekbom T, et al.
Reference	a. Lancet 1999;354:1751-1756. b. Lancet 1991;1281-1285.
Disease	Hypertension.
Purpose	To compare the effects of older antihypertensive drugs (β-blockers and diuretics) to the newer agents (calcium channel blockers [isradipine and felodipine] and ACE inhibitors [enalapril and lisinopril]) on cardiovascular mortality in elderly patients with hypertension.
Design	Prospective, randomized, open-label, blinded end point evaluation, multicenter.
Patients	6614 patients, aged 70-84 years, with hypertension (≥180/105 mm Hg).
Follow-up	54 months. 33,249 patient-years.
Regimen	Randomization to conventional treatment (diuretics, β-blockers), ACE inhibitors (enalapril 10 mg/d or lisinopril 10 mg/d) or calcium antagonists (felodipine 2.5 mg/d or isradipine 2.5 mg/d).
Add'l Tx	If target blood pressure (<160/95 mm Hg) had not been achieved, diuretics were added to patients on β-blockers or on ACE inhibitors, and β-blockers to those on calcium antagonists or diuretics.

Results	The blood pressure lowering effects were comparable among the 3 groups. Total mortality was 33.1 per 1000 patient-years in the conventional therapy group, 34.4 per 1000 patient-years in the ACE inhibitors group and 32.8 per 1000 patient-years in the calcium antagonist group. Cardiovascular mortality was 19.8, 20.5, and 19.2 per 1000 patient-years, respectively. Sudden death occurred in 4.8 per 1000 patient-years of the conventional therapy group, 5.3 per 1000 patient-years of the ACE inhibitors group, and 4.7 per 1000 patient-years of the calcium antagonists group. Myocardial infarction occurred in 14.1, 12.8, and 16.7 per 1000 patient-years, respectively, whereas stroke occurred in 22.2, 20.2, and 19.5 per 1000 patient-years, respectively. Congestive heart failure occurred in 16.4, 13.9, and 17.5 per 1000 patient-years, respectively. The relative risk of congestive heart failure for ACE inhibitors vs calcium antagonists was 0.78 (95% CI=0.63-0.97; p=0.025), whereas the relative risk for acute myocardial infarction was 0.77 (95% CI=0.61-0.96; p=0.018). Otherwise, none of the comparisons in secondary end points of cardiovascular mortality and morbidity among the 3 treatment groups were statistically significant.
Concl.	ACE inhibitors and calcium antagonists have similar efficacy in prevention of cardiovascular mortality to the old antihypertensive agents (diuretics and β-blockers) in elderly patients with hypertension. ACE inhibitors were associated with less myocardial infarction and congestive heart failure than calcium antagonists, but not compared with conventional therapy.

SUCCESS-VII

Successive Celecoxib Clinical Efficacy and Safety Studies

Title	Effects of celecoxib and rofecoxib on blood pressure and edema in patients ≥65 years of age with systemic hypertension and osteoarthritis.
Authors	Whelton A, White WB, Bello AE, et al.
Reference	Am J Cardiol 2002;90:959-963.
Disease	Hypertension.
Purpose	To determine the effects of celecoxib and rofecoxib on blood pressure and edema in elderly OA patients being treated with established antihypertensive regimens.
Design	Multicenter, double-blind, randomized, controlled.
Patients	Patients ≥65 years of age with osteoarthritis of the hip, knee, or hand according to the American College of Rheumatology criteria and classified as having a functional capacity of I to III, with controlled, stable hypertension, and likely to gain benefit from daily treatment with nonsteroidal anti-inflammatory drugs (NSAIDS) for arthritis symptoms. Patients were eligible only if they had taken a fixed dose of the same antihypertensive medication for at least 3 months before study entry. Patients were required to have blood pressure ≤160/95 mm Hg at screening and at visits thereafter.
Follow-up	6 weeks.
Regimen	Patients were randomized to receive either celecoxib 200 mg/d or rofecoxib 25 mg/d for 6 weeks. Aspirin was used for cardioprophylaxis and permitted if the dose had been unchanged for at least 30 days before the first dose of study medication. Other NSAIDs, corticosteroids, intra-articular hyaluronic acid, or antiulcer drugs were not permitted.

Results	The primary end points of the study were: presence of elevated systolic BP (>20 mm Hg increase from study start and value ≥140 mm Hg); development of clinically significant edema defined as an increase from 1+ with a 3% weight gain, 2+ or greater increase in edema, or development of 4+ edema, or edema that requires medical treatment. Another primary end point was change in systolic BP from baseline. Secondary end points included mean change of diastolic BP from baseline, changes in diuretic or anti-hypertensive medications for treating edema or hypertension, new-onset or worsening heart failure, and a cardiorenal event. 549 patients were randomized to receive celecoxib and 543 were randomized to receive rofecoxib. The 2 study groups were well matched at baseline. Patients in the celecoxib group had a lower frequency of clinically significant elevated systolic BP at any visit vs patients in the rofecoxib group (6.9% vs 14.9%, RR 0.43; 95% CI=0.29-0.64; p<0.001). At each visit after baseline, the systolic BP of patients in the rofecoxib group increased approximately 3 mm Hg, and systolic BP was not significantly changed in the celecoxib group. Differences in the systolic BP between the groups were statistically significant at each time point (p<0.001). At study completion, significantly elevated mean systolic BP from baseline was seen in rofecoxib patients who used ACE inhibitor alone, b-blocker alone, or either with diuretics. Changes in BP were minimal and similar between the groups for patients on calcium-channel antagonists or diuretic monotherapy. Edema occurred more frequently in the rofecoxib group vs the celecoxib group during the study (7.7% vs 4.7%; p=0.045). The number of patients who required adjustments of their medications to control either hypertension or edema was similar between the groups. 2 patients (0.4%) in the celecoxib group had new-onset or worsening heart failure and 3 patients (0.6%) in the rofecoxib group, a nonsignificant difference.
Concl.	Rofecoxib was associated with a significantly increased frequency of elevated systolic BP during the 6-week study period vs celecoxib. New or worsening edema was also more frequently found in rofecoxib patients vs celecoxib patients. Patients who were taking either ACE inhibitor, β-blockers, or either combined with diuretic showed significant increases in BP with rofecoxib, but those taking either calcium channel blockers or diuretics did not experience an increase.

Syst-Eur

Systolic Hypertension-Europe

Title	Randomized double-blind comparison of placebo and active treatment for older patients with isolated systolic hypertension.
Authors	Staessen JA, Fagard R, Thijs L, et al.
Reference	Lancet 1997;350:757-764.
Disease	Hypertension.
Purpose	To evaluate the effectiveness of antihypertensive therapy in prevention of cardiovascular complications in patients >60 years old with isolated systolic hypertension.
Design	Randomized, double-blind, placebo-controlled, multicenter.
Patients	4695 patients, ≥60 years old, with sitting systolic blood pressure 160-219 mm Hg, and diastolic blood pressure <95 mm Hg when treated with masked placebo. Standing systolic blood pressure should have been ≥140 mm Hg. Patients with secondary systolic hypertension that needed special medical or surgical correction, retinal hemorrhage or papilledema, congestive heart failure, aortic dissection, renal failure, stroke or myocardial infarction in the preceding year, dementia, substance abuse, or severe concomitant disease were excluded.
Follow-up	A median of 2 years (range 1-97 months).
Regimen	Nitrendipine 10-40 mg/d (if necessary replaced or combined with enalapril 5-20 mg/d, hydrochlorothiazide 12.5-25 mg/d or both) or matching placebo. Goal of systolic blood pressure: <150 mm Hg, with a reduction of at least 20 mm Hg.

Results   After 2 years, 58.9% of the patients who had been assigned to nitrendipine and 39.6% of the patients assigned to placebo still received the study drug as the only treatment. Among the patients who withdrew from the study treatment, but continued to be followed, 36.5% of the patients assigned to active treatment and 58.1% of the patients in the placebo group were on antihypertensive medications. By intention-to-treat analysis, the sitting systolic and diastolic blood pressure decreased after 2 years by 13 and 17 mm Hg, respectively in the placebo group, and by 23 and 7 mm Hg in the active treatment group. Standing systolic and diastolic blood pressure decreased by 10 and 2 mm Hg in the placebo group, and by 21 and 7 mm Hg in the active treatment group. At median follow-up, more patients from the active treatment group (43.5%) than the placebo group (21.4%) had reached the target blood pressure (p<0.001). The between group differences in sitting blood pressure (the mean change from baseline in the active treatment group minus the mean change in the placebo group) were 10.1 mm Hg (95% CI=8.8-11.4) systolic and 4.5 mm Hg (95% CI=3.9-5.1) diastolic at 2 years, and 10.7 mm Hg (95% CI=8.8-12.5) and 4.7 mm Hg (95% CI=3.7-5.6) at 4 years. Heart rate was not changed with active treatment. Withdrawal from the study due to uncontrolled hypertension occurred in 5.5% of the placebo group vs 0.5% of the active treatment group (p<0.001). Total mortality per 1000 patient years was 24.0 in the placebo and 20.5 in the active treatment group (-14% difference; 95% CI=-33-+9%; p=0.22). Cardiovascular mortality was 13.5 vs 9.8, respectively (-27% difference; 95% CI=-48-+2%; p=0.07). Fatal myocardial infarction occurred at a rate of 2.6 and 1.2 per 1000 patient years in the placebo and active treatment, respectively (-56% difference; 95% CI=-82-9%; p=0.08). Non cardiovascular and cancer mortality were comparable between the 2 groups. The cumulative stroke rates were 13.7 and 7.9 per 1000 patient years (-42% difference; 95% CI=-60-17%; p=0.003). Non fatal cardiac end points (heart failure, fatal and non fatal myocardial infarction, and sudden death) occurred at a rate of 20.5 per 1000 patient years in the placebo group vs 15.1 in the active treatment group (-26% difference; 95% CI=-44-3%; p=0.03). The rate of all cerebrovascular events was 18.0 and 11.8 per 1000 patient years in the placebo and active treatment group, respectively (-34% difference; 95% CI=-51-11%; p=0.006). Angina pectoris occurred less frequently in the active treatment group (18.1 vs 23.9 per 1000 patient years; -24% difference; 95% CI=-41-2%; p=0.04). The cumulative rate of all fatal and nonfatal cardiovascular end points was 33.9 per 1000 patient years in the placebo group and 23.3 in the active treatment group (-31% difference; 95% CI=-45-14%; p<0.001).

Concl.   Nitrendipine therapy reduced the rate of cardiovascular complications and cerebrovascular events in patients ≥60 years old with isolated systolic hypertension. However, the decrease in total mortality was not statistically significant.

Syst-Eur (Substudy)

Systolic Hypertension-Europe

Title	Response to antihypertensive therapy in older patients with sustained and nonsustained systolic hypertension.
Authors	Fagard RH, Staessen JA, Thijs L, et al.
Reference	Circulation 2000;102:1139-1144.
Disease	Hypertension.
Purpose	To determine effect of antihypertensive therapy on clinic vs ambulatory blood pressures on ECG voltage, stroke, and cardiovascular events in older patients with sustained vs nonsustained systolic hypertension.
Design	As per Syst-Eur.
Patients	Patients ≥60 years old with systolic clinic blood pressure of 160-219 mm Hg and diastolic pressure of <95 mm Hg. Subgroup of patients enrolled in Ambulatory Blood Pressure Monitoring Side Project.
Follow-up	As per Syst-Eur.
Regimen	As per Syst-Eur

Results   695 patients had successful baseline ambulatory blood pressure measurements. Mean of 6 clinic blood pressures was 174±11/86±6 mm Hg while 24 hour ambulatory blood pressure averaged 147±16/80±9 mm Hg. ECG voltage at baseline increased from nonsustained hypertension to mild sustained hypertension, to moderate sustained hypertension defined as daytime systolic ambulatory blood pressure averaged <140 mm Hg, 140-159 mm Hg or ≥160 mm Hg, respectively. Patients with nonsustained hypertension at baseline had a lower incidence of stroke (p<0.05) and of cardiovascular complications vs the other groups (p=0.01). More patients in the sustained hypertensive groups progressed to dual and triple antihypertensive therapy than patients in the nonsustained hypertensive groups. In the active therapy group, daytime and nighttime ambulatory blood pressures were reduced in patients with sustained but not nonsustained hypertension; while clinic blood pressures were reduced in all 3 groups. Active therapy reduced ECG voltage, stroke and cardiovascular events, more favorably than placebo only in patients with moderate sustained high blood pressure.

Concl.   Sustained hypertension was associated with higher ECG voltage and cardiovascular events than nonsustained hypertension. Active therapy had favorable effects on cardio and cerebrovascular events primarily in patients with moderate sustained hypertension.

TOHP-II

Trials of Hypertension Prevention-II

Title	Long-term weight loss and changes in blood pressure: results of the trials of hypertension prevention, phase II.
Authors	Stevens VJ, Obarzanek E, Cook NR, et al.
Reference	Ann Intern Med 2001;134:1-11.
Disease	Hypertension.
Purpose	To investigate whether dietary sodium restriction, weight loss alone, or a combination of both, may be effective in reducing blood pressure in patients with high-normal blood pressure.
Design	Randomized, multicenter.
Patients	1191 overweight (a body mass index of 26.1 to 37.4 kg/m^2 for men and 24.4 to 37.4 kg/m^2 for women) adults, 30-54 years old, with diastolic blood pressure 83-89 mm Hg and systolic blood pressure <140 mm Hg without medications. Patients on medications that might alter blood pressure, and those with cardiovascular disease, diabetes mellitus, renal failure, and current or planned pregnancy were excluded.
Follow-up	3 years.
Regimen	Randomization to weight loss alone, sodium restriction only, combined weight loss and sodium restriction, or usual care.

Results	This report concentrates on the effect of weight loss. 595 patients were assigned to the weight loss group and 596 patients to the usual care group. Mean weight change at 6 months was -4.4 kg in the weight loss group and +0.1 kg in the control group. At 18 months and 36 months the changes were -2.0 kg vs +0.7 kg and -0.2 kg vs +1.8 kg, respectively ($p<0.001$ for each time point). Diastolic blood pressure was significantly lower in the weight reduction group than in the control group (-2.7 mm Hg at 6 months [$p<0.001$]; -1.3 mm Hg at 18 months [$p<0.001$]; and -0.9 mm Hg at 36 months [$p<0.05$]). The systolic blood pressure was also lower in the weight reduction group (-3.7 mm Hg at 6 months [$p<0.001$]; -1.8 mm Hg at 18 months [$p<0.001$]; and -1.3 mm Hg at 36 months [$p<0.01$]). Patients who had the greatest body weight loss had the largest reduction in blood pressure. Regression analysis revealed that for every 1 kg of body weight reduction, a 0.36 mm Hg reduction in diastolic blood pressure and 0.45 mm Hg in systolic blood pressure was expected. Hypertension (blood pressure >140/90 mm Hg) or prescription of antihypertensive medications occurred less often in the weight reduction group (RR 0.58; 95% CI=0.36-0.94 at 6 months; RR 0.78; 95% CI=0.62-1.00 at 18 months; and RR 0.81; 95% CI=0.70-0.95 at 36 months). Patients who lost ≥4.5 kg during the first 6 months and maintained their body weight for the next 30 months had the greatest reduction in blood pressure and a lower risk for developing hypertension compared with the control group (RR 0.35; 95% CI=0.20-0.59). For those who lost ≥4.5 kg at 6 months, but at 36 months their weight loss was <2.5 kg, the RR was 0.75 (95% CI=0.53-1.04) compared with the control group.
Concl.	Modest weight reduction was associated with a reduction in systolic and diastolic blood pressure and a lower risk for developing hypertension in overweight patients with high-normal blood pressure.

TONE

Trial of Nonpharmacologic Interventions in the Elderly

Title	Effect of reduced sodium intake on hypertension control in older individuals. Results from the trial of nonpharmacologic interventions in the elderly (TONE).
Authors	Appel LJ, Espeland MA, Easter L, et al.
Reference	Arch Intern Med 2001;161:685-693.
Disease	Hypertension.
Purpose	To determine the effects of decreased sodium intake in elderly patients and African Americans with hypertension.
Design	Randomized, multicenter.
Patients	681 patients with hypertension; aged 60-80 years, with systolic blood pressure less than 45 mm Hg and diastolic blood pressure less than 85 mm Hg while on 1 anti-hypertensive medicine.
Follow-up	Mean follow-up was 27.8 months.
Regimen	Reduced sodium intervention vs control. Reduced sodium goal was 24-hour dietary sodium intake of 80 mmol/L or less of sodium as measured by 24-hour urine collections.
Add'l Tx	3 months after start of intervention, medication was withdrawn.

Results	Primary end point was occurrence of average systolic blood pressure of 150 mm Hg or more, average diastolic blood pressure of 90 mm Hg or more, resumption of medicines, or a cardiovascular event. During follow-up, end point occurred in 59% of reduced sodium group vs 73% of control group (relative hazard ratio=0.68; p<0.001). The relative hazard ratio in African Americans was 0.56 (p=0.005). End points were progressively less frequent with greater sodium reduction (p=0.002). Urinary sodium excretion was reduced by 40 mmol/d in the reduced sodium group (p<0.001). Effect of reduced sodium on blood pressure was determined by comparing the change in blood pressure from baseline with blood pressure at the visit prior to withdrawal of medicine. Reduced sodium intervention was associated with a 4.3 mm Hg (p<0.001) and 2.0 mm Hg (p=0.001) drop in systolic and diastolic pressures, respectively. At the end of follow-up, 43% of reduced sodium group did not have blood pressure elevation vs 27% in the control group.
Concl.	Reduced sodium intake can lower blood pressure and control hypertension in older patients.

6. Hypertension

Eplerenone vs Enalapril in Hypertension

Title	Efficacy of eplerenone vs enalapril as monotherapy in systemic hypertension.
Authors	Williams GH, Burgess E, Kolloch RE, et al.
Reference	Am J Cardiol 2004;93:990-996.
Disease	Hypertension.
Purpose	To compare the long-term efficacy and safety of eplerenone and enalapril in patients with hypertension.
Design	Randomized, double-blind, parallel-group, multicenter.
Patients	499 men and nonpregnant women, ≥18 years old, with stage 1 or stage 2 hypertension (seated diastolic blood pressure 90-110 mm Hg and systolic blood pressure <190 mm Hg) and serum potassium 3.0-5.0 mmol/L. Patients with orthostatic hypotension, secondary, malignant, or severe hypertension were excluded. Patients on hormone replacement therapy, and those with diabetes or liver disease were not included. In addition, those who had a history of heart failure, myocardial infarction, coronary revascularization, unstable angina, stroke or arrhythmia in the preceding 6 months were excluded. Patients were also excluded if seated diastolic blood pressure remained >90 mm Hg after receiving the highest dose of the study drug for 4 weeks or if additional antihypertensive medications were needed.
Follow-up	1 year.
Regimen	1-2 week pretreatment screening, followed by 2-4 weeks, single-blind, placebo run-in phase. Then, patients were randomized to double-blind treatment with enalapril (initial dose 10 mg qd) or eplerenone (starting dose 50 mg qd). The dose was increased at 4, 8, and 12 weeks if seated blood pressure was ≥90 mm Hg. The maximal dose of enalapril was 40 mg qd and of eplerenone 200 mg qd. After 6 months, the doses of the study drugs were reduced by 1 level (ie, eplerenone 200 mg to 100 mg).
Add'l Tx	Additional antihypertensive medications were prohibited.

Results	253 patients were randomized to eplerenone and 246 to enalapril. During the first 24 weeks of the study, 36.4% of the patients in the eplerenone and 36.6% in the enalapril group were withdrawn from the study. After 6 months, 63.6% of the patients in the eplerenone vs 63.4% in the enalapril group were still taking the study drugs. After 6 months, systolic BP was reduced by 14.5 mm Hg in the eplerenone and by 12.7 mm Hg in the enalapril group (p=0.20) and the diastolic BP was reduced by 11.2 mm Hg and 11.3 mm Hg, respectively (p=0.91). Eplerenone was noninferior to enalapril (p<0.001). Treatment failure occurred in 23.3% and 22.8% of the patients in the eplerenone and enalapril groups, respectively (p=NS). There were no differences in the diastolic BP and systolic BP reductions between the groups at 12 months. 46% and 52% of the eplerenone and enalapril patients (p=NS) were able to maintain BP control after the down-titration phase. Plasma active renin after 12 months of therapy was 16.0 pg/mL in the eplerenone and 23.3 pg/mL in the enalapril group (p=NS). 12-month aldosterone levels were 20.9 ng/dL and 9.3 ng/dL in the eplerenone and enalapril group, respectively. Among patients with baseline urinary albumin/creatinine ratio (UACR) of <30 mg/g, mean change in UACR was -8.4% in the eplerenone group (n=163) and -10.5% in the enalapril group (n=164) (p=0.742). Among those with baseline UACR ≥30 mg/g, treatment resulted in mean change of -61.5% (n=34) and -25.7% (n=30), respectively (p=0.010). Adverse events occurred at similar rates between the groups.
Concl.	Eplerenone was well tolerated and as effective as enalapril when given qd for treating stage 1 and 2 hypertension. When given qd, eplerenone was more effective than enalapril in reducing albuminuria.

6. Hypertension

Title	Clinical efficacy of sildenafil in primary pulmonary hypertension: a randomized, placebo-controlled, double-blind, crossover study.
Authors	Sastry BK, Narasimhan C, Reddy NK, et al.
Reference	J Am Coll Cardiol 2004;43:1149-1153.
Disease	Pulmonary Hypertension.
Purpose	To compare the efficacy of sildenafil with placebo for treatment of primary pulmonary hypertension.
Design	Randomized, double-blind, placebo-controlled, crossover trial.
Patients	22 patients (men and women) with primary pulmonary hypertension.
Follow-up	12 weeks.
Regimen	Sildenafil 25 to 100 mg tid (on the basis of body weight) or placebo.
Results	Exercise time increased by 44%, from 475±168 seconds to 686±224 seconds after 6 weeks of sildenafil treatment (p<0.0001). Cardiac index improved from 2.8±0.9 L/m^2 to 3.5±1.1 L/m^2 (p<0.0001), while pulmonary artery systolic pressure decreased insignificantly, from 105.23±17.82 mm Hg to 98.5±24.38 mm Hg. Dyspnea and fatigue improved significantly as measured on a quality of life questionnaire. During placebo treatment, 1 patient died and another had syncope. Sildenafil did not cause any serious side effects.
Concl.	In this short-term study, sildenafil improved exercise tolerance, cardiac index, and quality of life in patients with primary pulmonary hypertension.

INVEST

International Verapamil-Trandolapril Study

Title	A calcium antagonist vs a non-calcium antagonist hypertension treatment strategy for patients with coronary artery disease. The International Verapamil-Trandolapril Study (INVEST): a randomized controlled trial.
Authors	Pepine CJ, Handberg EM, Cooper-DeHoff RM, et al.
Reference	JAMA 2003;290:2805-2816.
Disease	Hypertension, coronary artery disease.
Purpose	To evaluate mortality and morbidity in patients with hypertension and coronary artery disease treated with a calcium antagonist strategy vs a non-calcium antagonist strategy.
Design	Multicenter, randomized, open-label, blinded end point study.
Patients	22,576 patients, age ≥50 years, with coronary artery disease, and hypertension.
Follow-up	24 months; 61,835 patient-years (mean 2.7 yr/patient).
Regimen	Verapamil sustained release 240 mg/d (calcium antagonist strategy) or atenolol 50 mg/d (non-calcium antagonist strategy).
Add'l Tx	If target blood pressure was not achieved, patients in calcium antagonist strategy group could also receive trandolapril (an angiotensin-converting enzyme inhibitor) and those in the non-calcium antagonist strategy group could also receive hydrochlorothiazide.

Results	Primary outcome was the first occurrence of death (all cause), nonfatal MI, or nonfatal stroke by intention-to-treat analysis. These components individually were the secondary outcomes. Other outcomes examined: cardiovascular death, angina, adverse experiences, hospitalizations, and BP control end of trial. At 24 months, 6391 patients (81.5%) in the calcium antagonist strategy (CAS) group were taking verapamil sustained release, 4934 (62.9%) were taking trandolapril, and 3430 (43.7%) hydrochlorothiazide. In the non-calcium antagonist strategy (NCAS) group, 6083 patients (77.5%) were taking atenolol, 4733 (60.3%) hydrochlorothiazide, and 4112 (52.4%) trandolapril. At follow-up, 2269 patients had a primary outcome event, with no significant difference between CAS and NCAS groups (9.93% in CAS and 10.17% in NCAS, relative risk 0.98; 95% CI=0.90-1.06). BP control was similar between the groups: 71.7% of CAS and 70.7% of the NCAS group achieved a BP of <140/90 mm Hg. Similar results were observed comparing treatment strategies for all-cause mortality, cardiovascular death, and cardiovascular hospitalization. Both treatment strategies were well tolerated.
Concl.	CAS and NCAS treatment strategies yielded equivalent outcomes in prevention of the outcome of all-cause mortality, nonfatal MI, or nonfatal stroke. These findings support the use of either strategy in clinically stable patients with CAD who require BP control. The results indicate that lower targets for BP can be achieved in most hypertensive patients with CAD using a multidrug strategy.

SCOPE

Study on Cognition and Prognosis in the Elderly

Title	The Study on Cognition and Prognosis in the Elderly (SCOPE): principal results of a randomized double-blind intervention trial.
Authors	Lithell H, Hansson L, Skoog I, et al.
Reference	J Hypertens 2003;21:875-886.
Disease	Hypertension.
Purpose	To assess whether antihypertensive treatment with the angiotensin II receptor blocker candesartan in elderly patients with hypertension yields a reduction in cardiovascular events, cognitive decline, and dementia.
Design	Multicenter, international, prospective, double-blind, randomized, parallel-group.
Patients	4964 patients, aged 70-89 years, with systolic blood pressure 160-179 mm Hg and/or diastolic blood pressure 90-99 mm Hg; Mini Mental State Examination test score ≥24. Mini Mental State Examination is a brief, standardized measure of mental status. A score of 24 is considered normal (maximum score 30).
Follow-up	Mean 3.7 years.
Regimen	Candesartan 8 or 16 mg/d or placebo.
Add'l Tx	Open-label antihypertensive therapy (diuretic, β-blocker, calcium antagonist, angiotensin-converting enzyme inhibitor, angiotensin II receptor blocker added as needed).

Results	BP decreased by 21.7/10.8 mm Hg in the candesartan group and by 18.5/9.2 mm Hg in the control group. The primary outcome measure was major cardiovascular events, a composite of cardiovascular death, nonfatal stroke and nonfatal MI. Secondary outcome measures included cardiovascular death, nonfatal and fatal stroke, MI, cognitive function Mini Mental State Examination (MMSE), and dementia. In the candesartan group, 242 patients had a first major cardiovascular event, vs 268 in the control group; risk reduction with candesartan was 10.9% (p=0.19; 95% CI=-6 to 25.1). The candesartan group had a marked 27.8% reduction in nonfatal stroke (p=0.04; 95% CI=1.3-47.2) and a 23.6% reduction in all stroke (p=0.056; 95% CI=-0.7 to 42.1). There were no significant differences in MI and cardiovascular mortality. Mean MMSE decreased only very slightly in both groups, from 28.5 to 28 with candesartan and from 28.5 to 27.9 in the control group (p=0.20). The proportions of patients who had a significant cognitive decline or who developed dementia were similar between groups. Both treatment regimens were well tolerated.
Concl.	Candesartan-based therapy resulted in a slightly greater BP reduction vs control therapy, yielding a modest, nonsignificant reduction in major cardiovascular events and a marked reduction in nonfatal stroke. It is not clear whether the stroke reduction in the candesartan group is due to the slightly greater BP reduction or to other effects of angiotensin II receptor blockade. Cognitive function was well maintained in both groups in the presence of substantial BP reductions.

VALUE

Valsartan Antihypertensive Long-Term Use Evaluation

Title	Outcomes in hypertensive patients at high cardiovascular risk treated with regimens based on valsartan or amlodipine: the VALUE randomised trial.
Authors	Julius S, Kjeldsen SE, Weber M, et al.
Reference	http://image.thelancet.com/extras/04art4187web.pdf (published online).
Disease	Hypertension.
Purpose	To determine whether, at the same level of blood pressure control, valsartan would reduce cardiac morbidity and mortality more than amlodipine in hypertensive patients at high risk of cardiovascular events.
Design	Prospective, international, double-blind, randomized, active-controlled, parallel-group trial.
Patients	15,245 patients, aged ≥50 years, with treated (upper limit blood pressure 210/115 mm Hg) or untreated (160-210/<115 mm Hg) hypertension and at high risk of cardiac events.
Follow-up	Mean 4.2 years, range 4-6 years.
Regimen	Valsartan 80 mg/d or amlodipine 5 mg/d; both titrated upward as needed to reach target blood pressure of <140/90 mm Hg.
Add'l Tx	Hydrochlorothiazide, other antihypertensives as needed to reach target blood pressure. Angiotensin-converting enzyme inhibitors or calcium antagonists allowed only if clinically indicated for reasons other than hypertension.

Results   Both treatments caused a reduction in BP, but the effects of the amlodipine-based regimen were more pronounced, especially early in the trial (BP 4/2.1 mm Hg lower in the amlodipine than in the valsartan group after 1 month and 1.5/1.3 mm Hg lower after 1 year [p<0.001 between groups]). The primary end point was a composite of sudden cardiac death, fatal MI, death during or after PCTA or CABG, death due to heart failure, and death associated with recent MI on autopsy, heart failure requiring hospitalization, nonfatal MI, and emergency procedures to prevent MI. End point events occurred in 810 patients in the valsartan group (10.6%; 25.5 per 1000 patient-years) and 789 in the amlodipine group (10.4%; 24.7 per 1000 patient-years; hazard ratio 1.04; 95% CI=0.94-1.15; p=0.49). Rates of MI were lower in the amlodipine group (p<0.02). Rates of heart failure admissions and strokes did not differ significantly between the groups. There was no difference in rate of death between groups. Valsartan was associated with fewer cases of new-onset diabetes than amlodipine (p<0.0001).

Concl.   The main outcome of cardiac events did not differ between the amlodipine- and valsartan-based treatment groups. The unequal reductions in BP may account for differences between the groups in cause-specific outcomes. The results draw attention to the clinical relevance of small differences in BP within the high to normal range. They also emphasize the importance of rapid BP control, ie, weeks rather than months.

7. Congestive Heart Failure

Metoprolol vs Carvedilol in Heart Failure

Title	Differential effects of β-blockers in patients with heart failure: a prospective, randomized, double-blind comparison of the long-term effects of metoprolol vs carvedilol.
Authors	Metra M, Giubbini R, Nodari S, et al.
Reference	Circulation 2000;102:546-551.
Disease	Heart failure.
Purpose	To assess the hemodynamic and clinical differences between metoprolol and carvedilol in heart failure patients.
Design	Randomized, double-blind.
Patients	150 patients with chronic heart failure; New York Heart Association class II-IV symptoms for ≥6 months and left ventricular ejection fraction ≤0.35.
Follow-up	44 months.
Regimen	Randomized to metoprolol or carvedilol. Metoprolol started at 5 mg bid; carvedilol started at 3.125 mg bid Doses increased every 1-2 weeks if tolerated over 8 weeks to 10, 25, 50 mg bid for metoprolol and 6.25 mg, 12.5 mg, and 25 mg bid for carvedilol. Weight adjustment for patients ≥75 kg.
Add'l Tx	Furosemide, ACE inhibitors, digoxin.

Results   After up-titration patients received average dose of 115 mg/d
            metoprolol and 44 mg/d of carvedilol. Primary outcome was
            comparison of drug-therapy on LVEF by radionuclide ventricu-
            lography. Secondary end points were to assess hemodynamic
            variables at rest and peak exercise, exercise tolerance, quality of
            life, NYHA functional class, frequency of death and urgent trans-
            plantation. Patients treated with carvedilol had greater increases
            in LVEF at rest (10.9%±11.0%) vs metoprolol (7.2%±7.7%),
            p=0.038). While both drugs increased stroke volume and stroke
            work and decreased mean pulmonary artery wedge pressure and
            heart rate; increases in stroke volume were greater with carvedilol
            (32 to 43 mL/m^2) vs metoprolol (35 to 42 mL/m^2; p=0.016) as
            were increases in stroke work index during exercise. Decreases
            in mean pulmonary artery pressure were greater with carvedilol
            (33 to 24 mm Hg) vs metoprolol (32 to 26; p=0.049); decreases
            in pulmonary wedge pressure were greater with carvedilol (27
            to 17 mm Hg) than metoprolol (25 to 20 mm Hg; p=0.002)
            during rest, and also during exercise. Metoprolol showed greater
            increases in maximal exercise capacity than carvedilol (p=0.035).
            Both drugs improved symptoms, submaximal exercise tolerance,
            and quality of life to equal degrees. 17 patients in the carvedilol
            group and 21 in the metoprolol group died or underwent heart
            transplantation at a mean of 23 months follow-up.

Concl.   Carvedilol improved LVEF to a greater degree than metoprolol
            during long-term therapy of heart failure.

Title	Outcome of patients with congestive heart failure treated with standard vs high-doses of enalapril: a multicenter study.
Authors	Nanas JN, Alexopoulos G, Anastasiou-Nana MI, et al.
Reference	J Am Coll Cardiol 2000;36:2090-2095.
Disease	Congestive heart failure.
Purpose	To compare the outcome of patients with congestive heart failure treated with high-dose vs standard dose of enalapril.
Design	Randomized, open-label, multicenter.
Patients	248 patients with congestive heart failure, left ventricular ejection fraction ≤35%.
Follow-up	1 year.
Regimen	Randomization to enalapril with a target dose of 10 mg bid (n=122) or 30 mg bid (n=126). All patients started with a dose of 2.5 mg bid that was gradually up-titrated to the target dose.
Add'l Tx	All patients received digoxin, nitrates and diuretics. If blood pressure was <90 mm Hg, or there were symptoms of hypotension, the dose of enalapril was not increased.

Results	The mean LVEF of the patients in the standard-dose group was 20.0%±9.8% and in the high-dose group 18.8%±8.1% (p=0.424). The mean total daily dose of enalapril was 17.9±4.4 mg in the standard dose group and 42.5±19.4 mg in the high-dose group (p=0.000). 72.5% of the patients in the standard-dose group and 32.5% of the patients in the high-dose group reached their target drug doses by the end of 3-month follow-up, and 79.6% and 45.5%, respectively, by the end of the first year. 1-year mortality was 18.03% in the standard-dose group and 18.25% in the high-dose group (p=0.995). The hazard ratio was 0.998 (CI=0.556-1.790). There were 32 and 28 hospital admissions in the standard- and high-dose groups, respectively (p=0.556). Hospitalizations for heart failure decompensation occurred in 17 and 19 patients, respectively (p=0.940), for angina pectoris in 3 and 4 patients, respectively (p=0.999) and for noncardiogenic causes in 4 and 1 patients, respectively (p=0.208). After 1 year, LVEF had increased to 31.5%±19.2% in the standard-dose group and to 30.1%±12.3% in the high-dose group (p=NS). NYHA class at 1 year was 1.9±0.7 and 1.9±0.7 in the standard- and high-dose groups, respectively (p=NS). Systolic blood pressure and heart rate did not change significantly from baseline in either group.
Concl.	There were no differences in survival and clinical and hemodynamic outcomes between patients with heart failure treated with standard and high-doses of enalapril.

Title	Comparison of the occurrence of ventricular arrhythmias in patients with acutely decompensated congestive heart failure receiving dobutamine vs nesiritide therapy.
Authors	Burger AJ, Elkayam U, Neibaur MT, et al.
Reference	Am J Cardiol 2001;88:35-39.
Disease	Congestive heart failure.
Purpose	To compare the arrhythmogenicity of dobutamine with the human B-type natriuretic peptide, nesiritide, a known arterial and venodilator that inhibits sympathetic activity, in patients with decompensated congestive heart failure (CHF).
Design	Randomized, active-control, multicenter.
Patients	305 patients with decompensated CHF requiring intravenous vasoactive therapy.
Follow-up	Acute, in-hospital.
Regimen	Patients randomized to 1 of 3 treatments for a maximum of 7 days. Standard care (n=102) defined as single IV vasoactive drug (eg, IV nitroglycerin, dobutamine, milrinone, or nitroprusside); nesiritide 0.015 mg/kg/min after an IV loading dose of 0.3 mg/kg (n=103); nesiritide 0.030 mg/kg/min (n=100) after an IV loading dose of 0.6 mg/kg. Note: dobutamine was the drug most often given for initial parenteral therapy (n=58).

Results	Total durations of infusions of parenteral vasoactive therapy were 3.7±4.1 days for dobutamine, 2.1±1.8 for 0.015 mg/kg/min nesiritide group (p<0.001 vs dobutamine), and 1.8±1.6 days for 0.030 mg/kg/min nesiritide group (p<0.001 vs dobutamine). Groups were similar regarding baseline use of antiarrhythmic agents. Sustained ventricular tachycardia occurred in 4 (7%) dobutamine patients vs 2 (1%) on nesiritide. Nonsustained ventricular tachycardia occurred in 10 (17%) of dobutamine vs 23 (11%) of nesiritide patients, respectively (p=0.029). Cardiac arrest occurred in 3 (5%) of dobutamine vs zero nesiritide patients (p=0.011).
Concl.	The incidence of serious ventricular arrhythmias was lower in patients receiving nesiritide vs those receiving dobutamine for decompensated CHF.

Immunosuppressive Treatment of Inflammatory Dilated Cardiomyopathy

Title	Randomized, placebo-controlled study for immunosuppressive treatment of inflammatory dilated cardiomyopathy. 2-year follow-up results.
Authors	Wojnicz R, Nowalany-Kozielska E, Wojciechowska C, et al.
Reference	Circulation 2001;104:39-45.
Disease	Congestive heart failure, dilated cardiomyopathy.
Purpose	To determine whether patients with increased expression of HLA in cardiac biopsy specimens as a marker of chronic myocarditis would benefit from treatment with immunosuppression.
Design	Randomized, prospective.
Patients	Of 202 patients with dilated cardiomyopathy, 84 with increased expression of HLA were randomized to placebo or immunosuppression for 3 months.
Follow-up	2 years.
Regimen	43 patients received placebo and 41 immunosuppression-steroids and azathioprine. Prednisone started at 1 mg/kg/d and after 12 days the dose was tapered until reaching a maintenance dose of 0.2 mg/kg/d for 90 days. Azathioprine given as 1 mg/kg/d for a total of 100 days.
Add'l Tx	Usual therapy such as digitalis, diuretics, angiotensin-converting enzyme (ACE) inhibitors, nitrates, amiodarone.

Results	Primary composite end point was cardiac death, heart transplantation, readmission to hospital. At 2 years there was no difference in the primary end point between groups: 20.5% in the placebo vs 22.8% for the immunosuppressed group. However there were improvements in secondary end points in the treated group. At 3 months, mean ejection fraction (EF) (by echocardiography) had increased in the immunosuppressive group vs placebo (95% CI=4.2-13.1; p<0.001). At 6 months LVEF was 30.2%±12.4% in the placebo group vs 39.5%±10.7% in the immunosuppressive therapy group (95% CI=3.79-14.83; p=0.001). At 6 months LV end diastolic volume was smaller in the treated group (162.7±55.4 mL) vs the placebo group (208.4±63.9; 95% CI=17.22-74.25; p=0.002); LV end systolic volume was also smaller in the treated group (111.6±44.3 mL vs the control group at 158.3±63.2 mL; 95% CI=20.73-72.80; p=0.001). There was a trend, although not statistically significant toward better New York Heart Association (NYHA) class in the treated group (1.0) vs placebo group (2.0). At 2 years, improvement in EF, end diastolic and systolic volumes remained significant (p ≤0.001) and NYHA class remained improved (1.0 vs 2.0).
Concl.	Immunosuppressive therapy benefited patients with inflammatory dilated cardiomyopathy (HLA upregulated on biopsy) in terms of LV function and NYHA class (at 2 years) but did not alter a composite of death, heart transplantation, or readmission.

Randomized, Controlled Trial of Long-Term Moderate Exercise Training in Chronic Heart Failure. Effects of Functional Capacity, Quality of Life, and Clinical Outcome

Title	Randomized, controlled trial of long-term moderate exercise training in chronic heart failure. Effects of functional capacity, quality of life, and clinical outcome.
Authors	Belardinelli R, Georgiou D, Cianci G, et al.
Reference	Circulation 1999; 99:1173-1182.
Disease	Congestive heart failure.
Purpose	To determine whether long-term moderate exercise training in CHF patients improves functional capacity, quality of life, and outcome.
Design	Control, randomized, prospective.
Patients	99 patients with stable CHF, average age 59 years; 88 men; 11 women. Patients had to have clinical heart failure with LVEF ≤40% and sinus rhythm.
Follow-up	14 months.
Regimen	Patients were randomized to 2 groups: exercise (n=50) and control (n=49). Initial exercise consisted of exercise 3 times a week for 8 weeks at 60% of peak VO_2; followed by a second phase, a 12 month maintenance program with same intensity of exercise but for 2 sessions per week. Sessions lasted about an hour with a warm up phase followed by 40 minutes of cycling.
Add'l Tx	Standard anti CHF medicines.

Results   Peak VO$_2$ and thallium scores improved at 2 months (18% and 24%, respectively; p<0.001). These parameters did not change further after 1 year. 75% of exercise trained vs 2% of untrained patients with ischemic heart disease had an improvement in thallium uptake (p<0.001). Patients did not experience significant cardiovascular events during the training session; some had supraventricular arrhythmias and ventricular premature beats during exercise. Quality of life questionnaires showed improved scores in the trained patients after 2 months that remained stable during the subsequent 12 months. Improvements in score paralleled the improvements in peak VO$_2$ in trained patients (r=0.80; p<0.001). Mortality was lower in trained patients (n=9) vs those without training (RR 0.37; 95% CI=0.17-0.84; p=0.01). Hospitalization for heart failure was lower in trained (n=5) than untrained patients (n=14; RR 0.29; 95% CI=0.11-0.88; p=0.02).

Concl.   Moderate exercise training in patients with heart failure improved functional capacity, quality of life, and improved outcome.

ALPHABET

Arterial Pulmonary Hypertension and Beraprost European Trial

Title	Effects of beraprost sodium, an oral prostacyclin analogue in patients with pulmonary arterial hypertension: a randomized, double-blind, placebo-controlled trial.
Authors	Galiè N, Humbert M, Vachièry JL, et al.
Reference	J Am Coll Cardiol 2002;39:1496-1502.
Disease	Pulmonary artery hypertension.
Purpose	To test the efficacy and safety of beraprost sodium (orally active prostacyclin analogue) in New York Heart Association (NYHA) class II and III pulmonary artery hypertension patients.
Design	Randomized, double-blind, placebo-controlled.
Patients	130 patients with pulmonary artery hypertension due to primary pulmonary hypertension, due to collagen vascular disease, congenital shunts, portal hypertension, and human immunodeficiency virus infection. Baseline 6-minute walking distance had to be between 50-500 m, mean pulmonary artery pressure >25 mm Hg and pulmonary capillary wedge pressure <15 mm Hg.
Follow-up	12 weeks.
Regimen	20 mg tablets of beraprost sodium or matching placebo 4 times a day for first week. Dose was increased by 20 mg 4 times a day each week to a maximum dose of 120 mg 4 times a day by week 6. Up-titration was based on tolerability due to side effects (moderate to severe flushing, headache, diarrhea). Median dose was 80 mg 4 times a day (n=65); 65 patients were randomized to placebo.

Results	Primary efficacy parameter was exercise capacity measured by distance patient could walk in 6 minutes (baseline vs week 12) and dyspnea score. There was a 25.1 m increase in 6-minute walking distance at 12 weeks in the beraprost-treated group vs the placebo group (95% CI=1.8-48.3; p=0.036). Difference in mean change in Borg dyspnea index was -0.94 (95% CI=-1.63 to -0.24; p=0.009). Results were even more striking in the subgroup of patients with primary pulmonary hypertension in which there was a mean improvement of 46.1 m (95% CI= 3.0-89.3; p=0.035) in the 6-minute walking distance. The Borg dyspnea index decreased -1.46 in this subgroup. At 12 weeks 25% in the beraprost and 15% in the placebo group had improvement in NYHA functional class (p=0.190). Beraprost resulted in a nonsignificant trend toward a decrease in systolic pulmonary artery pressure by 2 mm Hg whereas it increased by 2 mm Hg in the placebo group (assessed by right heart catheterization).
Concl.	Exercise capacity and symptoms of dyspnea were improved by oral beraprost in patients with pulmonary hypertension, especially in those patients with primary pulmonary hypertension.

ATLAS

Assessment of Treatment with Lisinopril and Survival

Title	Comparative effects of low and high doses of the ACE inhibitor, lisinopril, on morbidity and mortality in chronic heart failure.
Authors	Packer M, Poole-Wilson PA, Armstrong PW, et al.
Reference	Circulation 1999;100:2312-2318.
Disease	Chronic congestive heart failure.
Purpose	To compare the efficacy and safety of low and high doses of ACE inhibitor on the risk of death and hospitalization in patients with congestive heart failure.
Design	Randomized, double-blind, multicenter.
Patients	3164 patients with NYHA Class II-IV and LVEF ≤30%. Patients with an acute coronary ischemic event, revascularization procedure within the preceding 2 months, a history of sustained ventricular tachycardia, intolerance to ACE inhibitors, serum creatinine >2.5 mg/dL, or severe noncardiac disease were excluded.
Follow-up	39-58 months (median 45.7).
Regimen	All patients received open-label lisinopril for 4 weeks. Only patients who could tolerate 12.5-15 mg/d for ≥2 weeks were further randomized to either low dose (2.5-5.0 mg/d) or high dose (32.5-35 mg/d) lisinopril.

Results   Of the 3793 patients who entered the open-label phase, 176
           patients experienced adverse effects or had laboratory abnor-
           malities that prevented their randomization to the double-blind
           phase. 1596 patients were included in the low dose group and
           1568 in the high dose group. Target doses were achieved in
           92.7% and 91.3% of the patients in the low dose and high
           dose groups, respectively. During follow-up 30.6% and 27.2%
           of the patients in the low and high dose groups stopped taking
           the study medications. Open-label ACE inhibitors were initi-
           ated in 22.1% and 18.3% of the patients, respectively. The high
           dose group had an insignificant 8% lower risk of total mortality
           (42.5% vs 44.9%; p=0.128) and a 10% lower risk of cardiovas-
           cular mortality (37.2% vs 40.2%; p=0.073) than the low dose
           group. The combined end point of all cause mortality and hos-
           pitalization was significantly 12% lower in the high dose group
           (79.7% vs 83.8%; p=0.002). The high dose group had 13%
           fewer hospitalizations for any cause (3819 vs 4397; p=0.021),
           16% fewer hospitalization for a cardiovascular cause (2456 vs
           2923; p=0.05), and 24% fewer hospitalization for heart failure
           (1199 vs 1576; p=0.002). During follow-up 18.0% of the low
           dose vs 17.0% of the high dose group had to stop the study
           medication due to side effects.

Concl.   High dose lisinopril was more effective than low dose lisinopril
           therapy for patients with heart failure. Patients with heart fail-
           ure should receive the high doses found effective in randomized
           studies, unless high doses cannot be tolerated.

BEST

The β-Blocker Evaluation of Survival Trial

Title	A trial of the β-blocker bucindolol in patients with advanced chronic heart failure.
Authors	The β-Blocker Evaluation of Survival Trial Investigators.
Reference	N Engl J Med 2001;344:1659-1667.
Disease	Congestive heart failure.
Purpose	To determine whether the nonselective β-adrenergic β-blocker and mild vasodilator bucindolol reduces mortality in patients with advanced heart failure and to assess its effects among various demographic and ethnic backgrounds.
Design	Randomized, double-blind, multicenter.
Patients	2708 patients with New York Heart Association functional class III (92% of patients) or IV (8% of patients) heart failure, left ventricular ejection fraction of ≤35% due to primary or secondary dilated cardiomyopathy.
Follow-up	Average 2.0 years.
Regimen	Randomized to initial oral dose of 3 mg of bucindolol or placebo, repeated twice daily for 1 week. Doses up-titrated on a weekly basis to 6.25 mg, 12.5 mg, 25 mg, 50 mg (for patients 75 kg or more) and 100 mg twice daily.
Add'l Tx	Other standard heart failure medicines.

Results	Primary end point was death. Secondary end points included death from cardiovascular cause, hospitalization, hospitalization for heart failure, composite of death or heart transplant, left ventricular ejection fraction at 3 and 12 months, MI, quality of life, change in need for concomitant therapy. There were 449 deaths in the placebo group (33%) and 41 in the bucindolol group (30%, adjusted p=0.13). Risk of death from cardiovascular cause was lower in bucindolol group (hazard ratio [HR] 0.86; 95% CI=0.74-0.99; p = 0.04). Bucindolol decreased proportion of patients hospitalized for illness due to heart failure (HR=0.78; 95% CI=0.69-0.88; p<0.001); there was a nonsignificant trend in favor of bucindolol for proportion of patients hospitalized for any reason (HR=0.92; CI=0.84-1.01; p=0.08). Bucindolol reduced the number of in-patient days per patient. The risk of death or heart transplantation was reduced by bucindolol (HR=0.87; CI=0.77-0.99; p=0.04). There was a significant survival benefit for non-black patients (HR=0.82; 95% CI=0.70-0.96; p=0.01). There was a lack of benefits in black patients (HR=1.17; 95% CI=0.89-1.53; p=0.27). There was a trend toward better survival with bucindolol for patients with less severe heart failure.
Concl.	In patients with class III and IV heart failure, bucindolol did not improve overall survival.

BREATHE-1

Bosentan Randomized Trial of Endothelin Antagonist Therapy-1

Title	Bosentan therapy for pulmonary arterial hypertension.
Authors	Rubin LJ, Badesch DB, Barst RJ, et al.
Reference	N Engl J Med 2002;346:896-903.
Disease	Pulmonary arterial hypertension.
Purpose	To determine the effect of the endothelin-1 antagonist, bosentan, on exercise capacity, in patients with pulmonary artery hypertension.
Design	Double-blind, placebo-controlled, multicenter.
Patients	213 patients with symptomatic, severe pulmonary hypertension despite treatment with anticoagulation, vasodilators, diuretics, cardiac glycosides, or oxygen.
Follow-up	28 weeks.
Regimen	Patients randomized to placebo (n=69) or 6.25 mg of bosentan (n=144) twice a day for 4 weeks followed by either of 2 doses of bosentan (125 or 250 mg twice daily) for a minimum of 12 weeks.

Results	64%-77% of the patients had primary pulmonary hypertension. Scleroderma was the cause in 18%-29% of cases and systemic lupus erythematosus was the cause in 5%-10% of cases. Primary end point was change from baseline to week 16 in exercise capacity. In the combined bosentan groups there was an increase in distance walked in 6 minutes, by 36 m; there was deterioration in the placebo group by 8 m (mean difference of 44 m; 95% CI=21-67; p<0.001). Patients treated with bosentan also had a decrease in the Borg dyspnea index. In the placebo group this index increased by 0.3±0.2. In the group receiving 125 mg bosentan twice daily, the index decreased by -0.1±0.2; in the group receiving 250 mg of bosentan twice daily the index decreased by -0.6±0.2. At baseline, 90% of the patients were in WHO (World Health Organization) class III. By week 16, 34%-38% of patients on bosentan had improved to class II and 1%-3% improved to class I. In the placebo group 28% improved to class II and no patients improved to class I.
Concl.	Endothelin-receptor antagonism with bosentan benefited exercise capacity in patients with pulmonary artery hypertension.

COPERNICUS

Carvedilol Prospective Randomized Cumulative Survival Study

Title	Effect of carvedilol on survival in severe chronic heart failure.
Authors	Packer M, Coats AJS, Fowler MB, et al.
Reference	N Engl J Med 2001;344:1651-1658.
Disease	Congestive heart failure.
Purpose	To determine the effects of the β-blocker carvedilol (blocks β1, β2 receptors; has a-adrenergic, antioxidant, and anti-endothelin properties) on survival of patients with severe CHF. Previous studies had shown that this drug was effective in patients with mild to moderate heart failure.
Design	Randomized, double-blind, placebo-controlled, multicenter.
Patients	2289 patients with heart failure symptoms at rest or minimal exertion for at least 2 months, and a left ventricular ejection fraction less than 25% despite conventional therapy.
Follow-up	Average of 10.4 months.
Regimen	Patients randomized to placebo (n=1133) vs carvedilol (n=1156). Initial carvedilol dose was 3.125 mg twice a day which was titrated up to a target dose of 25 mg twice a day.
Add'l Tx	Other standard heart failure medicines.

Results	Primary end point was death from any cause and combined risk of death or hospitalization. 190 patients in the placebo group died vs 130 in the carvedilol group. The 35% decrease in risk of death with carvedilol was highly significant (95% CI=19-48%; p=0.0014). There was a 24% decrease in combined risk of death or hospitalization in the carvedilol group (n=425) vs the placebo group (n=507) (95% CI=13-33%; p<0.001). At 4 months 78.2% of surviving patients in the placebo group and 65.1% in the carvedilol group were receiving target doses (mean dose of carvedilol=37 mg). The favorable effect of carvedilol on both end points was consistent across subgroups of patients including those at the highest risk (patients with recent or recurrent cardiac decompensation or severely depressed ventricular function). There were fewer patients in the carvedilol group who withdrew because of adverse effects or reasons other than death.
Concl.	Carvedilol improved mortality and morbidity in patients with severe heart failure.

COPERNICUS

Carvedilol Prospective Randomized Cumulative Survival Study

Title	Effect of carvedilol on the morbidity of patients with severe chronic heart failure: results of the carvedilol prospective randomized cumulative survival study.
Authors	Packer M, Fowler MB, Roecher EB, et al.
Reference	Circulation 2002;106:2194-2199.
Disease	Heart failure.
Purpose	To determine whether the α- and β-adrenergic blocker carvedilol is effective in patients with severe chronic heart failure.
Design	Randomized, placebo-controlled, double-blind, multicenter.
Patients	2289 patients, n=1133 in placebo and n=1156 in carvedilol groups. Patients were eligible if they had dyspnea or fatigue at rest or with minimal exertion for at least 2 months and a left ventricular ejection fraction less than 25%, occurring due to cardiomyopathy of ischemic or nonischemic origin.
Follow-up	Mean 10.4 months.
Regimen	The beginning dose of carvedilol or placebo was 3.125 bid, which was increased every 2 weeks, as tolerated, to 6.25 mg, 12.5 mg, and ultimately to a target dose of 25 mg bid. All patients received a diuretic and either an ACE inhibitor or an angiotensin II receptor antagonist. Usage of digitalis, spironolactone, vasodilators, and amiodarone were permitted, but not required. Patients could not have an active illness that required hospitalization, and were not to have been treated with an IV positive inotropic agent or vasodilator within the previous 4 days.

Results	The study primary end point was all-cause death. There were 4 prespecified secondary end points: 1) combined risk of death or hospitalization from any cause; 2) combined risk of death or hospitalization for a cardiovascular cause; 3) combined risk of death or hospitalization due to heart failure; and 4) patient global assessment. The rate of death at 1 year was 19.7%/patient-year at follow-up in the placebo group and 12.8% in the carvedilol group, a reduction of 35% (p=0.00013). There were fewer hospitalizations for any reason in the carvedilol group vs the placebo group (32.2% vs 38.1%; p=0.003). There were 395 patients in the placebo group who died or were hospitalized due to cardiovascular cause and 314 such patients in the carvedilol group; the Kaplan-Meier 1-year cumulative risks were 41.6% and 30.2%, respectively. This represented a 27% risk reduction (RR) with carvedilol (95% CI=16%-37%; p=0.00002). There were 357 patients in the placebo group who died or were hospitalized with heart failure and 271 patients in the carvedilol group; representing a 31% lower risk for the carvedilol group (95% CI=19%-41%; p=0.000004). Patients in the carvedilol group were more likely to consider themselves improved and less likely to consider themselves worse according to the global assessment; differences in favor of carvedilol were p<0.0001 and p=0.0009, respectively, according to whether or not patients missing in the follow-up were assigned the worst rank or not. Serious adverse events such as worsening heart failure, sudden death, cardiogenic shock, and ventricular tachycardia were less common in the carvedilol group vs the placebo group (each p<0.05). Events commonly attributed to α- or β-adrenergic blockade (ie bradycardia, hypotension, or syncope) occurred with a similar frequency in the 2 groups.
Concl.	Carvedilol reduces the risk of all-cause death, and hospitalizations due to heart failure, cardiovascular causes, or any cause, in patients with severe chronic heart failure.

COPERNICUS

Carvedilol Prospective Randomized Cumulative Survival Study

Title	Effects of initiating carvedilol in patients with severe chronic heart failure.
Authors	Krum H, Roecker EB, Mohacsi P, et al.
Reference	JAMA 2003;289:712-718.
Disease	Congestive heart failure.
Purpose	To determine the early effects of beginning therapy with the β-blocker carvedilol in patients with severe heart failure.
Design	Randomized, double-blind, placebo-controlled, multicenter.
Patients	2289 patients, n=1133 in placebo and n=1156 in carvedilol groups. Patients were eligible if they had dyspnea or fatigue at rest or with minimal exertion for at least 2 months and a left ventricular ejection fraction less than 25% occurring due to cardiomyopathy of ischemic or nonischemic origin. There were numerous exclusion criteria, including a reversible or correctable cause of heart failure, severe pulmonary, renal, or hepatic disease, contraindication to β-blocker therapy, cardiac surgery or angioplasty within the 2 months prior, and others.
Follow-up	8 weeks.
Regimen	Patients were randomized to placebo or carvedilol. The beginning dose of carvedilol was 3.125 mg bid, which was increased every 2 weeks, as tolerated, to 6.25 mg, 12.5 mg, and ultimately to a target dose of 25 mg bid. All patients received a diuretic and either an ACE inhibitor or an angiotensin II receptor antagonist. Use of digitalis, spironolactone, vasodilators, and amiodarone were permitted, but not required. Patients could not have an active illness that required hospitalization, and were not to have been treated with an IV positive inotropic agent or vasodilator within the previous 4 days.

Results   A major clinical event was death, hospitalization, or permanent withdrawal of the study medication. In addition to the analysis of all randomized patients, an analysis was also performed on a very high-risk subgroup of patients who had recent or recurrent cardiac decompensation or very depressed cardiac function. These high-risk patients had 1 or more of the following: pulmonary rales, ascites, or edema at study start, 3 or more hospitalizations for heart failure in the past year, hospitalization at study start, need for IV positive inotropic agent or vasodilator in the 14 days before randomization, or LVEF ≤15%. 27.3% of the randomized patients matched the criteria for the very high-risk subgroup. In the first 8 weeks, patients in the carvedilol group were less likely than those in the placebo group to die (hazard ratio [HR] 0.75; 95% CI=0.41-1.35); to die or be hospitalized for any reason (HR 0.85; 95% CI=0.67-1.07); or to die, be hospitalized, or withdraw from the study drug (HR 0.83; 95% CI=0.68-1.03). Similarly, in the high-risk patients, those in the carvedilol group were less likely than those in the placebo group to die (HR 0.20; 95% CI=0.06-0.70); to die or be hospitalized for any reason (HR 0.71; 95% CI=0.48-1.04); or to die, be hospitalized, or withdraw from the study drug (HR 0.67; 95% CI=0.47-0.96). 5.2% of patients in the placebo group and 4.4% of patients in the carvedilol group permanently withdrew from their medications for any reason other than death. The number of patients who withdrew for worsening heart failure was similar between the groups (0.7% in the placebo, 0.6% in the carvedilol, and 1.9% and 1.6%, respectively, in the high-risk groups). There were fewer patients who had a serious adverse event in the carvedilol group compared to placebo (13.8% vs 15.0%, and in the high-risk patients, 16.2% vs 22.2%). The frequency of worsening heart failure was similar in the 2 groups (6.4% vs 5.1%, placebo vs carvedilol; in high-risk patients, 11.4% vs 8.8%, respectively).

Concl.   In patients who have chronic heart failure and are clinically euvolemic, initiation of treatment with carvedilol is associated with a benefit-to-risk relationship in the first 8 weeks similar to that seen during long-term therapy.

DIAMOND-CHF

Danish Investigations of Arrhythmia and Mortality on Dofetilide in Congestive Heart Failure

Title	Dofetilide in patients with congestive heart failure and left ventricular dysfunction.
Authors	Torp-Pedersen C, Moller M, Bloch-Thomsen PE, et al.
Reference	N Engl J Med 1999;341:857-865.
Disease	Congestive heart failure, atrial fibrillation.
Purpose	To determine whether dofetilide, a novel class III antiarrhythmic drug, alters survival or morbidity in patients with decreased LV function and congestive heart failure.
Design	Randomized, double-blind, multicenter.
Patients	1518 patients with severe left ventricular dysfunction and symptomatic congestive heart failure.
Follow-up	18 months.
Regimen	Therapy was begun in-hospital with 3 days of dose adjustment and cardiac monitoring. 756 patients received placebo and 762 received dofetilide. Initially 500 µg of dofetilide twice-a-day to patients without atrial fibrillation, and 250 µg twice-a-day to patients with atrial fibrillation. Later in the study dose was based on creatinine clearance: those with a creatinine clearance of 40-<60 mL per minute received 250 µg twice-a-day; those with a clearance of 20-<40 mL per minute received 250 µg once-a-day. Additional changes if there was prolongation of QT interval.
Add'l Tx	Other usual therapy for congestive heart failure.

Results	Primary end point was death from any cause. There was no difference in incidence of death between groups (41% in the dofetilide group and 42% in the placebo group). Dofetilide decreased the risk of hospitalization for worsened congestive heart failure (RR 6.75; 95% CI=0.63-0.89) and at 1 month restored sinus rhythm in 22 of 190 patients with atrial fibrillation at baseline (12%) vs only 3 of 201 patients (1%) that were given placebo. Dofetilide was more effective than placebo in maintaining sinus rhythm once it had been restored. Torsade de pointes occurred in 25 patients receiving dofetilide (3.3%) vs none in the placebo group. While overall rates of adverse events and discontinuation of therapy did not differ significantly between dofetilide and placebo, prolongation of the corrected QT interval was a more common reason for discontinuation in the dofetilide (n=14) vs placebo patients (n=3). Increase in the corrected QT interval peaked within the first 2 days of treatment.
Concl.	In patients with congestive heart failure and reduced LV function dofetilide did not affect mortality. Dofetilide did convert atrial fibrillation to sinus rhythm better than placebo, maintained sinus rhythm better than placebo, and decreased hospitalizations for worsening congestive heart failure.

ELITE II

Evaluation of Losartan in the Elderly II

Title	1. Effect of losartan versus captopril on mortality in patients with symptomatic heart failure: rationale, design, and baseline characteristics of patients in the losartan heart failure survival study—ELITE II. 2. Effect of losartan compared with captopril on mortality in patients with symptomatic heart failure: randomized trial—the Losartan Heart Failure Survival Study ELITE II.
Authors	Pitt B, Poole-Wilson PA, Segal R, et al.
Reference	1. J Card Fail 1999;5:146-154. 2. Lancet 2000;355:1582-1587.
Disease	Congestive heart failure.
Purpose	To verify whether losartan is better than captopril in reducing mortality in patients with heart failure.
Design	Randomized, double-blind, multicenter.
Patients	3152 patients, >60 years old, with congestive heart failure (NYHA Class II-IV), LVEF ≤40%, who were not on ACE inhibitor or angiotensin II antagonist therapy, or were exposed to such therapy for ≤7 days. Patients with intolerance to the study drugs, systolic blood pressure <90 mm Hg, diastolic blood pressure >95 mm Hg, stenotic valvular disease, active pericarditis or myocarditis, AICD, recent PCI within a week prior to randomization, acute coronary syndrome or acute myocardial infarction within 2 weeks prior to enrollment, recent CABG, CVA or TIA within 6 weeks prior to enrollment, renal artery stenosis, renal failure, or hematuria were excluded.
Follow-up	Median follow-up 1.5 years.
Regimen	After a run-in of 1-28 days of single blind placebo phase, patients were randomized to losartan (initial dose 12.5 mg/d; dose was increased gradually up to 50 mg/d) + captopril-matched placebo (n=1578), or to captopril (initial dose 12.5 mg tid; dose was increased gradually up to 50 mg tid) + losartan matched placebo (n=1574).

Results   All cause mortality was 17.7% in the losartan group vs 15.9% in the captopril group (hazard ratio [HR] 1.13; 95.7% CI=0.95-1.35; p=0.16). The estimated average annual mortality rate was 11.7% and 10.4%, respectively. Sudden death or resuscitated cardiac arrest occurred in 9.0% in the losartan group vs 7.3% in the captopril group (HR 1.25; 95.7% CI=0.98-1.60; p=0.08). Sudden death occurred in 8.2% vs 6.4%, respectively (HR 1.30; 95.7% CI=1.00-1.69). Overall, 41.8% of the losartan group vs 40.5% of the captopril group were hospitalized (HR 1.04; 95.7% CI=0.94-1.16; p=0.45). Hospitalization for heart failure occurred in 17.1% vs 18.6%, respectively (HR 0.92; 95.7% CI=0.78-1.08; p=0.32). More patients in the captopril group than in the losartan group discontinued study medication because of adverse effects (14.7% vs 9.7%; p<0.001). Cough caused discontinuation of study medication in 2.7% of the captopril treated patients vs 0.3% of the losartan treated patients.

Concl.   Losartan was not superior to captopril in reducing mortality in patients >60 years old with congestive heart failure. However, losartan was better tolerated than captopril.

EPHESUS

Eplerenone Post-Acute Myocardial Infarction Heart Failure Efficacy and Survival Study

Title	Eplerenone, a selective aldosterone blocker, in patients with left ventricular dysfunction after myocardial infarction.
Authors	Pitt B, Remme W, Zannad F, et al.
Reference	N Engl J Med 2003;348:1309-1321.
Disease	Myocardial infarction/congestive heart failure.
Purpose	To determine if eplerenone, a selective aldosterone blocker, can result in better outcomes than placebo when added to standard care, including ACE inhibitors and beta blockers, in patients who are post-myocardial infarction with left ventricular dysfunction and evidence of heart failure.
Design	Multicenter, randomized, double-blind, placebo-controlled.
Patients	6642 patients, eligible if they were 3-14 days postmyocardial infarction with a left ventricular ejection fraction ≤40%, and heart failure, as demonstrated by pulmonary rales, pulmonary venous congestion on chest radiography, or third heart sound. Diabetic patients in whom the criteria for left ventricular dysfunction were met did not have to demonstrate heart failure to be included in the trial. Exclusion criteria included use of potassium-sparing diuretics, serum creatinine concentration greater than 2.5 mg/dL, and serum potassium concentration more than 5.0 mmol/L.
Follow-up	Mean 16 months (range 0-33).
Regimen	Patients were randomized to eplerenone (25 mg/d) or matched placebo for 4 weeks. The dose of the eplerenone was then increased to a maximum of 50 mg/d.

Results	The primary end points of the study were time to death from any cause, time to death from cardiovascular cause, or first hospitalization for a cardiac event such as heart failure, recurrent infarction, stroke, or ventricular arrhythmia. The secondary end points were death from cardiovascular causes and all-cause death or hospitalization. 3313 patients were assigned to placebo, and 3319 were assigned to eplerenone. 87% were taking ACE inhibitors or angiotensin receptor blockers, 75% were taking b-blockers, 88%% aspirin, and 60% diuretics. 478 patients in the eplerenone group and 554 patients in the placebo group died (relative risk [RR] 0.85; p=0.008). For the end point of cardiovascular death or hospitalization for cardiovascular causes, 885 patients in the eplerenone group reached this end point and 993 patients in the placebo group reached this end point (RR 0.87; p=0.002). The number of deaths due to cardiovascular causes was 407 in the eplerenone group and 483 in the placebo group (RR 0.83; p=0.005). The reduction in risk of sudden death from a cardiac cause was significantly lower in the eplerenone group (RR 0.79; p=0.03). There was 15% reduction in the risk of hospitalization for heart failure in the eplerenone group (RR 0.85; p=0.03), and there were 23% percent fewer episodes of hospitalization for heart failure in the eplerenone group vs the placebo group (RR 0.77; p=0.002). At 1 year, the mean BP was increased by 8/4 mm Hg in the placebo group and 5/3 mm Hg in the eplerenone group (p<0.01). At 1 year, the serum creatinine concentration was increased by 0.02 mg/dL in the placebo group and 0.06 mg/dL in the eplerenone group (p<0.001). Potassium levels increased in both groups at 1 year compared to baseline (0.2 mmol/L in the placebo group and 0.3 mmol/L in the eplerenone group; p<0.001). Serious hyperkalemia (potassium concentration ≥6.0 mmol/L) was noted in 5.5% of patients in the eplerenone group and 3.9% in the placebo group (p=0.002).
Concl.	Eplerenone therapy provides incremental reductions in death and hospitalization from cardiovascular causeswhen added to standard therapy, including ACE inhibitors and beta blocker, in patients with acute MI and LV dysfunction and heart failure.

IMPRESS

Inhibition of Metalloproteinase BMS-186716, Omipatrilat, in a Randomized Exercise and Symptom Study with Heart Failure

Title	Comparison of a vasopeptidase inhibitor, omapatrilat, and lisinopril on exercise tolerance and morbidity in patients with heart failure: IMPRESS randomised trial.
Authors	Rouleau JL, Pfeffer MA, Stewart DJ et al.
Reference	Lancet 2000; 356: 615-620.
Disease	Congestive heart failure.
Purpose	To compare the effects of omapatrilat with lisinopril on exercise tolerance in patients with congestive heart failure.
Design	Randomized, double-blind, multicenter.
Patients	573 patients, ≥18 years old, with stable symptomatic heart failure (New York Heart Association class II-IV), left ventricular ejection fraction ≤40%, who were receiving an ACE inhibitor for ≥4 weeks. Patients with systolic blood pressure <90 mm Hg, uncontrolled hypertension, acute coronary event or revascularization within 3 months, hypo- or hyperkalemia, renal failure, liver function disturbances, neutropenia or thrombocytopenia were excluded.
Follow-up	24 weeks. Patients underwent maximum exertion exercise test with a modified Naughton protocol at baseline, 12 weeks and 24 weeks.
Regimen	Randomization to omapatrilat (target dose 40 mg/d) (n=289) or lisinopril (target dose 20 mg/d) (n=284).
Add'l Tx	β-blockers were permitted only if they had been used for at least 6 months. ACE inhibitors, vasodilators other than nitrates, and inotropes other than digoxin were prohibited.

Results   Exercise time at 12 weeks increased by 24±6 seconds in the omapatrilat group and by 31±6 seconds in the lisinopril group (p=0.45). The week 24 adjusted change from baseline was 40 and 48 seconds for the omapatrilat and lisinopril groups, respectively (p=0.5). Both drugs were well tolerated. Serious cardiovascular adverse events were noted in 7% in the omapatrilat group vs 12% in the lisinopril group (p=0.04). Worsening of heart failure was noted in 10% in the omapatrilat and 26% in the lisinopril-treated patients (p=NS). Ischemic adverse events were noted in 35% and 4%, respectively (p=NS), whereas arrhythmic events in 4% and 5%, respectively (p=NS). Any serious adverse events were noted in 25% in the omapatrilat group vs 33% in the lisinopril group (p=NS). Mortality was 2% vs 4% in the omapatrilat and lisinopril groups (p=NS). Admissions for worsening of heart failure occurred in 3% and 5%, respectively (p=NS). Study-drug withdrawal due to worsening of heart failure occurred in 1% and 2%, respectively. The composite end point of death, admission or study drug discontinuation due to worsening of heart failure occurred in 6% vs 10%, respectively (p=0.035). After 24 weeks more patients in the omapatrilat group had an improvement in NYHA class than in the lisinopril group (p=0.059). This was noted among patients with NYHA class III-IV at baseline (p=0.035), but not among those with NYHA class II at baseline. The effects of the 2 drugs on plasma norepinephrine, angiotensin, and endothelin differed only slightly. Atrial natriuretic peptide levels were significantly lower with lisinopril than with omapatrilat.

Concl.   Omapatrilat and lisinopril did not differ in their effects on exercise tolerance. There were fewer cardiovascular serious adverse events with omapatrilat than with lisinopril, however, there was a trends toward more ischemic events with omapatrilat. Omapatrilat was associated with greater improvement in NYHA class, especially in patients with NYHA class III-IV at baseline.

LIDO

Levosimendan Infusion vs Dobutamine

Title	Efficacy and safety of intravenous levosimendan compared with dobutamine in severe low-output heart failure (the LIDO study): a randomised double-blind trial.
Authors	Follath F, Cleland JG, Just H, et al.
Reference	Lancet 2002; 360:196-202.
Disease	Congestive heart failure.
Purpose	To compare the effects of levosimendan, a calcium sensitizer, with dobutamine on hemodynamic parameters and clinical outcome of patients with low-output heart failure.
Design	Randomized, double-blind, double-dummy, multicenter.
Patients	203 patients, <21 years old, admitted to hospitals with low cardiac output heart failure who needed intravenous inotropic agent therapy and had LVEF <35%, cardiac index <2.5 L/min/m², and a mean pulmonary capillary wedge pressure of >15 mm Hg. Patients with restrictive or hypertrophic cardiomyopathy, heart failure due to stenotic valvular disease, chest pain, recent ventricular tachycardia or fibrillation, advanced atrioventricular block, heart rate >120 bpm, hypotension, serum creatinine >450 µmol/L, liver failure, ARDS, septic shock, and cardiac tamponade were excluded.
Follow-up	30 hours after start of infusion (24 hours of treatment and 6 hours thereafter). All patients had a flow-directed pulmonary-artery thermodilution catheter for hemodynamic follow-up. Clinical follow-up for 180 days.
Regimen	All patients received 2 simultaneous infusions (1 active and 1 placebo). Patients were randomized to levosimendan (loading dose of 24 µ/kg over 10 minutes, and an infusion of 0.1 µg/kg/min) (n=103) or dobutamine (5 µg/kg/min) (n=100). The rate of the infusions was doubled if cardiac index was not increased by 30% after 2 hours. The infusions were maintained at a constant rate for 24 hours.

Add'l Tx	Milrinone, amrinone or enoximone were prohibited.
Results	5 patients in the levosimendan and 6 in the dobutamine group had dose-limiting events leading to temporary discontinuation of the study medications. 6 patients in the levosimendan and 10 in the dobutamine did not receive study drugs for 24 hours. The primary end point of the study (a ≥30% increase in cardiac output and a ≥25% decrease in pulmonary capillary wedge pressure at 24 hours) was reached by 28% of the patients in the levosimendan vs only 15% in the dobutamine group (hazard ratio [HR] 1.9; 95% CI=1.1-3.3; p=0.022). Per protocol analysis showed that 31% of the 94 patients in the levosimendan vs 15% of the 88 patients in the dobutamine group reached the primary end point (p=0.021). β-blockers attenuated the effect of dobutamine, but did not interact with levosimendan. Termination of the infusion led to loss of the effects within 6 hours in the dobutamine group, but not in the levosimendan group. 3 patients in the dobutamine and 0 in the levosimendan group died within the first 24 hours (p=NS). Total serious adverse effects during infusion occurred in 5 and 1 patient(s), respectively (p=NS). 31-day mortality was 8% and 17% in the levosimendan and dobutamine group (HR 0.43; 95% CI= 0.18-1.00; p=0.049). 180-day mortality was 26% and 38%, respectively (HR 0.57; 95% CI=0.34-0.95; p=0.029).
Concl.	Levosimendan infusion was more efficacious than dobutamine infusion in improving hemodynamics in patients with low cardiac output heart failure. Levosimendan infusion for 24 hours was safe and associated with lower 180-day mortality than dobutamine.

MACH 1

Mortality Assessment in Congestive Heart Failure 1

Title	Effect of mibefradil, a T-type calcium channel blocker, on morbidity and mortality in moderate to severe congestive heart failure. The MACH 1 Study.
Authors	Levine TB, Bernink PJLM, Caspi A, et al.
Reference	Circulation. 2000;101:758-764.
Disease	Congestive heart failure.
Purpose	To assess the effect of mibefradil, a T-type calcium channel blocker, on mortality and morbidity of patients with CHF, New York Heart Association class II-IV.
Design	Randomized, double-blind, placebo-controlled, multicenter.
Patients	2590 patients, with stable CHF, NYHA class II-IV despite treatment with loop diuretics and angiotensin-converting enzyme inhibitors, and left ventricular ejection fraction <35%. Patients scheduled for revascularization, cardiac operation or transplantation, a myocardial infarction, coronary artery bypass graft or percutaneous coronary intervention in the preceding 1 month before randomization, high degree atrioventricular block without a permanent pacemaker, clinically significant arrhythmias, bradycardia <55 bpm, hypertension >160 mm Hg or hypotension <90 mm Hg, a cerebrovascular accident within 3 months before randomization, or any significant disease other than heart failure were excluded.
Follow-up	Planned 3 years (594±301 days for the placebo group and 565±324 days for the mibefradil group).
Regimen	After a 2-week placebo run-in, patients were randomized to mibefradil 50 mg/d or placebo. The dose was up-titrated after 1 month to 100 mg/d.
Add'l Tx	All patients received ACE inhibitors and diuretics. Vasodilators and digitalis were permitted. Calcium channel blockers were not permitted.

Results	Total mortality was 27.0% in the mibefradil group vs 24.6% in the placebo group (p=0.151). Mibefradil was associated with a 14% increased risk of death in the first 3 months of treatment (95% CI=from 2.2% reduction to 33% increase; p=0.093). Cardiovascular mortality was 24.0% in the mibefradil group vs 22.2% in the placebo group (p=0.246) and cardiovascular events (mortality and morbidity) occurred in 51.6% vs 53.4% of the patients, respectively (p=0.783). 9.5% of the patients in the mibefradil group vs 5.8% in the placebo group were hospitalized because of arrhythmia, and 4.6% vs 2.8%, respectively, were hospitalized because of syncope. There were slightly more hospitalizations because of worsening of heart failure in the placebo group (31.3% vs 26.7%). Patients with atrial fibrillation at baseline had a statistically significant greater risk for death with mibefradil. The effect of placebo and mibefradil on NYHA class was comparable. After 6 months of treatment, the increase in total exercise duration time was similar between the placebo and mibefradil groups. Mibefradil was associated with a statistically insignificant greater increase in Vo_2, Vco_2 and minute ventilation than placebo. Mibefradil did not cause a significant change in angiotensin II, endothelin-1, atrial natriuretic peptide, norepinephrine, IL-1b, IL-2R, IL-6, and TNF-a, compared with placebo. Quality of life measures were comparable between the groups (p=0.447 for treatment difference). 7.6% of the patients in the placebo group vs 10.3% in the mibefradil group withdew from the study because of adverse events. Patients who received digoxin, class I or III anti-arrhythmic agents or amiodarone had a significantly increased risk of death with mibefradil.
Concl.	Mibefradil did not reduce mortality and morbidity in patients with CHF. There is a potential interaction with digoxin and antiarrhythmic drugs, especially with amiodarone, and drugs associated with torsade de pointes arrhythmia, leading to increased risk of death.

MERIT-HF

Metoprolol CR/XL Randomised Intervention Trial in Congestive Heart Failure

Title	a. Effect of metoprolol CR/XL in chronic heart failure: Metoprolol CR/XL randomized intervention trial in congestive heart failure (MERIT-HF). b. Effects of controlled release metoprolol on total mortality, hospitalization, and well being in patients with heart failure. The metoprolol CR/XL randomized intervention trial in congestive heart failure (MERIT-HF).
Authors	a. MERIT-HF Study Group. b. Hjalmarson A, Goldstein S, Fagerberg B, et al.
Reference	a. Lancet 1999;353:2001-2007. b. JAMA 2000;283:1295-1302.
Disease	Congestive heart failure.
Purpose	To assess the effects of metoprolol CR/XL on mortality, hospitalization, quality of life, and symptoms in patients with congestive heart failure.
Design	Randomized, double-blind, placebo-controlled, multicenter.
Patients	3991 patients, aged 40-80 years, with LVEF ≤0.40 and stable chronic congestive heart failure (NYHA Class II-IV) despite optimal standard therapy (diuretics and an ACE inhibitor or hydralazine, long acting nitrate, or an angiotensin II receptor antagonist). Patients with acute coronary syndromes within 28 days before enrollment, indication or contraindication for β-blockers or drugs with β-blocking activity, heart failure secondary to systemic disease or alcohol abuse were excluded. Patients scheduled for or who had cardiomyoplasty, heart transplantation or AICD and patients scheduled for or who underwent within 4 months prior enrollment CABG or PTCA were not included. Other exclusion criteria were atrioventricular block, resting heart rate <68/minute, hypotension (<100 mm Hg), other serious disease, use of amiodarone within 6 months before enrollment, and use of calcium antagonists.

Follow-up	Mean 1 year.
Regimen	Randomization to metoprolol controlled release/ extended release (CR/XL) (n=1990) or placebo (n=2001). The initial dose was 12.5 mg or 25 mg/d. Every 2 weeks, the dose was doubled until the target dose of 200 mg/d was achieved.
Add'l Tx	Diuretics, ACE inhibitors (or hydralazine and nitrates or angiotensin II blockers in case of intolerance) and digoxin.
Results	a. Study drug was permanently stopped before the end of the study in 13.9% of the metoprolol assigned patients and in 15.3% of the placebo group. The mean daily dose of the study drug at the end of the study was 159 mg in the metoprolol group (with 64% receiving the target dose of 200 mg/d) and 179 mg in the placebo group (with 82% receiving the target dose). The study was terminated early by the international steering committee. Total mortality was 7.2% per patient year of follow-up in the metoprolol group vs 11.0% per patient year in placebo group (relative risk [RR] 0.66; 95% CI=0.53-0.81; p=0.00009). There were 128 cardiovascular deaths in the metoprolol group vs 203 in the placebo (RR 0.62; 95% CI=0.50-0.78; p=0.00003). Sudden death occurred less in the metoprolol group (79 vs 132; RR 0.59; 95% CI=0.45-0.78; p=0.0002). Death due to worsening of heart failure occurred in 30 patients in the metoprolol group vs 58 patients in the placebo group (RR 0.51; 95% CI=0.33-0.79; p=0.0023).
	b. The combined end point of total mortality or all cause hospitalization occurred in 641 patients of the metoprolol group vs 767 patients in the placebo group (19% risk reduction; 95% CI=1-27; p<0.01). Total mortality or hospitalization due to worsening heart failure occurred in 311 vs 439 patients, respectively (31% risk reduction; 95% CI=20-40; p<0.001), and cardiac death or non-fatal acute myocardial infarction occurred in 139 vs 225 patients (39% risk reduction; 95% CI=25-51; p<0.001). 581 (29.1%) patients of the metoprolol vs 668 (33.3%) patients of the placebo group were hospitalized (p=0.004). Days in hospital were 10,172 in the metoprolol vs 12,262 in the placebo group (p=0.004). 394 patients (19.8%) of the metoprolol vs 494 patients (24.7%) of the placebo group were hospitalized due to cardiovascular causes (p<0.001), and 200 (10.0%) vs 294 (14.7%), respectively

were hospitalized due to worsening of heart failure (p<0.001). Improvement in the NYHA Class was noted in 28.6% of the metoprolol group vs 25.8% of the placebo group, and deterioration in 6.0% vs 7.5%, respectively (p=0.003). There was an improvement in the McMaster Overall Treatment Evaluation score, as assessed by the patients, in the metoprolol group compared with the placebo group (p=0.009).

Concl.	a. Metoprolol controlled release/ extended release once daily, added to standard therapy, was well tolerated, safe, and reduced mortality in patients with mild to severe stable chronic congestive heart failure secondary to left ventricular systolic dysfunction of ischemic or on-ischemic etiology. b. Metoprolol CR/XR reduced the need for hospitalization, improved NYHA Functional Class, and had beneficial effects on patients well being.

MERIT-HF (Substudy)

Metoprolol CR/XL Randomized Intervention Trial in Chronic Heart Failure

Title	Metoprolol controlled release/extended release [CR/XL] in patients with severe heart failure. Analysis of the experience in the MERIT-HF Study.
Authors	Goldstein S, Fagerberg B, Hjalmarson A, et al.
Reference	J Am Coll Cardiol 2001;38:932-938.
Disease	Congestive heart failure (CHF).
Purpose	To determine whether β-blocker therapy was efficacious in a subgroup of patients in the MERIT-HF study that had severe heart failure (New York Heart Association [NYHA] functional class III/IV with left ventricular ejection fraction [LVEF] <0.25).
Design	As per MERIT-HF.
Patients	795 patients in the MERIT-HF study with severe heart failure, NYHA functional class III/IV and LVEF <0.25.
Follow-up	≈18 months.
Regimen	As per MERIT-HF.
Add'l Tx	As per MERIT-HF.

Results	Of the subgroup with severe CHF 399 were randomized to metoprolol CR/XL and 396 to placebo. Average EF was 0.19 for both groups. Metoprolol CR/XL therapy reduced all predefined mortality end points. 45 deaths occurred in the metoprolol CR/XL group vs 72 deaths in the placebo group (risk reduction 39%; 95% CI=11%-58%; p=0.0086). Death due to worsening heart failure occurred in 13 metoprolol CR/XL patients vs 28 in the placebo group (RR 55%; 95% CI=13%-17%; p=0.015). Sudden death occurred in 22 metoprolol CR/XL patients vs 39 placebo patients (RR 45%; 95% CI=7%-67%; p=0.024). The number of hospitalizations for worsening CHF was reduced by 45% with metoprolol CR/XL. Improvement in NYHA functional class occurred in 46.2% of metoprolol CR/XL patients vs 36.7% of placebo patients (p=0.0031). Treatment was well tolerated with 31% fewer withdrawals from metoprolol therapy than placebo (p=0.027). Total mortality, sudden death, and death due to worsening CHF was reduced by 34%, 41%, and 49%, respectively, by metoprolol CR/XL in the overall MERIT-HF study. In the subgroup of patients with severe CHF metoprolol CR/XL reduced these outcomes to a similar extent: 39%, 45% and 55% respectively.
Concl.	In the subgroup of patients with severe CHF in the MERIT-HF study patients with severe heart failure received similar mortality benefit and similar reductions in hospitalizations for worsening heart failure as patients in the entire study.

MERIT-HF (Substudy)

Metoprolol CR/XL Randomized Intervention Trial in Heart Failure

Title	Metoprolol CR/XL in female patients with heart failure. Analysis of the experience in metoprolol extended-release randomized intervention trial in heart failure.
Authors	Ghali JK, Pina IL, Gottlieb SS, et al.
Reference	Circulation 2002;105:1585-1591.
Disease	Congestive heart failure (CHF).
Purpose	Post-hoc analysis of MERIT-HF to determine the effect of metoprolol controlled release/extended-release (CR/XL) on outcome in women with heart failure and reduced left ventricular ejection fraction.
Design	As per MERIT-HF. Post-hoc analysis of female patients.
Patients	898 female patients, ages 40-80 years, left ventricular ejection fraction (LVEF) ≤0.40 and New York Heart Association (NYHA) class II-IV for ≥3 months prior to enrollment.
Follow-up	≈18 months.
Regimen	As per MERIT-HF. Metoprolol CR/XL vs placebo.
Add'l Tx	Diuretics, angiotensin-converting enzyme (ACE) inhibitors, digitalis; angiotensin receptor blockers if ACE inhibitors not tolerated.

Results   Female patients tended to be older, had higher systolic pressure, and were less likely to have previous MI. Therapy in women decreased the primary combined end point of all-cause mortality/all-cause hospitalizations by 21% (164 placebo vs 137 in the metoprolol CR/XL group; p=0.044). Metoprolol CR/XL decreased cardiovascular hospitalizations by 29% and decreased hospitalizations for worsening CHF by 42%. 183 women in the study had severe CHF with NYHA class III-IV and LVEF <0.25. In this subgroup of women metoprolol CR/XL decreased cardiovascular hospitalization by 57% and hospitalizations for worsening CHF by 72% (all significant). Metoprolol did not decrease the number of deaths (33 in the placebo group; 7.5% per patient-year of follow-up) vs 31 (6.9%) in the metoprolol CR/XL group.

Concl.   Metoprolol CR/XL was beneficial for women with heart failure, including those with severe heart failure.

MIRACLE

Multicenter InSync Randomized Clinical Evaluation

Title	Cardiac resynchronization in chronic heart failure.
Authors	Abraham WT, Fisher WG, Smith AL, et al.
Reference	N Engl J Med 2002;346:1845-1853.
Disease	Congestive heart failure.
Purpose	To determine whether cardiac resynchronization through atrial-synchronized biventricular pacing improves clinical outcome in patients with heart failure with intraventricular conduction delay.
Design	Randomized, double-blind, multicenter.
Patients	453 patients with moderate to severe congestive heart failure, ejection fraction (EF) of 35% or less, QRS interval of 130 msec or more.
Follow-up	6 months.
Regimen	Implantation of cardiac-resynchronization device with 3 pacing leads: right atrial, right ventricular, specialized left ventricular (LV) lead placed in distal cardiac vein via coronary sinus guiding catheter. Patients then randomized to atrial-synchronized biventricular pacing (resynchronization group, n=228) or to control (no pacing, n=225) for 6 months.
Add'l Tx	Medications for heart failure to be kept constant including diuretic, angiotensin-converting enzyme inhibitor or angiotensin receptor blocker, usually digitalis, and β-blockers.

Results   Primary end points were New York Heart Association (NYHA) class, quality of life, and distance walked in 6 minutes. Of 571 initial patients implantation of the device was unsuccessful in 8%. In 4 patients implantation of the device was complicated by hypotension, bradycardia or asystole; in 2 the coronary sinus was perforated requiring pericardiocentesis. 2 patients died. 453 patients were randomized. Of 225 patients in control group 16 died; of 228 in the resynchronization group, 12 died. 6-minute walking distance improved over 6 months to a greater extent in the resynchronization group (+39 m) vs the control group (+10 m; p=0.005). Quality of life improved in the treated group (-18.0 points) vs the control group (-9.0 points; p=0.001). NYHA functional class improved by a greater extent in treated vs control patients (p<0.001). 52% in the treated group improved by 1 class vs 32% in the control group. 16% in the treated group improved by 2 or more classes vs 6% in the control group. Resynchronization also was associated with improved time on treadmill during exercise testing (+81 vs +19 seconds; p=0.001). EF improved by 4.6% in the treated group vs -0.2% in the control group (p<0.001). Change in LV end-diastolic dimension was -3.5 in the resynchronization group vs 0 in the control group. Hospitalization was required in 8% of the treated vs 15% of control patients (p<0.05). Fewer in the treated group required intravenous medical therapy.

Concl.   Cardiac resynchronization improved exercise time, quality of life, and EF in heart failure patients with intraventricular conduction delay.

MUSTIC

Multisite Stimulation in Cardiomyopathies

Title	Effects of multisite biventricular pacing in patients with heart failure and intraventricular conduction delay.
Authors	Cazeau S, Leclerco C, Lavergne T, et al.
Reference	N Engl J Med 2001;344:873-880.
Disease	Congestive heart failure.
Purpose	To determine the clinical efficacy and safety of transvenous atriobiventricular pacing in patients with severe heart failure and intraventricular conduction delay.
Design	Single-blind, randomized, controlled, crossover study.
Patients	67 patients with severe heart failure, normal sinus rhythm, QRS interval of more than 150 msec.
Follow-up	30-week study.
Regimen	Patients received atriobiventricular pacemakers, all leads placed transvenously. Each patient randomized to 3 months of active pacing vs 3 months of inactive pacing (ventricular inhibited pacing, baseline rate 40 bpm) and then crossover to other therapy.
Add'l Tx	Patients stayed on their usual medicines.
Results	Primary end point was distance walked in 6 minutes. During active phase, mean distance walked was 23% longer (399 meters) compared to inactive pacing (326 meters; p<0.001). Quality of life score was improved by 32% (p<0.001) and peak oxygen uptake increased by 8% (p<0.03) during active pacing. There were 3 hospitalizations for heart failure during active pacing and 9 during inactive pacing (p<0.05). 85% of patients stated that they preferred the period that corresponded to active-pacing (p<0.001).
Concl.	Atriobiventricular pacing significantly improved exercise tolerance and quality of life in patients with heart failure and intraventricular conduction delay.

MUSTIC (Long-Term Analysis)

The Multisite Stimulation in Cardiomyopathies

Title	Long-term benefits of biventricular pacing in congestive heart failure: results from the MUSTIC study.
Authors	Linde C, Leclercq C, Rex S, et al.
Reference	J Am Coll Cardiol 2002; 40:111-118.
Disease	Congestive heart failure.
Purpose	To determine if benefits of biventricular pacing in congestive heart failure patients were sustained over 1 year.
Design	Randomized, controlled, multicenter.
Patients	131 patients with severe chronic heart failure due to idiopathic or ischemic LV systolic dysfunction, EF <35% by radionuclide study and LVEDD >60 mm by echocardiography. 75 patients were followed for 1 year.
Follow-up	12 months.
Regimen	Study had begun as a single-blind crossover comparison of biventricular pacing and inactive pacing each for 3 months or biventricular vs right univentricular pacing (adaptive ventricular inhibited pacing). After the end of a crossover phase, patients were asked which of the 3-month periods they preferred and were programmed according to preference. This analysis was a 12-month intrapatient analysis of baseline vs 12-month outcomes of the patients that were programmed to biventricular pacing (m=71).
Add'l Tx	Usual anti-heart failure medicines.

Results   A number of parameters were evaluated at baseline and at 12 months. At the end of the crossover phase more patients preferred the biventricular pacing. At 12 months all patients in sinus rhythm and 88% of those in atrial fibrillation received biventricular pacing. The 6-minute walked distance improved by 20% in the sinus rhythm group at 12 months (p=0.0001) and by 17% in the atrial fibrillation group (p=0.004). Peak Vo2 increased by 11% and 9% in the sinus rhythm and atrial fibrillation patients, respectively. NYHA class improved by 25% and 27% in the 2 groups (both p=0.0001). LV ejection fraction improved by 5% and 4% and mitral regurgitation was reduced by 45% and 50% in the sinus rhythm and atrial fibrillation groups, respectively. Quality of life also improved over 12 months.

Concl.   Biventricular pacing demonstrated clinical improvements in heart failure patients over a 12-month period.

OPTIME-CHF

Outcomes of a Prospective Trial of Intravenous Milrinone for Exacerbations of Chronic Heart Failure

Title	Short-term intravenous milrinone for acute exacerbation of chronic heart failure. A randomized controlled trial.
Authors	Caffe MS, Califf RM, Adams KF, et al.
Reference	JAMA 2002;287:1541-1547.
Disease	Congestive heart failure.
Purpose	To determine whether short-term use of milrinone on top of standard therapy improves clinical outcomes of hospitalized patients with exacerbation of congestive heart failure.
Design	Prospective, randomized, double-blind, placebo-controlled, multicenter.
Patients	951 patients with exacerbation of systolic heart failure not on inotropic support. Mean age 65; most with New York Heart Association class III or IV; mean left ventricular ejection fraction of 23%.
Follow-up	60 days.
Regimen	IV milrinone (n=477) at initial infusion of 0.5 mg/kg per minute for 48-72 hours. Rate could be adjusted downward to 0.375 mg/kg/min if hypertension occurred or upward to 0.75 mg/kg/min vs saline placebo (n=472).
Add'l Tx	Other therapy at discretion of physicians. Including angiotensin-converting enzyme inhibitors, diuretics.

Results	Primary end point was total number of days hospitalized for cardiovascular causes or deceased within 60 days of randomization. Median number of days hospitalized for cardiovascular causes was 6 in the milrinone group vs 7 in the placebo group (p=0.71). Death or readmission within 60 days occurred in 35% of patients in both groups. Patients who received milrinone had more sustained hypotension requiring intervention (10.7% vs 3.2%; p<0.001) and more new atrial arrhythmias (4.6% vs 1.5%; p=0.004). In hospital mortality was 3.8% in the milrinone group vs 2.3% in the placebo group (p=0.19). There was no difference in 60-day mortality between the groups (10.3% with milrinone vs 8.9% with placebo; p=0.41).
Concl.	The data do not support the routine use of IV milrinone in the treatment of patients hospitalized with exacerbations of heart failure.

OVERTURE

Omapatrilat vs Enalapril Randomized Trial of Utility in Reducing Events

Title	Comparison of omapatrilat and enalapril in patients with chronic heart failure: The Omapatrilat Versus Enalapril Randomized Trial of Utility in Reducing Events.
Authors	Packer M, Califf RM, Konstam MA, et al.
Reference	Circulation 2002;106:920-926.
Disease	Heart failure.
Purpose	To determine whether combined inhibition of angiotensin-converting enzyme and neutral endopeptidase would be more beneficial than ACE inhibition alone in patients with heart failure.
Design	Double-blind, randomized, multicenter.
Patients	Patients with New York Heart Association class II, III, or IV heart failure for ≥2 months or with left ventricular ejection fraction ≤30% and who were hospitalized for heart failure in the previous 12 months were eligible. Exclusion criteria included: surgically correctable or reversible cause of heart failure, previous or likely cardiac transplant or left ventricular assist device, severe primary pulmonary, renal, or hepatic disease, or history of intolerance to ACE inhibitor. Patients with an acute coronary syndrome within the past month or either coronary revascularization or acute cerebral ischemic event within the past 3 months were also excluded. Patients with a history of ventricular tachycardia, ventricular fibrillation, or sudden death were also excluded unless they had received an implantable cardioverter-defibrillator that had not fired within the past 2 months. Patients should not have been hospitalized or have received IV therapy for heart failure inotropic agent intravenously within the 2 weeks prior to study randomization. A systolic blood pressure >180 or <90 mm Hg, heart rate >130 bpm, serum creatinine >2.5 mg/dL, or serum potassium <3.5 or >5.2 mmol/L were also exclusion criteria.
Follow-up	Mean 14.5 months.

Regimen	Existing therapy with ACE inhibition or angiotensin receptor blocker was stopped, but other treatments were continued. Eligible patients were randomized to receive either omapatrilat 10 mg qd or enalapril 2.5 mg bid. After 2 weeks, the dosages were increased to omapatrilat 20 mg once a day and enalapril 5 mg twice a day, and 2 weeks thereafter, to the target dosages of omapatrilat 40 mg once a day and enalapril 10 mg twice a day.
Add'l Tx	All patients received diuretics and were not restricted from receiving all other appropriate medications.
Results	5770 patients were enrolled and randomized: 2886 to omapatrilat and 2884 to enalapril. The primary end point was the composite risk of all-cause mortality and hospitalization due to heart failure. The secondary end points were: all-cause mortality; the composite risk of cardiovascular death or cardiovascular hospitalization; and the composite risk of cardiovascular death, MI, stroke, or myocardial revascularization. The primary end point occurred in 973 patients in the enalapril group, compared to 914 in the omapatrilat group (hazard ratio [HR] 0.94; 95% CI=0.86-1.03; p=0.187), which showed noninferiority of omapatrilat to enalapril but not superiority. A post-hoc analysis of the data that included all hospitalizations for heart failure (the definition of heart failure used in the Studies of Left Ventricular Dysfunction [SOLVD] Treatment Trial) yielded a HR of 0.89 (95% CI=0.82-0.98; p=0.012). Differences between the 2 analyses were explained by hospitalizations for heart failure that were treated only with increased dosages of oral medication; such patients were classified under hospitalization for heart failure in the post-hoc analysis. There were 1275 cardiovascular deaths or cardiovascular hospitalizations in the enalapril group and 1178 in the omapatrilat group (HR 0.91; 95% CI=0.84-0.99; p=0.024). The combined numbers of cardiovascular death, MI, stroke, or myocardial revascularization were 578 in the enalapril group, and 537 in the omapatrilat group (HR 0.93; 95% CI=0.83-1.05; p=0.233). Study drug was withdrawn in 17.9% of the omapatrilat group vs 17.0% of the enalapril group, for adverse events. Angioedema occurred in 24 (0.8%) omapatrilat-treated and 14 (0.5%) enalapril-treated patients.
Concl.	Compared to ACE inhibition alone, omapatrilat reduced the number of deaths and rehospitalizations due to heart failure but did not produce substantial benefit in reducing all-cause mortality or the risk of primary clinical events.

PRAISE

Prospective Randomized Amlodipine Survival Evaluation

Title	Effect of amlodipine on morbidity and mortality in severe chronic heart failure.
Authors	Packer M, O'Connor CM, Ghali JK, et al.
Reference	N Engl J Med 1996;335:1107-1114.
Disease	Congestive heart failure.
Purpose	To evaluate the long-term effect of amlodipine, a calcium channel blocker, on mortality and morbidity in patients with advanced congestive heart failure.
Design	Randomized, double-blind, placebo-controlled, multicenter.
Patients	1153 patients with congestive heart failure (NYHA class IIIB or IV) and left ventricular ejection fraction <0.30, despite therapy with digoxin, diuretics, and an ACE inhibitor. Patients with uncorrected primary valvular disease, active myocarditis, constrictive pericarditis, history of cardiac arrest or who had sustained ventricular fibrillation or tachycardia within the previous year, unstable angina or acute myocardial infarction within the previous month, cardiac revascularization or stroke within 3 months, severe concomitant disease, hypotension or hypertension, or serum creatinine >3.0 mg/dL were excluded.
Follow-up	6 to 33 months (median 13.8 months).
Regimen	Randomization to amlodipine or placebo. The initial dose of amlodipine was 5 mg X1/d for 2 weeks and than increased to 10 mg/d.
Add'l Tx	Diuretics, digoxin, and an ACE inhibitor. Nitrates were permitted, but other vasodilators, β-blockers, calcium channel blockers, and, class IC antiarrhythmic agents were prohibited.

Results	Of the patients with ischemic heart disease, 370 were assigned to placebo and 362 to amlodipine. Of the patients with nonischemic cardiomyopathy, 212 were assigned to placebo and 209 patients to amlodipine. A primary end point of the study (mortality from all causes or cardiovascular morbidity, defined as hospitalization for ≥24 hours for pulmonary edema, severe hypoperfusion, acute MI, or ventricular tachycardia/fibrillation) was reached by 39% of the amlodipine treated patients and in 42% of the placebo group. Amlodipine therapy was associated with insignificant risk reduction of primary end points (9%; 95% CI=24% reduction to 10% increase; p=0.31). 33% vs 38% of the amlodipine and control groups died, respectively (16% risk reduction; 95% CI=31% reduction to 2% increase; p=0.07). Among patients with ischemic etiology, amlodipine therapy did not affect mortality or the combined end point of mortality and cardiovascular morbidity. 45% of the patients in both groups had a fatal or non fatal event, and 40% of the patients in both groups died. However, in patients with nonischemic cardiomyopathy amlodipine was associated with better outcome. Primary end point was reached by 36.8% of the placebo, but in only 27.8% of the amlodipine group (31% risk reduction; 95% CI=2% to 51% reduction; p=0.04). Mortality was 34.9% vs 21.5% in the placebo and amlodipine group, respectively (46% risk reduction; 95% CI=21% to 63% reduction; p<0.001). Subgroup analysis revealed that amlodipine therapy was not associated with adverse effects in any of the subgroups. A favorable effect on survival was found only in patients without a history of angina. Total adverse effects that mandated discontinuation of double-blind therapy was comparable between the groups. However, peripheral edema (27% vs 18%; p<0.001) and pulmonary edema (15% vs 10%; p=0.01) occurred more frequently in the amlodipine group, while uncontrolled hypertension (2% vs <1%; p=0.03) and symptomatic cardiac ischemia (31% vs 25% among patients with ischemic heart disease; p=0.07) was more frequent in the placebo than amlodipine group. The frequencies of MI, arrhythmias, and worsening of heart failure were similar.
Concl.	Amlodipine was not associated with increased mortality and morbidity among patients with severe CHF. Amlodipine was associated with better outcome in patient with nonischemic cardiomyopathy, whereas in patients with ischemic heart disease there was no difference in outcome.

PRAISE (Substudy)

Prospective Randomized Amlodipine Survival Evaluation

Title	Circadian rhythm and sudden death in heart failure.
Authors	Carson PA, O'Connor CM, Miller AB, et al.
Reference	J Am Coll Cardiol 2000;36:541-546.
Disease	Congestive heart failure.
Purpose	To determine the timing of sudden death in advanced heart failure.
Design	As per PRAISE.
Patients	A study of 185 sudden deaths among the 1,153 patients in PRAISE.
Follow-up	As per PRAISE.
Regimen	As per PRAISE.
Add'l Tx	As per PRAISE.
Results	Sudden death defined as "death from cardiac or unknown causes that occurred instantaneously or within 60 minutes of symptom onset." This included patients resuscitated from cardiac arrest who remained comatose and were pronounced dead within 72 hours. There was a striking peak of sudden death at 4 p.m.-8 p.m. and unlike previous reports, a morning peak was not observed. This 4 p.m.-8 p.m. peak was due to sudden deaths in the patients with heart failure due to ischemia but not in those with nonischemic heart failure. The distributions of sudden death were not altered by amlodipine, aspirin, or warfarin.
Concl.	Sudden death in patients with advanced heart failure did not show an expected morning peak suggesting that circadian sympathetic activation at this time did not influence sudden death. Heart failure patients with an ischemic etiology were more likely to experience sudden death between 4 p.m.-8 p.m.

RALES

Randomized Aldactone Evaluation Study Investigators

Title	The effect of spironolactone on morbidity and mortality in patients with severe heart failure.
Authors	Pitt B, Zannad F, Remme WJ, et al.
Reference	N Engl J Med 1999;341:709-717.
Disease	Congestive heart failure.
Purpose	To determine whether spironolactone would decrease the risk of death in patients with severe heart failure due to systolic dysfunction who were also receiving standard therapy including an ACE inhibitor.
Design	Randomized, double-blind, placebo-controlled, multicenter.
Patients	1663 patients with NYHA Class III-IV heart failure at time of enrollment who were receiving ACE inhibitor (if tolerated), loop diuretic, and had an LV ejection fraction of no more than 35%.
Follow-up	Mean of 24 months.
Regimen	25 mg spironolactone orally once daily vs placebo. Patents were excluded if serum creatinine was >2.5 mg/dL and if serum potassium was >5.0 mmol/L.
Add'l Tx	Digitalis and vasodilators were allowed as well as ACE inhibitors; potassium sparing diuretics were not allowed. Potassium supplements not recommended unless hypokalemia present.

Results	The primary end point was death from all causes. 841 patients assigned to placebo and 822 to spironolactone. 200 patients in placebo and 214 in spironolactone discontinued therapy for lack of response, adverse events, or other reasons. The study was stopped early because interim analysis showed a lower death rate among spironolactone treated patients. 386 patients died in the placebo group (46%) vs 284 in the spironolactone group (35%; RR 0.70; 95% CI=0.60-0.82; p<0.001). The 30% decrease in death among treated patients was due to a lower rate of death from progressive heart failure and sudden cardiac death. There was a 30% reduction in risk of hospitalization for cardiac causes in the spironolactone group (RR 0.70; 95% CI=0.59-0.82; p<0.001). There was a significant improvement in NYHA Functional Class among patients who received spironolactone. The median creatinine concentration in the spironolactone patients increased by 0.05-0.10 mg/dL, median potassium concentration increased by 0.30 mmol/L. The incidence of serious hyperkalemia was 1% in the placebo group and 2% in the spironolactone group (n=NS). Gynecomastia was more common in the spironolactone group (10%) vs the placebo group (1%; p<0.001).
Concl.	The aldosterone receptor blocker spironolactone, in addition to standard therapy, reduced morbidity and mortality in patients with severe heart failure.

REMATCH

Randomized Evaluation of Mechanical Assistance for the Treatment of Congestive Heart Failure

Title	Long-term use of a left ventricular assist device for end-stage heart failure.
Authors	Rose EA, Gelijns AC, Moskowitz AJ, et al.
Reference	N Engl J Med 2001;345:1435-1443.
Disease	Congestive heart failure.
Purpose	To investigate the use of the HeartMate left ventricular assist device (LVAD) for long-term myocardial replacement therapy for patients with severe heart failure who were ineligible for cardiac transplantation.
Design	Randomized, open-label, multicenter.
Patients	129 patients, ≥18 years old, with chronic end-stage heart failure (New York Heart Association (NYHA) class IV for ≥90 days), LV ejection fraction ≤25%, and a peak oxygen consumption of ≤12 mL/kg/min or a continued need for IV inotropic therapy. All patients were ineligible for cardiac transplantation.
Follow-up	Enrollment ended once the predetermined number of 92 deaths had occurred.
Regimen	Patients were randomized to receive optimal medical therapy (n=61) or to undergo a vented electric LVAD implantation (n=68).
Add'l Tx	All patients received angiotensin-converting enzyme inhibitors, diuretics, and digoxin before randomization. Continuation of β-blocker use (if administered for ≥60 of the 90 days before randomization) was permitted.

Results	All patients who were assigned to receive an LVAD received the device. There was no cross over and none of the patients underwent cardiac transplantation. The Kaplan-Meier survival curves showed a 48% reduction in the risk of death in the LVAD group (relative risk 0.52; 95% CI=0.34-0.78; p=0.001). The estimated survival at 1 year was 52% in the LVAD group vs only 25% in the medical therapy group (p=0.002). The estimated survival at 2 years was 23% and 8%, respectively (p=0.09). Median survival was 408 and 150 days, respectively. Terminal heart failure was the major reason for death in the medical therapy group (50 patients), whereas sepsis (17 patients) and failure of the device (7 patients) were the most common causes of death in the LVAD group. Quality of life was significantly improved at 1 year in the LVAD group. The Medical Outcomes Study Short form 36 physical function score was 46±19 in the LVAD and 21±21 in the medical therapy group (p=0.01), and the emotional role score was 64±45 vs 17±28, respectively (p=0.03). The Minnesota Living with Heart Failure score was better in the LVAD group than in the medical treatment group (41±22 vs 58±21; p=0.11). The median NYHA class at 1 year was II in the LVAD group and IV in the medical therapy group (p<0.001). Serious adverse events occurred more often in the LVAD group (6.45 events/patient-year) than in the medical therapy group (2.75 events/patient-year) (rate ratio 2.35; 95% CI=1.86-2.95). There was a predominance of infection, bleeding, and malfunction of the device in the LVAD group.
Concl.	Long-term use of an LVAD improved survival and quality of life in patients with severe chronic heart failure who were ineligible for cardiac transplantation.

RESOLVD

Randomized Evaluation of Strategies for Left Ventricular Dysfunction

Title	Comparison of candesartan, enalapril, and their combination in congestive heart failure. RESOLVD Pilot Study.
Authors	McKelvie RS, Yusuf S, Pericak D, et al.
Reference	Circulation 1999;100:1056-1064.
Disease	Congestive heart failure.
Purpose	To determine the effects of the angiotensin II antagonist candesartan alone, enalapril alone, and their combination on various parameters of congestive heart failure.
Design	Randomized, double-blind, parallel, placebo-controlled, multicenter.
Patients	768 patients with NYHA Functional Class II-IV with ejection fraction <0.40 and 6 minute walk distance <500 m.
Follow-up	43 weeks.
Regimen	Candesartan (4, 8, or 16 mg daily) vs enalapril 10 mg twice-a-day, vs combination of candesartan at either 4 or 8 mg daily plus enalapril 10 mg twice-a-day.
Add'l Tx	After 19 weeks, patients were eligible for randomization to metoprolol vs placebo. No interactions occurred across outcomes between use of metoprolol and the other groups.

Results	Primary end points included change in 6 minute walking distance, ejection fraction, ventricular volumes, neurohormone levels, quality of life, NYHA Functional Class at 17 or 18 weeks and 43 weeks. There were no differences in walking distance, functional class, or quality of life among the groups. There was a nonsignificant increase in ejection fraction assessed by radionuclide angiography in the combination group (0.025 ± 0.004) compared with the candesartan (0.015 ± 0.004) or enalapril group (0.015 ± 0.005). Combination of candesartan and enalapril had less increase ($p<0.01$) in end diastolic volume (8 ± 4 mL), than with candesartan alone (27 ± 4 mL) or enalapril alone 23 ± 7 mL). Also the increase in end systolic volumes increased less ($p<0.01$) with combination therapy (1 ± 4 mL), than with candesartan alone (18 ± 3 mL) or enalapril alone (14 ± 6 mL). Blood pressure decreased more with combination therapy ($-6/-4$ mm Hg) than with either therapy alone. Combination therapy decreased aldosterone levels at 17 but not 43 weeks compared to candesartan or enalapril alone. Combination therapy was also associated with a greater decrease in brain natriuretic peptide. Death, hospitalization for heart failure, and any hospitalizations did not differ among the groups. Death occurred in 8.7% with combination therapy, 6.1% in candesartan, and 3.7% in enalapril alone groups ($p=NS$). Heart failure hospitalizations occurred in 9.3%, 13.1%, and 6.4% in combination, candesartan, and enalapril groups respectively ($p=0.09$).
Concl.	Both candesartan and enalapril were effective, safe, and tolerable for treating heart failure. Combination of candesartan and enalapril reduced left ventricular dilation greater than either agent alone.

7. Congestive Heart Failure

RESOLVD (Metoprolol Study)

Randomized Evaluation of Strategies for Left Ventricular Dysfunction

Title	Effects of metoprolol CR in patients with ischemic and dilated cardiomyopathy. The RESOLVD Pilot Study.
Authors	The RESOLVD Investigators.
Reference	Circulation 2000;101:378-384.
Disease	Congestive heart failure.
Purpose	To determine the effects of controlled release metoprolol on clinical status, LV volumes and function, and neurohumoral activation in patients with congestive heart failure.
Design	Randomized, double-blind 3 x 2 partial factorial design, 2 stage randomization.
Patients	426 eligible patients from Stage 1 (see RESOLVD: candesartan vs enalapril). NYHA Class II-IV, 6 minute walk distance of <500 m, LVEF of <40%, had to tolerate 12.5 mg metoprolol once daily for 1 week.
Follow-up	From randomization into Stage II (metoprolol vs placebo) until end of this study was 24 weeks.
Regimen	Metoprolol CR (25 mg) once daily or placebo.
Add'l Tx	As per RESOLVD: candesartan, enalapril, or both.

Results   Metoprolol CR attenuated an increase in LV end diastolic volumes (+6±61 mL metoprolol vs +23±65 mL placebo; p=0.01). Metoprolol also attenuated an increase in LV end systolic volumes (-2±51 mL metoprolol vs +19±55 mL in placebo; p<0.001). LV ejection fraction increased by 2.4% in metoprolol patients vs -0.05% in the placebo group (p=0.001). 6 minute walk distance, NYHA, and quality of life were not changed by metoprolol. Metoprolol was associated with fewer deaths (3.4%) vs placebo (8.1%) but no difference in number of patients with composite end point of death or any hospitalization. Greater decreases in angiotensin II and renin occurred with metoprolol; but it increased N-terminal natriuretic and brain natriuretic peptide.

Concl.   Metoprolol CR improved LV function, reduced LV dilation, and resulted in fewer deaths in heart failure patients who were already on an ACE inhibitor, angiotensin II receptor antagonist, or both.

RITZ-4

Randomized Intravenous Tezosentan Study-4

Title	Tezosentan in patients with acute heart failure and acute coronary syndromes. Results of RITZ-4.
Authors	O'Connor CM, Gattis WA, Adams KF, et al.
Reference	J Am Coll Cardiol 2003;41:1452-1457.
Disease	Congestive heart failure, acute coronary syndrome.
Purpose	To determine whether tezosentan (dual endothelin receptor antagonist) had beneficial effects on patients with acute severe heart failure associated with acute coronary syndromes.
Design	Randomized, double-blind, placebo-controlled, multicenter.
Patients	193 patients with acute heart failure and acute coronary syndromes (including Q-wave and non Q-wave myocardial infarction or unstable angina).
Follow-up	72 hours.
Regimen	Patients were randomized to tezosentan (25 mg/h IV for 1 hour followed by 50 mg/h for 23 hours up to 48 hours) or placebo.
Add'l Tx	Increase in dose or new therapy with inotropes, sympathomimetics, or vasodilators during first 24 hours done only if necessary. IV diuretics were not given within 2 hours before randomization or 6 hours after unless absolutely necessary.
Results	Primary end point was composite of death, worsening CHF, recurrent ischemia, recurrent or new MI within 72 hours. The primary end point was reached in 24.2% of placebo patients and 28.9% of tezosentan patients (p=NS). There was no difference in outcome of the individual components of the composite outcome between the 2 groups. Vasodilator adverse effects (headache, hypotension, dizziness) were more common in the tezosentan group. There was a trend toward worsening heart failure in the tezosentan group (19.6%) vs the placebo group (11.6%; p=0.16).
Concl.	Tezosentan did not result in clinical improvement in patients with acute heart failure and acute coronary syndromes.

RUSSLAN

Randomized Study on Safety and Effectiveness of Levosimendan in Patients with Left Ventricular Failure Due to an Acute Myocardial Infarct

Title	Safety and efficacy of a novel calcium sensitizer, levosimendan, in patients with left ventricular failure due to an acute myocardial infarction. A randomized, placebo-controlled, double-blind study (RUSSLAN).
Authors	Moiseyev VS, Poder P, Andrejevs N, et al.
Reference	Eur Heart J 2002;23:1422-1432.
Disease	Acute myocardial infarction, heart failure.
Purpose	To evaluate the safety and efficacy of levosimendan, a calcium sensitizer that increases the contractility of the myocardium by enhancing the sensitivity of myofilaments to calcium without increasing intracellular calcium concentration at therapeutic doses, in patients with left ventricular dysfunction after acute myocardial infarction.
Design	Randomized, double-blind, placebo-controlled, multicenter.
Patients	504 patients within 5 days of an acute myocardial infarction, evidence of pulmonary venous congestion or pulmonary edema on chest X-ray, and a clinical need for inotropic support. Patients with right ventricular infarction, hypotension, ventricular tachycardia, atrial fibrillation, immediate need for cardiac pacing, PCI or CABG, severe mitral regurgitation, cardiac rupture or cardiac tamponade, use of b agonists within 30 minutes of initiation of the study, acute respiratory distress syndrome, septic shock, renal or hepatic insufficiency, and women with childbearing potential were excluded.
Follow-up	180 days.

Regimen	Patients were randomized to placebo (n=102) or to 1 of 4 regimens of levosimendan: 1) 6 µg/kg bolus and 0.1 µg/kg/min infusion (n=103); 2) 12 µg/kg bolus and 0.2 µg/kg/min infusion (n=100); 3) 24 µg/kg bolus and 0.2 µg/kg/min infusion (n=99); or 24 µg/kg bolus and 0.4 µg/kg/min infusion (n=100). The bolus was administered over 10 minutes and the infusion was maintained for 5 hours and 50 minutes.
Results	Clinically significant ischemia or hypotension occurred in 10.8% of the patients in the placebo group and in 10.7%, 12.0%, 12.1%, and 19.0% in the 4 levosimendan groups (p=0.319). There was a weak relationship between the levosimendan dose and the risk of hypotension and ischemia (p=0.054), which was attributed to the highest dose. 6-hour mortality was 3.9% in the placebo and 1.9%, 1.0%, 0, and 0 in the 4 levosimendan groups (p=0.015). 24-hour mortality was 4.9% in the placebo and 3.9%, 1.0%, 1.0%, and 2.0% with the 4 groups of levosimendan (p=0.127). 180-day mortality was 31.4% in the placebo group and 26.2%, 16.0%, 27.3%, and 21.0% in the 4 levosimendan groups (p=0.088). The combined end point of death or worsening of heart failure at 6 hours occurred in 5.9% of the patients in the placebo group and in 2.9%, 2.0%, 1.0%, and 2.0% in the 4 levosimendan groups (p=0.094). Death or worsening of heart failure at 24 hours occurred in 8.8% in the placebo group and in 5.8%, 3.0%, 3.0%, and 4.0% in the 4 levosimendan groups (p=0.089). When all 4 levosimendan groups were considered together, 14-day mortality was 19.6% in the placebo group and 11.7% in the levosimendan groups (hazard ratio [HR] 0.56; 95% CI=0.33-0.95; p=0.031), and 180-day mortality was 31.4% vs 22.6%, respectively (HR 0.67; 95% CI=0.45-1.00; p=0.053). Levosimendan induced dose-dependent decreases in systolic and diastolic BP and increases in heart rate. During the 6-hour infusion, adverse effects were noted in 23.4% of the patients in the levosimendan groups and in 17.6% in the placebo group (p=0.233).
Concl.	Levosimendan at an infusion rate of 0.1 to 0.2 µg/kg/min was safe and reduced the risk of worsening heart failure and mortality in patients with evidence of heart failure shortly after acute MI.

SOLVD

Studies of Left Ventricular Dysfunction (Substudy)

Title	Efficacy of angiotensin-converting enzyme inhibition in reducing progression from asymptomatic left ventricular dysfunction to symptomatic heart failure in black and white patients.
Authors	Dries DL, Strong MH, Cooper RS, et al.
Reference	J Am Coll Cardiol 2002;40:311-317.
Disease	Congestive heart failure.
Purpose	To determine whether enalapril was equally effective in preventing the development of symptomatic heart failure in black and white patients with asymptomatic left ventricular dysfunction.
Design	Retrospective analysis of a randomized, double-blind, placebo-controlled trial.
Patients	4228 patients with known heart disease with ejection fraction <0.35 and not receiving diuretics, digoxin, or vasodilators.
Follow-up	Mean 34 months (as per SOLVD trial, N Engl J Med 1999;340:609-616).
Regimen	Enalapril (2.5 or 5 mg bid) with gradual increase to 10 mg bid vs placebo (as per SOLVD). Patients were permitted to use diuretic therapy for hypertension, digoxin for atrial fibrillation, or nitrates for angina.

Results   There were 403 black patients and 3651 white patients. No significant differences in the baseline characteristics of white patients were found. In black patients, the enalapril group had more women, as well as hypertensives, and a higher systolic BP. Overall, white patients had fewer women, were less likely to have a history of diabetes or hypertension, but were more likely to have an ischemic etiology of systolic dysfunction and baseline β-blocker use. The primary end points (indicators of progression of asymptomatic left ventricular dysfunction [ALVD]) were: development of heart failure (HF) symptoms, development of HF symptoms and addition of HF medications, death or development of HF symptoms, first hospitalization for HF, death or first hospitalization for HF. Black patients showed an increased incidence of the primary end points vs white patients in both enalapril and placebo groups. Patients in the enalapril groups had a decreased risk of progression of ALVD vs placebo; the decreased risk was similar for black and white patients (relative risk [RR] for primary end point vs placebo: 0.61-0.86 in black patients, 0.62-0.81 in white patients). In black patients, enalapril significantly reduced the risk of: development of HF symptoms (RR 0.69; 95% CI=0.51-0.93; p=0.02), development of HF symptoms and adding HF medications (RR 0.61; 95% CI=0.41-0.89; p=0.01), and death or development of HF symptoms (RR 0.74; CI=0.56-0.97; p=0.03). Adjustment of the analyses to account for differences in baseline characteristics between black patients randomized to enalapril and placebo revealed similar results.

Concl.   Enalapril was equally effective in reducing progression of heart failure in black and white patients with asymptomatic LV dysfunction.

SOLVD

Insights From Studies of Left Ventricular Dysfunction

Title	Enalapril decreases the incidence of atrial fibrillation in patients with left ventricular dysfunction: insight from the Studies of Left Ventricular Dysfunction (SOLVD) trials.
Authors	Vermes E, Tardif JC, Bourassa MG, et al.
Reference	Circulation 2003;107:2926-2931.
Disease	Heart failure, arrhythmia.
Purpose	To assess the impact of the angiotensin-converting enzyme inhibitor enalapril on the incidence of atrial fibrillation in patients with left ventricular dysfunction.
Design	Retrospective analysis.
Patients	374 patients from the Montreal Heart Institute randomly assigned in SOLVD who did not have significant arrhythmia on the baseline electrocardiogram.
Follow-up	2.9±1 years.
Regimen	Enalapril 5-20 mg/d or placebo.

Results   A total of 1491 ECGs were examined: 693 in the placebo
          group and 798 in the enalapril group (3.7±4.1 and 4.1±5 per
          patient, respectively). 55 patients had atrial fibrillation (AF)
          during follow-up: 10 (5.4%) in the enalapril group and 45
          (24%) in the placebo group (p<0.0001), yielding an abso-
          lute risk reduction of 18.6%. By Cox multivariate analysis,
          enalapril was the most powerful predictor for risk reduction
          of AF (hazard ratio 0.22; 95% CI=0.11-0.44; p<0.0001). The
          majority of AF episodes were paroxysmal and required hos-
          pitalization for worsening heart failure. Only a few patients
          required electrical cardioversion.

Concl.   ACE inhibitor therapy with enalapril markedly and signifi-
          cantly reduced the risk of development of AF in patients with
          LV dysfunction.

STRETCH

Symptom, Tolerability, Response to Exercise Trial of Candesartan Cilexetil in Heart Failure

Title	Improvement in exercise tolerance and symptoms of congestive heart failure during treatment with candesartan cilexetil.
Authors	Riegger GAJ, Bouzo H, Petr P, et al.
Reference	Circulation 1999;100:2224-2230.
Disease	Congestive heart failure.
Purpose	To determine the effect of the angiotensin II type 1 receptor antagonist, candesartan, on exercise tolerance and symptoms in patients with congestive heart failure.
Design	Prospective, randomized, double-blind, placebo-controlled, multicenter, parallel group.
Patients	844 patients with congestive heart failure; NYHA Class II or III; ejection fraction of 30%-45%.
Follow-up	12 weeks.
Regimen	Candesartan 4, 8, or 16 mg orally once-a-day or matching placebo.
Add'l Tx	Diuretics, long acting nitrates, cardiac glycosides. Patients were not on ACE inhibitors during the trial.

Results   Primary efficacy data was total exercise time assessed by bicycle ergometry. Other measures were NYHA Functional Class, signs and symptoms of congestive heart failure, and cardiothoracic ratio on chest x-ray. Candesartan cilexetil 16 mg resulted in significantly greater exercise time (47.2 seconds) compared to placebo (30.8 seconds, $p = 0.046$), and there was a dose related improvement in exercise time (39.7 seconds at 4 mg and 45.8 seconds at 8 mg). Dyspnea Fatigue Index scores were improved on candesartan compared with placebo and there was a trend toward improved NYHA Class. There was a small but significant decrease in cardiothoracic ratio. Candesartan was associated with an increase in plasma renin activity and angiotensin II levels and a decrease in aldosterone levels. The drug was well tolerated.

Concl.   In patients with mild to moderate congestive heart failure, candesartan improved exercise tolerance times, symptoms and signs of congestive heart failure, and cardiothoracic ratio.

The MIRACLE ICD Trial

The Multicenter InSync Randomized Clinical Evaluation-Implantable Cardioverter Defibrillator Trial

Title	Combined cardiac resynchronization and implantable cardioversion defibrillator in advanced chronic heart failure.
Authors	Young JB, Abraham WT, Smith AL, et al.
Reference	JAMA 2003;289:2685-2694.
Disease	Congestive heart failure.
Purpose	To determine efficacy and safety of combined cardiac resynchronization therapy (CRT) through biventricular pacing and implantable cardioversion defibrillation (ICD) therapy in patients with NYHA Class III or IV CHF.
Design	Randomized, double-blind, parallel-controlled.
Patients	369 patients with NYHA Class III or IV CHF, LVEF ≤35%, left ventricular end diastolic diameter ≥55 mm, QRS duration of ≥130 ms, at high risk of ventricular arrhythmias.
Follow-up	6 months.
Regimen	182 patients were randomized to receive an implantable cardioverter-defibrillator (ICD) plus optimal medical treatment. 187 patients received ICD plus CRT plus optimal medical therapy.
Add'l Tx	ACE inhibitor or angiotensin receptor blocker; β-blocker allowed if patient on it at least 3 months prior to enrollment.

Results	Primary efficacy end points were NYHA functional class, quality of life score, and distance achieved during 6-minute walking test. Secondary end points included peak Vo_2, treadmill exercise duration, LVEF, plasma neurohormones, overall heart failure status, and others. Patients assigned to CRT had a greater improvement in median quality of life score (-17.5; 95% CI=-21 to -14) vs ICD alone (-11.0; 95% CI=16 to -7; p=0.02). There was also greater improvement in functional class in CTR group vs ICD alone (-1 [-1 to -1] vs 0 [-1 to 0]; p=0.007). There was no difference in 6-minute walking distance between CTR vs ICD alone (55 m [44-79] vs 53 m [43-75]; p=0.36). However, exercise treadmill duration increased by 56 seconds in the CRT group and decreased by 11 seconds in the ICD alone group (p<0.001). Vo_2 max increased by 1.1 mL/kg/min in the CRT group vs 0.1 mL/kg/min in the ICD alone group (p=0.04). There were no significant differences in LV function, size, heart failure status, survival, or hospitalization rates. Proarrhythmia was not observed with biventricular pacing, nor did CRT compromise ICD arrhythmia termination capability.
Concl.	Cardiac resynchronization therapy through biventricular pacing improved quality of life, NYHA functional class, and exercise capacity in patients with moderate-to-severe heart failure, wide QRS, and life-threatening ventricular arrhythmias.

Val-HeFT

Valsartan Heart Failure Trial

Title	A randomized trial of the angiotensin-receptor blocker valsartan in chronic heart failure.
Authors	Cohn JN, Tognoni G, for the Valsartan Heart Failure Trial Investigators.
Reference	N Engl J Med 2001;345:1667-1675.
Disease	Congestive heart failure (CHF).
Purpose	To assess the long-term effects of valsartan in patients with CHF receiving standard therapy.
Design	Randomized, placebo-controlled, double-blind, multicenter.
Patients	5010 patients, ≥18 years old, with stable CHF for ≥3 months. Patients should have been on a fixed dose drug regimen for ≥2 weeks and have left ventricular (LV) ejection fraction <40% and LV dilatation. 93% of the patients received angiotensin-converting enzyme (ACE) inhibitors and 35% received β-blockers at baseline. Only 5% of the patients received spironolactone.
Follow-up	Mean follow-up 23 months (range 0-38 months).
Regimen	After 2-4 weeks assessment while taking placebo, patients were randomized to valsartan (n=2511) or placebo (n=2499). Valsartan was initiated at a dose of 40 mg bid. The dose was gradually increased to 160 mg bid.

Results	The target dose of 160 mg bid was achieved by 84% of the patients in the valsartan vs 93% in the placebo group. Systolic blood pressure was reduced by 5.2±16.0 mm Hg in the valsartan group vs 1.3±15.9 mm Hg in the placebo group after 1 year. Mortality was 19.7% in the valsartan group vs 19.4% in the placebo group (relative risk 1.02; 95% CI=0.88-1.18; p=0.80). The combined end point of death, hospitalization for heart failure, cardiac arrest with resuscitation, or administration of IV inotropic or vasodilator therapy for heart failure occurred in 28.8% in the valsartan group vs 32.1% in the placebo group (RR 0.87; 95% CI=0.77-0.97; p=0.009). The difference was related to less hospitalization for heart failure worsening in the valsartan group (13.8% vs 18.2%, respectively; p<0.001). There were 3106 hospitalizations in the placebo group vs 2856 in the valsartan group (p=0.14). More patients in the valsartan group had improvement in their NYHA class (23.1% vs 20.7%) and fewer had worsening (10.1% vs 12.8%) (p<0.001). Valsartan significantly reduced mortality in the 226 patients who did not receive β-blockers or ACE-inhibitors (p=0.012). Among the 1610 patients who received both β-blockers and ACE inhibitors, valsartan treatment was associated with increased mortality (p=0.009). Among the 3034 patients who received ACE inhibitors without β-blockers, valsartan was not beneficial. Among the 140 patients who received β-blockers but not ACE inhibitors, the effect of valsartan was not statistically significant. Among all 366 patients who did not receive ACE inhibitors (irrespective of β-blocker therapy), there were less combined end point events in the valsartan group (RR 0.56; 95% CI=0.39-0.81) and lower mortality (RR 0.67; 95% CI=0.42-1.06). Discontinuation of the study drug due to adverse effects occurred in 9.9% in the valsartan group vs 7.2% in the placebo (p<0.001).
Concl.	Valsartan reduced the combined end point of death and morbidity and improved clinical signs and symptoms of heart failure. However, the beneficial effect was restricted to patients who were not receiving ACE inhibitors. Among patients who received ACE inhibitors and β-blockers, valsartan was associated with increased mortality.

Val-HeFT Echocardiographic Study:

Valsartan Benefits Left Ventricular Structure and Function in Heart Failure

Title	Echocardiographic study: valsartan benefits left ventricular structure and function in heart failure.
Authors	Wong M, Staszewsky L, Latini R, et al.
Reference	J Am Coll Cardiol 2002;40:970-975.N Engl J Med 2001;345:1667-1675.
Disease	Congestive heart failure.
Purpose	To determine the effect of addition of an angiotensin receptor blocker to standard heart failure therapy on left ventricular structure and function.
Design	Randomized, double-blind, placebo-controlled, prospective, multicenter.
Patients	5010 patients with New York Heart Association (NYHA) Class II-IV heart failure, currently on angiotensin-converting enzyme inhibitor and/or b-blocker. Entry criteria were: a left ventricular internal diastolic diameter >2.9 cm/m^2 and ejection fraction (EF) <40%.
Follow-up	Up to 24 months.
Regimen	Patients were randomized to receive valsartan (n=2511) or placebo (n=2499). Valsartan was initiated at a dose of 40 mg bid and gradually increased to 160 mg bid. Left ventricular internal diastolic (LVID) diameter and EF were measured by echocardiography at 4, 12, 18, and 24 months, as well as at the end point (last post-randomization was carried forward).
Add'l Tx	Other appropriate anti-heart failure medicines including ACE inhibitors, β-blockers, diuretics, and digoxin.

Results | LVID diameter/BSA and EF were adjusted for effects of treatment group, pooled center, baseline, use of ACE inhibitors or b-blockers, and analysis of covariance. LVID diameter/body surface area (BSA) and EF values were similar between the valsartan and placebo groups at baseline. EF increased from baseline starting at 4 months and demonstrated a consistent, statistically significant increase in the valsartan group at each of the measurement points (4, 12, 18, 24 months, and end point) compared with placebo ($p < 0.03$ at all points). Similarly, LVID diameter/BSA decreased from baseline starting at 4 months and a statistically significant decrease was found in the valsartan group vs placebo at each measurement point ($p < 0.03$ at all points). LVID diameter was reduced by 0.12 ± 0.4 cm/m^2 in the valsartan group vs 0.05 ± 0.4 in the placebo group ($p < 0.00001$) at 18 months. EF increased by $4.5\% \pm 8.9\%$ in valsartan vs $3.2\% \pm 8.6\%$ in the placebo group at 18 months ($p < 0.00001$). Statistically significant decreases in LVID diameter/BSA and increases in EF were found in all subgroups categorized by use or nonuse of ACE inhibitors and/or β-blockers except in the subgroup using both ACE inhibitors and β-blockers, in which there were no differences between the valsartan and placebo groups.

Concl. | Valsartan, when taken with either ACE inhibitors or β-blockers, is beneficial in reversing LV remodeling in heart failure.

VMAC

Vasodilation in the Management of Acute Congestive Heart Failure

Title	Intravenous nesiritide vs nitroglycerin for treatment of decompensated congestive heart failure. A randomized controlled trial.
Authors	Publication Committee for the VMAC Investigators.
Reference	JAMA 2002;287:1531-1540.
Disease	Congestive heart failure (CHF).
Purpose	To compare the acute efficacy and safety of IV nesiritide, nitroglycerin vs placebo in hospitalized patients with decompensated CHF in patients older than 65 years.
Design	Randomized, double-blind, multicenter.
Patients	489 hospitalized patients with dyspnea at rest from decompensated CHF. 246 of these patients received pulmonary artery catheterization.
Follow-up	Acute hemodynamic study; mortality assessed through 6 months.
Regimen	IV nesiritide (a recombinant human brain natriuretic peptide; n=204); IV nitroglycerin (n=143) or placebo (n=142) added to standard therapy for 3-24 hours. Various doses of nesiritide were used.
Add'l Tx	Usual medicines for CHF including dobutamine or dopamine.

Results   Primary end point was comparison of hemodynamic and clinical effects of nesiritide vs placebo when added to standard therapy—including absolute change in pulmonary capillary wedge
pressure (PCWP) in catheterized patients and patients' self evaluation of dyspnea. Mean decrease in PCWP at 3 hours vs baseline was -5.8±6.5 mm Hg (mean±SD) in the nesiritide group vs
-3.8±5.3 mm Hg for nitroglycerin vs -2±4.2 mm Hg for placebo
(p<0.001 for nesiritide vs placebo and p=0.03 for nesiritide vs
nitroglycerin; and p=0.09 for nitroglycerin vs placebo). Also, at
3 hours, nesiritide improved dyspnea vs placebo (p=0.03) but
did not improve dyspnea, or global clinical status vs nitroglycerin. Nesiritide resulted in a greater reduction in PCWP at 24
hours (-8.2 mm Hg) vs nitroglycerin (-6.3 mm Hg) but at this
time, patients did not report significant differences in dyspnea
between these 2 groups.

Concl.   Nesiritide improved hemodynamic function and some self-
reported symptoms better than nitroglycerin or placebo in
patients hospitalized with acutely decompensated CHF already
receiving standard care.

ACTIV in CHF

Acute and Chronic Therapeutic Impact of a Vasopressin Antagonist in Congestive Heart Failure

Title	Effects of tolvaptan, a vasopressin antagonist, in patients hospitalized with worsening heart failure: a randomized controlled trial.
Authors	Gheorghiade M, Gattis WA, O'Connor CM, et al.
Reference	JAMA 2004;291:1963-1971.
Disease	Congestive heart failure.
Purpose	To evaluate the short- and intermediate-term effects of tolvaptan in patients hospitalized with heart failure.
Design	Multicenter, randomized, double-blind, placebo-controlled, parallel-group, dose-ranging, phase 2 study.
Patients	319 patients with left ventricular ejection fraction <40% hospitalized for congestive heart failure with persistent signs and symptoms of systemic congestion despite standard therapy.
Follow-up	60 days.
Regimen	Tolvaptan 30, 60, or 90 mg/d orally or placebo for up to 60 days.
Add'l Tx	Standard congestive heart failure therapy, including diuretics.
Results	The study had 2 primary end points: acute (in-hospital) change in body weight at 24 hours after randomization and outpatient outcome. Median (interquartile range) body weight at 24 hours decreased by 1.80 (3.85-0.50), 2.10 (3.10-0.85), 2.05 (2.80-0.60), and 0.60 (1.60-0.00) kg, respectively, in the patients receiving 30, 60, and 90 mg/d of tolvaptan and placebo. The decrease in body weight with tolvaptan was not associated with changes in heart rate or BP, nor did it result in hypokalemia or worsening renal function. There were no differences in worsening CHF at 60 days between tolvaptan and placebo. 60-day mortality was lower in tolvaptan-treated patients with renal dysfunction or severe systemic congestion.

Concl.   Arginine vasopressin levels are elevated in CHF and may result in myocardial fibrosis/hypertrophy and vasoconstriction. Tolvaptan, a vasopressin antagonist, may hold promise for management of systemic congestion in patients hospitalized for CHF. It increased net fluid loss, resulting in decreased body weight, more effectively than standard therapy alone. These effects were achieved without adverse effects on BP, heart rate, electrolyte levels, and renal function. Tolvaptan also improved serum sodium levels in patients with hyponatremia. Tolvaptan did not reduce the rate of worsening CHF after discharge; however, post hoc analysis suggests that mortality may be reduced in high-risk patients treated with tolvaptan.

ATTACH

Anti-TNF Therapy Against Congestive Heart Failure

Title	Randomized, double-blind, placebo-controlled, pilot trial of infliximab, a chimeric monoclonal antibody to tumor necrosis factor-α, in patients with moderate-to-severe heart failure: results of the Anti-TNF Therapy Against Congestive Heart Failure (ATTACH) trial.
Authors	Chung ES, Packer M, Lo KH, et al.
Reference	Circulation 2003;107:3133-3140.
Disease	Congestive heart failure.
Purpose	To investigate the efficacy and safety of infliximab, a chimeric monoclonal antibody to tumor necrosis factor-α, in patients with moderate to severe congestive heart failure.
Design	Multicenter, randomized, double-blind trial.
Patients	150 patients with stable New York Heart Association class III or IV congestive heart failure and left ventricular ejection fraction $\leq 35\%$.
Follow-up	28 weeks.
Regimen	Infliximab 5 mg/kg (n=50) or 10 mg/kg (n=51) or placebo (n=49) at 0, 2, and 6 weeks after randomization.

Results	The primary end point of the study was clinical status at 14 weeks. Neither dose of infliximab improved clinical status at 14 or at 28 weeks despite suppression of inflammatory markers (C-reactive protein and interleukin-6) and a slight improvement in LVEF in patients receiving 5 mg/kg. Patients receiving 10 mg/kg were more likely than those receiving the smaller dose or placebo to have worsening of clinical status at 14 and 28 weeks. The worsening clinical status in the 10-mg/kg group was related primarily to an increased risk of major adverse clinical events, ie, they were more likely to die or be hospitalized for CHF than patients in the placebo group (hazard ratio 2.84; 95% CI=1.01-7.97; nominal p=0.043). There were no differences in quality of life scores among the 3 groups. The rate of adverse events was likewise similar, although patients receiving infliximab 10 mg/kg reported more worsening heart failure. Serious infections occurred in 8% of the patients receiving infliximab 10 mg/kg, 5.9% of those receiving 5 mg/kg, and 2.1% of those receiving placebo.
Concl.	Short-term TNF-α antagonism with infliximab did not improve clinical status, and the larger dose adversely affected clinical status, in patients with moderate to severe chronic heart failure. Infliximab did produce the expected biological effects, ie, suppression of C-reactive protein and interleukin-6; however, improvements in physiologic variables often do not translate into measurable clinical benefits, although the lack of benefit may be related to the relatively short duration of the trial.

CHARM

The Candesartan in Heart Failure Assessment of Reduction in Mortality and Morbidity

Title	Effects of candesartan on mortality and morbidity in patients with chronic heart failure: the CHARM overall programme.
Authors	Pfeffer MA, Swedberg K, Granger CB, et al.
Reference	Lancet 2003;362:759-766.
Disease	Chronic heart failure.
Purpose	To determine whether the angiotensin receptor blocker, candesartan, could reduce the mortality and morbidity in patients with chronic heart failure.
Design	Parallel, randomized, double-blind, controlled, multicenter in 3 distinct trials.
Patients	Patients aged 18 years and older with symptomatic heart failure (Class II-IV) for at least 4 weeks. Patients entered into 1 of 3 trials: 1) Patients with left ventricular ejection fraction ≤40% on an angiotensin-converting enzyme inhibitor (CHARM-Added); 2) ≤40% or lower and not on an angiotensin-converting enzyme inhibitor because of intolerance (CHARM-Alternative); or 3) in patients with preserved left ventricular ejection fraction (>40%; CHARM-Preserved). Exclusion criteria included serum creatinine of 265 mmol/L or more, serum potassium of 5.5 mmol/L or more, known bilateral renal artery stenosis, symptomatic hypotension, and others.
Follow-up	Median follow-up was 37.7 months.
Regimen	3803 patients randomized to candesartan (starting at 4 or 8 mg titrated to a target dose of 32 mg qd) vs placebo (n=3796). Blood pressure, serum potassium, and creatinine were monitored.

Results	There were 886 (23%) deaths in the candesartan group vs 945 (25%) in the placebo group (unadjusted hazard ratio [HR] 0.91; 95% CI=0.83-1.00; p=0.055); covariate adjusted 0.90; 95% CI=0.82-0.99; p=0.032. The candesartan group had fewer cardiovascular deaths at 691 (18%) compared to the placebo group at 769 (20%) (unadjusted HR 0.88; 95% CI=0.79-0.97; p=0.012; covariate adjusted HR 0.87; 95% CI=0.78-0.96; p=0.06). There was also a significant reduction in admissions for heart failure in the candesartan group (20%) vs the placebo group (24%; p<0.0001). Incidence of cardiovascular death or hospitalization for worsened heart failure was lower with candesartan (30%) than placebo (35%; p<0.0001). Importantly, there was no significant heterogeneity for the results of candesartan across the 3 trials for the impact of candesartan on all-cause mortality or cardiovascular deaths or hospital admissions. Baseline use of other heart failure drugs (β-blockers, spironolactone, diuretics, digitalis) did not negate candesartan's advantage. Cancer deaths were slightly higher in the candesartan group (2.3%) than in the placebo group (1.6%), but incidence of nonfatal neoplasms was similar between the 2 groups (5.1% vs 4.6% for candesartan vs placebo, respectively). In the 2 trials including patients with an LVEF ≤40%, the primary composite end point of cardiovascular death or unplanned hospitalization for worsening heart failure and its components was lower in the candesartan group vs placebo. In the trial with LVEF >40%, candesartan did decrease hospitalizations for worsening heart failure but did not show a significant benefit for cardiovascular death alone or the composite end point. Discontinuation for adverse events or abnormal laboratory values were more frequent with candesartan including concerns about renal function, hypotension, and hyperkalemia.
Concl.	In patients with chronic heart failure, candesartan reduced cardiovascular deaths and hospital admissions for heart failure. LVEF and therapies at baseline did not affect these benefits.

CHARM-Added

Candesartan in Heart Failure: Assessment of Reduction in Mortality and Morbidity (with Addition of an ACE Inhibitor)

Title	Effects of candesartan in patients with chronic heart failure and reduced left-ventricular systolic function taking angiotensin-converting-enzyme inhibitors: the CHARM-Added trial.
Authors	McMurray JJ, Ostergren J, Swedberg K, et al.
Reference	Lancet 2003;362:767-771.
Disease	Congestive heart failure.
Purpose	To investigate whether combining the angiotensin receptor blocker candesartan with angiotensin-converting enzyme inhibitors improves clinical outcome.
Design	Prospective, parallel, randomized, double-blind, controlled multicenter in 3 distinct trials.
Patients	2548 patients with New York Heart Association class II-IV congestive heart failure and left ventricular ejection fraction ≤40% who were being treated with angiotensin-converting enzyme inhibitors (usually enalapril, lisinopril, captopril, or ramipril).
Follow-up	Median 41 months.
Regimen	Angiotensin-converting enzyme inhibitors + candesartan (target dose 32 mg/d) (n=1276) or angiotensin-converting enzyme inhibitors + placebo (n=1272).
Add'l Tx	At baseline, 55% of patients were also treated with β-blockers and 17% with spironolactone.

Results	The primary outcome was the composite of cardiovascular death or hospital admission for CHF. Analysis was by intention to treat. A total of 483 patients in the candesartan group (38%) and 538 in the placebo group (42%) had a primary outcome event (unadjusted hazard ratio 0.85; 95% CI=0.75-0.96; p=0.011; covariate adjusted p=0.010). Annual event rates were 14.1% in the candesartan group and 16.6% in the placebo group. Candesartan reduced cardiovascular mortality and the risk of admission to hospital for CHF individually as well. There were 302 (24%) cardiovascular deaths in the candesartan group vs 347 (27%) in the placebo group; p=0.029. 44 patients receiving candesartan and 69 placebo had an MI (p=0.012), 47 receiving candesartan and 41 placebo had a stroke (p=0.62), and 69 receiving candesartan and 75 receiving placebo underwent coronary revascularization. The benefits of candesartan were similar in all predefined subgroups, including patients receiving β-blockers at baseline.
Concl.	The addition of candesartan to ACE inhibitor therapy results in clinically important reductions in cardiovascular events in patients with CHF and reduced ejection fraction. These results are consistent with the evidence that angiotensin II continues to be produced despite chronic ACE inhibitor treatment, and with mechanistic studies showing beneficial neurohumoral, homodynamic, and LV remodeling effects of angiotensin receptor blockers.

CHARM-Alternative

Candesartan in Heart Failure: Assessment of Reduction in Mortality and Morbidity-Alternative

Title	Effects of candesartan in patients with chronic heart failure and reduced left-ventricular systolic function intolerant to angiotensin-converting enzyme inhibitors: the CHARM-Alternative trial.
Authors	Granger CB, McMurray JJ, Yusuf S, et al.
Reference	Lancet 2003;362:772-776.
Disease	Congestive heart failure.
Purpose	To determine whether the angiotensin receptor blocker candesartan could improve outcome in patients intolerant to angiotensin-converting enzyme inhibitors.
Design	Prospective, parallel, randomized, double-blind, controlled, multicenter study comprising 3 distinct trials.
Patients	2028 patients with symptomatic congestive heart failure and left ventricular ejection fraction <40% who were not receiving angiotensin-converting enzyme inhibitors because of previous intolerance.
Follow-up	Median 33.7 months.
Regimen	Candesartan (target dose 32 mg/d) (n=1013) or placebo (n=1015).
Add'l Tx	At baseline, 55% of patients were taking β-blockers and 24% spironolactone.

Results	The most common manifestations of ACE-inhibitor intolerance were cough (72%), symptomatic hypotension (13%), and renal dysfunction (12%). During follow-up, 334 patients in the candesartan group (33%) and 406 in the placebo group (40%) died from cardiovascular causes or were hospitalized for CHF (unadjusted hazard ratio [HR] 0.77; 95% CI=0.67-0.89; p=0.0004; covariate adjusted HR 0.70; 95% CI=0.60-0.81; p<0.0001). The average annual event rates were 13.8% in the candesartan group and 18.2% in the placebo group. There was a 23% relative risk reduction in the primary end point with candesartan treatment. Each component of the primary end point was reduced, as was the total number of hospital admissions for CHF, in the candesartan group. Study drug discontinuation rates were similar with candesartan and placebo.
Concl.	Candesartan was generally well tolerated and reduced cardiovascular mortality and morbidity in patients with symptomatic chronic CHF and intolerance to ACE inhibitors. The absolute reduction of 7 major events per 100 patients treated corresponds to the need to treat 14 patients with candesartan to prevent 1 patient from dying from cardiovascular causes or being admitted for heart failure.

CHARM-Preserved

Candesartan in Heart Failure: Assessment of Reduction in Mortality and Morbidity-Preserved LVEF

Title	Effects of candesartan in patients with chronic heart failure and preserved left-ventricular ejection fraction: the CHARM-Preserved trial.
Authors	Yusuf S, Pfeffer MA, Swedberg K, et al.
Reference	Lancet 2003;362:777-781.
Disease	Congestive heart failure.
Purpose	To determine the effect of adding the angiotensin receptor blocker candesartan to current treatments in patients with congestive heart failure and preserved left ventricular function.
Design	Prospective, parallel, randomized, double-blind, controlled multicenter in 3 distinct trials.
Patients	3023 patients with congestive heart failure and preserved left ventricular function. Patients had to have a New York Heart Association congestive heart failure class of II-IV but left ventricular ejection fraction of greater than 40%.
Follow-up	Median 36.6 months.
Regimen	Candesartan (target dose 32 mg/d) (n=1514) or placebo (n=1509).
Add'l Tx	At baseline, 296 patients in the candesartan group (20%) and 280 in the placebo group (19%) were taking angiotensin-converting enzyme inhibitors; 847 (56%) and 837 (56%), respectively, were taking β-blockers.

Results	Cardiovascular death or admission to hospital for CHF (the primary outcome) occurred in 333 patients (22%) in the candesartan group and 366 (24%) in the placebo group (relative risk reduction [RR] 11%, adjusted hazard ratio [HR] 0.89; 95% CI=0.77-1.03; p=0.118; covariate adjusted HR 0.86; 95% CI=0.74-1.00; p=0.051). Annual event rates were 8.1% in the candesartan group and 9.1% in the placebo group. 170 patients in each group died from cardiovascular causes; the number of non-cardiovascular deaths was similar (74 vs 67). Fewer patients in the candesartan group were admitted to the hospital for CHF (230 vs 279; p=0.017), and fewer were admitted more than once (98 vs 122; p=0.093). Therefore, the total number of admissions for CHF was 402 in the candesartan group and 566 in the placebo group (p=0.014).
Concl.	Candesartan has a modest impact on admissions for CHF among patients with CHF and well preserved LV function.

CHRISTMAS

Carvedilol Hibernating Reversible Ischemia Trial: Marker of Success

Title	Myocardial viability as a determinant of the ejection fraction response to carvedilol in patients with heart failure (CHRISTMAS trial): randomised, controlled trial.
Authors	Cleland JGF, Pennell DJ, Ray SG, et al.
Reference	Lancet 2003;362:14-21.
Disease	Congestive heart failure.
Purpose	To determine whether improvement in left ventricular ejection fraction is associated with the volume of hibernating myocardium in patients with congestive heart failure.
Design	Randomized, placebo-controlled, double-blind trial.
Patients	387 patients with chronic heart failure due to ischemic left ventricular systolic dysfunction. Patients designated as "hibernators" or "non-hibernators" according to the volume of hibernating myocardium.
Follow-up	189 days.
Regimen	Carvedilol, initial dose 3.125 mg bid, titrated as necessary to 25 mg bid or 50 mg bid (in patients weighing ≥85 kg) or placebo.

Results   The primary end point was change in LVEF, measured by radio-
           nuclide ventriculography, in hibernators vs nonhibernators, on
           carvedilol compared with placebo. Analysis was by intention
           to treat. 82 patients dropped out because of adverse events,
           withdrawal of consent, or failure to complete the investigation,
           yielding 305 patients (79%) for analysis. Mean change in LVEF
           was not significant between groups (mean change -0.4±0.9 in
           the nonhibernators and -0.4±0.8 in the hibernators). However,
           LVEF increased with carvedilol (2.5±0.9 and 3.2±0.8 for non-
           hibernators and hibernators, respectively; p<0.001 vs baseline).
           The mean placebo-subtracted change in LVEF was 3.2% (95%
           CI=1.8-4.7; p=0.0001) overall and 2.9% (95% CI=0.7-5.1;
           p=0.011) and 3.6% (95% CI=1.7-5.4; p=0.0002) in nonhiber-
           nators and hibernators, respectively. Patients with more myocar-
           dium affected by hibernation or by hibernation and ischemia
           had a greater increase in LVEF with carvedilol.

Concl.   The effect of carvedilol on LVEF may be mediated, in part, by
           improved function of hibernating or ischemic myocardium, or
           both. Medical treatment may be a useful adjunct or alternative
           to revascularization for patients with hibernating myocardium.

COMET

Carvedilol or Metoprolol European Trial

Title	Comparison of carvedilol and metoprolol on clinical outcomes in patients with chronic heart failure in the Carvedilol Or Metoprolol European Trial (COMET): randomised controlled trial.
Authors	Poole-Wilson PA, Swedberg K, Cleland JG, et al.
Reference	Lancet 2003;362:7-13.
Disease	Congestive heart failure.
Purpose	To compare the effects of carvedilol (blocks β 1, β 2, and α 1 adrenergic receptors) vs metoprolol (blocks β 1 adrenergic receptor) in patients with chronic congestive heart failure already on diuretics and angiotensin-converting enzyme inhibitors.
Design	Randomized, parallel-group trial, double-blind, multicenter.
Patients	1511 patients with chronic heart failure (New York Heart Association class II-IV), previous admission for a cardiovascular etiology, ejection fraction ≤0.35, and to have been optimally treated with diuretics and angiotensin-converting enzyme inhibitors (unless not tolerated).
Follow-up	Mean follow-up was 58 months.
Regimen	Patients were randomized to receive either 3.125 mg carvedilol bid (n=1511) or to 5 mg metoprolol tartrate bid (n=1518). The dose of each β blocker was increased during a titration phase (≈6 weeks) to a target of carvedilol 25 mg twice daily or metoprolol 50 mg twice daily. Patients then entered a maintenance phase and were assessed every 4 months.

Results	The primary end points included all-cause mortality as well as the composite end point of all-cause mortality or all-cause admission. Mean age was 62 years and mean ejection fraction was 0.26. All-cause mortality was 34% (512 of 1511) in the carvedilol group vs 40% (600 of 1518) in the metoprolol group (hazard ratio 0.83; 95% CI=0.74-0.93; p=0.0017. The decrease in mortality was similar across predefined subgroups by age, New York Heart Association class, cause of CHF, LVEF, diabetes, and others. The benefit of carvedilol over metoprolol on mortality first appeared at about 6 months into therapy. Sudden death was the mode of death in 14% of the carvedilol patients and 17% of the metoprolol patients. There were 438 (29%) cardiovascular deaths in the carvedilol group vs 534 (35%) in the metoprolol group [hazard ratio 0.80; 95% CI=0.70-0.90; p=0.0004]. The composite of mortality or all-cause admission was 74% in the carvedilol group vs 76% in the metoprolol group (p=0.122). There were small differences in side effects between the two groups, favoring carvedilol.
Concl.	Carvedilol was superior to metoprolol for extending survival in heart failure patients.

COMPANION

Comparison of Medical Therapy, Pacing, and Defibrillation in Heart Failure

Title	Cardiac-resynchronization therapy with or without an implantable defibrillator in advanced chronic heart failure.
Authors	Bristow MR, Saxon LA, Boehmer J, et al.
Reference	N Engl J Med 2004;350:2140-2150.
Disease	Arrhythmia, congestive heart failure.
Purpose	To test the hypothesis that prophylactic cardiac-resynchronization therapy (biventricular stimulation with a pacemaker with or without a defibrillator) reduces the risk of death and hospitalization among patients with advanced chronic congestive heart failure and intraventricular conduction delays.
Design	Multicenter, controlled clinical trial.
Patients	1520 patients with advanced congestive heart failure (New York Heart Association class III or IV) due to ischemic or nonischemic cardiomyopathies and a QRS interval ≥120 milliseconds.
Follow-up	12 months.
Regimen	Optimal pharmacologic therapy (diuretics, angiotensin-converting enzyme inhibitors, β-blockers, spironolactone) alone or in combination with cardiac-resynchronization therapy with a pacemaker or a pacemaker-defibrillator.

Results	The primary composite end point was time to death from or hospitalization for any cause. Compared with optimal pharmacologic therapy alone, cardiac-resynchronization therapy with a pacemaker decreased the risk of the primary end point (hazard ratio [HR] 0.81; p=0.014), as did cardiac-resynchronization with a pacemaker-defibrillator (HR 0.80; p=0.01). The risk of the combined end point was reduced by 34% with pacemaker therapy (p<0.002) and by 40% with pacemaker-defibrillator therapy (p<0.001 vs pharmacologic therapy group). A pacemaker reduced the risk of the secondary end point (death from any cause) by 24% (p=0.059), and a pacemaker-defibrillator reduced the risk by 36% (p=0.003). A total of 61% of patients receiving pharmacologic therapy had moderate or severe adverse events vs 66% receiving a pacemaker and 69% receiving a pacemaker-defibrillator. Moderate or severe adverse events related to implantation occurred in 10% of patients receiving a pacemaker and 8% receiving a pacemaker-defibrillator.
Concl.	In patients with advanced CHF and a prolonged QRS interval, cardiac-resynchronization therapy with a pacemaker or a pacemaker-defibrillator can improve the clinical course of chronic CHF.

RAD B253

Everolimus in Cardiac Transplant Recipients

Title	Everolimus for the prevention of allograft rejection and vasculopathy in cardiac-transplant recipients.
Authors	Eisen HJ, Tuzcu EM, Dorent R, et al.
Reference	N Engl J Med 2003;349:847-858.
Disease	Vasculopathy.
Purpose	To evaluate the effect of the combination of everolimus and cyclosporine on rejection and vasculopathy in recipients of a first cardiac allograft.
Design	Randomized, double-blind clinical trial.
Patients	634 recipients of a first heart transplant.
Follow-up	12 months.
Regimen	1.5 mg/d (n=209) or 3 mg/d (n=211) of everolimus or 1-3 mg/kg/d of azathioprine (n=214).
Add'l Tx	Cyclosporine, corticosteroids, and statins.

Results   The primary end point was a composite of death, graft loss
            or retransplantation, loss to follow-up, biopsy-proved acute
            rejection, or rejection with hemodynamic compromise. At 6
            months, 27% of the patients receiving 3 mg of everolimus
            (p<0.001) and 36.4% receiving 1.5 mg (p=0.03) had reached
            the end point, compared with 46.7% of those receiving aza-
            thioprine. The average increase in maximal intimal thickness
            (by intravascular ultrasound) was significantly smaller in the
            2 everolimus groups (0.04 mm with 1.5 mg; p=0.01, 0.03
            mm with 3 mg; p=0.003) than in the azathioprine group (0.1
            mm). Vasculopathy was less common with everolimus (35.7%
            with 1.5 mg; p=0.045, and 30.4% with 3 mg; p=0.01) than
            with azathioprine (52.8%). The rates of cytomegalovirus
            were significantly lower with everolimus (7.7% with 1.5 mg;
            p<0.001, and 7.6% with 3 mg; p<0.001) than with azathio-
            prine (21.5%). Rates of bacterial infection were significantly
            higher in the 3-mg group than in the azathioprine group.
            Everolimus therapy was associated with a significant increase
            in serum creatinine levels.

Concl.   Everolimus, a novel proliferation inhibitor and immunosuppres-
            sant, was more effective than azathioprine for suppressing car-
            diac-allograft vasculopathy. The 3-mg dose yielded better results
            than the 1.5-mg dose.

RENEWAL

Randomized Etanercept Worldwide Evaluation

Title	Targeted anticytokine therapy in patients with chronic heart failure: results of the Randomized Etanercept Worldwide Evaluation (RENEWAL).
Authors	Mann DL, McMurray JJ, Packer M, et al.
Reference	Circulation 2004;109:1594-1602.
Disease	Congestive heart failure.
Purpose	To test the effect of etanercept, a tumor necrosis factor antagonist, on patient functional status and morbidity/mortality.
Design	Two double-blind, randomized, placebo-controlled, multicenter clinical trials, RECOVER and RENAISSANCE.
Patients	Patients with New York Heart Association class II to IV congestive heart failure and left ventricular ejection fraction ≤30% (RECOVER, n=1123; RENAISSANCE, n=925).
Follow-up	24 weeks.
Regimen	RECOVER: placebo (n=373) or SC etanercept 25 mg/wk (n=375) or twice weekly (n=375). RENAISSANCE: placebo (n=309), etanercept 25 mg twice weekly (n= 308) or 3 times weekly (n=308).
Results	The primary end point of each trial was clinical status at 24 weeks. Analysis of the effect of the 2 larger doses of etanercept on the combined outcome of death or hospitalization due to CHF from the 2 studies was also planned (RENEWAL). However, on the basis of prespecified stopping rules, both trials were terminated prematurely owing to lack of benefit. Etanercept had no effect on clinical status in RENAISSANCE or RECOVER and had no effect on the death or chronic CHF hospitalization end point in RENEWAL.
Concl.	The RENEWAL trial revealed no clinically relevant benefit of etanercept on the rate of death or hospitalization due to chronic CHF.

8. Lipid-Lowering Studies

Cerivastatin in Primary Hypercholesterolemia

Title	Efficacy and safety of cerivastatin, 0.2 mg and 0.4 mg, in patients with primary hypercholesterolemia: A multinational, randomised, double-blind study.
Authors	Ose L, Luurila O, Eriksson J, et al.
Reference	Curr Med Res Opin 1999;15:228-240.
Disease	Hyperlipidemia.
Purpose	To compare the efficacy and safety of cerivastatin 0.2 mg/d and 0.4 mg/d in patients with primary hypercholesterolemia.
Design	Randomized, double-blind, parallel group, multicenter.
Patients	494 patients, 18-75 years old, with primary hypercholesterolemia (LDL cholesterol ≥160 mg/dL or ≥130 mg/dL and either a history of coronary heart disease or ≥2 cardiovascular risk factors). All patients had triglyceride levels ≤350 mg/dL. Patients with obesity, diabetes mellitus, other endocrine disorders, clinically significant ophthalmic abnormalities, a history of hepatic disease, renal failure or malignancy, alcohol abuse, a history of myocardial infarction, unstable angina, stroke, transient ischemic attack or uncontrolled hypertension were excluded.
Follow-up	24 weeks.
Regimen	After a 6 week placebo run-in phase patients were randomized in a 2:1 ratio to cerivastatin 0.4 mg/d (n=332) or 0.2 mg/d (n=162).
Add'l Tx	Treatment with hypoglycemic agents, corticosteroids, androgens, erythromycin, oral anticoagulants, immunosuppressants, and other lipid lowering agents was not permitted.

Results   By intention to treat analysis, LDL cholesterol was lowered by 37.9%±0.7% with cerivastatin 0.4 mg/d and by 30.3%±1.0% by cerivastatin 0.2 mg/d (p<0.0001). Maximal treatment effect was noticed after 4 weeks of therapy and sustained for the 24 weeks of the study. 97% and 94% of the patients in the cerivastatin 0.4 and 0.2 mg/d, respectively, had ≥15% decrease in their LDL cholesterol. Total cholesterol decreased by 25.6%±0.5% and 20.6%±0.7% with cerivastatin 0.4 and 0.2 mg/d (p<0.0001). There were no statistically significant differences between the groups in the change in HDL cholesterol and in serum triglycerides. With per protocol analysis, cerivastatin was more effective in women than men in lowering LDL cholesterol. Adverse effects were noted in 65.5% of the patients in the cerivastatin 0.4 mg/d vs 60.5% in the cerivastatin 0.2 mg/d, 21.4% and 19.8% were probably or possibly related to the drug. Minor increase (≤3 X ULN) in creatine kinase levels was noted in 19.9% and 14.8% of the patients in the cerivastatin 0.4 and 0.2 mg/d, respectively, and >3 X ULN elevation in creatine kinase occurred in 2.7% and 0%, respectively. Minor ALT elevations (≤3 X ULN) were noted in 18.7% and 13.6%, respectively, whereas >3 X ULN elevations occurred in 0.3% and 0%, respectively. Overall, 2.4% and 3.1% of the patients in the cerivastatin 0.4 and 0.2 mg/d, respectively, withdrew from the study due to adverse effects.

Concl.   Cerivastatin was safe and effective in lowering LDL cholesterol levels in a dose-dependent manner.

Extended Release Niacin vs Gemfibrozil for the Treatment of Low Levels of High-Density Lipoprotein Cholesterol

Title	Extended release niacin vs gemfibrozil for the treatment of low levels of high density lipoprotein cholesterol.
Authors	Guyton JR, Blazing MA, Hagar J, et al.
Reference	Arch Intern Med 2000;160:1177-1184.
Disease	Lipid abnormality: low HDL cholesterol.
Purpose	To compare the effect of extended release niacin (Niaspan) vs gemfibrozil on high density lipoprotein cholesterol (HDL-C) in patients with baseline low levels of HDL-C.
Design	Randomized, double-blind, placebo-controlled, multicenter.
Patients	173 patients with an HDL-C level of ≤40 mg/dL, LDL ≤160 mg/dL, or <130 mg/dL with atherosclerotic disease, and a triglyceride level of ≤400 mg/dL.
Follow-up	16 weeks after an initial titration phase.
Regimen	Gemfibrozil 600 mg or its placebo given twice daily. Niaspan or its placebo given once at bedtime (after low fat snack). Niaspan was titrated during an initial 3 week titration phase from 375 mg daily up to 1000 mg for 4 weeks; 1500 mg for 4 weeks; and 2000 mg for 8 weeks.
Add'l Tx	Aspirin a half hour before bedtime study medication.

Results	72 patients assigned to Niaspan completed the protocol; 68 assigned to gemfibrozil completed the study. Niaspan raised HDL-C level by 21% at the 1500 mg dose and 26% at the 2000 mg dose which was >13.3% increase achieved with gemfibrozil ($p=0.01$; $p<0.001$). Niaspan at 1500 and 2000 mg raised apolipoprotein A-1 level by 9% and 11%, respectively, vs 4% with gemfibrozil ($p=0.02$; $p=0.001$). Niaspan reduced lipoprotein (a) by -7% and -20% while gemfibrozil did not affect it. Niaspan had no adverse effects on LDL (2% and 0%); gemfibrozil was associated with a 9% increase in LDL. Triglycerides were decreased by gemfibrozil (-40%) to a greater extent than Niaspan 1000 mg (-16%; $p<0.001$); or Niaspan 2000 mg (-29%; $p=0.02$). Niaspan tended to decrease fibrinogen levels while gemfibrozil tended to increase fibrinogen levels.
Concl.	At higher doses extended release niacin increased HDL to a greater extent than gemfibrozil. Niaspan also decreased lipoprotein (a), and lowered fibrinogen levels compared to gemfibrozil. Gemfibrozil reduced triglyceride levels to a greater extent than Niaspan.

8

Statin, Restenosis and the PlA2 Polymorphism of the Platelet Glycoprotein IIIa Gene

Title	Statin therapy is associated with reduced restenosis rates after coronary stent implantation in carriers of the PlA2 allele of the platelet glycoprotein IIIa gene.
Authors	Walter DH, Schachinger V, Elsner M, et al.
Reference	Eur Heart J 2001;22:587-595.
Disease	Coronary artery disease, percutaneous coronary intervention, restenosis.
Purpose	To study whether statin therapy will reduce restenosis and clinical events at 6 months after successful coronary artery stenting in patients with and without the glycoprotein IIb/IIIa PlA2 allele.
Design	Observational study.
Patients	650 consecutive patients undergoing successful coronary stent implantation.
Follow-up	6-month clinical follow-up with repeated coronary angiography at 6 months.
Regimen	19% of the patients (n=63) were already receiving statin therapy before PCI and continued their treatment and in 263 patients with hypercholesterolemia, statin therapy was started 1 day after PCI.
Add'l Tx	All patients were pretreated with aspirin 100 mg/d for ≥10 days prior to stent implantation, or received aspirin 500 mg IV before PCI. All patients received IV 15,000 U heparin with a target activated clotting time of >250s. 2.5% of the patients received IV IIb/IIIa inhibitors. Patients received ticlopidine 250-500 mg/d for 4 weeks and aspirin 100 mg/d indefinitely.

Results   21.8% of the 650 patients had the PlA2 allele and 78.2% were
           homozygous for the PlA1 allele (7 patients [1%] were homozy-
           gous for the PlA2 allele). The restenosis rate was higher among
           patients with the PlA2 allele than in patients homozygous for
           the PlA1 allele (39.2% vs 30.3%; p=0.06). Multivariate analy-
           sis revealed postprocedure minimal lumen diameter (p<0.001),
           stent length (p=0.001), and statin therapy (p=0.02) to be inde-
           pendent risk factors for restenosis, whereas the PlA2 allele was not
           (p=0.2). Among patients homozygous to the PlA1 allele, resteno-
           sis occurred in 27% of those receiving statin therapy (n=233) vs
           34% of those not on statin therapy (n=209) (p=0.13). Among
           patients carrying the PlA2 allele, restenosis occurred in 28.6%
           of those receiving statin therapy vs 50.9% of those not receiv-
           ing statins (p=0.01). Among patients not receiving statin therapy,
           the PlA2 allele was associated with a significant increase in the
           risk for restenosis (50.9% vs 34%; p=0.01). Among patients
           receiving statin therapy, the PlA2 allele was not associated with
           increased risk (28.6% vs 27%; p=NS). In carriers of the PlA2
           allele, angiographic late loss during the follow-up angiography
           was significantly reduced by statin therapy to values observed in
           patients homozygous for the PlA1 allele. Among patients with the
           PlA2 allele, major end point events (target vessel revascularization,
           myocardial infarction due to target vessel occlusion and death)
           occurred in 28.2% and 49.3% of those receiving or not receiving
           statins (p<0.01), whereas among the patients homozygous for the
           PlA1 allele, major end point events occurred in 32.1% and 37.5%
           of the patients receiving or not receiving statins (p=0.38). The
           lipid levels were comparable between patients with the PlA2 allele
           and those homozygous to the PlA1 allele in both the statin and
           the no-statin groups, both at baseline and at 6 months. The extent
           of cholesterol lowering by statin therapy was comparable between
           the carriers of the PlA2 allele and those who were homozygous for
           the PlA1 allele.

Concl.   Statin therapy was effective in reducing the rates of restenosis
           and clinical events following coronary stenting in patients carry-
           ing the PlA2 allele, and was less effective in patients homozygous
           for the PlA1 allele. This effect was unrelated to the magnitude of
           lowering lipid levels. The interaction with the PlA2 allele sug-
           gests that statins interfere with the functional consequence of a
           genetically determined platelet-mediated risk factor related to
           the PlA2 polymorphism.

Comparison of Effects on Low-Density Lipoprotein Cholesterol and High-Density Lipoprotein Cholesterol with Rosuvastatin vs Atorvastatin in Patients with Type IIa or IIb Hypercholesterolemia

Title	Comparison of effects on low-density lipoprotein cholesterol and high-density lipoprotein cholesterol with rosuvastatin vs atorvastatin in patients with type IIa or IIb hypercholesterolemia.
Authors	Davidson M, Ma P, Stein EA, et al.
Reference	Am J Cardiol 2002;89:268-275.
Disease	Hypercholesterolemia.
Purpose	To compare lipid-lowering effects of 2 doses of rosuvastatin with 1 dose of atorvastatin over 12 weeks.
Design	Randomized, double-blind, placebo-controlled, multicenter.
Patients	516 patients with type IIa or IIb hypercholesterolemia; low-density lipoprotein (LDL) cholesterol had to be ≥160 mg/dL and <250 mg/dL; triglycerides had to be ≤400 mg/dL.
Follow-up	12 weeks.
Regimen	Patients randomized to placebo (n=132), rosuvastatin 5 mg (n=128), rosuvastatin 10 mg (n=129), or atorvastatin 10 mg (n=127).
Add'l Tx	Diet therapy.

Results	Primary end point was change in LDL cholesterol from baseline to week 12. Secondary end points were achievement of National Cholesterol Education Program (NCEP), Adult Treatment Panel (ATP) II Guidelines and European Atherosclerosis Society LDL cholesterol goals at 2, 6, and 12 weeks, and changes in high-density-lipoprotein (HDL), total cholesterol, triglycerides, and others. No significant changes occurred over 12 weeks in the placebo group. Percent decrease in the rosuvastatin 5 mg group was -40%; in the rosuvastatin 10 mg group it was -43%; in the atorvastatin group it was -35% (p<0.01 and p<0.001 for rosuvastatin 5 and 10 mg vs atorvastatin 10 mg). HDL cholesterol was increased by 13% and 12% in the rosuvastatin 5 and 10 mg group vs 8% in the atorvastatin 10 mg group (p<0.01 and p<0.05). Total cholesterol was reduced by -28% and -30% with the 5 and 10 mg rosuvastatin groups vs -25% with atorvastatin (p<0.05 and p<0.001, respectively). Apolipoprotein B reductions and apolipoprotein A increases were also greater with rosuvastatin whereas triglyceride reductions were similar. 84% of patients achieved NCEP-ATPII goals with rosuvastatin vs 73% with atorvastatin. 84% and 82% of rosuvastatin patients achieved ATP III LDL goals vs 72% with atorvastatin. The 10 mg rosuvastatin dose was more effective than atorvastatin at achieving European Atherosclerosis Society LDL goals. Overall safety profile was similar among groups.
Concl.	At the doses used (rosuvastatin 5 and 10 mg) and atorvastatin 10 mg, rosuvastatin provided at least a 5% greater LDL cholesterol reduction. However, it is uncertain whether similar results would have been seen had higher doses of atorvastatin been compared.

Atorvastatin vs Cerivastatin

Title	Comparison of the efficacy of atorvastatin vs cerivastatin in primary hypercholesterolemia.
Authors	Hunninghake D, Insull W, Kropp R, et al.
Reference	Am J Cardiol 2001;88:635-639.
Disease	Hypercholesterolemia.
Purpose	To compare efficacy and safety of atorvastatin with cerivastatin in hypercholesterolemic patients.
Design	Prospective, randomized, open-label blinded end point (PROBE), multicenter.
Patients	215 patients with hypercholesterolemia (low-density lipoprotein [LDL] cholesterol ≥160 mg/dL; triglycerides ≤400 mg/dL).
Follow-up	6 weeks.
Regimen	Atorvastatin 10 mg once daily (n=108) vs cerivastatin 0.3 mg once daily (n=107).
Add'l Tx	National Cholesterol Education Program step 1 diet.

Results   Primary efficacy measure was percent change in LDL cho-
          lesterol from baseline to week 6. Reduction in LDL was
          greater with atorvastatin (37.7%) vs cerivastatin (30.2%;
          p<0.0001). Atorvastatin also produced greater reductions
          in total cholesterol (27.5% vs 22.2%) and apolipoprotein B
          (28.6% vs 21.1%); both p<0.0001. Atorvastatin increased
          HDL by 6.8% vs cerivastatin at 4.3%; p<0.05. There was
          a nonsignificant trend toward a greater reduction in tri-
          glycerides with atorvastatin (17.5% vs 12.5%; p=0.098).
          National Cholesterol Education Program LDL cholesterol
          goal was achieved in 73% of patients on atorvastatin vs 66%
          of patients on cerivastatin. Drug related adverse events were
          mostly mild to moderate and related to the digestive system
          and were less common with atorvastatin (5%) vs cerivastatin
          (14%; p<0.05). 2 patients in the cerivastatin group and 1 in
          the atorvastatin group had creatine phosphokinase values >3
          times upper limit of normal. No patients had alanine ami-
          notransferase or aspartate aminotransferase values >3 times
          upper limit of normal.

Concl.   Atorvastatin (10 mg/d) is more effective than cerivastatin (0.3
          mg/d) at lowering LDL cholesterol. (Cerivastatin was taken off
          US markets due to myositis/rhabdomyolysis.)

Title	Comparison of effect of intensive lipid lowering with atorvastatin to less intensive lowering with lovastatin on C-reactive protein in patients with stable angina pectoris and inducible myocardial ischemia.
Authors	Kinlay S, Timms T, Clark M, et al.
Reference	Am J Cardiol 2002;89:1205-1207.
Disease	Angina pectoris, coronary artery disease.
Purpose	To determine how rapidly reduction of low-density lipoprotein (LDL) cholesterol with statins could lower C-reactive protein (CRP) levels in patients with stable angina and inducible myocardial ischemia.
Design	Randomized, double-blind, placebo-controlled trial.
Patients	110 patients in the Vascular Basis for the Treatment of Myocardial Ischemia Study. Nonsmoking patients with stable angina pectoris with coronary artery disease and myocardial ischemia on an exercise treadmill test and 48-hour ambulatory monitor.
Follow-up	12 months.
Regimen	Patients randomized to: 1) intensive LDL lowering with a goal of <80 mg/dL and antioxidant vitamins C and E; 2) intensive LDL reduction (<80 mg/dL) alone; and 3) LDL reduction goal of <130 mg/dL. The 72 patients in intensive LDL lowering group received atorvastatin 10 mg/d with dose titration every 4 weeks to achieve goal. Modest LDL reduction group received placebo and 33 of 38 patients required lovastatin 5-10 mg/d to achieve LDL <130 mg/dL.

Results   In all of the cohorts most of the change in LDL occurred within the first 6 months. Intensive LDL lowering brought LDL to a level of 85±17 mg/dL while modest LDL lowering brought it to 122±18 mg/dL (p<0.001). Reduction of CRP was significant in the intensive LDL lowering group (2.6 to 1.7 mg/L; p=0.002) but was not significantly lowered in the modest LDL lowering group (2.6 to 2.4 mg/L; p=0.9). In the intensive LDL lowering group, half of the reduction in CRP occurred by 1 month.

Concl.   Atorvastatin reduced CRP more rapidly and to a greater extent than low-dose lovastatin. Intensive LDL lowering (<80 mg/dL) may offer greater plaque stability in high-risk patients.

Title	Long-term safety and efficacy of a once-daily niacin/lovastatin formulation for patients with dyslipidemia.
Authors	Kashyap ML, McGovern ME, Berra K, et al.
Reference	Am J Cardiol 2002;89:672-678.
Disease	Dyslipidemia.
Purpose	To assess the efficacy of safety of 1-year treatment with a combination of niacin extended-release (ER) and lovastatin.
Design	Open-label, multicenter.
Patients	814 patients, ≥21 years old, with type IIA or IIB hyperlipidemia. Patients were required to have either coronary artery disease (CAD) or diabetes + low-density lipoprotein cholesterol (LDL-C) ≥130 mg/dL; 2 CAD risk factors + LDL-C >160 mg/dL; or <2 CAD risk factors + LDL-C >190 mg/dL. Patients whose LDL-C levels were unstable (>12% at 2 consecutive tests within 10 days in the baseline evaluation phase) were excluded. Patients with triglyceride levels >800 mg/dL, liver dysfunction, recent myocardial infarction, recent stroke, recent coronary artery bypass graft surgery, recent arterial bleeding, severe hypertension, significant cardiac arrhythmia, type 1 or uncontrolled type 2 diabetes, active gallbladder disease, active peptic ulcer disease, uncontrolled hypothyroidism, or recent gout attack were not included. Patients that received dyslipidemic medication within the past year and those receiving cyclosporin, troglitazone, macrolide antibiotics, and anti-fungal medications were excluded.
Follow-up	600 patients were followed for 6 months and 200 for 12 months.
Regimen	Patients were enrolled after a 4-week dietary lead-in or drug washout phase and a 2-week baseline evaluation phase. In the first 16 weeks of the study the dose was increased gradually from 500 mg niacin-ER/10 mg lovastatin once daily. It was followed by 36-week dose-maintenance phase. The target dose was 2000 mg niacin-ER/ 40 mg lovastatin once daily.

Results	At the end of the 16-week dose escalating phase LDL-C was reduced by 47% and triglycerides by 41%. HDL-C increased by 30% (all p<0.001). LDL/HDL-C ratio decreased by 58% and total/HDL-C ratio was decreased by 48%. These effects on total cholesterol, LDL-C, and triglycerides persisted through the 36-week maintenance phase. At the end of the maintenance phase there was a 41% increase in HDL-C. Lipoprotein(a) and C-reactive protein decreased by 25% and 24%, respectively (p<0.01). 49% of the patients with CAD reached the National Cholesterol Education Program target of LDL-C <100 mg/dL level. 75% of the patients with >2 risk factors but without diabetes or established CAD and 85% of the patients with <2 risk factors reached their NCEP targets. Treatment was well tolerated. Flushing caused 10% of patients to withdraw from the study. An additional 13% of the patients withdrew from the study due to miscellaneous adverse events or laboratory abnormalities. Another 7% withdrew for administrative or unrelated medical reasons. Gastrointestinal adverse events were reported by 24% of the patients. Headache was reported by 7% of the patients and dizziness by 5% of the patients. Drug-induced myopathy was not observed. In 7 patients, elevations of creatine kinase led to discontinuation of treatment. 3 patients withdrew from the study because of elevated liver function tests. The incidence of liver enzyme elevation (>3 times the upper limit of normal) was 0.5%.
Concl.	Once-daily niacin/lovastatin combination was effective in reducing lipid levels. However, a substantial number of patients (23%) had to withdraw from the study due to medical reasons.

Comparison of the Effects of Atorvastatin Versus Simvastatin on Subclinical Atherosclerosis in Primary Prevention as Determined by Electron Beam Tomography

Title	Comparison of the effects of atorvastatin versus simvastatin on subclinical atherosclerosis in primary prevention as determined by electron beam tomography.
Authors	Hecht HS, Harman SM.
Reference	Am J Cardiol 2003;91:42-45.
Disease	Coronary artery disease.
Purpose	To determine the comparative effects of atorvastatin and simvastatin on progression of calcified plaque as determined by electron beam tomography (EBT) in patients without symptomatic coronary artery disease.
Design	Observational.
Patients	103 patients in the atorvastatin group and 46 in the simvastatin group. No patients had a history of symptomatic CAD. In each group, mean age was approximately 59 years, approximately 27% had hypertension, approximately 5% were smokers, and 60% had a family history of CAD. 2% and 9% of patients in the atorvastatin and simvastatin groups were diabetic, respectively. All differences between the 2 groups were nonsignificant. Total cholesterol and LDL cholesterol were significantly higher in the atorvastatin group at study start than in the simvastatin group (p<0.05). Dosages of the statins and niacin were determined by the treating physicians of the patients and were not established in the protocol. The mean dose of atorvastatin was 14.2±8.1 mg and simvastatin was 23.7±11.8 mg. Approximately half of all patients were taking niacin, and the average dose was 1890 and 1875 mg in the atorvastatin and simvastatin groups, respectively.

Follow-up	1.2 years.
Regimen	Statin treatment to lower LDL cholesterol as described above and niacin treatment to increase HDL and lower triglycerides as above. Diet, weight loss, exercise, smoking cessation, and aspirin were recommended to all patients.
Results	The EBT calcium score and volume score at study start were similar between the 2 groups. The baseline LDL cholesterol, total, and non-HDL cholesterol levels were significantly higher in the atorvastatin group. The EBT percentile was significantly higher in the atorvastatin cohort. The change in total cholesterol in the atorvastatin and simvastatin groups, respectively, was -26.2% and -22.2%; for LDL cholesterol: -39.8% and -34.7%; for HDL: +15.6% and +14.9%; for triglycerides: -22.1% and -18.8%; none of these differences were significant between the statin groups. The change in calcium scores was +10.8% and +7.5%, and the change in volume scores was +8.5% and +7.8% in the atorvastatin and simvastatin groups, respectively, with no significant differences between the groups. The calcium score and volume score were similar between the groups at the end of the study.
Concl.	Treatment with atorvastatin and simvastatin in patients who are asymptomatic for CAD produced an equal progression of calcified plaques as determined by EBT.

Efficacy and Safety of a Potent New Selective Cholesterol Absorption Inhibitor, Ezetimibe, in Patients with Primary Hypercholesterolemia

Title	Efficacy and safety of a potent new selective cholesterol absorption inhibitor, ezetimibe, in patients with primary hypercholesterolemia.
Authors	Dujovne CA, Ettinger MP, McNeer JF, et al.
Reference	Am J Cardiol 2002;90:1092-1097.
Disease	Hypercholesterolemia.
Purpose	To determine whether ezetimibe, a new cholesterol absorption inhibitor, is safe and effective in patients with primary hypercholesterolemia.
Design	Multicenter, randomized, double-blind, placebo-controlled.
Patients	892 patients, ≥18 years of age, with diagnosed primary hypercholesterolemia (having LDL cholesterol 130-250 mg/dL and triglycerides ≤350 mg/dL after wash-out phase). Exclusion criteria were numerous and included: pregnancy or lactation, New York Heart Association class III or IV congestive heart failure, uncontrolled arrhythmias, myocardial infarction, coronary artery bypass surgery or angioplasty in the previous 6 months, unstable angina, known renal or hepatic disease, and others.
Follow-up	12 weeks.
Regimen	After a 2-12 week screening/drug wash-out period during which lipid-lowering medications were stopped, patients were randomized to receive either ezetimibe 10 mg or identical-appearing placebo qd.

Add'l Tx	Oral corticosteroids, cyclosporine, and orlistat were not permitted during the study. Psyllium or other fiber-based laxatives were allowed if the patient had been on the medication >4 weeks prior to study start. Cardiovascular medications were allowed if the patients had been on the medication for at least 8 weeks before study start. Aspirin ≤325 mg/d was allowed.
Results	The primary outcome was the percent change in LDL cholesterol from baseline to the end point. The secondary outcomes included changes in total cholesterol, triglycerides, HDL cholesterol, HDL subfractions HDL2 and HDL3, apolipoprotein A-I, apolipoprotein B, and lipoprotein (a) (Lp[a]). The 2 treatment groups were comparable in baseline characteristics. Patients in the ezetimibe group had a mean percent reduction of 17% in LDL cholesterol vs 0.4% in the placebo group (p<0.01). 60% of patients in the ezetimibe group had a reduction in LDL ≥15% vs only 10% in the placebo group. The reduction of LDL levels in the ezetimibe group occurred early in the treatment (2 weeks) and was maintained until the end of follow-up. Compared to placebo, ezetimibe also reduced the calculated LDL cholesterol, apolipoprotein B, total cholesterol, and triglycerides, while increasing HDL cholesterol and HDL3 cholesterol (p<0.01 for each). The frequency of adverse events was similar between the groups, with upper respiratory infection and headache being the most common. There was no complaint that was particularly common in either group. Laboratory results such as blood chemistry, prothrombin time, hematology, urinalysis, and liver function tests were generally similar between the 2 groups.
Concl.	Ezetimibe is safe and effective for lowering LDL cholesterol and improving other lipid parameters in patients with primary hypercholesterolemia.

Efficacy and Safety of Ezetimibe Added to Ongoing Statin Therapy for Treatment of Patients with Primary Hypercholesterolemia

Title	Efficacy and safety of ezetimibe added to ongoing statin therapy for treatment of patients with primary hypercholesterolemia.
Authors	Gagné C, Bays HE, Weiss SR, et al.
Reference	Am J Cardiol 2002;90:1084-1091.
Disease	Hypercholesterolemia.
Purpose	To determine if ezetimibe is safe and effective when added to existing statin therapy in patients with primary hypercholesterolemia.
Design	Randomized, double-blind, placebo-controlled.
Patients	769 patients, age ≥18 years, with primary hypercholesterolemia, who were currently taking a statin at a stable dose for at least 6 weeks. Patients should already have received instruction regarding a cholesterol-lowering diet. A patient's LDL level was required to be at or above the target level recommended for that person's risk category according to the National Cholesterol Education Program Adult Treatment Panel II (NCEP ATP II) guidelines. Serum triglyceride levels had to be ≤350 mg/dL. There were numerous exclusion criteria which included: heart failure, uncontrolled arrhythmias, myocardial infarction, coronary bypass surgery, coronary angioplasty, unstable angina, poorly controlled or new-onset diabetes mellitus, impaired renal or hepatic function, alanine aminotransferase and aspartate transferase concentration greater than 2 times the upper limit of normal, malignancy, and others.
Regimen	Patients were randomized 1:1 to receive either ezetimibe 10 mg/d (n=379) or matched placebo (n=390). Study investigators attempted to achieve an equal distribution of patients taking simvastatin, atorvastatin, and all other statins. Patients were to continue taking their open-label statin as previously prescribed.

Results	The primary end point was the mean percent change of LDL cholesterol concentration from study start to the end point. The 2 groups were generally well balanced. Patients in the placebo group had a 3.7% reduction in their LDL levels at end point vs baseline, whereas patients in the ezetimibe group had a 25.1% reduction (p<0.001 for difference between groups). LDL levels were lowered mostly in the first 2 weeks of treatment and were maintained through the 8-week treatment period. Ezetimibe reduced LDL cholesterol similarly regardless of the type of statin being used concurrently. Response to ezetimibe was generally similar across subgroups defined by gender, age, race, NCEP ATP II category, BMI, and waist circumference. During the 8-week follow-up, 75.5% of the ezetimibe plus statin group reached the prespecified NCEP ATP II target LDL cholesterol levels vs 27.3% in the placebo plus statin group (OR 19.6; p<0.001). In patients whose LDL levels were above NCEP ATP II LDL target levels, 71.5% in the ezetimibe and statin group reached their target LDL cholesterol vs 18.9% in the statin plus placebo group (OR 23.7; p<0.001). Patients in the ezetimibe group had an increase in HDL cholesterol of 2.7% vs 1.0% in the placebo group (p<0.05), and triglycerides decreased 14.0% in the ezetimibe group vs 2.9% in placebo (p<0.001). Other measures of coronary heart disease risk, such as total cholesterol, non-HDL cholesterol, apolipoprotein B, LDL cholesterol:HDL cholesterol, and total cholesterol:HDL cholesterol, as well as C-reactive protein (p<0.05), were significantly lowered with ezetimibe vs placebo (p<0.001). The rate of adverse events attributed to treatment was similar in both groups (21% in ezetimibe and 17% in placebo). The most commonly involved body system was gastrointestinal. There were 5 patients who had elevated levels of either alanine aminotransferase or aspartate aminotransferase at least 3 times the upper limit of normal (4 on statin plus ezetimibe, 1 on statin plus placebo), all of which resolved upon termination of statin and study drug. There were no cases of rhabdomyolysis or death.
Concl.	Ezetimibe is safe and effective when added to existing statin therapy in patients with primary hypercholesterolemia.

Long-Term Persistence in Use of Statin Therapy

Title	Long-term persistence in use of statin therapy in elderly patients.
Authors	Benner JS, Glynn RJ, Mogun H, et al.
Reference	JAMA 2002;288:455-461.
Disease	Coronary artery disease, atherosclerosis, hypercholesterolemia.
Purpose	To elucidate the long-term patterns and predictors of statin use in elderly patients.
Design	Retrospective cohort.
Patients	34,501 patients, ≥65 years, who started statin therapy between 1990 and 1998.
Follow-up	Until death, disenrollment, or December 31, 1999.
Regimen	Patients age >65 who initiated therapy with a statin (atorvastatin, cerivastatin, fluvastatin, lovastatin, pravastatin, or simvastatin) were included in the retrospective analysis.

Results   The specific goals of the study were: 1) investigate long-term patterns of statin use; 2) elucidate patient characteristics that are predictors of poor long-term compliance; and 3) determine whether statin compliance has improved over time in accordance with growing evidence of statin usefulness. Usage of statins was determined quarterly during the first year and every 6-months thereafter. The term "adherence" was designated to mean the extent of prescription-filling in a given time period, and "persistence" was defined as the length of time during which a patient continued to fill statin prescriptions. The "proportion of days covered" [PDC] was calculated from the number of pills dispensed and the number of supplied days from each filled prescription. Patients were divided into 3 groups at each interval: adherent, patients with a PDC ≥80% in that interval; partially adherent, patients with a PDC between 20% and 79%; and nonadherent, PDC <20%. Patients generally became less adherent with statin therapy over time: adherence rates were 60%, 43%, 26%, and 32% after 3, 6, 60, and 120 months, respectively. Nonadherent patients composed 29% of the group at 6 months but 56% at 60 months, with slight improvement during the final 2 years of follow-up. Many patients were partially adherent at treatment start, but this group became smaller, making up 40%, 29%, and 18% of the group at 3, 6, and 60 months, respectively; most of these patients became non-adherent. Age, black race, other non-white race, enrollment in Medicaid, depression, and dementia were significant (p<0.001 for each) predictors of suboptimal long-term use (less than 80% of days with available statin), while patients with hypertension, stroke, CHF, or diabetes were more likely to persist in statin use vs those without those conditions (p<0.001 for each). Generally, patients with increasing severity of coronary heart disease (CHD) were more likely to persist with statin use, except for the category of patients who had an acute MI; these patients had a 20% greater chance of suboptimal persistence. Patients who started therapy recently (1996-1998) were 21%-25% less likely to discontinue or decrease their statin use (p<0.001).

Concl.   Statin use decreases significantly over time in elderly patients. Certain patient characteristics are associated with increased risk of treatment non-compliance.

Ezetimibe

Title	Effects of ezetimibe, a new cholesterol absorption inhibitor, on plasma lipids in patients with primary hypercholesterolemia.
Authors	Knopp RH, Gitter H, Truitt T, et al.
Reference	Eur Heart J 2003;24:729-741.
Disease	Hypercholesterolemia.
Purpose	To assess the safety and efficacy of ezetimibe 10 mg/d in patients with primary hypercholesterolemia.
Design	Randomized, double-blind, placebo-controlled, multicenter.
Patients	827 patients, ≥18 years old, with primary hypercholesterolemia (LDL cholesterol 130-250 mg/dL; and plasma triglycerides ≥350 mg/dL). Pregnant or lactating women were not included. Patients with congestive heart failure (NYHA class III or IV), uncontrolled arrhythmia, recent (6 months) myocardial infarction or revascularization procedure, severe peripheral artery disease, unstable angina, gastrointestinal, hepatic, renal, hematological or central nervous system disorders, uncontrolled diabetes, uncontrolled endocrine or metabolic disease, and HIV positive were excluded.
Follow-up	12 weeks.
Regimen	After 2-12 week drug wash-out phase, patients underwent a 4-week single-blind placebo run-in phase and then randomized to double-blind treatment for 12 weeks. Patients were randomized to ezetimibe 10 mg/d (n=622) or placebo (n=205) in a 3:1 ratio.

Add'l Tx	All patients received dietary counseling for NCEP Step 1 diet. All prior lipid-altering medications, including corticosteroids, cyclosporine and orlistat, were discontinued.
Results	766 patients (93%) completed the study. 8% of the patients in the ezetimibe and 6% in the placebo group discontinued the study drug. LDL cholesterol increased by 0.8%±0.9% in the placebo and decreased by 17.7%±0.6% in the ezetimibe group (p<0.01). HDL cholesterol decreased by 1.3%±0.8% in the placebo group and increased by 1.0%±0.5% in the ezetimibe group (p<0.01). Total cholesterol increased by 0.6%±0.6% in the placebo group and decreased by 12.4%±0.4% in the ezetimibe group (p<0.01). Triglycerides increased by 2.4%±2.2% in the placebo group and decreased by 1.7%±1.4% in the ezetimibe group (p=0.09). Apolipoprotein B decreased by 1.0%±0.8% in the placebo group and by 15.4%±0.5% in the ezetimibe group (p<0.01). Lipoprotein (a) increased by 1.8%±2.9% in the placebo group and decreased by 7.5%±1.9% in the ezetimibe group (p<0.01). Response to ezetimibe was consistent across all subgroups tested. Ezetimibe did not affect the serum levels of lipid-soluble vitamins or altered cortisol production. Ezetimibe was safe and well tolerated. Adverse effects were reported in 61% of the patients in the ezetimibe group and in 65% in the placebo group. The adverse event profiles were comparable between the placebo and the ezetimibe groups. 5 patients in the ezetimibe group vs 0 in the placebo group discontinued treatment because of an increase in liver enzymes.
Concl.	Ezetimibe was safe and well tolerated and reduced total cholesterol, LDL cholesterol, apolipoprotein B, and lipoprotein (a).

Title	Efficacy and safety of ezetimibe coadministered with pravastatin in patients with primary hypercholesterolemia: a prospective, randomized, double-blind trial.
Authors	Melani L, Mills R, Hassman D, et al.
Reference	Eur Heart J 2003;24:717-728.
Disease	Hypercholesterolemia.
Purpose	To assess the safety and efficacy of ezetimibe (10 mg/d) combined with pravastatin (10-40 mg/d) in patients with primary hypercholesterolemia.
Design	Randomized, double-blind, placebo-controlled, 2 × 4 factorial design, multicenter.
Patients	538 adult patients with primary hypercholesterolemia (LDL cholesterol 3.8-6.5 mmol/L and triglycerides ≤4.0 mmol/L). Patients with concomitant diseases including congestive heart failure (NYHA class III or IV), uncontrolled arrhythmia, severe peripheral artery disease, recent (6 months) myocardial infarction, unstable angina or revascularization procedure, uncontrolled diabetes, renal or hepatic impairment, coagulopathy, uncontrolled endocrine disorder, and treatment with immunosuppressant agents or corticosteroids were excluded.
Follow-up	12 weeks.
Regimen	After an initial 2-12 week wash-out phase, patients underwent a 4 week single-blind, placebo treatment run-in phase and then randomized in a 2 ′ 4 factorial design to ezetimibe 10 mg/d or placebo and to pravastatin 10, 20, or 40 mg/d or placebo. The treatment phase lasted 12 weeks.

Results	492 patients (91%) completed the treatment phase. LDL cholesterol increased by $1.3\% \pm 1.6\%$ in the placebo group, decreased by $18.7\% \pm 1.6\%$ in the ezetimibe group, decreased by $24.3\% \pm 0.9\%$ in the pravastatin alone group; and decreased by $37.7\% \pm 0.9\%$ in the ezetimibe plus pravastatin group (combined therapy vs pravastatin alone $p<0.01$; combined therapy vs ezetimibe $p<0.01$). Total cholesterol increased by $0.2\% \pm 1.2\%$ in the placebo group, decreased by $13.2\% \pm 1.2\%$ in the ezetimibe alone group, decreased by $17.2\% \pm 0.6\%$ in the pravastatin alone group, and decreased by $27.1\% \pm 0.6\%$ in the ezetimibe plus pravastatin group (combined therapy vs pravastatin alone $p<0.01$; combined therapy vs ezetimibe $p<0.01$). Triglycerides increased by $2.0\% \pm 1.5\%$ in the placebo group, decreased by $2.1\% \pm 3.8\%$ in the ezetimibe group, decreased by $7.6\% \pm 2.1\%$ in the pravastatin group, and decreased by $17.6\% \pm 2.1\%$ in the combination group (combined therapy vs pravastatin alone $p<0.01$; combined therapy vs ezetimibe $p<0.01$). Apolipoprotein B decreased by $2.2\% \pm 1.8\%$ in the placebo group, decreased by $14.8\% \pm 1.8\%$ in the ezetimibe group, decreased by $20.0\% \pm 1.0\%$ in the pravastatin group, and decreased by $30.2\% \pm 1.0\%$ in the combination group (combined therapy vs pravastatin alone $p<0.01$; combined therapy vs ezetimibe $p<0.01$). There was no significant effect of either ezetimibe or the combination therapy on lipoprotein (a) levels. The combination therapy was safe and well tolerated.
Concl.	Coadministration of ezetimibe and pravastatin was safe and well tolerated and had a synergistic effect, resulting in a significant reduction of LDL cholesterol and triglycerides compared to either ezetimibe alone or pravastatin alone.

Rosuvastatin vs Pravastatin and Simvastatin

Title	Efficacy and safety of rosuvastatin compared with pravastatin and simvastatin in patients with hypercholesterolemia: a randomized, double-blind, 52-week trial.
Authors	Brown WV, Bays HE, Hassman DR, et al.
Reference	Am Heart J 2002;144:1036-1043.
Disease	Hyperlipidemia.
Purpose	To compare the efficacy of rosuvastatin with that of pravastatin and simvastatin in lowering LDL-Cl levels in patients with hypercholesterolemia.
Design	Randomized, double-blind, multicenter.
Patients	477 patients, ≥18 years old, with LDL-C between 160-250 mg/dL and triglycerides ≤400 mg/dL after a 6-week lead-in phase in which all lipid-altering medications were discontinued, fasting serum glucose ≤180 mg/dL or HbA1c ≤9%. Patients with active liver disease, active arterial disease within the preceding 3 months, history of cancer in the preceding 10 years, uncontrolled hypertension, history of ketoacidosis within the previous 5 years, uncontrolled hypothyroidism, renal failure, creatine kinase >3 times the upper limit of normal, familial hypercholesterolemia, alcohol or drug abuse, use of lipid-altering medications, and hypersensitivity to statins were excluded.
Follow-up	52 weeks.
Regimen	Randomization to rosuvastatin 5 or 10 mg/d, pravastatin 20 mg/d, or simvastatin 20 mg/d for 12 weeks. Thereafter, 40-week dose titration phase to try to maintain LDL-C within National Cholesterol Education Program Adult Treatment Panel II (ATP-II) guidelines. Rosuvastatin maximal dose was 80 mg/d, pravastatin was 40 mg/d, and simvastatin was 80 mg/d.
Add'l Tx	NCEP Step I diet.

Results	82% of the randomized patients completed the 52-week treatment. After 2 weeks LDL-C was reduced by 37.6% and 44.8% in the rosuvastatin 5 mg/d and 10 mg/d groups, by 24.2% in the pravastatin group, and by 32.1% in the simvastatin group (p<0.001 for both rosuvastatin groups vs pravastatin or simvastatin). After 12 weeks, LDL-C was reduced by 39.1% and 47.4% in the rosuvastatin 5 mg/d and 10 mg/d groups, respectively; 26.5% in the pravastatin group; and 34.6% in the simvastatin group (p<0.05 for both rosuvastatin groups vs pravastatin or simvastatin). At 12 weeks, triglycerides were reduced by 17.6% with rosuvastatin 5 mg/d, 21.5% by rosuvastatin 10 mg/d, 11.4% by pravastatin, and 10.2% by simvastatin. HDL-C increased by 8.2% with rosuvastatin 5 mg/d, 11.9% by rosuvastatin 10 mg/d, 8.3% by pravastatin, and 8.8% by simvastatin. After 12 weeks 80.2% of the patients in the rosuvastatin 5 mg/d group, 89.6% in the rosuvastatin 10 mg/d group, 53.4% in the pravastatin group, and 68.9% in the simvastatin group reached ATP-II goals. After 52 weeks, 88.1% of the patients in the rosuvastatin 5 mg/d group, 87.5% in the rosuvastatin 10 mg/d group, 60.0% in the pravastatin group, and 72.53% in the simvastatin group reached ATP-II goals. 65% of the patients in the rosuvastatin 5 mg/d group, 79% in the rosuvastatin 10 mg/d group, 31% in the pravastatin group, and 50% in the simvastatin group reached their ATP-II goals without increasing the starting dose. All 3 drugs were well tolerated and safe.
Concl.	At the doses tested in the study, rosuvastatin reduced LDL-C more than pravastatin and simvastatin did in patients with primary hypercholesterolemia. All 3 drugs were safe.

Rosuvastatin vs Atorvastatin

Title	Effects of rosuvastatin and atorvastatin compared over 52 weeks of treatment in patients with hypercholesterolemia.
Authors	Olsson AG, Istad H, Luurila O, et al.
Reference	Am Heart J 2002;144:1044-1051.
Disease	Hypercholesterolemia.
Purpose	412 patients, ≥18 years old, with hypercholesterolemia who had fasting LDL-C of 160-250 mg/dL and triglycerides ≤400 mg/dL after a 6-week lead-in phase during which all cholesterol-modifying drugs were discontinued.
Design	Randomized, double-blind, multicenter.
Patients	412 patients, ≥18 years old, with hypercholesterolemia who had fasting LDL-C of 160-250 mg/dL and triglycerides ≤400 mg/dL after a 6-week lead-in phase during which all cholesterol-modifying drugs were discontinued.
Follow-up	52 weeks.
Regimen	Randomization to rosuvastatin 5 mg/d (n=138), rosuvastatin 10 mg/d (n=134), or atorvastatin 10 mg/d (n=140) for 12 weeks. Thereafter, the study drug dose was titrated up to 80 mg/d to achieve the National Cholesterol Education Program Adult Treatment Panel II (ATP-II) LDL-C goal.
Add'l Tx	NCEP Step I diet.

Results	After 12 weeks, LDL-C decreased by 46%, 50%, and 39% in the rosuvastatin 5 mg/d, rosuvastatin 10 mg/d, and atorvastatin 10 mg/d groups, respectively (p<0.001 for rosuvastatin 5 mg/d vs atorvastatin and for the rosuvastatin 10 mg/d vs atorvastatin). HDL-C increased by 6%, 8%, and 6%, respectively (p=NS). Triglyceride levels decreased by 15%, 19%, and 16%, respectively (p=NS). After 12 weeks 86%, 89%, and 73% of the patients in the rosuvastatin 5 mg/d, rosuvastatin 10 mg/d and atorvastatin 10 mg/d groups reached the ATP-II LDL-C goal. After 52 weeks, LDL-C was decreased by 47%, 53%, and 44% in patients in the rosuvastatin 5 mg/d, rosuvastatin 10 mg/d, and atorvastatin 10 mg/d groups, respectively (p<0.05 rosuvastatin 5 mg/d vs atorvastatin; p<0.001 rosuvastatin 10 mg/d vs atorvastatin). HDL-C increased by 2% and 3% and decreased by 1%, respectively (p=NS rosuvastatin 5 mg/d vs atorvastatin; p<0.05 rosuvastatin 10 mg/d vs atorvastatin). Triglyceride levels decreased by 20%, 21%, and 19%, respectively (p=NS). After 52 weeks, 88% of patients in the rosuvastatin 5 mg/d group, 98% in the rosuvastatin 10 mg/d group, and 87% in the atorvastatin group reached their ATP-II LDL-Cl goals. 82% of patients in the rosuvastatin 10 mg/d group vs only 59% in the atorvastatin group reached their ATP-II LDL-C goal without the need for increasing the dose. Rosuvastatin and atorvastatin were well tolerated.
Concl.	With the initial doses used in this study, rosuvastatin reduced LDL-C to a greater extent than atorvastatin. Both drugs were safe and well tolerated.

4S

Scandinavian Simvastatin Survival Study

Title	Scandinavian Simvastatin Survival Study.
Authors	a + b. Scandinavian Simvastatin Survival Study Group. c. Kjekshus J, Pedersen TR, for the Scandinavian Simvastatin Survival Study Group d. Miettinen TA, Pyorala K, Olsson AG, et al. e. Johannesson M, Jonsson B, Kjekshus J, et al. f. Pedersen TR, Olsson AG, Faergeman O, et al. g. Pedersen TR, Kjekshus J, Pyorala K, et al.
Reference	a. Lancet 1994;344:1383-1389. b. Lancet 1995;345:1274-1275. c. Am J Cardiol 1995;76:64C-68C. d. Circulation 1997; 96:4211-4218. e. N Engl J Med 1997; 336:332-336. f. Circulation 1998;97:1453-1460. g. Am J Cardiol 1998; 81:333-335.
Disease	Coronary artery disease, hyperlipidemia.
Purpose	To assess the effect of simvastatin therapy on mortality and morbidity of patients with coronary artery disease and serum cholesterol 5.5-8.0 mmol/L. e. To determine the cost effectiveness of lowering cholesterol in relationship to age, sex, and the cholesterol level from the 4S study. f. To determine which baseline lipoproteins are predictive of coronary events. To determine which changes in lipoproteins accounted for the reduction in coronary events in the 4S. g. To determine effect of lipid intervention with simvastatin on noncoronary ischemic symptoms and signs over 5.4 years.
Design	Randomized, double-blind, placebo-controlled, multicenter. e. As per 4S trial. Estimation of cost per year of life gained with simvastatin therapy.

Patients	4444 patients, aged 35-70 years, with a history of angina pectoris or myocardial infarction, and serum cholesterol 5.5-8.0 mmol/L, (213-209 mg per deciliter) and serum triglyceride ≤2.5 mmol/L. Premenopausal women and patients with secondary hypercholesterolemia were excluded. Patients with myocardial infarction within 6 months, congestive heart failure, planned coronary artery surgery, or angioplasty were not included.
Follow-up	Clinical follow-up for 4.9-6.3 years (median 5.4 years).e. 5 years. f. 5.4 years.
Regimen	Simvastatin 20 mg/d or placebo. If serum cholesterol did not reach the target range of 3.0-5.2 mmol/L by simvastatin 20 mg/d, the dose was increased to 40 mg/d, or decreased to 10 mg/d. f. Placebo vs simvastatin 20 mg/d with titration to 40 mg. Target serum total cholesterol 116-201 mg/dL.
Add'l Tx	Dietary advice.
Results	Lipid concentrations changed only little in the placebo group, whereas simvastatin resulted in -25%, -35%, +8%, and -10% change from baseline of total, LDL, and HDL cholesterol, and triglycerides. After 1 year, 72% of the simvastatin group had achieved total cholesterol <5.2 mmol/L. During the follow-up mortality was 12% in the placebo and 8% in the simvastatin group (RR 0.70; 95% CI=0.58-0.85; p=0.0003). The Kaplan-Meier 6 year probability of survival was 87.7% in the placebo vs 91.3% in the simvastatin group. Coronary mortality was 8.5% vs 5.0%, respectively (RR 0.58; 95% CI=0.46-0.73). There was no difference in noncardiovascular death. 28% of the placebo and 19% of the simvastatin group had 1 or more major coronary events (coronary death, myocardial infarction, or resuscitated cardiac arrest (RR 0.66; 95% CI=0.59-0.75; p<0.00001). The relative risk of having any coronary event in the simvastatin group was 0.73 (95% CI=0.66-0.80; p<0.00001). Simvastatin also reduced the risk of undergoing coronary artery bypass surgery or angioplasty (RR 0.63; 95% CI=0.54-0.74; p<0.00001). The overall rates of adverse effects were not different between the groups. Simvastatin significantly reduced the risk of major coronary events in all quartiles of baseline total, HDL, and LDL cholesterol, by a similar amount in each quartile.d. A recent post hoc analysis showed that patients ≥65 years of age who received simvastatin had a reduced relative risk (RR) for clinical events. The RRs (95% confidence intervals)

were 0.66 (0.40-0.90) for all cause mortality; 0.57 (0.39-0.83) for coronary heart disease mortality; and 0.66 (0.52-0.84) for major coronary events. The RR was also reduced for any atherosclerotic-related events and revascularization procedures. In women the RRs were 1.16 (0.68-1.99), 0.86 (0.42-1.74), and 0.66 (0.48-0.91) for all cause mortality, coronary heart disease mortality, and major coronary events. Any atherosclerotic related event and revascularization procedures also were reduced in women on simvastatin. e. The cost of each year of life gained ranged from $3,800 for 70 year old men with cholesterol levels of 309 mg/dL to $27,400 for 35 year old women with 213 mg/dL. With indirect costs included, the costs ranged from youngest patients exhibiting a savings in money while 70 year old women with 213 cholesterol levels cost $13,300 per year of life gained.f. Simvastatin reduced cholesterol by 25% and LDL cholesterol by 34%. Three fourths of patients on simvastatin had reduction of LDL cholesterol by 30%; a quarter had reduction by > 45%. Reduction in coronary events on simvastatin correlated with on-treatment levels and changes in total, LDL cholesterol, and apolipoprotein B. There was less of a correlation with triglyceride levels. Each 1% reduction in LDL cholesterol reduced coronary risk by 1.7%. There was no evidence for any % reduction or on-treatment threshold below which further reduction of LDL cholesterol did not have benefit.g. Risk of claudication, bruits, and angina were decreased by simvastatin. The risk of new or worsening carotid bruits was significantly decreased. Fatal plus nonfatal cerebral events (stroke or transient ischemic attacks) was reduced by 28% with simvastatin. New or worsening intermittent claudication was decreased by 38% with the statin; new or worsening angina was decreased by 26%.

| Concl. | Long-term therapy with simvastatin is safe and effective in improvement of survival and reduction of the rate of coronary events.d. Simvastatin produced similar reductions in relative risk for major coronary events in women vs men and in elderly vs younger patients.e. In patients with coronary artery disease, simvastatin is cost effective.f. The beneficial effect of simvastatin on major coronary events was dependent upon the magnitude of reduction in LDL cholesterol, without a threshold below which reduction was no longer beneficial.g. Cholesterol lowering with simvastatin 20-40 mg/d retards progression of atherosclerosis throughout the vascular system. |

4S (Substudy)

Scandinavian Simvastatin Survival Study

Title	Reduced coronary events in simvistatin treated patients with coronary heart disease and diabetes or impaired fasting glucose levels. Subgroup analysis in the Scandinavian Simvistatin Survival Study.
Authors	Haffner SM, Alexander CM, Cook TJ, et al.
Reference	Arch Intern Med 1999;159:2661-2667.
Disease	Coronary heart disease, hyperlipidemia, diabetes mellitus.
Purpose	To determine the effect of simvistatin on coronary events in patients with coronary heart disease and diabetes or impaired fasting glucose levels.
Design	As per 4S.
Patients	678 patients had plasma glucose levels ≥110 mg/dL but less than 126 mg/dL which is diagnostic for impaired fasting glucose; 281 patients had plasma glucose ≥126 mg/dL but did not have a previous clinical history of diabetes; and 202 had clinical histories of diabetes (total of 483 patients with diabetes as defined by 1997 American Diabetes Association criteria). 3237 patients had normal fasting glucose.
Follow-up	5.4 years.
Regimen	As per 4S.
Add'l Tx	As per 4S.

Results	Incidence of coronary events increased in the placebo group by baseline glucose status. Impaired fasting glucose group had a relative risk (RR) of 1.15; in diabetics with elevated fasting glucose but no prior history this was 1.19; in diabetics with a history the relative risk was increased to 1.83. The relative risk of having increased coronary heart events in the combined diabetic groups vs those with a normal fasting blood sugar was increased at 1.44 (95% CI=1.14-1.82). Diabetic patients treated with simvistatin had decreased number of major coronary events compared to the placebo group (RR 0.58 ; p=0.001) as well as revascularization procedures (RR 0.52; p=0.005). There was a nonsignificant trend toward a reduction in total and coronary mortality in diabetic patients that received simvistatin vs placebo. Simvistatin also decreased the incidence of major coronary events (RR 0.62; p=0.003), revascularizations (RR 0.57; p=0.009), and total (RR 0.57; p=0.02) and coronary (RR 0.45; p=0.007) mortality in patients with impaired fasting glucose but not overt diabetes.
Concl.	Cholesterol lowering with simvistatin decreased coronary events and revascularizations in patients with diabetes (as defined by 1997 American Diabetes Association) and decreased the incidence of coronary events, revascularization, and mortality in patients with impaired fasting glucose levels.

ADMIT

Arterial Disease Multiple Intervention Trial

Title	Effect of niacin on lipid and lipoprotein levels and glycemic control in patients with diabetes and peripheral arterial disease. The ADMIT Study: a randomized trial.
Authors	Elam MB, Hunninghake DB, Davis KB.
Reference	JAMA 2000;284:1263-1270.
Disease	Hyperlipidemia, diabetes.
Purpose	To assess efficacy and safety of lipid modifying dosages of niacin in patients with diabetes.
Design	Prospective, randomized, placebo-controlled, multicenter.
Patients	468 patients with peripheral arterial disease, including 125 diabetics.
Follow-up	Up to 60 weeks.
Regimen	After run-in period (12 weeks) randomization to niacin (crystal-line nicotinic acid), 3000 mg/d or maximum tolerated dose or placebo up to 60 weeks (48 week double-blind).
Add'l Tx	Also was part of larger study investigating antioxidant vitamin cocktail and warfarin; in diabetics oral hypoglycemic agents, insulin.

Results   Primary outcomes included plasma lipoprotein, glucose, hemo-globin A1c, alanine, aminotransferase, uric acid levels, hypogly-cemic drug use, compliance, adverse events. Niacin increased HDL-C by 29% in both diabetics and nondiabetics ($p<0.001$ for niacin vs placebo); it decreased triglycerides by 23% in dia-betics and 28% in nondiabetics ($p<0.001$ for niacin vs placebo); it decreased LDL-C by 8% in diabetics and 9% in nondiabetics ($p<0.001$ for niacin vs placebo). Placebo increased HDL-C by 0% in diabetics and 2% in nondiabetics. Placebo increased tri-glycerides by 7% in diabetics and 0% in nondiabetics; placebo increased LDL-C by 1% in both diabetics and nondiabetics. Niacin modestly increased glucose by 8.7 mg/dL in diabetics and 6.3 mg/dL in nondiabetics ($p=0.04$ and $p<0.001$), but did not change HbA1c levels in diabetics; while in patients with diabetes that received placebo, HbA1c decreased by 0.3% ($p=0.04$). There were no differences in niacin discontinuation, niacin dosage or hypoglycemic therapy in patients with diabetes assigned to niacin vs placebo.

Concl.   Niacin was safely used in patients with diabetes and may be con-sidered as an alternate to statins or fibrates in diabetics in whom these agents are not tolerated or fail to correct low HDL-C or hypertriglyceridemia.

ADVENT

The Assessment of Diabetes Control and Evaluation of the Efficacy of Niaspan Trial

Title	Efficacy, safety, and tolerability of once-daily niacin for the treatment of dyslipidemia associated with type 2 diabetes.
Authors	Grundy SM, Vega GL, McGovern ME, et al.
Reference	Arch Intern Med 2002;162:1568-1576.
Disease	Hyperlipidemia, hypercholesterolemia.
Purpose	To determine the efficacy and safety of treatment of dyslipidemia with once-daily extended-release niacin in diabetic patients.
Design	Double-blind, randomized, placebo-controlled, multicenter.
Patients	46 patients, ≥21 years with stable type 2 diabetes, defined as a fasting blood glucose (FBG) level ≤200 mg/dL and HbA1c ≤9% on 2 separate measurements. Study patients had diabetes controlled with diet, oral hypoglycemic agents (sulfonylureas, metformin, and/or acarbose; thiazolidinediones were excluded), or insulin. Patients currently on an 3-hydroxy-3-methylglutaryl coenzyme A (HMG-CoA) reductase inhibitor were required to have LDL cholesterol (LDL-C) of at least 130 mg/dL, HDL cholesterol (HDL-C) ≤40 mg/dL, or a triglyceride (TG) level of at least 200 mg/dL. Patients not receiving HMG-CoA reductase inhibitors were required to have LDL-C ≤130 mg/dL but could qualify for entry if they had HDL-C ≤40 mg/dL or a TG level of at least 200 mg/dL. Aspartate aminotransferase and alanine aminotransferase levels at baseline had to be less than 1.3 times the upper limit of normal. Patients with chronic stable conditions such as hypertension or previous myocardial infarction or stroke (>6 months before study entry) were eligible, unless they were taking medication that might affect lipid levels. Other exclusion criteria were a history of psychiatric illness, substance abuse, liver disease, gout, or peptic ulcer disease. Any products containing at least 30 mg/d of niacin were not permitted.
Follow-up	16 weeks.

Regimen	There was a minimum 4-week drug wash-out phase, during which all lipid-lowering medications other than HMG-CoA reductase inhibitors were discontinued. At randomization, patients were assigned to 1 of 3 groups: placebo, extended release (ER) niacin at 1000 mg/d, or ER niacin at 1500 mg/d. During week 1, all patients were given 375 mg/d of either ER niacin or placebo; during week 2, 500 mg/d ER niacin or placebo; during week 3, 750 mg/d ER niacin or placebo; during week 4, 1000 mg/d ER niacin or placebo. After this point patients who were in the 1000 mg/d group received two 500 mg tablets once a day at bedtime through the 16th week. Patients in the 1500 mg/d group received two 750 mg tablets once a day at bedtime through the 16th week. Aspirin, 325 mg, up to 1 half hour before study medication, was permitted to relieve flushing.
Add'l Tx	All patients were required to conform to a recommended diabetes dietary program as described by the American Diabetes Association for a minimum of 4 weeks. All hypoglycemic medications, including insulin, were allowed except troglitazone. HMG-CoA reductase inhibitors were prohibited.
Results	All patients were required to conform to a recommended diabetes dietary program as described by the American Diabetes Association for a minimum of 4 weeks. All hypoglycemic medications, including insulin, were allowed except troglitazone. HMG-CoA reductase inhibitors were prohibited. The primary end points were the changes in HDL-C and TG levels from baseline to 16 weeks follow-up. Other study end points were: ratio of total cholesterol to HDL-C; LDL particle size; and levels of total cholesterol, LDL-C, lipoprotein (a) (Lp[a]), and high-sensitivity C-reactive protein (hsCRP). The primary safety was the change in HbA1c level from baseline to week 16. Other safety measures were FBG levels, serum transaminase concentrations, and self-reported adverse events. Baseline characteristics among patients in the 3 groups were generally similar; however, patients in the 1000 mg/d ER niacin group had greater weight and BMI, and lower baseline HDL-C levels ($p<0.001$). Current use of medication for diabetes was common throughout all groups (81%), with metformin (54.8%) and sulfonylureas (47.9%) the usual medications.

Approximately 15% of patients were using insulin. There were 69 patients (47.3 %) receiving HMG-CoA reductase inhibitors: 29 (59%) in the placebo group, 19 (42%) in the 1000 g ER niacin group, and 21 (40%) in the 1500 mg ER niacin group. ER niacin had a significant effect on the primary end points. Levels of HDL-C increased from baseline in both 1000 mg and 1500 mg niacin groups vs placebo at all time points (p<0.05). The mean absolute increases in HDL-C levels were 1.6 mg/dL, 7.6 mg/dL, and 11.0 mg/dL in the placebo, 1000 mg, and 1500 mg ER niacin groups, respectively. Levels of TG were decreased in the niacin groups vs placebo, although this was only significant for the 1500 mg group, where the median percentage changes from baseline ranged from -28% to -36%, with p<0.05 vs placebo. Similarly, there were decreases in LDL-C levels in the niacin groups vs placebo, but these were only significant in the 1500 mg ER niacin group at weeks 12 and 16 (p< 0.05). A similar but nonsignificant trend was observed for measures of total cholesterol. Changes in the ratio of total cholesterol/HDL-C were favorable and statistically significant for both niacin groups vs placebo (-12% and -22% in the 1000 mg and 1500 mg niacin groups, respectively; p<0.01). Changes in Lp(a) and hsCRP were suggestive of a dose-related favorable relationship for niacin, but did not reach statistical significance. The primary safety end point was similar between the 3 groups. Changes in HbA1c were -0.02 %, +0.07%, and +0.29% in the placebo, 1000 mg, and 1500 mg ER niacin groups, respectively; the +0.29% change in the 1500 mg ER niacin group was marginally significant vs placebo (p=0.048). There was an initial rise in fasting blood glucose levels in both ER niacin groups, but these returned to baseline by week 16. Flushing was the only adverse event that was reported more frequently in the niacin groups (approximately 66% in the niacin groups, 10% in placebo). There were no elevations of liver enzymes >3 times the upper limit of normal for any study patient.

| Concl. | Niacin is safe and effective in treating dyslipidemia in diabetic patients. |

ADVOCATE

The Advicor vs Other Cholesterol-Modulating-Agents Trial Evaluation

Title	Comparison of once-daily, niacin extended-release/lovastatin with standard doses of atorvastatin and simvastatin (The Advicor Versus Other Cholesterol-Modulating-Agents Trial Evaluation [ADVOCATE]).
Authors	Bays HE, Dujovne CA, McGovern ME, et al.
Reference	Am J Cardiol 2003;91:667-672.
Disease	Hyperlipidemia.
Purpose	To compare the efficacy of niacin extended-release/lovastatin with standard doses of simvastatin and atorvastatin for lowering blood lipids in patients with dyslipidemia.
Design	Randomized, open label, multicenter.
Patients	315 patients, 18-70 years old, with LDL cholesterol levels ≥160 mg/dL if they did not have coronary artery disease, or ≥130 mg/dL if they had coronary artery disease. Triglycerides should have been <300 mg/dL and HDL cholesterol <45 mg/dL in men and <50 mg/dL in women. Patients with intolerability or allergy to the study drugs, history of substance abuse, alcohol consumption, active gallbladder disease, uncontrolled hypertension, serum creatinine ≥1.5 mg/dL, hepatic dysfunction, fasting glucose ≥115 mg/dL, diabetes mellitus, NYHA class III/IV heart failure, hyperuricemia or gout, active peptic disease, history of cancer, fibromyalgia, stroke within the preceding 6 months, and acute coronary syndrome or revascularization within the preceding 6 months were excluded.
Follow-up	16 weeks.

Regimen	Randomization to simvastatin (10 mg/d for 8 weeks and then 20 mg/d for 4 weeks and 40 mg/d for 4 weeks), atorvastatin (10 mg/d for 8 weeks and then 20 mg/d for 4 weeks and 40 mg/d for 4 weeks) or niacin/lovastatin in 2 doses (500 mg niacin and 20 mg lovastatin per day for 4 weeks and then 1000 mg niacin and 40 mg lovastatin /d for 12 weeks or 500 mg niacin and 20 mg lovastatin /d for 4 weeks and then 1000 mg niacin and 40 mg lovastatin /d for 4 weeks, 1500 mg and 50mg/d, respectively for 4 weeks and 2000 mg and 40mg/d, respectively for the last 4 weeks.
Add'l Tx	NCEP Step 1 diet. Other lipid-lowering medications were prohibited. All subjects randomized to niacin/lovastatin were advised to take aspirin 325 mg/d or NSAID to prevent flushing.
Results	After 8 weeks of therapy LDL cholesterol decreased by 28%, 38%, 40%, and 38% in the simvastatin 10 mg/d, atorvastatin 10 mg/d and the 2 groups of niacin 1000 mg/lovastatin 40 mg/d, respectively. HDL cholesterol increased in 7%, 3%, 20%, and 20%, respectively. Triglycerides decreased by 18%, 20%, 35%, and 30%, respectively. At the end of the 16-week treatment, LDL cholesterol was decreased by 39%, 49%, 42%, and 39% in the simvastatin 40 mg/d, atorvastatin 40 mg/d, niacin 2000 mg/lovastatin 40 mg/d, and niacin 1000 mg/lovastatin 40 mg/d, respectively. HDL cholesterol increased by 7%, 6%, 32%, and 17%, respectively. Triglycerides decreased by 19%, 31%, 49%, and 29%. A total of 6% of the patients assigned to niacin/lovastatin discontinued study drug because of flushing. No drug-induced myopathy or >5 upper limit increase in CK occurred. None of the patients had >3 upper limit increase in aspartate aminotransferase (AST) or alanine aminotransferase (ALT).
Concl.	Niacin extended-release/lovastatin and atorvastatin 10 mg/d and 20 mg/d were more effective than simvastatin 10 mg/d and 20 mg/d in reducing LDL cholesterol. Niacin/lovastatin was more effective than simvastatin and atorvastatin in increasing HDL cholesterol and decreasing triglycerides. All 3 drugs were safe.

8

AFCAPS/TexCAPS

AFCAPS/TexCAPS C-Reactive Protein Substudy: Air Force/Texas Coronary Atherosclerosis Prevention Study

Title	Measurement of C-reactive protein for the targeting of statin therapy in the primary prevention of acute coronary events.
Authors	a. Downs JR, Beere PA, Whitney E, et al. b. Downs JR, Clearfield M, Whitney E, et al. c. Ridker PM, Rifai N, Clearfield M, et al.
Reference	a. Am J Cardiol 1997;80:287-293. b. JAMA 1998;279:1615-1622. c. N Engl J Med 2001;344:1959-1965.
Disease	Coronary artery disease.
Purpose	To determine whether statins prevent coronary artery events in persons with elevated C-reactive protein levels but with no hyperlipidemia.
Design	As per AFCAPs/TexCAPS. C-reactive protein measured at baseline and after 1-year follow-up.
Patients	5742 patients enrolled in AFCAPS/TexCAPS with average levels of cholesterol and below average levels of high-density lipoproteins.
Follow-up	Average 5.2 years.
Regimen	Lovastatin 20-40 mg/d vs placebo.

Results	Patients divided into 4 groups: LDL cholesterol lower than median (less than 149.1 mg/dL) and C-reactive protein lower than median (less than 0.16 mg/dL); LDL lower than median and C-reactive protein higher than median; LDL higher than median and C-reactive protein lower than median; LDL and C-reactive protein higher than median. Lovastatin reduced C-reactive protein by 14.8% (p<0.001). Lovastatin prevented coronary events (defined as fatal or nonfatal MI, unstable angina, or sudden death from cardiac causes) in patients whose baseline ratio of total cholesterol to HDL was higher than median ratio irrespective of C-reactive protein. The striking finding of this analysis was that lovastatin was effective in decreasing cardiac events in patients with a ratio of total to HDL lower than the median and a C-reactive protein higher than the median. (Number of patients needed to treat for 5 years to prevent 1 event=43; p=0.02). In patients with LDL <median, C reactive protein >median there were 22 events in 718 patients in the lovastatin group vs 37 events in 710 patients in the placebo group (RR 0.58; 95% CI=0.34-0.98). Lovastatin was not effective in patients with ratio of total to HDL and C-reactive protein lower than median.
Concl.	Lovastatin was effective in reducing cardiac events among people with elevated C-reactive protein but low lipid levels.

ALLHAT-LLT

Antihypertensive and Lipid-Lowering Treatment to Prevent Heart Attack Trial—Lipid Lowering Trial

Title	Major outcomes in moderately hypercholesterolemic, hypertensive patients randomized to pravastatin vs usual care. The Antihypertensive and Lipid-Lowering Treatment to Prevent Heart Attack Trial (ALLHAT-LLT).
Authors	The ALLHAT Officers and Coordinators for the ALLHAT Collaborative Research Group.
Reference	JAMA 2002;288:2998-3007.
Disease	Hyperlipidemia, Hypercholesterolemia.
Purpose	To assess the differential effects of pravastatin and usual care on all-cause mortality in older, moderately hypercholesterolemic, hypertensive patients with one other coronary artery disease risk factor.
Design	Randomized, nonblind, multicenter.
Patients	10,355 patients, age ≥55 years, with stage 1 or 2 hypertension, and at least 1 additional coronary heart disease (CHD) risk factor, fasting low density lipoprotein cholesterol (LDL-C) 120-189 mg/dL for those without known CHD or 100-129 mg/dL for those with known CHD, fasting triglycerides <350 mg/dL. Exclusion criteria included current use of lipid-lowering medications or large doses of niacin, use of probucol in the prior year, and known intolerance to statins, or significant liver or kidney disease.
Follow-up	Mean 4.8 years.
Regimen	Patients were randomized to receive pravastatin, 40 mg/d, or usual care. Patients were started on 20 mg/d each evening, and dosage was increased to 40 mg/d as necessary to reduce LDL-C by 25%. After the enrollment of 1000 participants, a dosage of 40 mg/d was instituted for all patients. Patients in the usual care group received treatment for lowering of LDL-C by their primary care physicians.

Results	The primary study was all-cause death. Secondary study end points included: composite of fatal CHD and nonfatal MI (CHD events), mortality due to specific cause, total and specific cancers, Q-wave MI, quality of life measures, costs. Other end points (not prespecified) were incidence of stroke and heart failure. At baseline, the mean total cholesterol was 224 mg/dL; LDL-C was 146 mg/dL, and high density lipoprotein cholesterol (HDL-C) was 48 mg/dL; triglycerides were 152 mg/dL. The mean age was 66 years. The study group consisted of 49% women, 38% black, 23% Hispanic, 35% with type 2 diabetes, and CHD in 13% of the pravastatin group and 15 % in the usual care group. At 4 years follow-up, total cholesterol had been lowered by 17.2% in the pravastatin group and 7.6% in the usual care group. The LDL-C levels had been lowered by 27.7% in the pravastatin group and 11.0% in the usual care group. HDL-C cholesterol increased by 3.3% and 2.4% in the pravastatin and usual care groups, respectively. During follow-up 70-75% of the patients in the pravastatin group took ≥80% of the pravastatin. 17% of the patients in the usual care group were taking non-study statins after 4 years (32% of those with CHD at baseline). The primary end point, all-cause mortality, was not significantly different between the 2 groups (mortality rate at 6 years: pravastatin 14.9% vs usual care 15.3%; relative risk [RR] 0.99; 95% CI=0.89-1.11; p=0.88). Rates of cardiovascular (CVD) deaths overall (RR 0.99; 95% CI=0.84-1.16; p=0.91) as well as deaths from CHD (RR 0.99; 95% CI=0.80-1.24; p=0.96), stroke (RR 0.95; 95% CI=0.66-1.39; p=0.81), and other CVD death (RR 1.01; 95% CI=0.74-1.37; p=0.96) were similar between the 2 study groups. CHD events, defined as fatal CHD or nonfatal MI, occurred at a rate of 9.3% and 10.4% in the pravastatin and usual care groups, respectively (RR 0.91; 95% CI=0.79-1.04; p=0.16). The rate of death due to cancer and other medical conditions were similar between the 2 groups. Results for mortality and CHD events were similar in the prespecified subgroups of age (≥65 or <65 years), sex, race (black vs nonblack), and diabetics and non-diabetics. Pravastatin had a significantly favorable effect on CHD events in blacks vs nonblacks (RR 0.73 vs 1.02; p=0.03). Results were also similar across subgroups defined by CHD status and levels of LDL-C.
Concl.	Compared to usual care, pravastatin did not reduce all-cause mortality or CHD events in older patients with moderately elevated LDL-C levels and well-controlled hypertension.

ASAP

Atorvastatin vs Simvastatin on Atherosclerosis Progression

Title	Effect of aggressive vs conventional lipid-lowering on athero-sclerosis progression in familial hypercholesterolaemia (ASAP): a prospective, randomised, double-blind trial.
Authors	Smilde TJ, van Wissen S, Wollersheim H, et al.
Reference	Lancet 2001;357:577-581.
Disease	Atherosclerosis.
Purpose	To compare the effects of high-dose atorvastatin and conventional dose simvastatin on carotid atherosclerosis.
Design	Randomized, double-blind, placebo-controlled.
Patients	325 patients, 30-70 years old, with familial hypercholesterolemia.
Follow-up	2 years.
Regimen	After an 8-week placebo run-in phase, patients were randomized to atorvastatin 40 mg/d or simvastatin 20 mg/d with matching placebo. After 4 weeks, dose of atorvastatin was increased to 80 mg/d and simvastatin to 40 mg/d.
Add'l Tx	A resin was added if serum total cholesterol remained >8.0 mmol/L.

Results	At baseline, lipid and lipoprotein concentrations were comparable between the groups. Atorvastatin and simvastatin reduced total cholesterol by 41.8% and 33.6%, respectively (p=0.0001); LDL-cholesterol by 50.5% and 41.2%, respectively (p=0.0001). HDL-cholesterol increased by 13.2% and 13.4%, respectively (p=0.8541); whereas triglycerides were reduced by 29.2% and 17.7%, respectively (p=0.0023); lipoprotein(a) was reduced by 14.3% and 15.2%, respectively (p=0.7705); and apolipoprotein B was reduced by 44.1% and 34.9%, respectively (p=0.0001). Carotid intima media thickness, as measured by quantitative B-mode ultrasound, was comparable at baseline. After 2 years, IMT decreased by 0.031 mm in the atorvastatin group, whereas it increased by 0.036 mm in the simvastatin group (p=0.0001). In 66% of the atorvastatin vs only 42% of the simvastatin-treated patients there was regression of the carotid IMT. The change in IMT after 2 years was correlated with baseline IMT and with % LDL-cholesterol reduction, but not with the change in HDL-cholesterol and lipoprotein(a) concentrations.
Concl.	Aggressive LDL-cholesterol reduction by 80 mg/d atorvastatin induced regression of carotid intima media thickness in patients with familial hypercholesterolemia, whereas 40 mg/d simvastatin did not.

ASCOT-LLA

Anglo-Scandinavian Cardiac Outcomes Trial—
Lipid Lowering Arm

Title	Prevention of coronary and stroke events with atorvastatin in hypertensive patients who have average or lower-than-average cholesterol concentrations, in the Anglo-Scandinavian Cardiac Outcomes Trial—Lipid Lowering Arm (ASCOT-LLA): a multicentre randomised controlled trial.
Authors	Sever PS, Dahlof B, Poulter NR, et al.
Reference	Lancet 2003;361:1149-1158.
Disease	Hypertension, hypercholesterolemia (mild).
Purpose	To study the cardiovascular effects of atorvastatin in hypertensive patients with total cholesterol of ≤6.5 mmol/L.
Design	Randomized, 2 x 2 factorial design, double-blind, multicenter. The antihypertensive arm is designed as Prospective Randomized Open Blinded end points (PROBE) trial.
Patients	10,305 patients, 40-79 years old, with untreated hypertension (≥160/100 mm Hg) or treated hypertension with blood pressure ≥140/90 mm Hg, who had also serum total cholesterol of ≤6.5 mmol/L and were not currently taking a fibrate or a statin. In addition, patients had to have ≥3 of the following risk factors (left ventricular hypertrophy, abnormal ECG, type 2 diabetes, peripheral vascular disease, previous TIA or stroke, male sex, age ≥55 years, microalbuminuria or proteinuria, smoking, total cholesterol/HDL cholesterol ratio of ≥6, or premature family history of coronary heart disease). Patients with previous myocardial infarction, angina, a stroke within the preceding 3 months, serum triglycerides >4.5 mmol/L, congestive heart failure, uncontrolled arrhythmia or any routine laboratory test showing important hematological or biochemical abnormality were excluded.

Follow-up	Median 3.3 years.
Regimen	After a 4-week run-in phase, 19,342 patients were randomized to b-blockers ± diuretics or to amlodipine ± ACE inhibitor. In addition, the eligible patients for the lipid-lowering arm were randomized to atorvastatin 10 mg/d (n=5168) or placebo (n=5137).
Results	The study was terminated prematurely by the Data and Safety Monitoring Board. Compared with placebo, atorvastatin reduced total cholesterol by 1.3 mmol/L, LDL cholesterol by 1.2 mmol/L, and triglycerides by 0.3 mmol/L at 1 year. HDL cholesterol levels were comparable between the groups. The primary end point of the study (nonfatal MI or coronary heart disease death) occurred in 1.9% in the atorvastatin group and in 3.0% in the placebo group (hazard ratio [HR] 0.64; 95% CI= 0.50-0.83; p=0.0005). All-cause mortality was 3.6% and 4.1%, respectively (p=0.165). Cardiovascular mortality was 1.4% and 1.6%, respectively (p=0.51). Stroke occurred in 1.7% and 2.4%, respectively (HR 0.73; 95% CI=0.56-0.96; p=0.024), and MI in 1.7% and 2.7%, respectively (HR 0.62; 95% CI= 0.47-0.81; p=0.0005). Total cardiovascular events and procedures occurred in 7.5% and 9.5% of the patients, respectively (HR 0.79; 95% CI=0.69-0.90; p=0.0005). Coronary events occurred in 3.4% in the atorvastatin and 4.8% in the placebo group (HR 0.71; 95% CI=0.59-0.86; p=0.0005). The rates of serious adverse events and liver-enzyme elevation were comparable between the atorvastatin and placebo groups.
Concl.	Atorvastatin 10 mg/d reduced major cardiovascular events and stroke in hypertensive patients with high-risk features for cardiovascular disease and normal or only mildly elevated serum cholesterol levels.

ASSET

Atorvastatin Simvastatin Safety and Efficacy Trial

Title	Comparison of efficacy and safety of atorvastatin (10 mg) with simvastatin (10 mg) at six weeks.
Authors	Insull W, Kafonek S, Goldner D, et al.
Reference	Am J Cardiol 2001;87:554-559.
Disease	Hyperlipidemia.
Purpose	To compare efficacy of atorvastatin and simvastatin in patients with mixed dyslipidemia.
Design	Randomized, open-label, multicenter.
Patients	1424 patients, 18-80 years old, with mixed hyperlipidemia (fasting triglyceride levels of 200-600 mg/dL, and an low-density lipoprotein cholesterol levels of 130-350 mg/dL), with or without type 2 diabetes mellitus. Patients with type 1 diabetes mellitus or uncontrolled type 2 diabetes mellitus, nephrotic syndrome, renal failure, uncontrolled hypothyroidism, liver disease, myocardial infarction, revascularization or severe or unstable angina within 1 month before screening were excluded.
Follow-up	54 weeks.
Regimen	Randomization to atorvastatin 10 mg/d (n=730) or simvastatin 10 mg/d (n=694).
Add'l Tx	All patients were instructed to follow the National Cholesterol Education Program step I or II diet.

Results   This trial reports the primary efficacy analysis at 6 weeks. The intention-to-treat analysis includes 712 patients in the atorvastatin group and 666 patients in the simvastatin group. Atorvastatin was associated with greater reduction in LDL cholesterol (37.2% vs 29.6%; p<0.0001), triglyceride (22.1% vs 16.0%; p<0.0001), total cholesterol (27.6% vs 21.5%; p<0.0001), and apolipoprotein B (28.3% vs 21.2%; p<0.0001). HDL cholesterol increased by 7.4% in the atorvastatin group and by 6.9% in the simvastatin group (p=0.38). 55.6% of the patients in the atorvastatin group vs 38.4% of the patients in the simvastatin group achieved the NCEP LDL cholesterol goal for the combined risk categories (p<0.0001). Atorvastatin reduced LDL cholesterol more than simvastatin both in patients without diabetes (37.3% vs 29.5%; p<0.0001) and in patients with diabetes (37.1% vs 29.7%; p<0.0001). Treatment-associated adverse events occurred in 5.8% of the patients in the atorvastatin group vs 2.9% in the simvastatin group. Most adverse events were mild or moderate and only <1% of the patients in both groups withdrew treatment due to adverse events.

Concl.   Atorvastatin 10 mg/d was more effective than simvastatin 10 mg/d in lowering blood lipids and reaching LDL cholesterol goals in patients with mixed hyperlipidemia. Both drugs were safe and well tolerated.

BIP

Bezafibrate Infarction Prevention

Title	Secondary prevention by raising HDL cholesterol and reducing triglycerides in patients with coronary artery disease. The BIP study.
Authors	The BIP Study Group.
Reference	Circulation 2000;102:21-27.
Disease	Coronary artery disease, low high-density lipoprotein; high triglycerides.
Purpose	To determine whether raising HDL-cholesterol and reducing triglycerides would decrease coronary artery disease mortality and nonfatal MI rates in patients with known CAD, low HDL and moderately elevated cholesterol.
Design	Double-blind, randomized, placebo-controlled, multicenter.
Patients	3090 patients with previous myocardial infarction or unstable angina, HDL-C ≤45 mg/dL, triglycerides ≤300 mg/dL, total cholesterol of 180-250 mg/dL, LDL ≤180 mg/dL.
Follow-up	Mean of 6.2 years
Regimen	400 mg bezafibrate daily (n=1548) vs placebo (n=1542).
Add'l Tx	Diet; patients could take other prescription cardiac medicines but not other lipid-lowering medicines.

Results	Bezafibrate caused an 18% increase in HDL-C and a decrease of 21% in triglycerides. The crude rate of the primary outcome (nonfatal and fatal MI and sudden death) was 13.6% in the bezafibrate group and 15.0% in the placebo group (p=0.26). At 6.2 years the reduction in cumulative probability of the primary end point was 7.3% with treatment (p=0.24). Post hoc analysis revealed that in patients with triglycerides <150 mg/dL at baseline there was no clear benefit of bezafibrate treatment. In a subgroup of patients with baseline triglycerides of greater or equal to 200 mg/dL the decrease in cumulative probability of the primary end point was 39.5% (p=0.02) with bezafibrate. Overall incidence of any adverse event was similar between groups.
Concl.	While bezafibrate was safe and effective in lowering triglyceride and elevating HDL-C it did not significantly decrease the primary cardiac event rate. In a post hoc subgroup analysis it did decrease the incidence of total or nonfatal MI or sudden death in coronary patients with a high baseline triglyceride (≥200 mg/dL).

CARE

Cholesterol and Recurrent Events

Title	a. The effect of pravastatin on coronary events after myocardial infarction in patients with average cholesterol levels. b. Relationship between plasma LDL concentrations during treatment with pravastatin and recurrent coronary events in the cholesterol and recurrent events trial. c. Reduction of stroke incidence following myocardial infarction with pravastatin: the CARE study.
Authors	a. Sacks FM, Pfeffer MA, Moye LA, et al. b. Sacks FM, Moye LA, Davis BR, et al. c. Plehn JF, et al.
Reference	a. 1. Am J Cardiol 1991;68:1436-1446.2. Am J Cardiol 1995;75:621-623.3. Am J Cardiol 1995;76:98C-106C.4. N Engl J Med 1996;335:1001-1009. b. Circulation 1998; 97:1446-1452. c. Presentation at the American Heart Association's 23rd International Joint Conference on Stroke and Cerebral Circulation. February 5-7, 1998, Orlando, Florida.
Disease	a. Coronary artery disease, myocardial infarction. b. Myocardial infarction, hypercholesterolemia.
Purpose	a. To evaluate the effectiveness of lowering blood cholesterol levels with pravastatin in patients after myocardial infarction and its effect on subsequent cardiac events. b. To determine the relationship between the LDL concentration during therapy, absolute reduction in LDL, and percent reduction in LDL and outcome.c. To analyze the effect of lipid lowering with pravastatin on the risk of stroke and transient ischemic attacks in the CARE trial.
Design	Randomized, double-blind, placebo-controlled, multicenter.
Patients	4159 patients, 21-75 years old, who have experienced myocardial infarction 3-20 months before randomization, had plasma total cholesterol <240 mg/dL, LDL cholesterol 115-174 mg/dL, triglycerides <350 mg/dL, fasting glucose levels ≤220 mg/dL, left ventricular ejection fraction ≥25%, and no symptomatic congestive heart failure.

Follow-up	Median follow-up 5 years (4-6.2 years).
Regimen	Pravastatin 40 mg/d or placebo. For patients with LDL cholesterol >175 mg/dL at follow-up, dietary counseling, and then cholestyramine.
Results	a. Pravastatin therapy lowered the mean LDL cholesterol of 139 mg/dL by 32% and maintained mean levels of 98 mg/dL. During follow-up LDL cholesterol was 28% lower, total cholesterol was 20% lower, HDL 5% higher, and triglycerides level 14% lower in the pravastatin than placebo group (p<0.001 for all comparisons). Primary end points (death from coronary artery disease or nonfatal myocardial infarction) occurred in 13.2% vs 10.2% in the placebo and pravastatin group, respectively (risk reduction 24%; 95% CI=9-36%; p=0.003). Cardiovascular death occurred in 5.7% in the placebo vs 4.6% in the pravastatin group (risk reduction 20%; 95% CI=-5-39%; p=0.10), and non fatal myocardial infarction occurred in 8.3% vs 6.5%, respectively (risk reduction 23%; 95% CI=4-39%; p=0.02). However, total mortality was comparable (9.4% vs 8.6% in the placebo and pravastatin group, respectively; 9% risk reduction; 95% CI=-12-26%; p=0.37). There was no difference in mortality from noncardiovascular causes. The risk of myocardial infarction was 25% lower in the pravastatin group (7.5% vs 10.0%; 95% CI=8-39%; p=0.006). The rate of coronary artery bypass surgery or PTCA was lower in the pravastatin group (14.1% vs 18.8%; risk reduction 27%; 95% CI=15-37%; p<0.001). The pravastatin group had also a 31% lower incidence of stroke (2.6% vs 3.8%; 95% CI=3-52%; p=0.03). There was also a trend toward less unstablangina in the pravastatin group (15.2% vs 17.3%; risk reduction 13%; 95% CI=-1-25%; p=0.07). The effect of pravastatin was greater among women then among men (46% vs 20% risk reduction for women and men respectively). Patients with baseline LDL cholesterol >150 mg/dL had a 35% reduction in major coronary events, as compared with a 26% reduction in those

with baseline LDL cholesterol of 125-150 mg/dL, and a 3% increase in those with baseline levels < 125 mg/dL (p=0.03 for the interaction between baseline LDL cholesterol level and risk reduction). The overall incidence of fatal or nonfatal cancer was comparable (161 in the placebo vs 172 in the pravastatin group). However, breast cancer occurred in 1 patient in the placebo and in 12 in the pravastatin group (p=0.002). Of the 12 cases in the pravastatin group, 3 occurred in patients who had previously had breast cancer. There was no other significant differences between the groups in the occurrence of other types of cancer.

b. Coronary death or recurrent MI were reduced by 24% with pravastatin. Coronary event rate declined as LDL was reduced from 174 to about 125 mg/dL; however, no further decline occurred in the LDL range of 71-125 mg/dL. LDL concentration achieved during follow-up was a significant but nonlinear predictor of coronary event rate; the extent of LDL reduction as absolute amount or percentage of LDL reduction was not a significant predictor of event rate. Triglycerides but not HDL weakly but significantly were associated with coronary event rate.

c. The stroke incidence was 3.7% in placebo patients and 2.5% in patients on pravastatin. Stroke or transient ischemic attack occurred in 6% of patients on placebo and 4.4% of patients on pravastatin. Thus, pravastatin decreased strokes by 32%; it decreased either strokes or transient ischemic attacks by 27% over 5 years. Unlike the CARE findings for reduced risk of myocardial infarction, (whereby lowering LDL below 125 mg/dL did not further reduce myocardial infarction), the investigators did not observe a threshold effect of LDL's below 125 mg/dL for stroke. Patients with LDL's above 150 had a 44% lower rate of strokes; those between 125-150, a 28% lower stroke rate; and under 125, a 25% reduction in stroke rate with pravastatin.

Concl.   a. Pravastatin therapy lowered cardiac mortality, the need for revascularization, and occurrence of stroke in both men and women with coronary artery disease, plasma total cholesterol of <240 mg per deciliter and plasma LDL cholesterol >125 mg per deciliter. In this study, no reduction in event rate was found in patients with LDL cholesterol <125 mg per deciliter. There was no reduction in overall mortality.

b. Reduction of LDL down to a concentration of about 125 mg/dL was associated with a reduction in coronary events. Further reduction to <125 mg/dL with therapy was not associated with additional benefit.

c. In the population of patients in the CARE study, pravastatin reduced the rates of stroke and stroke or transient ischemic attacks.

CARE (Substudy)

Cholesterol and Recurrent Events

Title	Long-term effects of pravastatin on plasma concentration of C-reactive protein.
Authors	Ridker PM, Rifai N, Pfeffer MA, et al.
Reference	Circulation 1999;100:230-235.
Disease	Post myocardial infarction patients with total cholesterol <240 mg/dL and LDL cholesterol between 115-175 mg/dL.
Purpose	To determine whether long-term therapy with pravastatin reduces the levels of the inflammatory marker, C-reactive protein.
Design	As per CARE.
Patients	472 randomly selected participants in CARE in whom C-reactive protein was measured at baseline and at 5 years and who had remained free of recurrent vascular events during follow-up.
Follow-up	5 years.
Regimen	As per CARE.
Add'l Tx	As per CARE.

Results	While C-reactive protein levels increased over time in placebo patients (median change = +4.2%; p=0.2 and mean change =+0.07 µg/dL; p=0.04), they decreased in pravastatin patients (median change =-17.4%; p=0.004 and mean change =-0.07 mg/dL; p=0.002). Median, mean, and absolute change in C-reactive protein were significantly lower in the pravastatin group at 5 years (-21.6%; p=0.007; -37.8%; p=0.002; and -0.137 µg/dL; p=0.003, respectively). The changes in C-reactive protein over time did not correlate with change in LDL cholesterol among pravastatin or placebo treated patients. There was also a lack of a correlation between change in C-reactive protein and changes in total cholesterol or HDL levels. Pravastatin reduced C-reactive protein levels at all LDL change increments.
Concl.	In post myocardial infarction patients, C-reactive protein levels tended to increase over 5 years in patients receiving standard therapy plus placebo; pravastatin decreased C-reactive protein levels independent of the degree of lipid improvement.

CARE (Substudy)

Cholesterol and Recurrent Events

Title	Low-density lipoprotein size, pravastatin treatment, and coronary events.
Authors	Campos H, Moye LA, Glasser SP, et al.
Reference	JAMA 2001;286:1468-1474.
Disease	Hyperlipidemia.
Purpose	To determine whether low-density lipoprotein (LDL) size independently predicts recurrent coronary events in coronary artery disease (CAD) patients.
Design	Prospective, nested case-control study within the CARE trial.
Patients	837 patients who survived myocardial infarction (MI) and had typical LDL concentrations of 115-174 mg/dL.
Follow-up	5 years.
Regimen	Patients were randomized to placebo vs pravastatin.
Add'l Tx	As per care.
Results	Primary outcome was subsequent MI or coronary death during 5 years of follow-up analyzed by quintile of LDL particle size and therapy. Mean LDL size at baseline was the same in cases and controls at 25.6 nm. LDL size was not measured at follow-up. In the placebo group, large LDL predicted coronary events in models adjusted for age (RR 1.79; 95% CI=1.01-3.17) and for age, lipid, and nonlipid risk factors (RR 4.00; 95% CI=1.81-8.82) in which LDL size was analyzed from lowest (24.5 nm) to highest (26.6 nm) quintile. In patients taking pravastatin there was no increased risk of LDL particle size with MI or coronary death. Previous studies had stressed small LDL particle size as a risk factor for coronary events—but these studies primarily investigated populations that had not yet experienced a coronary event while the current study focused on recurrent coronary events following an MI.

Concl. Large LDL size predicted recurrent coronary events in a population that had experienced an MI and were not on pravastatin.
This adverse predictive effect was not observed in patients on
pravastatin. The authors postulated that identifying patients on
the basis of LDL size might not be that useful since treating
elevated LDL also treated the risks associated with large LDL.

CHALLENGE

Comparison of Efficacy and Safety of Atorvastatin and Simvastatin in Patients with Dyslipidemia with and Without Coronary Heart Disease

Title	Comparison of efficacy and safety of atorvastatin and simvastatin in patients with dyslipidemia with and without coronary heart disease.
Authors	Karalis DG, Ross AM, Vacari RM, et al.
Reference	Karalis DG, Ross AM, Vacari RM, et al.
Disease	Hypercholesterolemia.
Purpose	To compare the efficacy and safety of 2 doses of simvastatin and atorvastatin.
Design	Randomized, open-label, blind end point, multicenter.
Patients	1732 patients, 18-80 years old, with dyslipidemia, with or without coronary heart disease. Pregnant or breast-feeding women, patients with body mass index >32 kg/m², fasting triglyceride levels ≤600 mg/dL, known hypersensitivity to statins, uncontrolled hypothyroidism, nephrotic syndrome, type 1 or uncontrolled type 2 diabetes mellitus, renal failure, hepatic dysfunction, elevated baseline creatine kinase levels, recent myocardial infarction, unstable angina or revascularization (within 3 months preceding enrollment) were excluded. In addition, patients taking systemic steroids, isotretinoin, cyclosporin, erythromycin and immunosuppressive drugs were not included.
Follow-up	6 weeks.
Regimen	After a 4-week run-in phase, patients were randomized to simvastatin 20 mg/d (n=650) vs atorvastatin 10 mg/d (n=650), or simvastatin 80 mg/d (n=216) or atorvastatin 40 mg bid (n=216).
Add'l Tx	National Cholesterol Education Program step I or II diet.

Results	1694 patients were included in the final analysis. Compliance was 93.0% for the atorvastatin 10 mg/d, 93.2% for the simvastatin 20 mg/d, 91.6% for the atorvastatin 80 mg/d, and 91.5% for the simvastatin 80 mg/d. After 6 weeks of therapy LDL cholesterol was reduced by 37.1% in the atorvastatin 10 mg/d vs 35.4% in the simvastatin 20 mg/d (p<0.025). Atorvastatin 80 mg/d and simvastatin 80 mg/d resulted in 53.4% and 46.7% reduction in LDL cholesterol, respectively (p<0.0001). Triglycerides were reduced by 18% and 14% in the atorvastatin 10 and simvastatin 20 groups, respectively (p<0.025), and by 28% and 23% in the atorvastatin 80 and simvastatin 80 groups, respectively (p<0.025). HDL cholesterol increased by 5% and 6% in the atorvastatin 10 and simvastatin 20 groups, respectively (p=NS), and by 2% and 6.5% in the atorvastatin 80 and simvastatin 80 groups, respectively (p<0.0001). Total cholesterol decreased by 27% and 25%, in the atorvastatin 10 and simvastatin 20 groups, respectively (p<0.025), and by 40% and 34% in the atorvastatin 80 and simvastatin 80 groups, respectively (p<0.001). 59% of the patients in the atorvastatin 10 mg/d vs 53% in the simvastatin 20 mg/d reached their NCEP LDL cholesterol goal (p=0.0125). 89% of the patients in the atorvastatin 80 vs 82% in the simvastatin 80 group reached their NCEP LDL cholesterol goal (p=0.0698). All 4 study regimens were well tolerated and safe. Elevation in creatine kinase was noted in 2/181 patients in the simvastatin 80 mg/d and in none of the patients in the other 3 groups. Increase in aspartate aminotransferase occurred in 1/203 of the patients in the atorvastatin 80 mg vs 1/187 in the simvastatin 80 mg group, and an increase in alanine aminotransferase in 1/198 and 1/186 of the patients, respectively. Adverse effects occurred in 46% of the patients in the atorvastatin groups vs 39% in the simvastatin groups.
Concl.	Atorvastatin resulted in a significantly greater decrease in total cholesterol, LDL cholesterol, and triglycerides than simvastatin. However, high-dose atorvastatin resulted in less of an increase in HDL cholesterol than high-dose simvastatin. Both drugs were safe.

FAST

Fukuoka Atherosclerosis Trial

Title	Effects of probucol and pravastatin on common carotid atherosclerosis in patients with asymptomatic hypercholesterolemia. Fukuoka Atherosclerosis Trial (FAST).
Authors	Sawayama Y, Shimizu C, Maeda N, et al.
Reference	J Am Coll Cardiol 2002;39:610-616.
Disease	Hypercholesterolemia.
Purpose	To evaluate the effects of probucol and pravastatin on the carotid artery intima-media thickness (IMT) in asymptomatic patients with hypercholesterolemia.
Design	Randomized, open-label.
Patients	246 asymptomatic patients, 30-89 years old, with primary hypercholesterolemia (total cholesterol ≥220 mg/dL) and treatment with either pravastatin or probucol. Patients with serum triglycerides ≥350 mg/dL, uncontrolled heart failure, recent myocardial infarction, severe or unstable angina, hypo- or hyperthyroidism, secondary hyperlipidemia, uncontrolled diabetes mellitus, uncontrolled hypertension, heavy alcohol abuse, obese patients on weight reduction programs, any severe disease, or steroid treatment were excluded.
Follow-up	2 years.
Regimen	Patients were randomized to probucol 500 mg bid (n=82), pravastatin 10 mg/d (n=83), or control (n=81).

Results	21% (34 patients) from the probucol and pravastatin groups did not complete the study. Total serum cholesterol was reduced by 20.0% and 20.1% in the probucol and pravastatin groups after 12 months of treatment (both p<0.001), and by 24.1% and 23.0%, respectively, after 24 months (both p<0.001). In the control group, total cholesterol was reduced at the end of follow-up, but the difference was not significant. After 12 months of therapy, LDL cholesterol (LDL-C) was reduced by 24.2% in the probucol group (p<0.001), by 32.7% in the pravastatin group (p<0.001) and by 5.1% in the control group. After 24 months, LDL-C was reduced by 28.6% (p<0.001), 35.9% (p<0.001) and 8.5% (p<0.05) compared to baseline, respectively. After 24 months, HDL-C reduced by 20.7% (p<0.05) in the probucol group and increased by 6.4% (p<0.05) and 5.4% (p=NS) in the pravastatin and control groups, respectively. There was no significant change in the triglyceride levels in all 3 groups. After 12 and 24 months, the intimal-media thickness (IMT) was reduced compared to baseline by 8.3% (p<0.01) and 13.9% (p<0.01) in the probucol group. In the pravastatin group there was no significant change in the IMT in the first 18 months; however, after 24 months there was a 13.9% reduction in the IMT (p<0.01). In the control group IMT increased by 23.3% after 24 months (p<0.05). There was no significant difference in IMT at 24 months between the probucol and pravastatin groups. There was a weak correlation between the absolute change in IMT and the change in LDL cholesterol in the pravastatin group (r=0.363; p=0.0051), but not in the probucol (r=0.065; p=0.5892) or control (r=0.130; p=0.3321) groups. There was no correlation between the absolute change in HDL-C cholesterol and the change in IMT in any of the 3 groups. Major cardiovascular events (cardiovascular death, myocardial infarction, or coronary revascularization) occurred in 2.4%, 4.8%, and 13.6% in the probucol, pravastatin, and control groups, respectively (p<0.05 for the difference between the probucol and control groups). Total mortality was 2.4%, 6.0%, and 11.1%, respectively.
Concl.	Probucol treatment was associated with a reduction in total cholesterol and LDL-C levels and a decrease in HDL-C levels. Both probucol and pravastatin reduced the carotid IMT. Probucol, but not low-dose pravastatin, reduced the incidence of cardiac events.

GAIN

German Atorvastatin Intravascular Ultrasound Study

Title	Use of intravascular ultrasound to compare effects of different strategies of lipid-lowering therapy on plaque volume and composition in patients with coronary artery disease.
Authors	Schartl M, Bocksch W, Koschyk DH, et al.
Reference	Circulation 2001;104:387-392.
Disease	Hyperlipidemia; coronary artery disease.
Purpose	To determine whether reducing low-density lipoprotein cholesterol (LDL-C) <100 mg/dL with atorvastatin vs moderate treatment with other lipid-lowering drugs led to less progression of coronary atherosclerosis and altered ultrasound appearance.
Design	Randomized, open-label, multicenter.
Patients	131 patients were recommended for and had successfully undergone an intracoronary intervention. The plaque studied for intravascular ultrasound (IVUS) analysis had to have a stenosis <50% on quantitative coronary angiography. If there was no such plaque visible in the vessel that underwent an intervention, then another coronary artery was imaged. LDL-C had to be >160 mg/dL for patients off lipid therapy and >130 for patients on lipid therapy.
Follow-up	12 month angiographic, IVUS measurements.
Regimen	Atorvastatin 20-80 mg to reach a target LDL-C of less than 100mg/dL (n=65); vs usual care (n=66) consisting of a heterogeneous mix of lipid-lowering agents, excluding atorvastatin.

Results   Mean daily dose of atorvastatin was 33 mg. In the usual care
           group 49% received statins, 44% fibrates, and 36% cholestyr-
           amine. At 12 months reduction in LDL-C was 42% with atorv-
           astatin and 16% in the usual care group (p<0.0001). Mean LDL
           fell from 155 to 86 mg/dL with atorvastatin and 166 to 140
           mg/dL in the usual care group. Plaque volume assessed by IVUS
           at 12 months vs baseline showed a nonsignificant trend toward a
           greater increase in the usual care group (9.6±28.1 mm^3) vs ator-
           vastatin (1.2±30.4 mm^3; p=0.191). Hyperechogenicity index
           was increased to a greater extent for atorvastatin (1.9%±8.3%)
           vs usual care (0.3%±7.5%; p=0.178). The percent change
           in hyperechogenicity index was greater with atorvastatin
           (42.2%±97.8%) vs usual care (10.1%±68.5%; p=0.021). It is
           assumed that hyperechogenicity correlates with a greater pres-
           ence of dense fibrous or elastic tissue in the plaque; whereas
           hypoechogenicity is associated with more lipid, loose fibrotic,
           and necrotic tissue.

Concl.   Lipid lowering with LDL-C <100 mg/dL with atorvastatin
           appeared to lead to some slow down of plaque growth of minor
           lesions and an increase in plaque hyperechogenicity.

GREACE

Greek Atorvastatin and Coronary Heart Disease Evaluation

Title	Treatment with atorvastatin to the National Cholesterol Educational Program goal vs "usual" care in secondary coronary heart disease prevention.
Authors	Athyros VC, Papageorgiou AA, Mercouris BR, et al.
Reference	Curr Med Res Opin 2002;18:220-228.
Disease	Hyperlipidemia.
Purpose	To assess the effect of atorvastatin on morbidity and mortality in patients with established coronary artery disease.
Design	Prospective, randomized, open-label, intention-to-treat.
Patients	1600 consecutive patients with established coronary heart disease: history of prior myocardial infarction (MI) or >70% stenosis of at least 1 coronary artery assessed by angiography, age <75 years, low-density lipoprotein cholesterol (LDL-C) >100 mg/dL, triglycerides (TG) <400 mg/dL.
Follow-up	Mean of 3 years.
Regimen	Patients randomized to atorvastatin (n=800) vs usual care (n=800). Usual care included lifestyle modification, and all necessary drug treatment including lipid-lowering agents (atorvastatin was not excluded from "usual" care group). Patients randomized to the atorvastatin group received 10 mg/d, which could be titrated up to 80 mg/d for patients not achieving LDL-C goal of <100 mg/dL at lower doses. Mean dose of atorvastatin was 24 mg/d. In the usual care group only 26% of patients received hypolipidemic drugs and then 12% discontinued this therapy.

Results	Primary end points were death, nonfatal MI, unstable angina, CHF, coronary revascularization, and stroke. Atorvastatin reduced LDL-C by 46%, total cholesterol by 36% and TGs by 31% and increased HDL by 7%. 95% of patients had LDL-C <100 mg/dL; only 3% in the usual care group achieved this goal. 196 (24.5%) patients in the usual care group had a recurrent coronary heart disease event or died vs 96 (12%) in the atorvastatin group (RR 0.49; CI=0.27-0.73; p<0.0001). Atorvastatin decreased total mortality by 43%; from 40 (5%) of patients in the usual care group to 23 (2.9%) in the atorvastatin group (p=0.0021); atorvastatin reduced coronary mortality by 47% (p=0.0017) and nonfatal MI rate by 59% (p=0.0001). Coronary morbidity was significantly reduced (RR 0.46; CI=0.25-0.71; p<0.0001) and stroke (RR 0.53; CI=0.30-0.82; p=0.0018) was also reduced with atorvastatin. Atorvastatin reduced unstable angina by 52%, (p=0.0032), need for PTCA/CABG by 51% (p=0.0011), and CHF by 50% (p=0.021). The benefit of atorvastatin was observed in all subgroups, including women, diabetics, hypertensives, patients aged 60-75, in those with CHF, recent unstable angina, or prior revascularization. Withdrawal due to side effects occurred in 0.75% of atorvastatin patients and 0.4% of patients in usual care group. 7 patients in the atorvastatin group had an increase in liver enzymes >3-fold upper limit of normal and in 3 patients dose reduction corrected the liver enzyme elevation. No patients had myalgia plus increase of creatine kinase (CK) activity 5-10 times upper limit of normal or myalgia without CK elevation. Treatment with atorvastatin was shown to be cost effective.
Concl.	Attaining LDL-C goal as per NCEP ATP III guidelines with atorvastatin in patients with coronary artery disease reduced total and coronary mortality, coronary morbidity, and stroke vs patients who received "usual" medical care.

HATS

HDL-Atherosclerosis Treatment Study

Title	Simvastatin and niacin, antioxidant vitamins, or the combination for the prevention of coronary disease
Authors	Brown BG, Zhao X-Q, Chait A, et al.
Reference	N Engl J Med 2001;345:1583-1592.
Disease	Coronary artery disease.
Purpose	To evaluate whether lipid-lowering therapy and antioxidant vitamin therapy, alone and together, are efficacious for cardiovascular protection in patients with coronary artery disease (CAD) and low high-density lipoprotein cholesterol (HDL-C).
Design	Randomized, double-blind, placebo-controlled, 2 × 2 factorial.
Patients	160 patients (men younger than 63 years and women younger than 70 years of age) with confirmed coronary artery disease, ≥3 coronary lesion with ≥30% of diameter stenosis or ≥1 coronary lesion with ≥50% diameter stenosis. Patients had to have low-density lipoprotein cholesterol (LDL-C) ≤145 mg/dL and triglyceride ≤400 mg/dL. All men had to have HDL-C ≤35 mg/dL and women, ≤40 mg/dL. Patients who underwent previous coronary artery bypass grafting (CABG) and those with severe hypertension, recent gout, liver disease, thyroid disease, renal disease, or uncontrolled diabetes were not included.
Follow-up	Repeated angiography after 3 years.
Regimen	Patients were randomized to simvastatin + niacin or placebo and to antioxidant vitamins or placebo. Simvastatin was started at a dose of 10-20 mg/d. Dose was adjusted to achieve LDL-C of 40-90 mg/dL. The placebo-treated patients also received simvastatin 10 mg/d if their LDL-C was ≥140 mg/dL. Niacin was administered at a dose of 500 mg-4g/d. The antioxidant therapy included vitamin E 800 IU, vitamin C 100 mg, β-carotene 25 mg, and selenium 100 µg/d.
Add'l Tx	All patients received counseling for weight loss, diet, smoking cessation, and exercise.

Results   146 patients completed the angiographic protocol, 2 patients died and 12 withdrew from the study. The mean doses of simvastatin taken by the patients was 13±6 mg/d and the niacin 2.4±2.0 g/d. Flushing was reported by 30% of the niacin treated patients vs 23% in the placebo (p=0.35). Antioxidant therapy did not alter lipid levels, except for lowering HDL2 levels by 15%. The simvastatin + niacin therapy reduced LDL-C by 42% and increased HDL-C by 26%. HDL2 was increased by 65% in the simvastatin + niacin alone group and by only 28% in the simvastatin + niacin + antioxidant group (p=0.02). Mean coronary lumen diameter stenosis increased by 3.9% in the placebo group, 1.8% in the antioxidant group (p=0.16 vs. placebo), and 0.7% in the simvastatin + niacin + antioxidant group (p=0.004). In contrast, mean diameter stenosis decreased by 0.4% in the simvastatin + niacin group (p<0.001). Clinical events (coronary mortality, myocardial infarction, stroke or revascularization) occurred in 24% of the placebo group, 21% in the antioxidant group, 14% in the simvastatin + niacin + antioxidant, and in 3% in the simvastatin + niacin group (p=0.03).

Concl.   Simvastatin + niacin reduced the rate of clinical events and prevented progression of CAD in patients with CAD, low HDL-C and without markedly elevated levels of LDL-C. The concomitant use of antioxidant vitamins seems to attenuate these effects.

L-CAD

Lipid-Coronary Artery Disease Study

Title	Beneficial effects of pravastatin (+/- cholestyramine/niacin) initiated immediately after a coronary event. (The randomized lipid-coronary artery disease [L-CAD] study).
Authors	Arntz H-R, Agrawal R, Wunderlich W, et al.
Reference	Am J Cardiol 2000;86:1293-1298.
Disease	Coronary artery disease, hyperlipidemia, acute myocardial infarction, unstable angina.
Purpose	To compare effects of cholesterol-lowering therapy initiated immediately after an acute coronary event with the effects of usual therapy.
Design	Prospective, open-label, randomized, single-center.
Patients	126 patients with acute MI and/or percutaneous transluminal coronary angioplasty secondary to unstable angina randomized within 6 days of acute event. Total cholesterol was >200 to <400 mg/dL and low-density lipoprotein-cholesterol >130 to <300 mg/dL to enter.
Follow-up	24 months.
Regimen	Randomized to pravastatin up to 40 mg/d (combined when necessary with cholestyramine, 4-32 g/d and or nicotinic acid, 1.5-6 g/d), to achieve LDL-C of ≤130 mg/dL (n=70) vs antilipidemic therapy by family physician (n=56).
Add'l Tx	All patients received dietary counseling.

Results   End points included quantitative coronary angiography. Combined clinical end points were total mortality, cardiovascular death, nonfatal MI, need for coronary intervention, stroke, and new onset peripheral vascular disease. In patients receiving pravastatin and/or cholestyramine/ niacin minimal lumen diameter increased by 0.05 ± 0.20 mm after 6 months and 0.13 ± 0.29 mm after 24 months; however, in the group that received routine therapy it decreased by 0.08 ± 0.20 mm and 0.18 ± 0.27 mm at 6 and 24 months ($p=0.004$ at 6 months and $p<0.001$ at 24 months). At 24 months 29/56 patients receiving routine therapy but only 16/70 patients receiving pravastatin +/- cholestyramine/ niacin experienced a clinical end point ($p=0.005$; OR=0.28; CI=0.13-0.60). Total cholesterol was reduced by an average of 20% in intensive therapy group and LDL was reduced by 28% ($p<0.001$) over entire study; in the routine therapy group these values remained close to baseline. Triglycerides, HDL-C, Lp(a) remained unchanged in both groups.

Concl.   Pravastatin-based therapy to lower lipids immediately after an acute coronary syndrome lessened angiographic evidence of coronary atherosclerosis and reduced composite clinical events.

LIPID (Incidence of Stroke)

Long-Term Intervention with Pravastatin in Ischemic Disease

Title	Pravastatin therapy and the risk of stroke.
Authors	White HD, Simes RJ, Anderson N, et al.
Reference	N Engl J Med 2000;343:317-326.
Disease	Stroke, hyperlipidemia.
Purpose	To determine whether patients with a history of myocardial infarction or unstable angina who received the lipid-lowering drug pravastatin had a reduction in stroke.
Design	As per LIPID trial. Definitions of stroke based upon clinical findings, brain imaging with computed tomography or magnetic resonance imaging, results of duplex ultrasound, or angiography, or autopsy findings.
Patients	9014 patients with a history of MI or unstable angina and a total cholesterol level of 155-271 mg/dL.
Follow-up	6 years.
Regimen	Patients randomized in double-blind manner to either 40 mg pravastatin or placebo.

Results	In the placebo patients 231 strokes occurred in 204 of 4502 patients (4.5%); in the pravastatin group, 188 strokes occurred in 169 of the 4512 patients (3.7%; relative reduction in risk of 19%; 95% CI=0-34%; p=0.05). Nonhemorrhagic strokes occurred in 4.4% of placebo and 3.4% of pravastatin patients (relative reduction in risk of 23%; 95% CI=5%-38%; p=0.02). Hemorrhagic stroke occurred in 0.2% of placebo and 0.4% of pravastatin group; p=0.28). With pravastatin therapy total cholesterol decreased from 218 mg/dL to 179 mg/dL an 18% reduction. LDL decreased by 27%. Pravastatin reduced the relative risk of death due to coronary heart disease by 24% (from 8.3% in the placebo group to 6.4% in the pravastatin-treated group; p<0.001). Pravastatin resulted in a 22% relative risk reduction for all causes of death.
Concl.	Pravastatin caused a moderate reduction in all strokes and in the risk of nonhemorrhagic strokes in patients who previously had MI or unstable angina.

LIPID (Substudy)

Long-Term Intervention with Pravastatin in Ischemic Disease

Title	Long-term effectiveness and safety of pravastatin in 9014 patients with coronary heart disease and average cholesterol concentrations: the LIPID trial follow-up.
Authors	The LIPID Study Group.
Reference	Lancet 2002;359:1379-1387. N Engl J Med 1998;339:1349-1357.
Disease	Coronary artery disease.
Purpose	To assess the long-term (up to 8 years) effects of initial treatment with pravastatin on cardiovascular mortality and morbidity.
Design	Open-label phase of follow-up of a randomized, double-blind, placebo-controlled multicenter trial.
Patients	7680 patients who participated in the original LIPID trial (3766 assigned placebo and 3914 assigned pravastatin) had 2 years of extended follow-up.
Follow-up	2 years after the initial mean 6-year follow-up of the LIPID trial.
Regimen	Originally patients were randomized to placebo or pravastatin treatment for 6 years. All patients still alive at the end of the placebo-controlled trial (both the placebo and pravastatin arms) were offered open-label pravastatin 40 mg/d.

Results	At the beginning of the open-label phase, 88% of the original pravastatin group and 86% of the original placebo group initiated open-label pravastatin. Additional patients received other lipid-lowering medications. Overall 90% of the patients received lipid-lowering therapy. During the open-label follow-up period total cholesterol, low-density lipoprotein cholesterol (LDL-C), high-density lipoprotein cholesterol (HDL-C), and triglyceride levels were comparable between the 2 groups. All-cause mortality during the open-label phase was 5.6% in the original pravastatin group vs 6.8% in the original placebo group (relative risk [RR] reduction 18%; 95% CI=2%-32%; p=0.029). Coronary heart disease mortality was 2.8% vs 3.6%, respectively (RR reduction 24%; 95% CI=12%-35%; p=0.026), and the combined end point of coronary heart disease mortality or myocardial infarction occurred in 4.5% vs 5.2%, respectively (RR reduction 16; 95% CI=-2% to 32%; p=0.08). Over the total 8-year follow-up, total mortality was 19.7% in the placebo group and 15.9% in the pravastatin group (RR reduction 21%; 95% CI=13%-29%; p<0.0001), and coronary heart disease mortality was 11.3% vs 8.8%, respectively (RR reduction 24%; 95% CI=14%-34%; p<0.0001). Fewer patients in the pravastatin group needed revascularization over the 8-year follow-up period (19.9% vs 16.8%; RR reduction 19%; 95% CI=11%-26%; p<0.0001). Stroke occurred less often in the pravastatin group (6.0% vs 5.0%; RR reduction 20%; 95% CI=4%-33%; p=0.015). Subgroup analysis revealed that pravastatin was equally effective in all subgroups, including both men and women, patients ≥70 years old, and patients with baseline total cholesterol of <5.5 mol/L. Long-term pravastatin treatment was safe and was not associated with significant adverse effects.
Concl.	The beneficial effects of pravastatin treatment were sustained for 2-year follow-up, even though the majority of the original placebo-assigned patients were started on lipid-lowering therapy. This study reinforces the importance of long-term lipid-lowering therapy for almost all patients with a history of coronary heart disease.

LIPID Substudy (Effect in Women)

Long-Term Intervention with Pravastatin in Ischemic Disease

Title	Effect of pravastatin on cardiovascular events and mortality in 1516 women with coronary heart disease: results from the LIPID study.
Authors	Hague W, Forder P, Simes J, et al.
Reference	Am Heart J 2003;145:643-651.
Disease	Coronary artery disease.
Purpose	To assess whether long-term treatment with pravastatin reduces coronary heart disease events in women.
Design	Sub-analysis of a randomized, double-blind, placebo-controlled, multicenter trial.
Patients	1516 women who were enrolled in the LIPID study.
Follow-up	6 years.
Regimen	Randomized to pravastatin 40 mg/d (n=756) or placebo (n=760).
Add'l Tx	See above.
Results	Mortality was lower in women than in men (10.3% vs 14.8%; p<0.01). Pravastatin reduced the risk of coronary events (relative risk reduction [RRR] 11%; 95% CI=18% reduction-33% increase; p=0.42), and coronary death in women (RRR 18%; 95% CI=25% reduction-46% increase; p=0.35), although the results are not statistically significant. However, the relative effects of treatment did not differ between women and men for most of the outcomes (p>0.05 for heterogeneity). Pravastatin treatment reduced hospitalization and duration of hospitalization among men, but the effect in women was smaller and did not reach statistical significance.
Concl.	The study was not adequately powered to show a significant effect of pravastatin in women. However, the results in women are consistent with the main results of the LIPID study.

LISA

Lescol in Severe Atherosclerosis

Title	The effect of fluvastatin on cardiac events in patients with symptomatic coronary artery disease during one year of treatment.
Authors	Riegger G, Abletshauser C, Ludwig M, et al.
Reference	Atherosclerosis 1999;144:263-270.
Disease	Hypercholesterolemia, coronary artery disease.
Purpose	To determine whether aggressive therapy with fluvastatin reduces cardiac events within 1 year in patients with hyperlipidemia and symptomatic coronary artery disease.
Design	Randomized, placebo-controlled, multicenter.
Patients	365 patients with symptomatic coronary artery disease and hypercholesterolemia. LDL cholesterol had to be >160 mg/dL.
Follow-up	1 year.
Regimen	Fluvastatin (40 mg daily; increased to twice daily if LDL cholesterol did not decrease more than 30%) vs placebo.
Add'l Tx	Antianginal drugs including nitrates, calcium blockers, β-blockers, aspirin.
Results	Primary outcome was major cardiac events (fatal MI, sudden death, nonfatal MI, CABG, unstable angina pectoris). Ten major cardiac events occurred in patients on placebo vs 3 in fluvastatin patients. Fluvastatin also demonstrated a trend towards less angina; fluvastatin improved exercise tolerance. Fluvastatin caused a 17% decrease in total cholesterol, a 27% decrease in LDL cholesterol, and a 25% decrease in triglycerides (in patients whose triglycerides were >227 mg/dL). The drug was well tolerated.
Concl.	Although overall event rates were low over 1 year, fluvastatin was associated with less cardiac events, less angina, and better exercise tolerance.

MIRACL

Myocardial Ischemia Reduction with Aggressive Cholesterol Lowering

Title	Effects of atorvastatin on early recurrent ischemic events in acute coronary syndromes. The MIRACL study: a randomized controlled trial.
Authors	Schwartz GG, Olsson AG, Ezekowitz MD, et al.
Reference	JAMA 2001;285:1711-1718.
Disease	Acute coronary syndrome.
Purpose	To assess the effects of atorvastatin, 80 mg/d, on mortality and morbidity of patients early after an acute coronary syndrome.
Design	Randomized, double-blind, placebo-controlled, multicenter.
Patients	3086 patients, ≥18 years old (65±12 years), within the first 24 hours of admission because of an acute coronary syndrome. Patients with serum total cholesterol >270 mg/dL, those scheduled for elective revascularization, evidence of Q-wave myocardial infarction within the preceding 4 weeks, coronary artery bypass graft surgery within the preceding 3 months, PCI within the preceding 6 months, left bundle branch block or paced rhythm, severe congestive heart failure, concurrent treatment with lipid-lowering agents, severe anemia, renal failure requiring dialysis, hepatic dysfunction, insulin-dependent diabetes, and pregnancy were excluded.
Follow-up	16 weeks.
Regimen	24-96 hours after hospitalization, patients were randomized to placebo or atorvastatin 80 mg/d for 16 weeks.
Add'l Tx	All patients received a National Cholesterol Education Program step I diet.

Results   1538 patients were included in the atorvastatin group and 1548 in the placebo group. The mean time from hospitalization and randomization was 63 hours in both groups. Treatment was discontinued prematurely in 11.2% of the atorvastatin vs 10.3% of the placebo group (p=NS). At baseline, serum lipid levels were comparable between the groups. Mean LDL cholesterol was 124 mg/dL, mean triglycerides 184 mg/dL, and mean HDL cholesterol 46 mg/dL. At the end of the study, mean LDL cholesterol had increased by 12% in the placebo group and decreased by 40% to 72 mg/dL in the atorvastatin group (p<0.001). Mean triglycerides increased by 9% in the placebo group and decreased by 16% in the atorvastatin group (p<0.001). Changes in HDL cholesterol were minor in both groups. The primary end point (death, acute MI, cardiac arrest with resuscitation, or recurrent symptomatic myocardial ischemia) occurred in 14.8% of the atorvastatin vs 17.4% of the placebo-treated patients (RR 0.84; 95% CI=0.70-1.00; p=0.048). Mortality was 4.4% in the placebo and 4.2% in the atorvastatin group (p=NS). Nonfatal MI occurred in 7.3% and 6.6%, respectively (p=NS), and resuscitated cardiac arrest in 0.6% and 0.5%, respectively (p=NS). Recurrent symptomatic myocardial ischemia occurred in 8.4% and 6.2% of the patients, respectively (RR 0.74; 95% CI=0.57-0.95; p=0.02). Stroke occurred in 1.6% of the placebo and 0.8% of the atorvastatin treated group (RR 0.50; 95% CI=0.26-0.99; p=0.045). There were no differences between the groups in the rates of revascularization or of worsening or new heart failure. There was no significant association between the percentage change in LDL cholesterol with atorvastatin from baseline to the end of the study and the occurrence of a primary end point event. The reduction of primary end point events by atorvastatin was independent of the baseline level of LDL cholesterol. Abnormal liver transaminases (>3 times upper limits of normal) were detected in 2.5% of the atorvastatin vs 0.6% of the placebo-treated patients (p<0.001).

Concl.   Atorvastatin 80 mg/d, started within 96 hours of hospitalization for acute coronary syndromes, reduced recurrent ischemic events, especially recurrent symptomatic angina requiring rehospitalization, in the first 16 weeks of therapy.

MIRACL

Myocardial Ischemia Reduction with Aggressive Cholesterol Lowering (Substudy)

Title	Effects of atorvastatin on stroke in patients with unstable angina or non-Q-wave myocardial infarction.
Authors	Waters DD, Schwartz GG, Olsson AG, et al.
Reference	Circulation 2002;106:1690-1695.
Disease	Hypercholesterolemia; unstable angina, non-Q-wave myocardial infarction; stroke.
Purpose	To determine whether aggressive lowering of lipid levels with a statin reduces the incidence of nonfatal stroke in patients who have had an acute coronary syndrome.
Design	Substudy of a randomized, placebo-controlled trial.
Patients	As per MIRACL.
Follow-up	16 weeks.
Regimen	Patients were randomized to atorvastatin (n=1538) 80mg/d or placebo (n=1548) for 16 weeks. All patients were counseled on adherence to the National Cholesterol Education Program Step I diet.

Results	The end point of this substudy was the incidence of fatal and nonfatal stroke. At study entry, the lipid levels between the 2 groups were similar; the mean level of total cholesterol was 206 mg/dL, 124 mg/dL for LDL cholesterol, 46 mg/dL for HDL cholesterol, and 182 mg/dL for triglycerides. The total and LDL cholesterol had increased slightly in the placebo group at the end of the study. LDL cholesterol had increased 12% in the placebo group, and decreased by 40% in the atorvastatin group. Nonfatal stroke occurred in 22 patients in the placebo group and 9 in the atorvastatin group (relative risk [RR] 0.40; 95% CI=0.19-0.88; p=0.02). Fatal and nonfatal stroke occurred in 24 patients in the placebo group and 12 in the atorvastatin group (RR 0.49; 95% CI=0.24-0.98; p=0.04). 3 strokes were classified as hemorrhagic; all were in the placebo group. 8 strokes were classified as either hemorrhagic or undetermined; 5 of these were in the placebo group. All other strokes were either thrombotic or embolic. Patients who developed stroke were older than those who did not, were more likely to be women, and more likely to have a history of heart failure, cerebrovascular disease, or MI. Lipid levels at baseline were similar in patients who developed stroke and those who did not. Cox proportional hazards analysis revealed that 2 variables were associated with an increased risk of nonfatal stroke: history of cerebrovascular disease (RR 3.44; 95% CI=1.50-7.87; p=0.004); and previous MI (RR 1.99; 95% CI=0.96-4.15; p=0.065). Treatment with atorvastatin had a RR of 0.41 (95% CI=0.19-0.89; p=0.024) and current smoking had a RR of 0.28 (95% CI=0.08-0.92; p=0.36). However, further analysis showed that current smokers in the study were younger and less likely to have diabetes, hypertension, history of heart failure, or previous coronary revascularization, which may account for this finding.
Concl.	Aggressive lowering of lipid levels with atorvastatin in patients with an acute coronary syndrome was associated with a significantly reduced risk of stroke in the short-term (16 weeks) follow-up period.

Post-CABG

Post-Coronary Artery Bypass Graft Trial (7.5-Year Follow-Up)

Title	Long-term effects on clinical outcomes of aggressive lowering of low-density lipoprotein cholesterol levels and low-dose anticoagulation in the post coronary artery bypass graft trial.
Authors	Knatterud GL, Rosenberg Y, Campeau L, et al.
Reference	Circulation 2000;102:157-165.
Disease	Coronary artery disease.
Purpose	To assess 7.5 years follow-up on post-CABG trial and determine effects of 2 lipid-lowering regimens and low-dose anticoagulation on development of atherosclerosis in saphenous vein grafts.
Design	Randomized (2 x 2 factorial design) to aggressive or moderate strategy to lower low-density lipoprotein cholesterol and either warfarin or placebo, multicenter.
Patients	Follow-up on 1351 patients who were part of post-CABG trial, who had undergone CABG 1-11 years prior to screening. Had to have LDL of 130-175 mg/dL and triglyceride <300 mg/dL after initiation of step 1 diet.
Follow-up	≈7.5 years.
Regimen	Aggressive LDL-C lowering patients received 40 or 80 mg per day of lovastatin (and 8 g cholestyramine per day if needed) to achieve LDL's of 60-85 mg/dL. Patients assigned to moderate LDL-C lowering received 2.5 or 5 mg per day of lovastatin and 8 g cholestyramine if needed to achieve LDL-C of 130-140 mg/dL. Patients were assigned to warfarin 1-4 mg/d to maintain international normalized ratio <2.0 or placebo.

Results	There was no significant difference in death rates between aggressive and moderate lipid-lowering. Patients on warfarin exhibited a survival benefit after 3-7.5 years; at end of follow-up there was a 35% decrease in mortality in the warfarin group (p=0.008). There was no difference in incidence of fatal or non-fatal MI between lipid-lowering strategies. At 7.5 years, rate of MI was 9.1% with warfarin vs 13.8% in the placebo group (p=0.01). Patients assigned to aggressive lipid-lowering had a 30% decrease in revascularization procedures (p=0.0006) and a 24% decrease in composite end point at follow-up (death, bypass surgery, or angioplasty; p=0.001).
Concl.	Aggressive lipid-lowering was associated with decreased need for repeat revascularization procedure (which is consistent with a prior observation of delayed atherosclerosis progression in grafts). There was also an unexplained long-term benefit of warfarin in these post-CABG patients.

8

PRINCE

Pravastatin Inflammation CRP Evaluation

Title	Effect of statin therapy on C-reactive protein levels. The pravastatin inflammation/CRP evaluation (PRINCE): a randomized trial and cohort study.
Authors	Albert MA, Danielson E, Rifai N, et al.
Reference	JAMA 2001;286:64-70.
Disease	Hyperlipidemia.
Purpose	To determine whether pravastatin has anti-inflammatory effects assessed by C-reactive protein (CRP). To determine whether any effects of pravastatin on CRP are dependent or independent of its changes on low-density lipoprotein cholesterol (LDL-C).
Design	Community-based, prospective, randomized, double-blind, primary prevention. Open-label secondary prevention cohort.
Patients	1702 patients with no history of cardiovascular disease (primary prevention cohort) and 1182 patients with known cardiovascular disease (secondary prevention cohort).
Follow-up	24 weeks.
Regimen	In primary prevention arm patients randomized to 40 mg/d of pravastatin (n=865) vs placebo (n=837) for 24 weeks. Patients in secondary prevention cohort received 40 mg/d open-label pravastatin for 24 weeks.

Results	Primary outcome was change in CRP from baseline to 24 weeks. Pravastatin decreased median CRP levels by 16.9% (p<0.001) at 24 weeks (a decrease of 0.02 mg/dL). At 12 weeks pravastatin reduced CRP by 14.7%; p<0.001. Placebo had no effect on CRP. There was no significant association between baseline CRP and baseline LDL-C levels; between CRP at end of study and LDL-C at end of study; or change in CRP and change in LDL-C over time. Change in CRP was predicted by randomization to pravastatin group and baseline CRP (p<0.001) for both. Pravastatin also reduced CRP levels in the secondary prevention cohort. CRP was reduced by 14.3% at 12 weeks and 13.1% at 24 weeks (p<0.005).
Concl.	Pravastatin reduced CRP levels at 12 and 24 weeks and this reduction appeared to be largely independent of LDL-C. The authors conclude that statins have anti-inflammatory effects in addition and independent of lipid lowering effects.

PROSPER

Prospective Study of Pravastatin in the Elderly at Risk

Title	Pravastatin in elderly individuals at risk of vascular disease (PROSPER): a randomised controlled trial.
Authors	Shepherd J, Blauw GJ, Murphy MB, et al.
Reference	Lancet 2002;360:1623-1630.
Disease	Hypercholesterolemia, coronary artery disease, atherosclerosis.
Purpose	To determine if pravastatin is beneficial in elderly patients who have or are at risk of developing cardiovascular disease or stroke.
Design	Randomized, double-blind, placebo controlled, multicenter.
Patients	5804 men and women, age 70-82 years, with a history of coronary, peripheral, or vascular disease or an increased risk of these due to smoking, hypertension, or diabetes. Total plasma cholesterol was required to be between 4.0-9.0 mmol/L, and triglycerides <6.0 mmol/L. Individuals with poor cognitive function (mini-mental state exam score <24) were excluded.
Follow-up	Mean 3.2 years (range 2.8 to 4.0 years).
Regimen	Patients eligible for study were started with a 4-week single-blind placebo lead-in period. Patients were then randomized to receive either pravastatin 40 mg/d or placebo for the remainder of the study.

Results	The primary end point was the composite of death due to definite or suspected CAD, nonfatal MI, and fatal or nonfatal stroke. The secondary end points were the coronary and cerebrovascular outcomes separately. Tertiary end points included transient ischemic attack, disability, and cognitive function. 10% of the patients in the clacebo and 5% in the pravastatin group received non-study statin therapy. At the 3-month follow-up, mean LDL cholesterol was 34% lower, HDL cholesterol 5% higher, and triglyceride 13% lower in the pravastatin-compliant group vs placebo. At the 2-year follow-up, LDL levels were 33% lower in the pravastatin-compliant group vs the placebo group. The risk of the primary end point was reduced by 15% in the pravastatin group vs placebo (placebo=473/2913, 16.2% vs pravastatin=408/2891, 14.1%, hazard ratio (HR) 0.85; 95% CI=0.74-0.97; p=0.014). Death due to CAD and non-fatal MI was reduced by 19% in the pravastatin group (356/2913, 12.2% vs 292/2891, 10.1%, HR 0.81; CI=0.69-0.94; p=0.006), but there were no differences noted in the incidence of fatal or non-fatal strokes (HR 1.03; CI=0.81-1.31; p=0.81). There was no difference in all-cause death (10.5% vs 10.3%; p=0.74). Decline in cognitive function occurred at the same rate in both groups. The rate of serious adverse events was similar between the groups, with no cases of rhabdomyolysis. There were 36 incidents of myalgia reported in the pravastatin group and 32 in the placebo group. Elevated levels of alanine and aspartate transaminases greater than 3 times the upper limit of normal occurred in 1 patient in each group.
Concl.	During a follow-up period of 3 years, pravastatin reduced the composite risk of coronary death, coronary events, and fatal or nonfatal stroke in an elderly patient population compared with placebo. There was no apparent reduction in all-cause mortality.

RIKS-HIA

Register of Information and Knowledge About Swedish Heart Intensive Care Admissions

Title	Early statin treatment following acute myocardial infarction and 1-year survival.
Authors	Stenestrand U, Wallentin L, for the Swedish Register of Cardiac Intensive Care (RIKS-HIA).
Reference	JAMA 2001;285:430-436.
Disease	Acute myocardial infarction, hyperlipidemia.
Purpose	To study the effects of early statin treatment after acute myocardial infarction and 1-year mortality.
Design	Prospective cohort, multicenter.
Patients	19,599 patients, <80 years old, with first registry-recorded acute myocardial infarction, and who were discharged alive from the hospital. Patients who died before hospital discharge were excluded.
Follow-up	1 year.
Regimen	5528 patients received statins at or before discharge were compared to 14,071 patients who did not receive statins.

Results	The statin-treated patients were younger (61.9 years vs 66.9 years; p<0.001), had less diabetes mellitus, were more often smokers, and had more history of prior myocardial infarction. Acute reperfusion therapy was administered to 41% of the patients in the statin group vs 38% in the no-statin group (p=0.001). The unadjusted 1-year mortality was 4.0% in the statin group, and 9.3% in the no-statin group. Regression analysis, adjusted for confounding factors, as well as the propensity score for statin prescription, revealed that early statin therapy was associated with a lower risk for 1-year mortality (RR 0.75; 95% 0.63-0.89; p=0.001). The decrease in 1-year mortality with early statin therapy was most apparent among patients 60-69 years of age (RR 0.50; 95% CI=0.36-0.69). Early statin therapy was associated with better 1-year survival both in males and in females, in patients with and without diabetes mellitus, in patients with and without prior myocardial infarction, in patients with and without heart failure, and in patients with and without ST-elevation myocardial infarction. The benefit of statins on survival was not dependent on the concomitant use of digitalis, diuretics, β-blockers, and anticoagulants.
Concl.	Early initiation of statin treatment at discharge or even before discharge of patients with acute myocardial infarction was associated with better 1-year survival.

STRRIDE

Studies of Targeted Risk Reduction Interventions Through Defined Exercise (Substudy)

Title	Effects of the amount and intensity of exercise on plasma lipoproteins.
Authors	Kraus WE, Houmard JA, Duscha BD, et al.
Reference	N Engl J Med 2002;347:1483-1492.
Disease	Hypercholesterolemia.
Purpose	To determine the changes in lipoprotein profile based on exercise amount and intensity.
Design	Prospective, randomized, controlled.
Patients	111 men and women who were overweight (body mass index between 25 and 35), had a sedentary lifestyle, and had dyslipidemia (LDL cholesterol 130-190 mg/dL or HDL cholesterol <40 mg/dL for men, <45 mg/dL for women).
Follow-up	Approximately 8 months.
Regimen	Patients were randomized to a nonexercising control group or 1 of 3 exercising groups. The exercising groups were: 1) high-amount-high-intensity, defined as the calorie equivalent of jogging approximately 20 miles each week for a 90-kg person at a peak oxygen consumption of 65%-80%; 2) low-amount/high-intensity exercise, the equivalent of jogging approximately 12 miles a week at a peak oxygen consumption of 65%-80%; and 3) low-amount/moderate-intensity, the equivalent of walking approximately 12 miles a week at a peak oxygen consumption of 40-55%. Patients in the high-amount/high-intensity group were to expend 23 kcal/kg of body weight/wk; patients in the 2 low-amount groups were to use 14 kcal/kg of body weight/wk. Machines that were used for

exercise were: cycle ergometers, treadmills, and elliptical
Patients were instructed to maintain body weight through
course of the study. Prespecified limits were set as to the a
ability of compliance rates; patients who did not do 74-1
of the assigned exercise were not included in the analysis. /
patients whose weight varied more than 5% from baseline at \
end of the study were excluded from the analysis. Results wei
reported using only fully compliant patients in the primary analysis, but an intention-to-treat analysis was also performed. P values
less than 0.0167 were considered statistically significant.

Results	Base-line characteristics of the groups were similar in terms of initial fitness, total caloric intake, and macronutrient intake. High-amount-high-intensity exercise was associated with signifi-cant reductions in small LDL particles (p=0.016), LDL particles (p=0.02), and increased average LDL particle size (p=0.002) vs the control group. The low-amount exercise groups also had improve-ment in concentration of small LDL cholesterol particles and LDL particles, but they were not significant. The low-amount-high-intensity group had a significant effect on the size of the LDL particles vs the control group. The effect of exercise on HDL level was significant in the high-amount/high-intensity group; the change in HDL concentration was increased vs the control group (p=0.015). All exercise groups demonstrated a significant benefit in concentrations of triglycerides, VLDL triglycerides, large VLDL particles, and size of VLDL particles (most p values significant vs control group). Ranking of the effects of exercise intensity and amount on 11 variables (which consisted of concentration and particle size of LDL, IDL, HDL, VLDL, and triglyceride con-centration) showed that high-amount/high-intensity had a great-er effect on 10 of 11 variables than low-amount/high-intensity exercise. In considering 22 variables for amount or intensity of exercise, 21/22 variables showed that a higher level of exercise (amount or intensity) had a greater effect on lipid levels. Amount of exercise was more important than intensity of exercise. The results from the intention-to-treat analysis were very similar to those in the primary analysis. There were no instances where a difference that was statistically significant in the primary analysis group was not significant in the intention-to-treat analysis.

Concl.   High amount of exercise has a beneficial effect on lipid parameters such as concentration of LDL particles, concentration of
small LDL cholesterol, size of LDL particles, and HDL concentration vs no exercise. The amount of exercise was more important than the intensity of exercise. Low amounts of exercise did
not result in significant improvement in lipid parameters but
did prevent weight gain and worsening of lipid levels seen in
control patients.

VA-HIT

Veterans Affairs High-Density Lipoprotein Cholesterol Intervention Trial

Title	Gemfibrozil for the Secondary Prevention of coronary heart disease in men with low levels of high density lipoprotein cholesterol.
Authors	Rubins HB, Robins SJ, Collins D, et al.
Reference	N Engl J Med 1999;341:410-418.
Disease	Patients with low levels of high density lipoprotein (HDL) levels, coronary artery disease.
Purpose	To determine whether increasing HDL with gemfibrozil would improve outcome in men with coronary artery disease, an HDL of ≤40 mg/dL and an LDL cholesterol of ≤140 mg/dL.
Design	Randomized, double-blind, matching placebo, mutlicenter.
Patients	2531 men with coronary artery disease (history of myocardial infarction, angina with objective evidence of ischemia, coronary revascularization, coronary stenosis >50% by angiography) and lipid parameters described above.
Follow-up	5.1 years.
Regimen	Slow release gemfibrozil at 1200 mg once daily vs placebo.
Add'l Tx	American Heart Association Step 1 diet.

Results	Primary end point was combined incidence of nonfatal myocardial infarction or death from coronary artery disease. Primary event developed in 275/1267 patients in the placebo group (21.7%) vs 219/1264 patients in the gemfibrozil group (17.3%) with an overall reduction in risk of 4.4%, and decrease in RR 22%; 95% CI=7%-35%; p=0.006. There was a 22% decrease in death from coronary artery disease (p=0.07) and 23% decrease in nonfatal myocardial infarction (p=0.02). The benefits did not become apparent until about 2 years of randomization. Gemfibrozil treatment resulted in a 24% relative risk reduction in the combined outcomes of death from coronary heart disease, nonfatal myocardial infarction, or confirmed stroke (95% CI=11%-36%; p<0.001). Gemfibrozil also reduced the incidence of transient ischemic attacks and need for carotid endarterectomy. At 1 year, mean HDL cholesterol was 6% higher and triglycerides were 31% lower, with no change in LDL cholesterol, in the gemfibrozil group.
Concl.	In men with coronary artery disease, whose main lipid abnormality was low HDL cholesterol, gemfibrozil, which increased HDL cholesterol and lowered triglycerides, reduced the risk of major cardiovascular events.

VA-HIT

Veterans Affairs High-Density Lipoprotein Intervention Trial (Substudy)

Title	Diabetes, plasma insulin, and cardiovascular disease.
Authors	Rubins HB, Robins SJ, Collins D, et al.
Reference	Arch Intern Med 2002;162:2597-2604.
Disease	Lipid abnormality, hyperlipidemia.
Purpose	To evaluate the efficacy of gemfibrozil in patients with various levels of glucose tolerance or insulin resistance, and to investigate the association between diabetic status, glucose and insulin levels, and risk of cardiovascular outcomes.
Design	Substudy of a randomized, controlled trial.
Patients	2531 men <74 years of age who had coronary heart disease and high-density lipoprotein cholesterol level ≤40 mg/dL, low-density lipoprotein level ≤140 mg/dL, and triglyceride level ≤300 mg/dL. Exclusion criteria included use of warfarin, clinical chronic heart failure, or left ventricular ejection fraction <35%.
Follow-up	5.1 years.
Regimen	Patients were randomized to gemfibrozil, 1200 mg/d, or matched placebo.

Results	The patients were categorized into 4 different groups according to their fasting blood glucose levels: diagnosed diabetic by history, undiagnosed diabetic with fasting blood glucose (FBG) level ≥ 126 mg/dL, impaired fasting glucose with FBG between 110 and 125 mg/dL, and normal with FBG less than 110 mg/dL. The primary outcome of the study was the combined end point of major cardiovascular events which included CHD death, nonfatal MI, or stroke. The incidence of the primary end point was 36.5% and 34.3% in the diagnosed and undiagnosed diabetic groups, respectively. The primary end point occurred in 23.8% and 21% in the impaired FBG and normal groups, respectively. The incidence rate for the 2 diabetic groups was significantly higher than the rates for the nondiabetic groups ($p<0.001$). After adjustment for several variables including age, race, smoking, medication use, and many others, the hazard ratio (HR) for a major cardiovascular event was 1.87 (95% CI=1.44-2.43; $p=0.001$) for patients with diagnosed diabetes, and 1.72 (95% CI=1.10-2.68; $p=0.02$) in patients with undiagnosed diabetes, while in subjects that had impaired fasting glucose, the HR was 1.15 (95% CI=0.80-1.66; $p=0.46$). After excluding diabetic patients, the risk of the primary end point was significantly higher in patients in the highest quarter of fasting plasma insulin (FPI) level vs the lower 3 quartiles. Use of gemfibrozil was associated with a significantly reduced risk in the end point in both diabetic and nondiabetic patients: diabetic group HR 0.68; 95% CI=0.53-0.88; $p=0.004$); nondiabetic group HR 0.82; 95% CI=0.67-1.02; $p=0.07$). The absolute risk reduction was 9.9% in the diabetic group and 3.6% in the nondiabetic group. Diabetic patients who were on gemfibrozil had larger reductions in the individual end points of CHD, death, and stroke vs nondiabetic patients. Diabetic patients had a 41% reduced risk of CHD death (HR 0.59; 95% CI=0.39-0.91; $p=0.02$), and a 40% reduced risk of stroke (HR 0.60; 95% CI= 0.37-0.99; $p=0.046$); persons without diabetes had nonsignificant 3% and 10% reductions in CHD, death, and stroke, respectively. In nondiabetic patients, gemfibrozil had the greatest effect in patients with the highest levels of FPI. Patients who had FPI ≥ 39 mU had a 35% reduced risk of the primary end point (HR 0.65; 95% CI=0.43-0.97; $p=0.04$).
Concl.	In patients with known CHD and low high-density lipoprotein cholesterol level, use of gemfibrozil was associated with a reduced risk of major cardiovascular events in diabetic patients and in nondiabetics with high FPI levels.

VA-HIT (Stroke Substudy)

Veterans Affairs HDL Intervention Trial

Title	Reduction in stroke with gemfibrozil in men with coronary heart disease and low HDL cholesterol.
Authors	Rubins HB, Davenport J, Babikian V, et al.
Reference	Circulation 2001;103:2828-2833.
Disease	Lipid abnormality. Low high-density lipoprotein cholesterol.
Purpose	To determine whether raising HDL cholesterol and lowering triglyceride would decrease stroke in men with CAD who had low levels of HDL and LDL cholesterol.
Design	Placebo-controlled, randomized, multicenter.
Patients	2531 men with CAD, mean HDL of 31.5 mg/dL and mean LDL cholesterol of 111 mg/dL.
Follow-up	5 years.
Regimen	Patients randomized to gemfibrozil 1200 mg/d vs placebo.
Results	There were 76 strokes in the placebo group (6%) and 58 in the gemfibrozil group (4.6%) representing an absolute risk reduction of 1.4% and relative risk reduction adjusted for baseline characteristics, of 31% (95% CI=2%-52%; p=0.036). 90% of the strokes were ischemic. Fatal stroke occurred in 9 placebo patients and 3 gemfibrozil patients. As previously shown, gemfibrozil caused a 59% decrease in transient ischemic attacks (p<0.001) and 65% decrease in carotid endarterectomies (p<0.001).
Concl.	Gemfibrozil significantly reduced the incidence of strokes in men with CAD, low HDL, and low LDL.

VA-HIT (Update)

Veterans Affairs High-Density Lipoprotein Cholesterol Intervention Trial

Title	Relation of gemfibrozil treatment and lipid levels with major coronary events. VA-HIT: a randomized controlled trial.
Authors	Robins SJ, Collins D, Wittes JT, et al.
Reference	JAMA 2001;285:1585-1591.
Disease	Low high-density lipoprotein.
Purpose	To evaluate whether the reduction in coronary heart disease morbidity and mortality with gemfibrozil is attributed to the changes in plasma lipid levels.
Design	Randomized, double-blind, placebo-controlled, multicenter.
Patients	2531 men with a history of coronary heart disease with low high-density lipoprotein-cholesterol levels (mean 32 mg/dL) and low low-density lipoprotein cholesterol (mean 111 mg/dL).
Follow-up	Median follow-up 5.1 years.
Regimen	Gemfibrozil, 1200 mg/d (n=1264) or placebo (n=1267).
Results	HDL cholesterol concentrations were 31.5±5.3 mg/dL at baseline. At follow-up, HDL cholesterol was 31.7±5.3 mg/dL with placebo and 33.4±5.8 mg/dL with gemfibrozil (p<0.001). Total cholesterol was 175±25 mg/dL at baseline and 177±25 mg/dL and 168±25 mg/dL after treatment with placebo and gemfibrozil, respectively (p<0.001). LDL cholesterol was 111±22 mg/dL at baseline and 113±23 mg/dL and 113±22 mg/dL after treatment with placebo and gemfibrozil, respectively (p=0.71). Triglycerides were 151±68 mg/dL at baseline and 156±70 mg/dL and 101±54 mg/dL after treatment with placebo and gemfibrozil, respectively (p<0.001). With placebo, the incidence of coronary heart disease events was inversely related to the on-treatment HDL cholesterol levels (log-rank test; p=0.01), but was unrelated to the triglyceride levels (log-rank test; p=0.93) and LDL cholesterol levels (log-rank

test; p=0.49). Gemfibrozil was associated with a significant reduction in events, compared with placebo, for the second through fourth quintiles of HDL cholesterol levels (p=0.02). The event rates were comparable between the placebo and gemfibrozil group in the lowest and highest quintiles of HDL cholesterol levels. In patients treated with gemfibrozil, there was no difference in the event rate among the lowest 4 quintiles of triglyceride levels. In the lowest 4 quintiles of triglycerides, the event rates were lower for the gemfibrozil than the placebo-treated patients. However, in the highest triglyceride level quintile, the event rates were comparable between the placebo and gemfibrozil treated patients. For all levels of LDL cholesterol, the gemfibrozil-treated patients had a lower event rate than in the placebo-treated patients. At baseline, the concentration of HDL cholesterol (for every 5 mg/dL RR 0.91; 95% CI=0.83-0.99; p=0.047); triglycerides (for every 50 mg/dL RR 1.07; 95% CI=1.00-1.15; p=0.045); LDL-cholesterol (for every 25 mg/dL RR 1.07; 95% CI=0.96-1.19; p=0.22) predicted the occurrence of nonfatal myocardial infarction or coronary heart disease mortality. However, during treatment, only HDL cholesterol levels (RR 0.89; 95% CI=0.81-0.97; p=0.01) significantly predicted an end point event. Multivariate analysis showed that during treatment, only HDL cholesterol level was independently associated with event rate (RR 0.89; 95% CI=0.81-0.98; p=0.02). By multivariate analysis, neither LDL cholesterol nor triglyceride levels at baseline or during treatment predicted coronary heart disease events. The magnitude of reduction of events with gemfibrozil was greater than what could be explained by the increases in HDL cholesterol levels.

| Concl. | HDL cholesterol levels during treatment with gemfibrozil predicted the magnitude of reduction in risk for coronary heart disease events in patients with low HDL cholesterol levels at baseline. However, changes in HDL cholesterol concentrations only partially explained the reduction in event rates by gemfibrozil. |

WATCH

Women's Atorvastatin Trial on Cholesterol

Title	Efficacy of atorvastatin in achieving National Cholesterol Education Program low-density lipoprotein targets in women with severe dyslipidemia and cardiovascular disease or risk factors for cardiovascular disease: The Women's Atorvastatin Trial on Cholesterol (WATCH).
Authors	McPherson R, Angus C, Murray P, et al.
Reference	Am Heart J 2001;141:949-956.
Disease	Hyperlipidemia.
Purpose	To study the efficacy and ability to achieve NCEP ATP II recommendations for target levels for low-density lipoprotein cholesterol with atorvastatin in women with either coronary heart disease or risk factors for coronary heart disease and the presence of mixed dyslipidemia with obesity.
Design	Nonrandomized, open-label, multicenter.
Patients	318 women, 18-75 years old, with either: 1) established cardiovascular disease and LDL cholesterol ≥130 mg/dl if not currently treated with hypolipidemic drugs or LDL cholesterol ≥100 mg/dL if treated with hypolipidemic drugs (n=198); 2) ≥2 cardiovascular disease risk factors and LDL cholesterol ≥160 mg/dL if not currently treated or ≥130 mg/dL if receiving hypolipidemic drugs (n=79); or 3) < 2 risk factors and LDL cholesterol ≥190 mg/dL if not treated or ≥160 mg/dL if on hypolipidemic drugs (n=41).
Follow-up	16 weeks.
Regimen	After a 3-week washout phase off medications, all patients received atorvastatin 10-80 mg/d.

Results	63% of the participants without cardiovascular disease reached target LDL cholesterol with atorvastatin 10 mg/d, 79% with up to 20 mg/d and 87% with atorvastatin up to 80 mg/d. 34% of the women with established cardiovascular disease reached the ≤100 mg/dL LDL cholesterol goal with atorvastatin 10 mg/d, 60% with up to 20 mg/d, and 80% with up to 80 mg/d. The presence of mixed dyslipidemia and obesity did not alter the efficacy of reaching LDL cholestrerol goals with atorvastatin. 87% of the women with obesity and mixed dyslipidemia vs 81% of the patients without this metabolic syndrome reached the NCEP LDL cholesterol goals. The most frequently adverse events were headache (5% of the women) and constipation (6% of the women). 4 patients had myalgia that resulted in withdrawal from the study. 1 patient had an increase in creatine kinase.
Concl.	Atorvastatin was safe and effective in achieving NCEP ATP II target LDL cholesterol levels in women with established cardiovascular disease or risk factors for cardiovascular disease.

8

WOSCOPS

Prevention of Coronary Heart Disease with Pravastatin in Men with Hypercholesterolemia: West of Scotland Coronary Prevention Study

Title	a. Prevention of coronary heart disease with pravastatin in men with hypercholesterolemia. b. Influence of pravastatin and plasma lipids on clinical events in the West of Scotland Coronary Prevention Study (WOSCOPS).
Authors	a. Shepherd J, Cobbe SM, Ford I, et al. b. West of Scotland Coronary Prevention Study Group.
Reference	a. N Engl J Med 1995;333:1301-1307. b. Circulation 1998; 97:1440-1445.
Disease	Hypercholesterolemia, coronary artery disease.
Purpose	a. To assess whether pravastatin therapy reduces the incidence of acute myocardial infarction and mortality from coronary heart disease in hypercholesterolemic men without a history of prior myocardial infarction. b. To determine the extent to which reduction of LDL influenced coronary heart disease risk reduction in the WOSCOPS.
Design	a. Randomized, double-blind, placebo-controlled, multicenter. b. Relationship between baseline lipid levels and rates of cardiovascular events; relationships between on-treatment lipid concentrations and risk reduction in patients taking pravastatin were examined by Cox regression models and division of cohorts into quintiles.
Patients	6595 men, 45-64 years of age, with fasting LDL cholesterol >252 mg per deciliter before diet and >155 mg per deciliter after 4 weeks of diet. None of the patients had a history of prior myocardial infarction. 78% of the patients were ex- or current smokers and 5% had angina pectoris.
Follow-up	a. The average follow-up was 4.9 years (32,216 subject years of follow-up). b. 5 years.

Regimen	Pravastatin (40 mg/d) or placebo.

Results	a. Compared to baseline values pravastatin reduced plasma total cholesterol levels by 20% and LDL cholesterol by 26%, whereas no such changes were observed in the placebo treated group. Pravastatin reduced coronary events by 31% (95% CI=17-43%; p<0.001). There were 174 (5.5%) and 248 (7.9%) coronary events in the pravastatin and control group, respectively. Pravastatin reduced the risk for nonfatal infarction by 31% (4.6% vs 6.5%; p<0.001; 95% CI=15-45%), and the risk for death from all cardiovascular causes by 32% (1.6 vs 2.3%; p=0.033; 95% CI=3-53%). There was no increase in mortality from noncardiovascular causes. b. Baseline LDL cholesterol was only a weak predictor of cardiac risk in both treated and untreated groups. The reduction in risk of a cardiac event by pravastatin was similar across all quintiles of baseline LDL levels. Baseline HDL showed a strong negative association with cardiovascular event rate, but reduction in risk with pravastatin was similar for all quintiles of HDL elevation. The fall in LDL level in the pravastatin group did not correlate with the reduction in risk of a cardiac event on multivariate regression. The maximum benefit of about a 45% risk reduction was observed in the middle quintile of LDL reduction, representing a 24% fall in LDL. Further decreases in LDL, up to 39%, did not result in further reduction in coronary heart disease risk reduction. When event rates between placebo and pravastatin treated subjects with the same LDL cholesterol level were compared, there was evidence for an LDL independent treatment benefit of pravastatin that remains to be determined.

Concl.	a. Primary prevention in moderately hypercholesterolemic men with 5 years Pravastatin therapy

WOSCOPS (Substudy)

West of Scotland Coronary Prevention Study

Title	Pravastatin and the development of diabetes mellitus. Evidence for a protective treatment effect in the West of Scotland Coronary Prevention Study.
Authors	Freeman DJ, Norrie J, Sattar N, et al.
Reference	Circulation 2001;103:357-362.
Disease	Hyperlipidemia, diabetes.
Purpose	To determine from the WOSCOPS database the effects of pravastatin therapy on risk of developing diabetes.
Design	As per WOSCOPS.
Patients	5974 of 6595 randomized subjects (excluded were subjects who reported diabetes at baseline or had baseline glucose levels of ≥7.0 mmol/L) and 139 of these subjects who became diabetic during the study.
Follow-up	3.5-6.1 years.
Regimen	As per WOSCOPS.
Add'l Tx	As per WOSCOPS.

Results   Of 5974 patients without diabetes at baseline, 139 developed it
            (defined by American Diabetes Association definition of diabetes
            mellitus-fasting blood glucose level of ≥7.0 mmol/L). Univariate
            predictors of developing diabetes mellitus included body mass
            index, HDL cholesterol, log triglycerides, total cholesterol, log
            WBC, baseline glucose and systolic blood pressure; and pravas-
            tatin treatment influenced the development of diabetes (hazard
            ratio=0.70; 95% CI=0.50-0.98; p=0.036). Multivariate Cox
            model predictor of diabetes showed baseline body mass index,
            log triglycerides and baseline glucose to be significant predictors
            as well as pravastatin treatment (multivariate hazard ratio of 0.70
            [95% CI=0.50-0.99; p=0.42]). It was estimated that pravastatin
            therapy resulted in a 30% reduction (p=0.042) in the hazard
            of developing diabetes during the study. Potential explanations
            included lowering plasma triglycerides, anti-inflammatory prop-
            erties, and beneficial endothelial effects.

Concl.   Pravastatin lowered the risk of developing diabetes in the
            WOSCOPS.

Ezetimibe Plus Simvastatin vs Simvastatin

Title	Treatment of high-risk patients with ezetimibe plus simvastatin co-administration vs simvastatin alone to attain National Cholesterol Education Program Adult Treatment Panel III low-density lipoprotein cholesterol goals.
Authors	Feldman T, Koren M, Insull W, et al.
Reference	Am J Cardiol 2004;93:1481-1486.
Disease	Hyperlipidemia.
Purpose	To compare the efficacy of ezetimibe + simvastatin and simvastatin alone to reach Adult Treatment Panel III low-density lipoprotein cholesterol goal (<100 mg/dL) in high-risk patients with hypercholesterolemia.
Design	Randomized, parallel-group, placebo-controlled, multicenter.
Patients	710 patients, 18-80 years old with coronary heart disease or coronary heart disease risk equivalent according to the Adult Treatment Panel III guidelines, low-density lipoprotein cholesterol ≥130 mg/dL and triglyceride ≤350 mg/dL. Pregnant women, or those likely to become pregnant, were not included. Patients with elevated liver enzymes or creatine kinase were excluded.
Follow-up	23 weeks.
Regimen	After a run-in 4 week placebo and diet, patients were randomized to: 1) simvastatin 20 mg/d (n=253); 2) ezetimibe 10 mg/d and simvastatin 10 mg/d (n=251); 3) ezetimibe 10 mg/d and simvastatin 20 mg/d (n=109); and 4) ezetimibe 10 mg/d and simvastatin 40 mg/d (n=97). Treatment was continued for 6 weeks and then the simvastatin dose was doubled every 6 weeks up to a maximum of 80 mg/d in patients whose low-density lipoprotein cholesterol was still ≥100 mg/dL. In patients in whom low-density lipoprotein cholesterol was <50 mg/dL in 2 consecutive tests, the simvastatin dose was halved. The ezetimibe treatment was blinded.

Results	616 patients (86.8%) completed the study. 94 patients (13.2%) discontinued the study because of adverse events (5.6%), lost to follow-up (1.7%), withdrawal of consent (3.5%), deviation from protocol (0.6%), and other (1.8%). The primary end point of the study (achieving LDL cholesterol <100 mg/dL) after 5 weeks of treatment was achieved by 46% of the patients in the simvastatin alone group and by 75%, 83%, and 87% in the ezetimibe + simvastatin 10, 20, and 40 mg/d (p<0.001 for each group vs simvastatin alone). Mean plasma LDL cholesterol was reduced by 38%±0.8% in the simvastatin-alone group, and by 47%±0.8%, 53%±1.2%, and 59%±1.3% in the 3 combination groups, respectively (p<0.001 for each group vs simvastatin alone). Total cholesterol was reduced by 27%±0.7% in the simvastatin alone, and by 33%±0.6%, 38%±0.9%, and 42%±1.0% in the 3 combination groups (p<0.001 for each group vs simvastatin alone). HDL cholesterol increased by 5.1%±0.7% in the simvastatin-alone group and by 6.2%±0.7%, 8.0%±1.0%, and 7.4%±1.1% in the 3 combination groups, respectively. Triglycerides were reduced by 19%±1.9% in the simvastatin alone group and by 19%±1.5%, 25%±2.7%, and 30%±2.6% in the 3 combination groups, respectively (p=NS, p<0.05, and p<0.001 vs simvastatin alone, respectively). At the end of the follow-up, more patients in the combination groups (78%, 83%, and 86%, respectively) reached their target LDL cholesterol than in the simvastatin-alone group (59%) (p<0.001 for each combination group vs the simvastatin-alone group). Treatment-related adverse events were noted in 7.5% of the patients in the simvastatin-alone and in 9.6%, 14%, and 10% in the 3 combination groups. Creatine kinase ≥10 × the upper limit of normal was noted in 0.8% of the patients in the simvastatin alone group and in 0, 0, and 1.0% in the combination groups, respectively. Increase in the alanine aminotransferase and/or aspartate aminotransferase ≥3 × the upper limit of normal was noted in 0, 0.4%, 0, and 1.0% of the patients, respectively.
Concl.	More patients reached their Adult Treatment Panel III LDL cholesterol goal when treated with a combination of ezetimibe + simvastatin than with simvastatin alone. The combination was safe and well tolerated.

Title	Efficacy and safety of ezetimibe co-administered with simvastatin compared with atorvastatin in adults with hypercholesterolemia.
Authors	Ballantyne CM, Blazing MA, King TR, et al.
Reference	Am J Cardiol 2004;93:1487-1494.
Disease	Hyperlipidemia.
Purpose	To compare the efficacy of atorvastatin and simvastatin + ezetimibe in lowering low-density lipoprotein cholesterol.
Design	Randomized, double-blind, active-controlled, multicenter.
Patients	788 patients, ≥18 years old, with a low-density lipoprotein cholesterol level ≥ the Adult Treatment Panel III threshold for initiation of treatment and with either: 1) established coronary artery disease or risk equivalent; 2) ≥2 risk factors and 10-year risk of >20% for coronary artery disease and LDL cholesterol ≥130 mg/dL; 3) no coronary heart disease and with ≥2 risk factors and 10-year risk of <20% and LDL cholesterol of ≥160 mg/dL; or 4) No coronary artery disease and <2 risk factors and LDL cholesterol ≥190 mg/dL. Patients with triglyceride levels >350 mg/dL were excluded. Patients with serum creatinine >1.5 mg/dL, active liver disease or elevated liver enzymes, creatine kinase ≥1.5 × the upper limit of normal, and hemoglobin A1c ≥9% were excluded.
Follow-up	28 weeks.
Regimen	After 4 week run-in phase of placebo and diet patients were randomized to: 1) atorvastatin (initial dose 10 mg/d, titrated to 20, 40, and 80 mg/d) (n=262); 2) ezetimibe 10 mg/d with simvastatin (initial dose 10 mg/d, titrated to 20, 40, and 80 mg/d) (n=263); and 3) ezetimibe 10 mg/d with simvastatin (initial dose 20 mg/d, titrated to 40, and to 80 mg/d) (n=263) for 24 weeks.

Add'l Tx	Fibrate therapy was discontinued at least 9 weeks before randomization. All lipid-lowering agents were discontinued 7 weeks before randomization.
Results	After the first 6 weeks of therapy-total cholesterol decreased by 28.1%±0.6% in the atorvastatin 10 mg/d, 33.9%±0.6% in the ezetimibe + simvastatin 10 mg/d (p≤0.05 vs atorvastatin), and 36.2%±0.6% in the ezetimibe + simvastatin 20 mg/d (p≤0.05 vs atorvastatin). LDL cholesterol was decreased by 37.2%±0.8%, 46.1%±0.8% (p≤0.05 vs atorvastatin), and 50.3%±0.8% (p≤0.05 vs atorvastatin), respectively. HDL cholesterol increased by 5.1%±0.8%, 8.0%±0.8% (p≤0.05 vs atorvastatin), 9.5%±0.8% (p≤0.05 vs atorvastatin), respectively. Triglycerides were decreased by 22.5%±1.8%, 26.3%±1.5% (p=NS vs atorvastatin), and 24.6%±2.0% (p=NS vs atorvastatin). Mean percent decrease in LDL cholesterol from baseline continued to be significantly greater in the ezetimibe + simvastatin groups than in the atorvastatin group when the medication doses were up titrated. At the end of the 24-week period, LDL cholesterol was reduced by 52.5%±1.0% in the atorvastatin 80 mg/d and by 59.4%±0.7% in the ezetimibe + simvastatin 80 mg/d (p<0.001). After 24 weeks HDL cholesterol increased by 6.5%±1.0% with atorvastatin 80 mg/d and by 12.3%±0.7% in the ezetimibe + simvastatin 80 mg/d (p<0.001). Clinical adverse events occurred at similar rates in all 3 groups. Drug-related adverse events occurred in 16.0% in the atorvastatin group and in 16.0% and 13.7% in the 2 combination groups. Increase in alanine aminotransferase ≥3 × the upper limit of normal occurred in 2.4%, 2.3%, and 2.0% of the patients, respectively. Increase in aspartate aminotransferase ≥3 × the upper limit of normal occurred in 0.8%, 1.2%, and 0% of the patients, respectively. Increase in creatine kinase ≥10 × the upper limit of normal occurred in 0, 0.4%, and 0.4% of the patients, respectively.
Concl.	A combination of simvastatin and ezetimibe decreased LDL cholesterol and increased HDL cholesterol more than atorvastatin alone. Both treatments were safe and well tolerated.

8

Rosuvastatin vs Atorvastatin in Heterozygous Familial Hypercholesterolemia

Title	Comparison of rosuvastatin vs atorvastatin in patients with heterozygous familial hypercholesterolemia.
Authors	Stein EA, Strutt K, Southworth H, et al.
Reference	Am J Cardiol 2003;92:1287-1293.
Disease	Hyperlipidemia, familial hypercholesterolemia.
Purpose	To compare the efficacy of high-dose atorvastatin and rosuvastatin to reduce low-density lipoprotein cholesterol in patients with heterozygous familial hypercholesterolemia.
Design	Randomized, double-blind, parallel-group, force-titration, multicenter.
Patients	623 patients with heterozygous familial hypercholesterolemia (documented low-density lipoprotein receptor gene defect or low-density lipoprotein cholesterol >190 mg/dL and/or total cholesterol >290 mg/dL and one of the following: 1) tendon xanthoma in the patient or close relative; 2) familial hypercholesterolemia in a close relative; 3) low-density lipoprotein cholesterol >190 mg/dL or total cholesterol >290 mg/dL in a close relative; or 4) a history of myocardial infarction at <55 years old in a close relative). Patients with hepatic disorder, active arterial disease in the preceding 3 months, uncontrolled hypertension, uncontrolled hypothyroidism, creatine kinase elevation >3× the upper limit of normal, renal insufficiency, use of cyclic hormonal therapy and use of medications that may affect serum lipid levels were excluded.
Follow-up	18 weeks.
Regimen	After a 6-week run-in drug wash-out phase, patients were randomized to rosuvastatin (n=436) or atorvastatin (n=187). The starting dose was 20 mg/d for 6 weeks, then the dose was increased to 40 mg/d for 6 weeks and then to 80 mg/d for 6 weeks.
Add'l Tx	National Cholesterol Education Program step I diet.

Results	After 6 weeks LDL cholesterol was reduced by 47.1%±0.8% with rosuvastatin 20 mg/d and by 38.0%±1.0% with atorvastatin 20 mg/d (-9.1% difference; 95% CI=-11.0 to -7.2; p<0.001). After 12 weeks, LDL cholesterol was reduced by 53.9%±0.8% in the rosuvastatin 40 mg/d and by 46.0%±1.1% in the atorvastatin 40 mg/d (-7.9% difference; 95% CI=-9.9 to -5.8; p<0.001). After 18 weeks LDL cholesterol was reduced by 57.9%±0.9% with rosuvastatin 80 mg/d and by 50.4%±1.2% with atorvastatin 80 mg/d (-7.5% difference; 95% CI=-9.8 to -5.1; p<0.001). After 18 weeks total cholesterol was reduced by 46.4%±0.8% with rosuvastatin 80 mg/d and by 42.1%±1.0% with atorvastatin 80 mg/d (p<0.001). Rosuvastatin 80 mg/d increased HDL cholesterol by 12.4%, whereas atorvastatin 80 mg/d by 2.9%±1.3% (p<0.001). Triglycerides were decreased by 27.8%±1.5% and by 31.6%±2.0% with rosuvastatin and atorvastatin 80 mg/d (p=NS). After 18 weeks of therapy, 58% of the patients in the rosuvastatin vs 44% in the atorvastatin reached their NCEP Adult Treatment Panel III LDL cholesterol goal (p<0.001). Both drugs reduced serum highly-sensitive C-reactive protein without difference between the groups. Both drugs were well tolerated. 4% of the patients in the rosuvastatin vs 3% in the atorvastatin group had adverse events that led to discontinuation of the study drug. >3 × the upper limit of normal increase in alanine aminotransferase was detected in <1% of the patients in both groups. >10 × the upper limit of normal increase in creatine kinase was not detected in both groups.
Concl.	Rosuvastatin was more effective than atorvastatin in reducing total cholesterol and LDL cholesterol and in increasing HDL cholesterol. Both drugs were safe and well tolerated.

8

ALERT

Assessment of Lescol in Renal Transplantation

Title	Effect of fluvastatin on cardiac outcomes in renal transplant recipients: a multicentre, randomised, placebo-controlled trial.
Authors	Holdaas H, Fellstrom B, Jardine AG, et al.
Reference	Lancet 2003;361:2024-2031.
Disease	Renal disease.
Purpose	To investigate the effects of fluvastatin on cardiac and renal events in renal transplant recipients.
Design	Multicenter, randomized, double-blind, placebo-controlled trial.
Patients	2102 renal transplant recipients with total cholesterol 4.0-9.0 mmol/L (155-348 mg/dL).
Follow-up	Mean 5.1 years, range 5-6 years.
Regimen	Fluvastatin 40 mg/d or placebo.
Add'l Tx	Cyclosporine for all patients; 81% received steroids and 95% cardiovascular drugs.

Results   Fluvastatin lowered mean LDL by 32% (95% CI=-33 to -30). Mean total cholesterol and mean triglyceride levels decreased significantly in the fluvastatin group vs placebo; HDL cholesterol did not differ. Two thirds of the patients in the fluvastatin group achieved a total cholesterol concentration <5 mmol/L (<193 mg/dL) and three fourths achieved an LDL cholesterol <3 mmol/L (<116 mg/dL). The primary end point was the occurrence of a major adverse cardiac event (MACE) (cardiac death, nonfatal MI, coronary intervention procedure). The reduction in MACE with fluvastatin was 17%, but this was not statistically significant vs placebo (p=0.139; risk ratio 0.83; 95% CI=0.64-1.06). Analysis of the secondary end points (individual cardiac events, combined cardiac death or nonfatal MI, cerebrovascular events, noncardiovascular death, all-cause mortality, graft loss, doubling of serum creatinine) was limited by the lack of a significant reduction in the primary end point. However, there was a 35% reduction in cardiac death and nonfatal MI with fluvastatin, a finding consistent with those of other statins.

Concl.   About half of renal transplant recipients are treated with statins, reflecting a widespread acceptance of data from other patient populations. However, fluvastatin did not generally reduce rates of coronary intervention procedures or mortality. The overall effects of fluvastatin were similar to those of statins in other populations.

ARBITER

Arterial Biology for the Investigation of the Treatment Effects of Reducing Cholesterol

Title	ARBITER: arterial biology for the investigation of the treatment effects of reducing cholesterol: a randomized trial comparing the effects of atorvastatin and pravastatin on carotid intima medial thickness.
Authors	Taylor AJ, Kent SM, Flaherty PJ, et al.
Reference	Circulation 2002;106:2055-2060.
Disease	Hypercholesterolemia.
Purpose	To compare the effect of pravastatin vs atorvastatin on carotid intima-media thickness (a surrogate cardiovascular end point).
Design	Single-center, randomized, open-label.
Patients	161 patients with known cardiovascular disease that met National Cholesterol Education Programs II criteria for lipid lowering.
Follow-up	12 months.
Regimen	Atorvastatin 80 mg/d (n=79) vs pravastatin 40 mg/d (n=82). Ultrasound studies of the carotid artery were performed at baseline, 6 months, and 12 months after randomization. Carotid intimal-medial thickness was read in a blinded fashion.

| Results | Mean baseline LDL cholesterol was 152±34 mg/dL. Mean carotid intimal thickening at baseline was 0.627±0.189 mm. At 12 months, LDL in the atorvastatin group was reduced by 48.5% to 76±23 mg/dL vs a 27.2% decrease (to 110±30 mg/dL) in the pravastatin group (p<0.001). C-reactive protein was reduced to a greater degree at 12 months in the atorvastatin group. At 12 months C-reactive protein was 0.21 mg/dL in the atorvastatin group vs 0.36 in the pravastatin group (p<0.005). Mean carotid intima-media thickness progressively decreased in patients taking atorvastatin. At baseline it was 0.625±0.188 mm; at 6 months it was 0.608±0.159, and at 12 months it was 0.591±0.145 in the atorvastatin group. In contrast, in the pravastatin group baseline intimal-media carotid artery thickness was 0.615±0.145, at 6 months it was 0.599±0.150 and at 12 months it was 0.640±0.150. Thus atorvastatin was associated with a progressive decrease or regression in the carotid intima-media thickness over 12 months of -0.034±0.021 mm, whereas this value was unchanged in the pravastatin group (0.025±0.017 mm; p=0.03 between groups). Carotid intima-media thickness regression at 6 months occurred in 38.6% of pravastatin patients vs 54.4% of atorvastatin patients (p=0.062). No patients developed liver enzyme elevations greater than 3 × the upper limit of normal. No patients developed myositis. 3 patients in each group had a cardiovascular event during the course of the study. |

| Concl. | Marked LDL lowering with atorvastatin was superior to moderate LDL lowering with pravastatin for regression of carotid artery intima-media thickness. |

HPS

Heart Protection Study (Simvastatin)

Title	MRC/BHF Heart Protection Study of cholesterol lowering with simvastatin in 20,536 high-risk individuals: a randomized placebo-controlled trial.
Authors	Heart Protection Study Collaborative Group.
Reference	Lancet 2002;360:7-22.
Disease	Atherosclerosis.
Purpose	To evaluate whether simvastatin will reduce morbidity and mortality in a large cohort of patients at substantial risk of death.
Design	Randomized, double-blind, 2 × 2 factorial, placebo-controlled, multicenter.
Patients	20,536 patients, 40-80 years old, with a history of coronary artery disease, peripheral vascular disease, stroke, diabetes, or hypertension and low-to-average total or low-density lipoprotein cholesterol (≥3.5 mmol/L [135 mg/dL]). Patients in whom statin therapy was considered indicated by their physicians were not included. Patients with chronic liver disease, creatinine >200 μmol/L, severe renal disease, inflammatory muscle disease, creatine kinase >750 IU/L, cyclosporine, fibrates, on niacin therapy, women with childbearing potential, severe heart failure, severe chronic lung disease, or other life-threatening disease were excluded.
Follow-up	5 years.
Regimen	After a run-in period of placebo treatment for 4 weeks and 4-6 weeks of fixed dose of simvastatin 40 mg/d, patients were randomized to either simvastatin (40 mg/d) (n=10,269) or placebo (n=10,267) and to vitamins (vitamin E 600 mg, vitamin C 250 mg, and β-carotene 20 mg) or placebo.
Add'l Tx	A nonstudy statin treatment was encouraged if the patient's physician thought it was indicated.

Results   Of the 63,603 patients screened, 32,145 patients were enrolled for the run-in phase and 20,536 patients were further randomized. In the simvastatin-allocated group, 85% of the patients were taking study or nonstudy statins at the end of the follow-up, whereas 32% of the patients allocated to placebo were receiving nonstudy statins. At the end of 5 years, the mean±standard error of the difference between the simvastatin and placebo groups was -1.2±0.02 mmol/L for total cholesterol, -1.0±0.02 mmol/L for LDL cholesterol, 0.03±0.01 mmol/L for HDL cholesterol, and -0.3±0.03 mmol/L for triglycerides. The absolute difference in LDL cholesterol between the simvastatin and placebo groups was -0.9, -1.0, and -1.0 mmol/L for patients with baseline LDL cholesterol <3.0, 3.0-3.5, and ≥3.5 mmol/L, respectively. Total mortality was 12.9% in the simvastatin group and 14.7% in the placebo group (rate ratio 0.87; 95% CI=0.81-0.94; p=0.0003), vascular mortality was 7.6% and 9.1%, respectively (rate ratio 0.83; 95% CI=0.75-0.91; p<0.0001), and nonvascular mortality 5.3% and 5.6%, respectively (rate ratio 0.95; 95% CI=0.85-1.07; p=0.4). Coronary mortality was 5.7% in the simvastatin group and 6.9% in the placebo group (p=0.0005). Stroke occurred in 4.3% of the patients in the simvastatin group vs 5.7% in the placebo (rate ratio 0.75; 95% CI=0.66-0.85; p<0.0001). Major coronary events occurred in 8.7% in the simvastatin group and 11.8% in the placebo group (rate ratio 0.73; 95% CI=0.67-0.79; p<0.001). Major vascular events occurred in 19.8% of the patients in the simvastatin group and in 25.2% in the placebo group (rate ratio 0.76; 95% CI=0.72-0.81; p<0.0001). A total of 5.0% vs 7.1% of the patients in the simvastatin and placebo groups, respectively, underwent coronary revascularization (p<0.0001), and 4.4% vs 5.2% underwent noncoronary revascularization (p=0.006). The benefit of simvastatin was irrespective of age, gender, and baseline total cholesterol or LDL cholesterol levels. The benefit of simvastatin was apparent even among the 6793 patients with baseline LDL cholesterol <3.0 mmol/L (major vascular events occurred in 17.6% and 22.2% of the patients in the simvastatin and placebo group, respectively; p<0.0001). There were no significant side effects. A significant elevation (>4 × upper limit of normal [ULN]) in alanine aminotransferase was detected in 0.42% of the patients in the simvastatin group vs 0.31% in the placebo group. Creatine kinase elevation 4-10 × ULN was detected in 0.19% and 0.13% of the patients, respectively, and >10 × ULN in 0.11% and 0.06% of the patients, respectively. Rhabdomyolysis was detected in 0.05% of the patients in the simvastatin group and 0.03% in the placebo group.

Concl.   Simvastatin 40 mg/d was safe and effective in reducing the incidence of death, MI, stroke, and revascularization in a wide range of high-risk patients, regardless of total or LDL cholesterol levels at baseline, age, or gender.

HPS

MRC/BHF Heart Protection Study of Cholesterol Lowering in Patients with Diabetes

Title	MRC/BHF Heart Protection Study of cholesterol-lowering with simvastatin in 5963 people with diabetes: a randomised placebo-controlled trial.
Authors	Heart Protection Study Collaborative Group.
Reference	Lancet 2003;361:2005-2016.
Disease	Diabetes, hypercholesterolemia.
Purpose	To determine the effects on vascular mortality and morbidity of intensive low-density lipoprotein cholesterol lowering over several years in persons with diabetes.
Design	Multicenter, double-blind, placebo-controlled trial.
Patients	5963 adults known to have diabetes and 14,573 with occlusive arterial disease but no diagnosed diabetes.
Follow-up	5 years.
Regimen	Simvastatin 40 mg/d or matching placebo.

8

Results   In study participants receiving simvastatin, both those with and those without diabetes, the first event rate for major coronary events, strokes, and revascularization was reduced by ≈25%. For the first occurrence of these major vascular events in patients with diabetes, there was a definite 22% reduction in the event rates (601 simvastatin-treated patients [20.2%] vs 748 placebo-treated patients [25.1%]) (p<0.0001; 95% CI=13%-30%), a rate similar to that for the nondiabetic high-risk patients. Among the 2912 diabetic patients who did not have diagnosed arterial disease at entry, the event rate was reduced by approximately one-third (p=0.0003; 95% CI=17%-46%). Among the 2426 diabetic patients whose pretreatment LDL-cholesterol level was below 116 mg/dL, the rate of events was reduced by 27% (p=0.0007; 95% CI=13%-40%). Risk was also reduced by about 25% in various subcategories of diabetic patients, among them those with different duration, type, or control of diabetes; those older than 65 years at entry; those with hypertension; and those with total cholesterol below 193 mg/dL.

Concl.   Lipid-modifying therapy may be beneficial in patients with diabetes, whether or not they have manifest coronary disease or dyslipidemia. Simvastatin therapy reduced the rate of first major vascular event by approximately one fourth in a wide range of diabetic patients. Statin therapy should be considered routinely for diabetic patients, irrespective of their initial cholesterol concentrations.

HPS Substudy

Heart Protection Study-Substudy

Title	Effects of cholesterol-lowering with simvastatin on stroke and other major vascular events in 20,536 people with cerebrovascular disease or other high-risk conditions.
Authors	Heart Protection Study Collaborative Group.
Reference	Lancet 2004;363:757-767.
Disease	Hyperlipidemia; atherosclerosis.
Purpose	To assess the efficacy of simvastatin on stroke rates in patients at high risk for vascular disease.
Design	Randomized, double-blind, placebo-controlled, 2 × 2 factorial, multicenter.
Patients	20,536 patients, 40-80 years old, with nonfasting total cholesterol of 135 mg/dL and history of cerebrovascular disease, coronary artery disease, peripheral arterial disease, diabetes mellitus or treated hypertension (if 65 years old). Patients with clear indications or contraindication to statins were excluded. Patients with stroke; myocardial infarction; or hospitalization for angina in the preceding 6 months; chronic liver disease; severe renal disease; muscle problems; treatment with cyclosporin, fibrates, or high-dose niacin were not included. In addition, patients with severe heart failure, nonvascular life-threatening conditions and women with childbearing potential were not included.
Follow-up	Mean 4.8 years for patients with established cerebrovascular disease and 5.0 years for the high-risk subgroup.
Regimen	All patients were subjected to a 4-week run-in phase with placebo treatment followed by 4-6 week phase of simvastatin 40 mg/d. Compliant patients were randomized to simvastatin 40 mg/d or placebo (and to antioxidant vitamins or placebo).
Add'l Tx	Nonstudy statin therapy was encouraged in patients with clinical indications.

Results   Overall, 3280 patients with cerebrovascular disease and 17,256 patients at high-risk but without established cerebrovascular disease were enrolled. Among patients randomized to simvastatin, 85% received statins, and among the patients randomized to placebo, 17% took nonstudy statins. Among patients with established cerebrovascular disease at enrollment there was 20% (95% CI=8%-29%; p=0.001) reduction in the incidence of major vascular events (coronary death, MI, stroke, or revascularization). Among the high-risk group, there was a 25% (95% CI=20%-30%; p<0.0001) reduction in major vascular events. Among the 1820 patients who had cerebrovascular disease but not CAD at enrollment, there was 23% (95% CI=6%-37%; p=0.01) reduction in major vascular events. Among patients with cerebrovascular disease, major coronary events occurred in 10.4% of the simvastatin and 13.3% in the placebo group. Among patients without prior cerebrovascular disease, such events occurred in 8.4% and 11.5% of the patients, respectively. Among patients with cerebrovascular disease, stroke occurred in 10.3% in the simvastatin and in 10.4% in the placebo group. Among patients without prior cerebrovascular disease, stroke occurred in 3.2% and 4.8% of the patients, respectively. Simvastatin reduced the revascularization rate in both the patients with (8.2% vs 11.7%) and without (9.3% vs 11.7%) cerebrovascular disease. Overall, simvastatin decreased the rate of coronary revascularization by 30% (95% CI=22%-38%; p<0.0001) and the rate of non-coronary revascularization by 16% (95% CI=5%-26%; p=0.006). Simvastatin reduced the rate of carotid endarterectomy or stenting (0.4% vs 0.8%; p=0.0003). Among patients with cerebrovascular disease, carotid endarterectomy or stenting was performed in 1.0% of the simvastatin-allocated patients vs 2.3% in the placebo-allocated patients (p=0.002). Simvastatin reduced the rate of ischemic stroke by 30% (2.8% vs 4.0%; p<0.0001). Simvastatin did not affect the rates of hemorrhagic stroke (0.5% vs 0.5%; p=0.8). The reduction in stroke was not significant during the first year of treatment, but became significant at the end of the second year (p=0.0004). Simvastatin was beneficial in all subgroups studied, including males and females, patients with and without diabetes, patients <65 years and >70 years, and in those with baseline LDL cholesterol levels of <3.0 mmol/L, 3.0-3.5 mmol/L, and ≥3.5mmol/L. The rate of stroke among patients with baseline LDL cholesterol ≥100 mg/dL was 4.4% in the simvastatin group vs 5.8% in the placebo group. Among those with LDL cholesterol <100 mg/dL the rates were 4.0% and 5.4%, respectively (p=0.9 for the interaction).

Concl.   Statins reduce the rate of ischemic strokes, without an effect on the incidence of hemorrhagic strokes. This protective effect was apparent in all ranges of baseline cholesterol levels. Although simvastatin did not reduce the rate of stroke among patients with preexisting cerebrovascular disease, it was beneficial in reduction of major coronary events and revascularizations in these patients, including the subgroup without known CAD.

LIPS-Substudy

Lescol Intervention Prevention Study-Substudy

Title	Effect of fluvastatin on long-term outcome after coronary revascularization with stent implantation.
Authors	Saia F, de Feyter P, Serruys PW, et al.
Reference	Am J Cardiol 2004;93:92-95.
Disease	Hyperlipidemia, coronary artery disease, percutaneous coronary intervention.
Purpose	To investigate if fluvastatin reduces major adverse cardiac events in patients who have undergone coronary stenting.
Design	A substudy of the Lescol Intervention Prevention Study (LIPS).
Patients	847 patients (50.5% of the total study group of LIPS), 18-80 years old, who underwent stent implantation during the index percutaneous coronary intervention. Only patients in whom all treated coronary lesions received stents were included. Baseline total cholesterol was 135-270 mg/dL and triglycerides <400 mg/dL. Patients with previous percutaneous coronary intervention or coronary artery bypass graft, blood pressure >180/100 mm Hg, left ventricular ejection fraction <30%, severe noncoronary heart disease, serum creatinine >1.8 mg/dL, body mass index >30 kg/m^2, and significant noncardiac systemic disease were excluded.
Follow-up	4 years.
Regimen	Randomized to fluvastatin 40 mg bid (n=417) or placebo (n=430) at hospital discharge (after successful percutaneous coronary intervention).
Add'l Tx	The decision regarding revascularization technique and stenting were done by the interventional cardiologist.

Results	After 6 weeks of therapy total cholesterol was decreased by 15.1% in the fluvastatin group and increased by 11.5% in the placebo group. LDL cholesterol decreased by 24.1% with fluvastatin and increased by 12.0% with placebo. There were no significant changes in the HDL cholesterol or triglyceride levels in both groups. Fluvastatin decreased the risk of first adverse cardiac event (16.3% vs 21.6%; relative risk [RR] 0.75; 95% CI=49%-3.4%; p=0.03). Mortality was 1.9% in the placebo group and 1.2% in the fluvastatin group (p=0.41). Q-wave MI occurred in 2.6% and 1.9% of the placebo and fluvastatin groups, respectively (p=0.49). There was no difference in the incidence of non-Q wave MI (1.7% vs 1.6%; p=1.00). 15.4% of the patients in the placebo group vs 11.6% in the fluvastatin group underwent revascularization (p=0.13). 7.9% vs 8.1% underwent target lesion revascularization (p=1.00), and 7.4% vs 3.5% underwent non-target vessel revascularization (RR 0.47; 95% CI=0.26-0.86; p=0.01).
Concl.	Long-term administration of fluvastatin 40 mg bid after successful coronary stenting reduced the risk of first adverse cardiac events by 30% compared with placebo in patients with average cholesterol levels. The difference was mainly due to reduction of non-target vessel revascularization rate, although there was a trend toward reduction of Q-wave MI and death rates.

PROVE IT-TIMI 22

*Pravastatin and Atorvastatin Evaluation and Infection
Therapy-Thrombolysis in Myocardial Infarction 22*

Title	Intensive vs moderate lipid lowering with statins after acute coronary syndromes.
Authors	Cannon CP, Braunwald E, McCabe CH, et al.
Reference	N Engl J Med 2004;350:1495-1504.
Disease	Acute myocardial infarction, unstable angina.
Purpose	To compare a regimen of moderate lipid lowering (low-density lipoprotein cholesterol approximately 100 mg/dL using pravastatin 40 mg/d with more intensive low-density lipoprotein cholesterol lowering [approximately 70 mg/dL with atorvastatin 80 mg/d]) as a means of preventing death or major cardiovascular events in patients with acute coronary syndrome.
Design	Multicenter, international, double-blind, double-dummy, randomized trial.
Patients	4162 patients at 349 sites who had been hospitalized for an acute coronary syndrome (acute myocardial infarction or high-risk unstable angina) within the preceding 10 days. Total cholesterol levels were ≤240 mg/dL; patients on long-term lipid-lowering therapy at the time of their acute event had to have a total cholesterol of ≤200 mg/dL at the time of screening.
Follow-up	18-36 months (mean 24 months).
Regimen	Pravastatin 40 mg/d (moderate lipid-lowering regimen) or atorvastatin 80 mg/d (aggressive lipid-lowering regimen).
Add'l Tx	Aspirin 75-325 mg/d, with or without clopidogrel or warfarin (standard therapy for acute coronary syndromes). Patients were also randomly assigned to receive a 10-day course of gatifloxacin or placebo every month during the trials (results not reported here).

Results	The median LDL cholesterol level achieved with pravastatin treatment was 95 mg/dL, vs 62 mg/dL with atorvastatin (p<0.001). The primary end point was death from any cause, MI, documented unstable angina requiring rehospitalization, or revascularization with coronary angioplasty or CABG, and stroke. Kaplan-Meier estimates of the rates of the primary end point at 2 years were 26.3% in the pravastatin group and 22.4% in the atorvastatin group, reflecting a 16% reduction in the hazard ratio in favor of atorvastatin (p=0.005; 95% CI=5%-26%). Among individual components of the primary end point, there was a 14% reduction in need for revascularization (p=0.04), a 29% reduction in the risk of recurrent unstable angina (p=0.02), and NS reductions in the rates of death from any cause (28%; p=0.07) and death or MI (18%; p=0.06). Strokes were infrequent and did not differ significantly between the groups. The risk of the secondary end point of death due to coronary heart disease, MI, or revascularization was reduced by 14% in the atorvastatin group (p=0.029); the 2-year event rate was 19.7% vs 22.3% in the pravastatin group. The risk of death, MI, or urgent revascularization was reduced by 25% in the atorvastatin group. Rates of discontinuation of treatment because of an adverse event or the patients' preference or for other reasons were similar in the 2 groups; 21.4% in the pravastatin group and 22.8% in the atorvastatin group at 1 year (p=0.3) and 33% and 30.4%, respectively, at 2 years (p=0.11). During treatment, the dose of pravastatin was halved among 1.4% of patients in the pravastatin group and 1.9% in the atorvastatin group (p=0.20) because of side effects or liver function abnormalities. Elevations of alanine aminotransferase levels >3× the upper limit of normal were higher in the atorvastatin group, 3.3%, vs 1.1% in the pravastatin group (p<0.001). Study treatment was discontinued because of a report of myalgias or muscle aches or creatine kinase elevations in 2.7% of pravastatin-treated patients vs 3.3% of atorvastatin-treated patients (p=0.23). No cases of rhabdomyolysis were reported in either group.
Concl.	In patients who have had an acute coronary syndrome, the intensive lipid-lowering regimen with In patients who have had an acute coronary syndrome. the intensive lipid-lowering regimen with atorvastatin provides greater protection against death or major cardiovascular events compared with the more conventional regimen. These patients benefit from early and continued lowering of LDL-C to levels well below current target levels recommended by the National Cholesterol Education Program.

REVERSAL

Reversal of Atherosclerosis with Aggressive Lipid Lowering

Title	Effect of intensive compared with moderate lipid-lowering therapy on progression of coronary atherosclerosis: a randomized controlled trial.
Authors	Nissen SE, Tuzcu EM, Schoenhagen P, et al.
Reference	JAMA 2004;291:1071-1080.
Disease	Coronary atherosclerosis.
Purpose	To determine whether aggressive lipid lowering therapy with atorvastatin is more effective than moderate lipid lowering with pravastatin in reducing progression of coronary atherosclerosis (as measured by intravascular ultrasound).
Design	Double-blind, randomized, active-control, multicenter trial.
Patients	654 patients aged 30-75 years with coronary atherosclerosis (at least 1 obstruction with angiographic luminal narrowing of ≥20%); 502 patients had evaluable intravascular ultrasound studies at baseline and at 18 months.
Follow-up	18 months.
Regimen	Patients were randomly assigned to pravastatin 40 mg/d (moderate lipid lowering) or atorvastatin 80 mg/d (aggressive lipid lowering).

Results	The baseline LDL cholesterol level in both groups was 150.2 mg/dL. LDL cholesterol was reduced to 110 mg/dL in patients receiving pravastatin and to 79 mg in the atorvastatin group (p<0.001). The progression rate was significantly lower in the atorvastatin group (p=0.02). Coronary atherosclerosis (change in atheroma volume) progressed in the pravastatin group (2.7%; 95% CI=0.2%-4.7%; p=0.001) vs baseline. Atherosclerosis did not progress in the atorvastatin group (-0.4%; CI=-2.4% to 1.5%) vs baseline (p=0.98). C-reactive protein decreased 5.2% with pravastatin and 36.4% with atorvastatin (p<0.001). Similar differences between groups were seen for secondary efficacy parameters, including change in total atheroma volume (p=0.02), change (%) in atheroma volume (p<0.001), and change in atheroma volume in the most severely diseased 10-mm vessel subsegment (p<0.01).
Concl.	For secondary prevention, intensive lipid-lowering therapy with 80 mg of atorvastatin in patients with moderate cholesterol elevations halted progression of atherosclerosis, whereas more moderate lipid-lowering therapy with 40 mg of pravastatin was associated with significant disease progression. The differences could be related to greater reduction in atherogenic lipoproteins and C-reactive protein in atorvastatin-treated patients.

STELLAR

Statin Therapies for Elevated Lipid Levels Compared Across Doses to Rosuvastatin

Title	Comparison of the efficacy and safety of rosuvastatin vs atorvastatin, simvastatin, and pravastatin across doses (STELLAR Trial).
Authors	Jones PH, Davidson MH, Stein EA, et al.
Reference	Am J Cardiol 2003;92:152-160.
Disease	Hyperlipidemia.
Purpose	To compare the efficacy of rosuvastatin, atorvastatin, simvastatin, and pravastatin in reducing low-density lipoprotein cholesterol.
Design	Randomized, open-label, parallel group, multicenter.
Patients	2431 men and nonpregnant women, ≥18 years old, with low-density lipoprotein cholesterol 160-250 mg/dL and triglycerides <400 mg/dL. Patients with intolerance to statins, serious or unstable psychological or medical conditions, heterozygous or homozygous familial hypercholesterolemia, history of drug or alcohol abuse, increase in creatine kinase or liver function tests were excluded.
Follow-up	6 weeks.
Regimen	After a 6-week dietary lead-in phase, compliant patients were randomized to: 1) rosuvastatin 10, 20, 40, or 80 mg/d; 2) atorvastatin 10, 20, 40, or 80 mg/d; 3) simvastatin 10, 20, 40, or 80 mg/d; and 4) pravastatin 10, 20, or 40 mg/d.

Results	Drug compliance was comparable among the groups, ranging from 90.5% to 95.3%. 94% of the patients completed the study. Among the patients randomized to rosuvastatin, atorvastatin, simvastatin, and pravastatin 10 mg/d, LDL cholesterol was decreased by 45.8%, 36.8%, 28.3%, and 20.1%, respectively (p<0.001 for each group vs rosuvastatin 10 mg/d). Among those randomized to 20 mg/d, LDL cholesterol was reduced by 52.4%, 42.6%, 35.0%, and 24.4%, respectively (p<0.001 for each group vs rosuvastatin 20 mg/d). Among those randomized to 40 mg/d, LDL cholesterol was reduced by 55.0%, 47.8%, 38.8%, and 29.7%, respectively (p<0.001 for each group vs rosuvastatin 40 mg). Among those randomized to 80 mg/d, LDL cholesterol decreased by 51.1% in the atorvastatin group and by 45.8% in the simvastatin group. Data on the rosuvastatin 80 mg/d is not provided, despite the fact that 146 patients in this group completed the protocol. At each dose, rosuvastatin reduced LDL cholesterol more than the other 3 drugs. The best LDL cholesterol reduction was seen with the rosuvastatin 40 mg/d group. HDL cholesterol increased by 7.7%, 9.5%, and 9.6% in the rosuvastatin 10, 20, and 40 mg/d groups. Again, data on rosuvastatin 80 mg/d are not provided. HDL cholesterol increased by 5.7%, 4.8%, 4.4%, and 2.1% in the atorvastatin 10, 20, 40, and 80 mg/d groups, respectively. HDL cholesterol increased by 5.3%, 6.0%, 5.2%, and 6.8% in the simvastatin 10, 20, 40, and 80 mg/d groups, respectively. HDL cholesterol increased by 3.2%, 4.4%, and 5.6% in the pravastatin 10, 20, and 40 mg/d groups, respectively. Thus, rosuvastatin resulted in a greater increase in HDL cholesterol than the other 3 agents. At each dose, rosuvastatin reduced total cholesterol more (p<0.001) than the other 3 agents. Adult Treatment Panel III LDL cholesterol goals were reached by 82%-89% of the rosuvastatin 10-40 mg/d patients, and by 69%-85% of the atorvastatin 10-80 mg/d patients. Drug tolerability was comparable among the 4 drugs.
Concl.	Rosuvastatin was more effective than atorvastatin, simvastatin, and pravastatin (at equivalent doses) in reducing LDL cholesterol and achieving Adult Treatment Panel III LDL cholesterol goals.

9. Arrhythmia

Oral d,l Sotalol Reduces the Incidence of Postoperative Atrial Fibrillation in Coronary Artery Bypass Surgery Patients: A Randomized, Double-Blind, Placebo-Controlled Study

Title	Oral d,l sotalol reduces the incidence of postoperative atrial fibrillation in coronary artery bypass surgery patients: a randomized, double-blind, placebo-controlled study.
Authors	Gomes JA, Ip J, Santoni-Rugiu F, et al.
Reference	J Am Coll Cardiol 1999;34:334-339.
Disease	Atrial fibrillation.
Purpose	To determine the efficacy of preoperative and postoperative oral d, l sotalol in preventing the occurrence of postoperative atrial fibrillation.
Design	Randomized, double-blind, placebo-controlled, 2 center study.
Patients	85 patients (73 to undergo CABG; 12 CABG plus valvular surgery). Ejection fraction had to be ≥28% and no clinical evidence of heart failure.
Follow-up	Hospital stay (≈7-8 days).
Regimen	Placebo (n=45) or sotalol (n=40; mean dose=190±43 mg/d) given 24-48 hours prior to surgery and continued for up to 4 days postoperatively. Sotalol was given as 80 mg orally twice daily and advanced to a dose of 120 mg orally twice daily if there was no bradycardia, CHF or QTc >500 msec. Study medicine was stopped if QTc was >500 msec, or if significant bradycardia with hypotension occurred.

Add'l Tx	Dose of β-blockers was halfed in those patients on ≥200 mg/d of metoprolol or its equivalent.
Results	The end point was occurrence of atrial fibrillation lasting ≥30 minutes or for any length of time requiring intervention secondary to symptoms of atrial fibrillation. 38% of patients in the placebo group developed atrial fibrillation vs 12.5% in the sotalol group (p=0.008). Drug was withdrawn for clinically significant bradycardia/hypotension in none of the placebo group and 5% of the sotalol patients (p=0.2). No patients that received sotalol developed torsade de pointes or sustained ventrical arrhythmias. QTc was prolonged on sotalol (458±38 msec) vs before sotalol (419±29 msec; p=0.0001). There was 1 death in the placebo group and none in the sotalol group. There was a nonsignificant trend toward shorter length of stay in the sotalol group (7 vs 8 days).
Concl.	Sotalol reduced the frequency of postoperative atrial fibrillation in patients undergoing CABG who did not have heart failure or significant LV dysfunction.

Efficacy and Safety of Ibutilide Fumarate for the Conversion of Atrial Arrhythmias After Cardiac Surgery

Title	Efficacy and safety of ibutilide fumarate for the conversion of atrial arrhythmias after cardiac surgery.
Authors	VanderLugt JT, Mattioni T, Denker S, et al.
Reference	Circulation 1999;100:369-375.
Disease	Atrial fibrillation, atrial flutter.
Purpose	To assess the efficacy and safety of ibutilide fumarate for rapid conversion of atrial fibrillation and flutter shortly after cardiac surgery.
Design	Randomized, double-blind, placebo-controlled, dose response, multicenter.
Patients	302 patients, ≥18 years old, <300 lbs body weight, hemodynamically stable, with atrial fibrillation (n=201) or flutter (n=101), 1 hour to 3 days in duration that had occurred 1-7 days after cardiac surgery. All patients were in normal sinus rhythm at the time of surgery with a corrected QT ≤440 ms. Patients with a history of torsade de pointes arrhythmia, a heart rate <60 bpm, myocardial infarction within 30 days, thyrotoxicosis, severe liver impairment, an electrolyte abnormality, recent treatment with antiarrhythmic agents or vasopressor drugs, and those who had been exposed to ibutilide were excluded.
Follow-up	72 hours.
Regimen	Patients were randomized to intravenous infusion of placebo or 0.25, 0.5, or 1.0 mg of ibutilide fumarate over 10 minutes. If the arrhythmia did not terminate within 10 minutes, an identical second dose was administered. The infusion was stopped after the arrhythmia terminated or if there was a fall in systolic blood pressure (<90 mm Hg), an increase in QTc (>600 ms), or the development of ventricular arrhythmia.

Add'l Tx	Other antiarrhythmic agents were not permitted within 4 hours after study drug failure and within 24 hours in cases who converted to sinus rhythm. Electrical cardioversion was permitted >90 minutes after treatment failure or in patients with recurrence of atrial arrhythmia after successful cardioversion by the study drug.
Results	The conversion to sinus rates within 90 minutes was 15% with placebo and 40%, 47%, and 57% with ibutilide 0.25 mg, 0.5 mg, and 1.0 mg, respectively ($p=0.0001$). The conversion rates were 20%, 28%, 42%, and 44% with placebo and 0.25, 0.5, and 1.0 mg ibutilide, respectively for patients with atrial fibrillation ($p=0.0055$) and 4%, 56%, 61%, and 78%, respectively, for patients with atrial flutter ($p=0.0001$). Mean time to cardioversion was 36 minutes for the 0.25 mg dose, 33 minutes for the 0.5 mg dose and 23 minutes for the 1.0 mg dose. Of the 104 patients successfully converted to sinus rhythm with ibutilide, 63% remained in sinus rhythm for 24 hours. 8 out of the 13 patients (62%) who converted spontaneously with placebo remained in sinus rhythm for 24 hours. Ibutilide 0.5 and 1.0 mg caused prolongation of the QTc. Ventricular arrhythmia was noted in 8.3% of the 218 patients randomized to ibutilide vs 1.2% of the 84 patients randomized to placebo. Nonsustained monomorphic ventricular tachycardia was noted in 3.2% and 0, respectively, nonsustained polymorphic ventricular tachycardia in 1.4% and 1.2%, respectively, and sustained polymorphic ventricular tachycardia in 0.9% and 0%, of the patients, respectively. There were no deaths, strokes, or myocardial infarctions.
Concl.	Ibutilide was safe and effective, when used in a carefully supervised clinical setting, for cardioversion of atrial fibrillation, and especially atrial flutter, in patients after a recent cardiac surgery.

Effective Prevention of Atrial Fibrillation by Continuous Atrial Overdrive Pacing After Coronary Artery Bypass Surgery

Title	Effective prevention of atrial fibrillation by continuous atrial overdrive pacing after coronary artery bypass surgery.
Authors	Blommaert D, Gonzalez M, Mucumbitsi J, et al.
Reference	J Am Coll Cardiol 2000;35:1411-1415.
Disease	Atrial fibrillation—after coronary artery bypass grafting.
Purpose	To determine the efficacy of an algorithm with continuous atrial dynamic overdrive pacing to prevent or reduce atrial fibrillation post CABG.
Design	Randomized, consecutive patients
Patients	96 consecutive patients undergoing CABG for severe, symptomatic coronary artery disease. Patients had to be in sinus rhythm without antiarrhythmic drugs and stable on second day following surgery.
Follow-up	In-hospital.
Regimen	2 sets of epicardial wire electrodes placed on the right ventricle and high right atrium in all patients. External pacemaker was connected to the atrial wires for 24 hours continuous atrial pacing with a lower rate of 80 bpm in an AAI pacing mode. The algorithm for dynamic overdrive was programmed to allow pacing above the patient's own rate. Patients were randomized to atrial stimulation vs no stimulation.
Add'l Tx	If necessary, atrial fibrillation was treated with antiarrhythmic drugs, usually an infusion of amiodarone.

Results	Primary end point was occurrence on 24 hour Holter ECG of an episode of atrial fibrillation when sustained for at least 15 minutes. 5 of 48 (10%) of patients in the paced group developed atrial fibrillation vs 13 of 48 (27%) in the control, nonpaced group. Duration of atrial fibrillation was 120 minutes (median) in paced and 378 minutes in nonpaced group. Mean heart rates were greater in the paced groups at 93 ± 11 bpm vs unpaced groups at 87 ± 11 bpm, as expected. A multivariate analysis revealed that atrial fibrillation increased with age. Atrial fibrillation decreased with a better left ventricular ejection fraction in patients undergoing atrial pacing. Atrial pacing was more effective when left ventricular ejection fraction was >50%.
Concl.	Continuous atrial pacing with an alogrithm for dynamic overdrive decreases atrial fibrillation after coronary artery bypass surgery.

Atrial Pacing for the Prevention of Atrial Fibrillation After Cardiovascular Surgery

Title	Atrial pacing for the prevention of atrial fibrillation after cardiovascular surgery.
Authors	Greenberg MD, Katz NM, Iuliano S, et al.
Reference	J Am Coll Cardiol 2000;34:1416-1422.
Disease	Atrial fibrillation (postoperative).
Purpose	To assess the efficacy of atrial pacing for prevention of atrial fibrillation after cardiovascular surgery.
Design	Randomized, single-center.
Patients	154 patients undergoing cardiac surgery (CABG: 88.3%; aortic valve replacement: 4.5%; both: 7.1%). Right and left atrial epicardial pacing electrodes placed at time of surgery.
Follow-up	In-hospital.
Regimen	Patients randomly assigned to no postoperative pacing: right atrial pacing, left atrial pacing, or bi-atrial pacing. Pacing rate varied from 100-110 bpm depending on the native heart rate.
Add'l Tx	Postoperative β-blockers were started in all patients without contraindications.
Results	Primary end point was atrial fibrillation lasting longer than 1 hour in duration or causing hemodynamic compromise requiring electrical or chemical cardioversion. Patients assigned to 1 of the 3 pacing strategies had a lower incidence of postoperative atrial fibrillation (17%) compared to patients that were not assigned to pacing (37.5%; p<0.005). The incidence of atrial fibrillation was 8% with right atrial pacing, 20% with left atrial pacing, and 26% with bi-atrial pacing vs patients that did not receive pacing (37.5%; p=0.002 for right atrial vs no pacing; p=NS for other pacing groups individually vs no pacing). Length of hospital stay was reduced by 22% in patients who received pacing (6.1±2.3 days) vs those that did not (7.8±3.7 days; p=0.003).

Concl.   Postoperative atrial pacing in the setting of postoperative β-blockade significantly decreased the incidence of atrial fibrillation and length of hospital stay. Right atrial pacing appeared to be the most beneficial but additional studies are needed to assess the most effective site for pacing.

Prevention of Implantable-Defibrillator Shocks by Treatment with Sotalol

Title	Prevention of implantable defibrillator or shocks by treatment with sotalol.
Authors	Pacifico A, Hohnloser SH, Williams JH, et al.
Reference	N Engl J Med 1999;340:1855-1862.
Disease	Sudden cardiac death, ventricular tachyarrhythmias.
Purpose	To assess the efficacy and safety of sotalol, an agent with Class III antiarrhythmic and β-blocking properties for prevention of appropriate and inappropriate shocks delivered to patients who had implantable cardioverter defibrillators.
Design	Double-blind, placebo-controlled, parallel group, randomized, multicenter.
Patients	302 patients with histories of life threatening ventricular arrhythmias who had received an implantable cardioverter defibrillator within 3 months of enrollment, and had undergone successful defibrillation at the time of implantation.
Follow-up	12 months.
Regimen	Patients were randomized to placebo (n=151) or 160-320 mg of sotalol per day (n=151); patients were stratified by LV ejection fraction (≤0.30 or >0.30).
Add'l Tx	Treatment with β-blockers, calcium blockers, and digoxin was allowed; other antiarrhythmic drugs were not allowed.

Results	Overall, 4 patients in the sotalol group died (2 of heart failure; 2 of noncardiac cause); 7 patients in the placebo group died (3 were cardiac). The primary end point was death from any cause or delivery of a first shock. End points were also analyzed regarding whether the first shock was appropriate (those delivered for ventricular tachycardia or fibrillation being deemed appropriate; those delivered for supraventricular arrhythmias or other events were deemed inappropriate). A secondary end point was frequency of shocks due to any cause. Treatment with sotalol resulted in a lower risk of death from any cause or delivery of a first shock for any reason (reduction in risk=48%; p<0.001); lower risk of death from any cause or delivery of a first appropriate shock (reduction in risk=44%; p=0.007). Sotalol also resulted in a lower rate of death from any cause or delivery of a first inappropriate shock (reduction in risk=64%; p=0.004). The mean of frequency of delivered shocks from any cause was reduced in the sotalol group (1.43 per year) vs the placebo group (3.89 per year). In the sotalol group, reduction in risk of death or delivery of first shock did not differ between those with higher vs lower ejection fractions.
Concl.	Sotalol was safe and effective in decreasing the risk of death or delivery of a first shock in patients with implantable defibrillators.

Facilitating Transthoracic Cardioversion of Atrial Fibrillation with Ibutilide Pretreatment

Title	Facilitating transthoracic cardioversion of atrial fibrillation with ibutilide pretreatment.
Authors	Oral H, Souza JJ, Michaud GF, et al.
Reference	N Engl J Med 1999;340:1849-1854.
Disease	Atrial fibrillation.
Purpose	To determine the effect of ibutilide on energy requirements for atrial defibrillation; to assess the ability of ibutilide to cardiovert patients with atrial fibrillation who are resistant to electrical transthoracic cardioversion.
Design	Randomized, single-center study.
Patients	100 patients referred for cardioversion for atrial fibrillation of at least 6 hours duration.
Follow-up	6 months.
Regimen	50 patients randomized to electrical transthoracic cardioversion with no ibutilide pretreatment; 50 assigned to undergo transthoracic cardioversion with ibutilide pretreatment. Ibutilide given as 1 mg infused over a 10 minute period. Cardioversion was performed with a step up protocol of 50, 100, 200, 300, and 360 J.
Add'l Tx	Patients on antiarrhythmic drug therapy at the time of cardioversion, continued on drug therapy after restoration of sinus rhythm. Anticoagulant therapy for 1 month post cardioversion in patients in atrial fibrillation for >48 hours.

Results	Cardioversion was successful in 36 (72%) of patients randomized to transthoracic cardioversion with no ibutilide. Of 50 patients in the ibutilide group, 10 (20%) cardioverted chemically. In the 40 remaining patients (80%), all cardioverted following transthoracic cardioversion. Overall efficacy of transthoracic electrical cardioversion was higher with ibutilide (100%) vs without the drug pretreatment (72%; $p<0.001$). Ibutilide pretreatment reduced the mean energy needed for defibrillation (166±80 J with ibutilide vs 228±93 J without ibutilide; $p<0.001$). Mean corrected QT interval was increased by ibutilide (482±49 msec vs 432±37 msec; $p<0.001$). In 2 of 64 patients that received ibutilide, both of whom had LV ejection fraction of ≤ 0.20, sustained polymorphic ventricular tachycardia occurred. There was no difference in the rate of freedom from recurrent atrial fibrillation at 6 months between the groups (57% in the no ibutilide group vs 64% who received ibutilide; $p=NS$).
Concl.	Pretreatment with ibutilide enhanced the efficacy of transthoracic electrical cardioversion for patients with atrial fibrillation. Ibutilide should be avoided in patients with very low left ventricular ejection fractions.

French Active Compression-Decompression Cardiopulmonary Resuscitation Study

Title	A comparison of standard cardiopulmonary resuscitation and active compression-decompression resuscitation for out-of-hospital cardiac arrest.
Authors	Plaisance P, Lurie KG, Vicaut E, et al.
Reference	N Engl J Med 1999;341:569-575.
Disease	Cardiac arrest.
Purpose	To evaluate the 1 year survival of patients undergoing active compression-decompression method of cardiopulmonary resuscitation.
Design	Randomized, multicenter.
Patients	750 patients who had cardiac arrest out-of-hospital; >80% had asystole.
Follow-up	1 year.
Regimen	Active compression-decompression resuscitation consisted of a hand held suction device. Active chest wall decompression reduces intrathoracic pressure, increasing venous blood return. Standard cardiopulmonary resuscitation (CPR, n=377); or active compression-decompression CPR (n=373), depending upon whether the arrest occurred on an even or odd day of the month.
Add'l Tx	Advanced life support, including epinephrine.

Results	The primary end point was 1 year survival; the secondary end point was survival to hospital discharge without neurologic impairment and neurologic outcome. 1-year survival rate was 5% in the active compression-decompression CPR group vs 2% in the standard CPR group (p=0.03). Rate of hospital discharge without neurologic impairment was 6% in the active compression-decompression CPR group vs 2% in the standard CPR group (p=0.01). In 12 of 17 survivors who had received active compression-decompression CPR, neurologic status at 1 year had returned to baseline vs 3 of 7 survivors that received the standard CPR (p=NS). 9 of 17 1-year survivors in the active compression-decompression CPR group and 2 of 7 in the standard CPR group had either asystole or cardiac electrical activity but no pulse. All of the survivors in both groups had a witnessed cardiac arrest.
Concl.	CPR using an active compression-decompression technique during advanced life support improved 1 year survival in patients with out-of-hospital cardiac arrest.

Cardiopulmonary Resuscitation by Chest Compression Alone or with Mouth-to-Mouth Ventilation

Title	Cardiopulmonary resuscitation by chest compression alone or with mouth-to-mouth ventilation.
Authors	Hallstrom A, Cobb L, Johnson E, Copass M.
Reference	N Engl J Med 2000;342:1546-1553.
Disease	Cardiac arrest.
Purpose	To compare cardiopulmonary resuscitation (CPR) with chest compression alone vs CPR with chest compression plus mouth to mouth ventilation.
Design	Randomized. Emergency medical services personnel blinded as much as possible.
Patients	520 patients with witnessed cardiac arrest.
Follow-up	Hospital discharge. Also follow-up of all survivors (enrollment began in 1992 and ended in 1998).
Regimen	Dispatcher instructed bystander CPR with chest compression alone vs dispatcher instructed chest compression plus mouth to mouth ventilation.
Results	64 patients survived to hospital discharge. 29/278 (10.4%) survived in the group receiving chest compression plus mouth to mouth ventilation vs 35/240 (14.6%) of patients who received chest compression only (p=0.18). 95/279 (34.1%) survived to hospital admission in the chest compression plus mouth to mouth ventilation group vs 97/241 (40.2%) in the chest compression alone group (p=0.15). Telephone instructions from dispatcher to bystander were completely delivered to 62% of episodes assigned to chest compression plus mouth to mouth ventilation vs 81% of episodes assigned to only chest compression (p=0.005).

Concl.   Hospitalization and survival to hospital discharge were similar among cardiac arrest victims who received bystander CPR with chest compression alone or with chest compression plus mouth to mouth ventilation.

Metoprolol CR/XL to Maintain Sinus Rhythm After Conversion From Atrial Fibrillation

Title	Use of metoprolol CR/XL to maintain sinus rhythm after conversion from persistent atrial fibrillation. A randomized, double-blind, placebo-controlled study.
Authors	Kuhlkamp V, Schirdewan A, Stangl K, et al.
Reference	J Am Coll Cardiol 2000;36:139-146.
Disease	Atrial fibrillation.
Purpose	To evaluate whether metoprolol CR/XL will reduce the risk of recurrence of atrial fibrillation after cardioversion.
Design	Randomized, double-blind, placebo-controlled, multicenter.
Patients	394 patients with persistent atrial fibrillation who were successfully converted to sinus rhythm either by class 1 antiarrhythmic drugs or by direct current. Patients with contraindications to β-blockers, sick sinus syndrome, chronic oral treatment with amiodarone, cardiac surgery within 2 months prior to randomization, concomitant therapy with β-blockers or antiarrhythmic drugs, and untreated thyroid dysfunction were excluded. Patients with paroxysmal atrial fibrillation were not included.
Follow-up	6 months.
Regimen	After cardioversion patients were randomized to metoprolol controlled release (CR/XL) 50-200 mg/d (n=197) or placebo (n=197).
Add'l Tx	All patients received anticoagulation before cardioversion and for ≥1 month after cardioversion. Class 1 or 3 antiarrhythmic drugs, β-blockers or calcium channel blockers were not permitted.

Results	Atrial fibrillation relapsed in 59.9% of the patients in the placebo group vs 48.7% in the metoprolol group (p=0.005). Among patients who were converted to sinus rhythm by direct current, 50.6% of the patients in the metoprolol group vs 65.0% of the patients in the placebo group relapsed (p=0.002). The median time to relapse was 13.0 days with metoprolol and 7.5 days with placebo (p=0.001). Mean heart rate of patients who had recurrence of atrial fibrillation or flutter was significantly lower in the metoprolol group (98±23 beats/min vs 107±27 bpm; p=0.015). Serious adverse events occurred in 20 patients in the metoprolol group vs 6 patients in the placebo group. However, the rate of adverse events reported was comparable between the groups when the difference in follow-up time was taken into account. 3 patients died, all in the metoprolol group. Bradycardia occurred in 7.1% of the patients in the metoprolol vs zero in the placebo group.
Concl.	Metoprolol CR/XL was effective in preventing recurrence of atrial fibrillation or flutter after cardioversion.

Title	Single-day loading dose of oral amiodarone for the prevention of new-onset atrial fibrillation after coronary artery bypass surgery.
Authors	Maras D, Boskovic SD, Popovic Z, et al.
Reference	Am Heart J 2001;141:E8.
Disease	Atrial fibrillation, coronary artery bypass grafting.
Purpose	To assess whether a single-day loading dose of oral amiodarone will prevent the occurrence of new onset atrial fibrillation during the first 7 days after CABG.
Design	Randomized, double-blind, single-center.
Patients	315 patients, >18 years old, who were referred for elective CABG surgery. Patients with a history of atrial fibrillation, uncontrolled thyroid dysfunction, elevated transaminases, bradycardia ($\leq$50 bpm), valvular heart disease requiring surgery, or congestive heart failure, and those receiving antiarrhythmic drugs or allergic to amiodarone were excluded.
Follow-up	7 days.
Regimen	Randomization to oral amiodarone (1200 mg) (n=159) or placebo (n=156) 1 day before surgery, and than 200 mg/d for 7 days.
Add'l Tx	If a patient had atrial fibrillation during the 7-day follow-up, therapy was directed to heart rate control with calcium channel blockers, digitalis or β-blockers and anticoagulation. Cardioversion or administration of other antiarrhythmic drugs were permitted only in patients with severe hemodynamic instability.

Results	New onset atrial fibrillation was detected in 19.5% of the patients in the amiodarone group and in 21.2% in the placebo group (p=0.78). Time to the first episode of atrial fibrillation was 3.4±2.0 days in the amiodarone group vs 3.1±1.4 days in the placebo group (p=0.52). The mean duration of atrial fibrillation was comparable (28.39±39.94 hours in the amiodarone group vs 21.09±29.06 hours in the placebo group; p=0.41). However, the ventricular response rate at the detection of atrial fibrillation was slower in the amiodarone group (102.6±10.3 bpm vs 128.4±16.2 bpm; p<0.001). Among patients who developed atrial fibrillation, hemodynamic compromise occurred in 48% and 54% of the patients in the amiodarone and placebo group, respectively (p=0.94). Among patients ≥60 years old, atrial fibrillation occurred in 26.7% of the patients in the amiodarone group vs 43.1% of the patients in the placebo group (p=0.05). The relative risk for the occurrence of atrial fibrillation in patients 50 years or older who received amiodarone was 0.62 (95% CI=0.39-0.99). Among patients younger than 60 years, atrial fibrillation occurred in 13.1% in the amiodarone group vs 5.6% in the placebo group (p=0.11). There were no differences between the amiodarone and placebo group regarding the rates of in-hospital morbidity and mortality and in the duration of hospitalization.
Concl.	A single-day loading dose of 1200 mg amiodarone did not prevent postoperative new onset atrial fibrillation in the general population of patients scheduled for elective CABG. However, among elderly patients, amiodarone may be effective in reducing the rate of postoperative atrial fibrillation.

Title	Tissue plasminogen activator in cardiac arrest with pulseless electrical activity.
Authors	Abu-Laban RB, Christenson JM, Inness GD, et al.
Reference	N Engl J Med 2002;346:1522-1528.
Disease	Cardiac arrest.
Purpose	To determine whether administration of tissue plasminogen activator (tPA) during cardiopulmonary resuscitation would improve outcome in patients with cardiac arrest.
Design	Randomized, double-blind, placebo-controlled.
Patients	1583 patients treated (233 enrolled) older than 16 years of age with more than 1 minute of pulseless electrical activity, not responsive to initial therapy outside the hospital or in the emergency ward.
Follow-up	Up to 1 year.
Regimen	Patients randomized to tPA (n=117) 100 mg over 15 minutes or placebo (n=116).
Add'l Tx	Heparin, aspirin to survivors at the discretion of the cardio-pulmonary resuscitation (CPR) leader. Other usual medicines given during CPR (including epinephrine, atropine, sodium bicarbonate, lidocaine).

Results   Primary outcome was survival to hospital discharge. Secondary outcomes included return of spontaneous circulation, length of hospital stay, hemorrhage, and neurologic outcome. 1 patient in the tPA group and zero in the placebo group survived to hospital discharge (p=NS). 21.4% in the tPA group and 23.3% in the placebo group had return of spontaneous circulation (p=NS). 62.4% of tPA patients and 63.8% of placebo patients died at the scene (p=NS). 1.7% in the tPA group and 0 in the placebo group had a major hemorrhage (p=NS). Mean length of hospital stay was 6.3 in the tPA group and 0.5 days in the placebo group.

Concl.   There was no benefit of tPA in patients with a cardiac arrest with pulseless electrical activity.

Hypothermia After Cardiac Arrest Study

Title	Mild therapeutic hypothermia to improve the neurologic outcome after cardiac arrest.
Authors	The Hypothermia After Cardiac Arrest Study Group.
Reference	N Engl J Med 2002;346:549-556.
Disease	Cardiac arrest due to ventricular fibrillation.
Purpose	To determine whether mild systemic hypothermia improves neurologic recovery following resuscitation from cardiac arrest due to ventricular fibrillation (VF).
Design	Blinded assessment of outcome, randomized, controlled, multi-center.
Patients	275 patients with restoration of spontaneous circulation following a witnessed cardiac arrest, VF or nonperfusing ventricular tachycardia, an estimated interval of 5-15 minutes from patient's collapse to first attempt at resuscitation and an interval of no more than 60 minutes from collapse to restoration of spontaneous circulation.
Follow-up	≈200 days.
Regimen	Patients randomized to hypothermia were cooled to a target temperature of 32-34 C with an external cooling device (mattress with a cover that delivers cold air over entire body). Ice packs used if needed. Cooling was maintained for 24 hours. Patients randomized to normothermia group were placed on conventional hospital bed.

Add'l Tx	Midazolam, fentanyl pancuronium to prevent shivering.
Results	Primary outcome was a favorable neurologic outcome at 6 months. The Pittsburgh cerebral-performance scale was used from 1 (good recovery), to 2 (moderate disability), 3 (severe disability), to 4 (vegetable state), and 5 (death). 75 of 136 (55%) patients in the hypothermia group had a favorable neurologic outcome (category 1 or 2) vs 54 of 137 (39%) in the normothermia group (risk ratio [RR] 1.40; 95% CI=1.08-1.81; p=0.009). 41% in the hypothermia group died vs 55% in the normothermic group (RR 0.74; 95% CI=0.58-0.95; p=0.02). Most patients with unfavorable neurologic outcomes died within 6 months after hospital discharge. Complication rates did not differ between groups.
Concl.	Therapeutic mild hypothermia improved favorable neurologic outcome and reduced mortality in patients successfully resuscitated following cardiac arrest due to VF.

Hypothermia in Cardiac Arrest

Title	Treatment of comatose survivors of out-of-hospital cardiac arrest with induced hypothermia.
Authors	Bernard SA, Gray TW, Buist MD, et al.
Reference	N Engl J Med 2002;346:557-563.
Disease	Cardiac arrest.
Purpose	To determine whether moderate induced hypothermia improves outcome in patients who remain unconscious after resuscitation from cardiac arrest.
Design	Prospective, controlled, multicenter.
Patients	77 patients with initial cardiac rhythm of ventricular fibrillation at time of arrival of ambulance, successful return of spontaneous circulation, but persistent coma.
Follow-up	Hospital discharge.
Regimen	Patients randomized to cooling (n=43) with extensive application of ice packs around the head, neck, torso, and limbs to reach a core temperature of 33°C. This temperature was maintained until 12 hours after hospital arrival. At 18 hours patients were actively rewarmed; or the patients were randomized to normothermia (n=34).
Add'l Tx	Midazolam, vecuronium (prevents shivering); thrombolytic therapy if ECG suggested myocardial infarction, IV heparin, lidocaine, potassium, insulin, aspirin.

Results	Primary outcome measure was survival to hospital discharge with neurologic function adequate enough to be discharged either home or to a rehabilitation facility. In this regard, 21 of 43 patients (49%) treated with hypothermia survived and had a good outcome vs 9 of 34 that received normothermia (26%; p=0.046). Adjusted (for age and time from collapse to return of spontaneous circulation) odds ratio for good outcome with hypothermia vs normothermia was 5.25 (95% CI=1.47-18.76; p=0.011). Death due to cardiac failure occurred in 5 of 22 patients who died in the hypothermia group and 4 of 23 in the normothermic group. 1 patient in each group was diagnosed as brain dead within 4 days. Remaining deaths resulted from severe neurologic injury between days 2-30. Overall mortality rate did not differ in hypothermia group (51%) vs normothermia group (68%; p=0.145). Cardiac index and systemic vascular resistance were higher in the hypothermia group.
Concl.	Moderate hypothermia improved outcome in patients with coma following resuscitation for cardiac arrest.

Delaying Defibrillation to Give Basic Cardiopulmonary Resuscitation to Patients with Out-of-Hospital Ventricular Fibrillation

Title	Delaying defibrillation to give basic cardiopulmonary resuscitation to patients with out-of-hospital ventricular fibrillation.
Authors	Wik L, Hansen TB, Fylling F, et al.
Reference	JAMA 2003;289:1389-1395.
Disease	Arrhythmia.
Purpose	To evaluate the administration of cardiopulmonary resuscitation before defibrillation on outcomes in patients who have ventricular fibrillation and a response time less than or longer than 5 minutes.
Design	Randomized, prospective.
Patients	200 patients, >18 years, with ventricular fibrillation or pulseless ventricular tachycardia, with cardiac arrest not witnessed by ambulance personnel.
Follow-up	1 year.
Regimen	Advanced cardiac life support was administered to all patients according to standard guidelines except for the duration of CPR, which was the investigated intervention. In the standard group, a 200 J shock was given immediately. If not successful, defibrillation was repeated at 200 J, and once more with 360 J if necessary. If no return of circulation was achieved, 1 minute of CPR was given for ventricular fibrillation/tachycardia or 3 minutes for nonventricular

fibrillation/tachycardia, followed by a new rhythm analysis, shock, and CPR as necessary. All patients received 100% oxygen and 1 mg epinephrine intravenously every 3 minutes until circulation was restored or until the resuscitation was terminated. In the CPR first group, the same procedure was followed, with the exception that CPR was given for 3 minutes before the first defibrillation, and if CPR was again necessary, it was given for 3 minutes. A 100 mg dose of lidocaine was given intravenously only after 9 defibrillation attempts. No other antiarrhythmic medications were given.

Results   The primary study end point was survival to hospital discharge. The secondary study outcome was return of spontaneous circulation (ROSC) and survival to the hospital, overall status determined by overall performance category (OPC) and neurological status as determined by cerebral performance category at discharge, and 1-year survival with neurological status. There were no significant differences between the 2 groups at baseline. There were 104 patients randomized to receive CPR first, and 96 randomized to receive standard treatment. Furthermore, there was no difference in the usage of epinephrine or lidocaine in the 2 groups. Overall, there was no difference between the 2 groups in survival rate to hospital discharge (CPR vs standard: 22% vs 15%, OR 1.66; 95% CI=0.80-3.46; p=0.20). There was also no difference in ROSC rates (56% vs 46%; p=0.16), and 1-year survival (20% vs 15%; p=0.30). In the 81 patients who had an ambulance response time of 5 minutes or less, there were no differences in ROSC, survival to hospital discharge, 1-year survival, or neurological outcome. However, in patients for whom the response time was longer than 5 minutes, there were more patients in the CPR group that had ROSC (58% vs 38%, OR 2.22 CI=1.06-4.63; p=0.04), survival to hospital discharge (22% vs 4%, OR 7.42 CI=1.61-34.3; p=0.006), and 1-year survival (20% vs 4%, OR 6.76 CI=1.42-31.4; p=0.01). The OR for survival in the CPR-before-defibrillation group increased from 0.4 (95% CI=0.08-1.80) for the less than 1-minute response group to 3.0 (95% CI=1.06-8.79) in the 7-minute response interval group and 6.1 (95% CI=1.34-27.80) in the 9-minute response interval group.

Concl.   There was no overall difference in survival in patients who had an out-of-hospital ventricular fibrillation when standard care and CPR first prior to defibrillation were compared. However, in patients who had longer response times (>5 minutes) there was a significant benefit in rates of hospital discharge and survival for those who were given CPR prior to defibrillation attempts.

AFFIRM

Atrial Fibrillation Follow-Up Investigation of Rhythm Management

Title	A comparison of rate control and rhythm control in patients with atrial fibrillation.
Authors	The Atrial Fibrillation Follow-up Investigation of Rhythm Management Investigators.
Reference	New Engl J Med 2002;347:1825-1833.
Disease	Atrial fibrillation.
Purpose	To determine the long-term effects of treatment of atrial fibrillation with a "rate-control" vs "rhythm-control" strategy.
Design	Randomized, multicenter.
Patients	4060 patients with atrial fibrillation who were at least 65 years of age or had other risk factors for stroke or death. Patients were eligible if investigators felt that the patient's atrial fibrillation was likely to recur, cause illness or death, if long-term treatment was appropriate, anticoagulant therapy was appropriate, the patient was able to undergo trials of at least 2 medications in either treatment strategy, and the patient could be started on treatment immediately after randomization.
Follow-up	Mean 3.5 years.

Regimen   Rhythm control group, n=2033. The choice of antiarrhythmic medication was left to the discretion of the treating physician. Cardioversion was used as necessary to maintain sinus rhythm. The medications acceptable for use were the following: amiodarone, disopyramide, flecainide, moricizine, procainamide, propafenone, quinidine, sotalol, dofetilide, and a combination of these. Rate control group, n=2027. The goal of this group was heart rate control. Acceptable medications were β-blockers, calcium channel blockers (verapamil and diltiazem), digoxin, and a combination of these. The target goal was heart rate less than 80 bpm at rest and less than 110 bpm during a 6-minute walk test. Patients who failed the standard treatment but had not yet failed at least 2 trials of either a rhythm-control or rate-control medication could be considered for nonpharmacologic therapy, such as radio-frequency ablation, a Maze procedure, and pacing, as allowed by their randomization strategy. Anticoagulation with warfarin was administered with a target INR of 2.0-3.0. Patients in the rhythm-control group had continuous anticoagulation that could be stopped if sinus rhythm was maintained between 4-12 consecutive weeks. Patients in the rate-control group had continuous mandatory anticoagulation.

Results	The primary end point was all-cause mortality. The secondary end point was a composite of death, severe stroke, disabling anoxic encephalopathy, major bleeding, and cardiac arrest. The 2 groups were balanced according to major characteristics at baseline. In the rate control group, the initial medication was a β-blocking drug in almost half of patients, and diltiazem was the most commonly used calcium channel blocker. Radiofrequency ablation to alter atrioventricular conduction was used in 5.2% of patients in this group after medication failure. 248 patients crossed over into the rhythm-control group during the study, and 86 of these patients had crossed back by the end of the study. In the rhythm-control group, most patients (>2/3) started with amiodarone or sotalol. 594 patients crossed over into the rate-control group, and 61 of these patients had crossed back by the end of the study. At the end of 5 years, there were 352 (24%) deaths in the rhythm-control group and 306 (21%) in the rate-control group. The primary end point, all-cause mortality, was similar between the 2 groups (hazard ratio [HR] 1.15; 95% CI=0.99-1.34; p=0.08). The secondary end point was also similar between the 2 groups (p=0.33). There were 77 and 80 patients who had ischemic strokes in the rate and rhythm-control groups, respectively. The numbers of patients with ischemic stroke, primary intracerebral hemorrhage, subdural or subarachnoid hemorrhage, or disabling anoxic encephalopathy were similar between both groups. Mini-Mental Status Examination scores and quality of life measurements were similar between the groups. The number of patients requiring hospitalization during the study was higher in the rhythm-control group vs the rate-control group (80.1% vs 73.0%; p<0.001). The rhythm-control group had a higher risk of death for patients who were older, did not have CHF, and had CAD. Torsade de pointes occurred rarely overall but more often in the rhythm-control group (12/2033 vs 2/2027; p=0.007).
Concl.	There is no survival advantage with the rhythm-control strategy for atrial fibrillation. The rate-control strategy has potential advantages such as decreased risk of adverse effects compare to the rhythm-control strategy. Anticoagulation therapy is needed in high-risk patients.

AFFIRM

Atrial Fibrillation Follow-Up Investigation of Rhythm Management

Title	The Atrial Fibrillation Follow-up Investigation of Rhythm Management (AFFIRM) study: approaches to control rate in atrial fibrillation.
Authors	Olshansky B, Rosenfeld LE, Warner AL, et al.
Reference	J Am Coll Cardiol 2004;43:1201-1208.
Disease	Arrhythmia.
Purpose	To evaluate approaches used to control rate, the effectiveness of rate control, and switches from 1 drug class to another in the AFFIRM study.
Design	Multicenter, randomized trial.
Patients	2027 patients randomly assigned to rate control in the AFFIRM study.
Follow-up	3.5±1.3 years.
Regimen	Rate-controlling drugs (β-blockers, calcium channel blockers, digoxin, alone or in combination).
Results	Initial treatment included a β-adrenergic blocker alone in 24% of patients, a calcium channel blocker alone in 17%, digoxin alone in 16%, a β-blocker and digoxin in 14% and a calcium channel blocker and digoxin in 14%. Overall rate control was achieved in 70% of patients who received β-blockers as the first drug, with or without digoxin; in 54% who received calcium channel blockers, with or without digoxin; and in 58% who received digoxin alone. In 58% of patients, adequate rate control was achieved with the first drug or combination. By multivariate analysis, there was an association between first drug class and several clinical variables. There were more changes to β-blocker therapy than to the other 2 drug therapies.
Concl.	Rate control can be achieved in the majority of patients with atrial fibrillation. β-blockers are the most effective agents. Frequent medication changes may be required to achieve adequate rate control.

AFFIRM Substudy

Atrial Fibrillation Follow-Up Investigation of Rhythm Management

Title	Maintenance of sinus rhythm in patients with atrial fibrillation: an AFFIRM substudy of the first antiarrhythmic drug.
Authors	AFFIRM First Antiarrhythmic Drug Substudy Investigators.
Reference	J Am Coll Cardiol 2003;42:20-29.
Disease	Arrhythmia.
Purpose	To compare the ability of different antiarrhythmic drugs to maintain sinus rhythm at 1 year.
Design	Multicenter, randomized substudy of AFFRIM, a study assessing rate control vs rhythm control for treatment of atrial fibrillation.
Patients	410 patients assigned to the rhythm control arm of AFFIRM.
Follow-up	1 year.
Regimen	Amiodarone, sotalol, or a class I or IC drug (quinidine, procainamide, disopyramide, moricizine, propafenone, flecainide).

Results	The primary end point was the proportion of patients alive, in sinus rhythm, with no additional cardioversions and still taking the assigned drug at 1 year. At 1 year, among 222 patients randomly assigned to amiodarone or a class I agent, 62% of patients were successfully treated with amiodarone vs 23% taking class I agents (p<0.001). Among 256 patients randomly assigned to amiodarone or sotalol, 60% vs 38% were successfully treated (p=0.002). In 183 patients randomly assigned to sotalol or class I agents, 34% vs 23% were successfully treated (p=0.488); however, this portion of the substudy was stopped early when amiodarone was shown to be better than class I agents. Nearly 80% of patients were in sinus rhythm at 1 year with serial therapy, regardless of initial therapy. By 1 year 29% of patients randomly assigned to amiodarone, 33% to sotalol, and 36% to class I agents had required cardioversion. There was only 1 case of torsades de pointes (in a patient taking quinidine for >1 year). Adverse effects leading to discontinuation of antiarrhythmic agents were common, occurring in 12.3% of patients taking amiodarone, 11.1% taking sotalol, and 28.1% taking class I agents.
Concl.	Amiodarone was more effective at 1 year than either sotalol or class I agents for the strategy of maintaining sinus rhythm without cardioversion. This substudy should be viewed in the context of the main AFFIRM results, which support rate control as an acceptable primary treatment.

AFIST

Atrial Fibrillation Suppression Trial

Title	Oral amiodarone for prevention of atrial fibrillation after open heart surgery, the Atrial Fibrillation Suppression Trial (AFIST): a randomized placebo-controlled trial.
Authors	Giri S, White CM, Dunn AB, et al.
Reference	Lancet 2001;357:830-836.
Disease	Atrial fibrillation, heart surgery.
Purpose	To evaluate the efficacy of oral amiodarone in preventing atrial fibrillation in patients ≥60 years of age undergoing open-heart surgery and already receiving β-blockers.
Design	Randomized, double-blind, placebo-controlled, single-center.
Patients	220 patients, ≥60 years old, candidates for elective heart surgery with systolic blood pressure >90 mm Hg, normal sinus rhythm, and corrected QT interval ≤440 ms. Patients with chronic atrial fibrillation, recent myocardial infarction, heart rate <45 beats per minute, advanced atrioventricular block, an automatic implantable cardioverter/ defibrillator, a history of amiodarone toxicity, untreated thyroid disease, liver function disturbances, treatment with cimetidine, phenytoin, cyclosporin, or class I and III antiarrhythmic drugs were excluded.
Follow-up	3-6 weeks after hospital discharge.
Regimen	Patients were randomized to placebo or amiodarone administered in a slow load (200 mg tid for 5 days before surgery and than 400 mg bid on postoperative days 1-4) or rapid load (400 mg X4/d for 1 day, 600 mg X2/d on the day of surgery and than 400 mg bid on postoperative days 1-4).
Add'l Tx	β-blockers were recommended unless contraindicated (89% of the patients received β-blockers preoperatively).

Results	Atrial fibrillation occurred in 38% of the patients in the placebo group (n=100) and in 23% of the patients in the amiodarone group (n=120) (15.5% difference; 95% CI=3.40-27.6%; p=0.01). Symptomatic atrial fibrillation occurred in 18% and 4% in the placebo and amiodarone groups, respectively (13.8% difference; 95% CI=5.5-22.2%; p=0.001). Amiodarone treatment prolonged the time to first episode of atrial fibrillation (3.37±2.5 days vs 2.68±1.3; p=0.009) and reduced the mean duration of fibrillation (8.7±20.2 hours vs 22.6±33.2 hours; p=0.0001). 3% of the patients in the amiodarone group vs 8% of the patients in the placebo group had atrial fibrillation at discharge (p=0.12). 7% of the patients in the placebo group vs 2% of the patients in the amiodarone group had a stroke (p=0.04), and 7% vs 2%, respectively had ventricular tachycardia (p=0.04). The effect of amiodarone on the prevention of atrial fibrillation was less obvious in patients with heart failure, those under 70 years of age, those receiving β-blockers, those with prior atrial fibrillation and in those with enlarged left atrium. Using a stepwise logistic regression model, it was found that amiodarone treatment was independently associated with reduced risk for atrial fibrillation (OR 0.39; 95% CI=0.18-0.88; p=0.023). Atrial fibrillation occurred in 19% and 70% of the patients in the placebo group who received or did not receive β-blockers (p=0.001), and in 16% vs 35% of the patients in the amiodarone group, respectively (p=0.02). 30-day mortality was comparable between the placebo and amiodarone groups (4% vs 3%; p=0.79). Length of stay was similar. The total costs accrued were U.S. $16,126 for the placebo group vs U.S. $15,574 for the amiodarone group (p=0.13).
Concl.	Oral amiodarone prophylaxis added to β-blockers therapy was safe and effective in preventing postoperative atrial fibrillation and reduced the risk of stroke and ventricular tachycardia.

AIRCRAFT

Australian Intervention Randomized Control of Rate in Atrial Fibrillation Trial

Title	The Australian intervention randomized control of rate in atrial fibrillation trial.
Authors	Weerasooriya R, Davis M, Powell A.
Reference	J Am Coll Cardiol 2003;41;1697-1702.
Disease	Atrial fibrillation.
Purpose	To compare atrioventricular junction ablation and pacing (AVJAP) to pharmacologic ventricular rate control in patients with permanent atrial fibrillation.
Design	Randomized, prospective, multicenter.
Patients	99 patients with symptomatic permanent atrial fibrillation (>12 months or with failed cardioversion or medical therapy), uncontrolled ventricular rate in which good rate control could be achieved by pharmacologic therapy.
Follow-up	12 months.
Regimen	Patients were randomized to pharmacologic therapy (n=50) for rate control of atrial fibrillation (digoxin, metoprolol, atenolol, verapamil, and diltiazem alone or in combination) or were randomized to AVJAP (n=49) in which patients underwent combined atrioventricular junction ablation and pacemaker insertion. Initial minimum pacing rate was 80-90 bpm for the first month following ablation followed by reprogramming to a lower rate as per the treating cardiologist.

Results	Primary end point was echocardiographically determined cardiac function and exercise tolerance; secondary end points were ventricular rate control and quality of life. At 12 months there was no difference in LVEF at 54%±17%, in the AVJAP vs 61%±13 % in the medical therapy group; p=NS. There was no difference in duration of exercise on treadmill testing between the 2 treatments (4.1±2 minutes vs 4.6±2 minutes; p=NS). Peak ventricular rate was lower during exercise in the AVJAP group (112) vs the medical group (153 bpm; p <0.05) as well as during activities of daily life assessed by ambulatory ECG monitoring (117 vs 152; p <0.05). Quality of life scores were better in the AVJAP group with fewer symptoms and a relative risk reduction in symptoms at 12 months of 18%.
Concl.	In patients with permanent, symptomatic atrial fibrillation, AVJAP had neutral effects on LV function and exercise duration but did improve quality of life measures.

ALIVE

Amiodarone vs Lidocaine in Prehospital Ventricular Fibrillation Evaluation

Title	Amiodarone as compared with lidocaine for shock-resistant ventricular fibrillation.
Authors	Dorian P, Cass D, Schwartz B, et al.
Reference	N Engl J Med 2002;346:884-890.
Disease	Out-of hospital cardiac arrest, arrhythmia.
Purpose	To compare the efficacy of lidocaine and amiodarone for patients with out-of-hospital ventricular fibrillation (VF).
Design	Randomized, double-blind.
Patients	347 adults, mean age 67±14 years, with ECG documented out-of-hospital VF or with documented other cardiac arrhythmia that deteriorated to VF. Only patients with resistant or recurrent VF after treatment (3 shocks, ≥1 dose of IV epinephrine, and a fourth shock) were included. Patients with VF due to trauma were not included.
Follow-up	Survival to admission to the hospital intensive care unit.
Regimen	Randomization to lidocaine (1.5 mg/kg) (n=167) or amiodarone (5 mg/kg) (n=180).

Add'l Tx	If ventricular fibrillation persisted after a further shock, a second dose of the study drug (1.5 mg/kg lidocaine or 2.5 mg/kg amiodarone) was given.
Results	22.8% of the patients in the amiodarone group vs only 12.0% in the lidocaine survived to hospital admission (unadjusted OR 2.17; 95% CI=1.21-3.83; p=0.009). After adjustment for other factors that may influence survival, the OR was 2.49 (95% CI=1.28-4.85; p=0.007). Among patients who had a transient return of spontaneous circulation before the study drug was administered, survival to hospital admission was 41.7% in the amiodarone treated and 27.3% in the lidocaine treated patients (p=0.48). Among patients who did not have transient return of spontaneous rhythm, survival to hospital admission was 19.9% and 10.9%, respectively (p=0.04). Among patients who had VF or pulseless ventricular tachycardia as their initial recorded rhythm, survival to hospital admission was 24.8% with amiodarone and 14.2% with lidocaine (p=0.03). Among patients who had other recorded initial rhythm, survival to hospital admission was 15.8% and 3.2%, respectively (p=0.08). Among patients for whom the time from dispatch to study drug administration was ≤24 minutes, the survival to hospital admission was 27.7% with amiodarone and 15.3% with lidocaine (p=0.05). 24% of the patients in the amiodarone vs 23% in the lidocaine group needed atropine for bradycardia. Asystole following defibrillation shock after administration of study drug occurred in 18.4% of the amiodarone treated patients vs 28.9% in the lidocaine treated patients (p=0.04). 5% of the amiodarone treated patients and 3% of the lidocaine treated patients were discharged alive from the hospital (p=0.34).
Concl.	Among patients with shock-resistant out of hospital VF, amiodarone was associated with better survival to hospital admission than lidocaine.

ALIVE

Azimilide Postinfarct Survival Evaluation

Title	The efficacy of azimilide in the treatment of atrial fibrillation in the presence of left ventricular systolic dysfunction: results from the Azimilide Postinfarct Survival Evaluation (ALIVE) trial.
Authors	Pratt CM, Singh SN, Al-Khalidi HR, et al.
Reference	J Am Coll Cardiol 2004;43:1211-1216.
Disease	Arrhythmia, coronary artery disease.
Purpose	To assess the effect of oral azimilide dihydrochloride vs placebo on the onset, termination, and prevalence of atrial fibrillation in a subpopulation of patients in the ALIVE trial.
Design	International, prospective, randomized, placebo-controlled, double-blind study.
Patients	Subpopulation of patients from the ALIVE trial (postmyocardial infarction patients with left ventricular ejection fraction of 15%-35%); patients in the subpopulation had atrial fibrillation on a baseline 12-lead electrocardiogram (n=93) or atrial fibrillation developed after randomization (n=27). The patients were identified on 12-lead electrocardiograms during routine visits at week 2 and months 1, 4, 8, and 12.
Follow-up	1 year.
Regimen	Placebo or azimilide dihydrochloride (a class III antiarrhythmic drug).
Results	Patients with atrial fibrillation (AF) at baseline had a higher mortality rate than those without (p=0.0006). Among patients with AF, there was no difference in mortality between those receiving azimilide and those receiving placebo. Fewer patients receiving azimilide had AF (0.5%) than those receiving placebo (1.2%; p=0.04). More patients receiving azimilide converted to sinus rhythm, although the difference was NS. Over 1 year of follow-up, more azimilide-treated patients than placebo patients were in sinus rhythm (p=0.04).

Concl.   Patients with CHF are at increased risk of AF and mortality. Azimilide was safe and effective therapy for AF in patients with depressed LV function after MI.

AMIOVIRT

Amiodarone vs Implantable Cardioverter-Defibrillator

Title	Amiodarone vs implantable cardioverter-defibrillator: randomized trial in patients with nonischemic dilated cardiomyopathy and asymptomatic nonsustained ventricular tachycardia.
Authors	Strickberger SA, Hummel JD, Bartlett TG, et al.
Reference	J Am Coll Cardiol 2003;41:1707-1712.
Disease	Nonsustained ventricular tachycardia, nonischemic dilated cardiomyopathy, heart failure.
Purpose	To determine whether implantable cardioverter-defibrillator decreases mortality greater than amiodarone in patients with nonischemic dilated cardiomyopathy and nonsustained ventricular tachycardia.
Design	Randomized, multicenter.
Patients	103 patients with nonischemic dilated cardiomyopathy and nonsustained ventricular tachycardia.
Follow-up	3 years.
Regimen	Amiodarone (800 mg/d for 7 days, then 400 mg/d. The dose was reduced to 300 mg/d after 1 year) (m=52) vs implanted defibrillator (m=51).
Results	Primary end point was total mortality and secondary end points were arrhythmia-free survival, quality of life and cost issues. The study was stopped when prospective stopping rule for futility was achieved. At 1 year there was no significant difference in survival in the amiodarone group (90%) vs the ICD group (96%). At 3 years there also was no significant difference in survival in the amiodarone group (87%) vs the ICD group (88%; p=0.8). There was no difference in quality of life between groups. Arrhythmia-free survival at 1 and 3 years were 82% and 73%, respectively, in the amiodarone group vs 78% and 63% in the ICD group (p=0.1). Total cost of medical care was lower in the amiodarone group vs the ICD group ($8,879 vs $22,079; p=0.1).

9.Arrhythmia

Concl.   There was no significant difference in mortality in patients with nonischemic dilated cardiomyopathy and asymptomatic non-sustained ventricular tachycardia who received amiodarone vs implantable cardioverterd efibrillator.

ARCH

Amiodarone Reduction in Coronary Heart Trial

Title	Intravenous amiodarone for the prevention of atrial fibrillation after open heart surgery: The ARCH Trial.
Authors	Guarnieri T, Nolan S, Gottlieb SO, et al.
Reference	J Am Coll Cardiol 1999;34:343-347.
Disease	Atrial fibrillation.
Purpose	To determine whether low dose IV amiodarone would prevent atrial fibrillation and shorten hospital stay in patients undergoing cardiac surgery.
Design	Randomized, double-blind, placebo-controlled, single-center.
Patients	300 patients undergoing standard open heart surgery with no evidence of preoperative atrial fibrillation.
Follow-up	1 month.
Regimen	Amiodarone IV 1 g over 24 hours for a total of 48 hours (2 g total) or placebo infusion.
Add'l Tx	About 50% of both groups were taking β-blockers before surgery.
Results	Primary end points were postoperative atrial fibrillation and length of stay in hospital. Atrial fibrillation occurred in 67 of 142 (47%) placebo patients and in 56 of 158 (35%) amiodarone patients (p=0.01). There was no difference in length of hospital stay in the placebo group (8.2±6.2 days) vs the amiodarone group (7.6±5.9 days). No deaths occurred in the amiodarone group; 2 in the placebo group. Drug effect appeared to occur during the first few days of treatment.
Concl.	Low dose IV amiodarone was effective in decreasing the frequency of atrial fibrillation following cardiac surgery.

ARREST

Amiodarone in Out-of-Hospital Resuscitation of Refractory Sustained Ventricular Tachyarrhythmias

Title	Amiodarone for resuscitation after out-of-hospital cardiac arrest due to ventricular fibrillation.
Authors	Kudenchuk PJ, Cobb LA, Copass MK, et al.
Reference	N Engl J Med 1999;341:871-878.
Disease	Cardiac arrest.
Purpose	To determine the effect of IV amiodarone in patients with out-of-hospital cardiac arrest with ventricular fibrillation or tachycardia who were refractory to precordial shocks.
Design	Randomized, double-blind, placebo-controlled.
Patients	504 patients who had out-of-hospital cardiac arrest with ventricular fibrillation or pulseless ventricular tachycardia and could not be resuscitated after receiving ≥3 defibrillator shocks.
Follow-up	Hospital discharge.
Regimen	300 mg IV amiodarone (n=246) or placebo (n=258) administered by paramedics on the scene of the cardiac arrest.
Add'l Tx	1 mg epinephrine IV.

Results	Primary end point was survival through admission to hospital with a spontaneously perfusing rhythm. 44% of the amiodarone group vs 34% of the placebo group survived to be admitted to the hospital (p=0.03). The adjusted odds ratio for survival to admission in amiodarone treated patients vs placebo patients was 1.6 (95% CI=1.1-2.4; p=0.02) and the benefit of amiodarone was observed across subsets of patients. Patients with ventricular fibrillation were more likely to survive to hospital admission (44%) than patients with initial rhythm of asystole or pulseless electrical activity (14%; p<0.001). Patients with transient return of spontaneous circulation before receiving amiodarone or placebo were more likely to survive to be admitted vs those who remained pulseless before getting study drug. Hypotension was more common with amiodarone (59%) vs placebo (48%; p=0.04); bradycardia was more common with amiodarone (41%) compared to placebo (25%; p=0.004). The percentage of patients discharged alive was 13.4% in the amiodarone group and 13.2% in the placebo group; the study was not powered to detect statistically significant differences in survival till hospital discharge between groups.
Concl.	Amiodarone resulted in a higher rate of survival to hospital admission in patients with out-of-hospital cardiac arrest and refractory ventricular arrhythmias.

AVID

Antiarrhythmics vs Implantable Defibrillators

Title	A comparison of antiarrhythmic drug therapy with implantable defibrillators in patients resuscitated from near fatal ventricular arrhythmias.
Authors	The antiarrhythmics vs implantable defibrillator (AVID) investigators.
Reference	N Engl J Med 1997; 337:1576-1583.
Disease	Ventricular fibrillation (VF), sustained ventricular tachycardia (VT).
Purpose	To determine survival of initial therapy of an implantable defibrillator vs amiodarone or sotalol in patients who were resuscitated from near fatal VF; or patients with symptomatic, sustained, and hemodynamically compromising VT.
Design	Randomized, multicenter, VT patients had to have sustained VT with syncope or an ejection fraction <0.40 and symptoms suggesting severe hemodynamic compromise (near syncope, heart failure, angina).
Patients	1016 patients; mean age 65 years; 79% male. 455 had VF; 561 had VT.
Follow-up	3 years plus.
Regimen	Implantable cardioverter defibrillator vs antiarrhythmic drug treatment (most took amiodarone followed by sotalol).
Results	There were fewer deaths among patients assigned to the implantable defibrillator (80) than antiarrhythmic drug group (122). Death rates at 18.2 months were 15.8% in the defibrillator group vs 24% in the antiarrhythmic group. There was a decrease in death rate at 1, 2, and 3 years of 39, 27, 31%, respectively, in patients receiving the device vs drug; hence patients receiving the defibrillator had a better survival throughout the course of the study (p<0.02). Automatic pacing or shocks were more common among patients who entered the study with VT compared to those that entered with VF.

Concl.   For survivors of VF or sustained, severely symptomatic VT, the implantable cardioverter defibrillator is superior to antiarrhythmic drugs regarding survival.

AVID (β-Blocker Substudy)

Antiarrhythmics vs Implantable Defibrillators

Title	β-blocker use and survival in patients with ventricular fibrillation or symptomatic ventricular tachycardia: The AVID Trial.
Authors	Exner DV, Reiffel JA, Epstein AE, et al.
Reference	J Am Coll Cardiol 1999;34:325-333.
Disease	Ventricular fibrillation, ventricular tachycardia.
Purpose	To determine whether β-blockers alone or in combination with other specific antiarrhythmics improve survival in patients with VT/VF.
Design	As per AVID.
Patients	Determination of survival of 1016 randomized and 2101 eligible but nonrandomized patients with VF or symptomatic VT in the AVID trial.
Follow-up	As per AVID.
Regimen	As per AVID.
Add'l Tx	As per AVID.

Results   There were 817 (28%) patients discharged from hospital on β-blockers. Patients discharged from hospital on β-blockers had fewer symptoms of heart failure and were less likely to be on a diuretic or ACE inhibitor. Metoprolol and atenolol were the 2 most commonly used β-blockers. β-blocker therapy was associated with improved survival in patients that did not receive amiodarone or an implantable defibrillator (relative risk [RR]=0.36; 95% CI=0.21-0.64; p=0.0004). However, β-blocker use at hospital discharge was not associated with improved survival in randomized amiodarone treated (RR 0.88; 95% CI=0.48-1.61; p=NS) or defibrillator patients (RR 0.69; 95% CI=0.39-1.24; p=0.22). β-blocker also was not associated with survival in eligible, nonrandomized patients that received amiodarone or defibrillator alone. Following adjustment, β-blockers were unrelated to survival in randomized and nonrandomized patients receiving amiodarone or defibrillator alone. β-blocker was independently associated with better survival in eligible, nonrandomized patients who were not treated with specific antiarrhythmic therapy (adjusted RR 0.47; 95% CI=0.25-0.88; p=0.018).

Concl.   β-blockers improved survival in patients with lethal ventricular arrhythmias who were not treated with amiodarone or implantable defibrillators, but did not have a protective effect on patients already receiving these specific forms of antiarrhythmic therapy.

BLOS

The β-Blocker Length of Stay

Title	Double-blind, placebo-controlled, randomized trial of prophylactic metoprolol for reduction of hospital length of stay after heart surgery: the BLOS study.
Authors	Connolly SJ, Cybulsky I, Lamy A, et al.
Reference	Am Heart J 2003;145:226-232.
Disease	Coronary artery bypass graft, atrial fibrillation.
Purpose	To evaluate whether metoprolol, started immediately after heart surgery, reduces hospital length of stay and cost.
Design	Randomized, double-blind, placebo-controlled.
Patients	1000 patients scheduled for heart surgery with cardiopulmonary bypass grafting who were residing at home before surgery. Patients with emergency surgery, history of intolerance to β-blockers, chronic obstructive lung disease, atrio-ventricular block, and long-term preoperative therapy with amiodarone were not included. Postoperative exclusion criteria were sinus bradycardia <50 bpm; cardiac index <2.3 L/min/m²; need for intravenous inotropic therapy other than low-dose dopamine; and bronchospasm.
Follow-up	Hospital stay.
Regimen	Within 12 hours of arrival to the ICU, eligible patients were randomized to oral (or nasogastric tube) metoprolol 50 mg bid or placebo for 14 days or until hospital discharge. After the initial 411 patients, the metoprolol was increased to 50 mg tid.

Add'l Tx	Nonstudy β-blockers and other medications were permitted.
Results	Nonstudy β-blockers were given to 40% of patients in the placebo group and to 29% of patients in the metoprolol group. Study medications were stopped at least once in 27% and 32% of the patients in the placebo and metoprolol groups, respectively (p=0.071). The incidence of atrial fibrillation was 39% in the placebo group and 31% in the metoprolol group (p=0.01). Hospital length of stay was comparable (152±61 hours in the placebo group, 155±90 hours in the metoprolol group; p=0.79). The ICU length of stay was 34±24 hours with placebo and 39±54 hours with metoprolol (p=0.10). 1.3% of patients in the metoprolol group vs 0 patients in the placebo group needed prolonged ventilation (p=0.03). Postoperative stroke occurred in 0.6% of patients in the placebo vs 1.4% in the metoprolol group (p=0.34). Costs were comparable between the placebo ($4,686) and metoprolol ($4,868) groups (p=0.27).
Concl.	Nonstudy β-blockers were given to 40% of patients in the placebo group and to 29% of patients in the metoprolol group. Study medications were stopped at least once in 27% and 32% of the patients in the placebo and metoprolol groups, respectively (p=0.071). The incidence of atrial fibrillation was 39% in the placebo group and 31% in the metoprolol group (p=0.01). Hospital length of stay was comparable (152±61 hours in the placebo group, 155±90 hours in the metoprolol group; p=0.79). The ICU length of stay was 34±24 hours with placebo and 39±54 hours with metoprolol (p=0.10). 1.3% of patients in the metoprolol group vs 0 patients in the placebo group needed prolonged ventilation (p=0.03). Postoperative stroke occurred in 0.6% of patients in the placebo vs 1.4% in the metoprolol group (p=0.34). Costs were comparable between the placebo ($4,686) and metoprolol ($4,868) groups (p=0.27).

CASH

Cardiac Arrest Study: Hamburg

Title	Randomized comparison of antiarrhythmic drug-therapy with implantable defibrillators in patients resuscitated from cardiac arrest: the Cardiac Arrest Study: Hamburg (CASH).
Authors	Kuck KH, Cappato R, Siebels J, et al.
Reference	Circulation 2000;102:748-754.
Disease	Ventricular arrhythmia, cardiac arrest.
Purpose	To compare the outcome of survivors of cardiac arrest due to documented ventricular arrhythmias receiving implantable cardioverter defibrillators (ICDs) vs drug treatment (amiodarone, metoprolol, and propafenone).
Design	Multicenter, randomized study.
Patients	288 patients who survived cardiac arrest due to documented ventricular arrhythmia.
Follow-up	Mean follow-up of 57 months.
Regimen	Randomized to ICD, amiodarone (loading dose of 1000 mg/d for 7 days; maintenance dose of 200-600 mg/d), metoprolol (12.5-25 mg/d increased within 7-14 days to maximum of 200 mg/d if tolerated). Assignment to propafenone discontinued secondary to a 61% higher all cause mortality than in ICD patients during 11 month follow-up. Thereafter study continued in remaining 3 groups: ICDs (n=99); amiodarone (n=92); metoprolol (n=97).

Results	Primary end point was all cause mortality. Secondary end points were sudden death and recurrence of cardiac arrest at 2-year follow-up. Over mean follow-up of 57 months, crude death rates were 36.4% in the ICD group, 44.4% in the amiodarone/metoprolol arm. There was a nonsignificant trend toward higher survival in patients receiving ICD vs those receiving drug-therapy (1-sided $p=0.081$), hazard ratio 0.766. Percent reductions in all cause mortality for year 1-9 in the ICD patients varied between 9.1% and 41.9%. Crude death rates were 43.5% for amiodarone and 45.4% for metoprolol ($p=NS$). Crude sudden death rates were 13% in the ICD arm and 33% in drug arm. Survival free of sudden death was significantly higher in patients assigned to ICD vs drug (1-sided $p=0.005$; hazard ratio 0.423). Crude rates of nonfatal cardiac arrest were 11.1% in ICD arm and 19.5% in drug arm and there was a nonsignificant trend toward higher survival free of cardiac arrest in the ICD group (1-sided $p=0.072$; hazard ratio of 0.481).
Concl.	During long-term follow-up there was a nonsignificant 23% reduction of all cause mortality with ICD therapy vs amiodarone/metoprolol in cardiac arrest survivors.

CAT

Cardiomyopathy Trial

Title	Primary prevention of sudden death in idiopathic dilated cardiomyopathy.
Authors	Bänsch D, Antz M, Boczor S, et al.
Reference	Circulation 2002;105:1453-1458.
Disease	Dilated, cardiomyopathy, congestive heart failure.
Purpose	To determine whether an implantable cardioverter defibrillator (ICD) improved survival in patients with dilated cardiomyopathy of recent onset (≤9 months) and impaired left ventricular ejection fraction (LVEF) (≤30%) without documented symptomatic ventricular tachycardia (VT).
Design	Randomized, primary prevention, multicenter.
Patients	104 patients with new onset dilated cardiomyopathy with impaired LV function. Coronary artery disease had to be excluded by angiography. Patients were excluded if they had symptomatic VT/ventricular fibrillation.
Follow-up	5.5 years.
Regimen	Patients were assigned to ICD (n=50); or control (n=54).
Add'l Tx	Most patients were on angiotensin-converting enzyme inhibitors, digitalis, and diuretics.
Results	Primary end point was all-cause mortality at 1 year. At 1 year all-cause mortality rate did not reach expected 30% in controls. At 1 year 4 patients died in the ICD group and 2 in the control group. Sudden death did not occur during first and second year of follow-up. After 5.5 years of follow-up there was no difference in death rates between groups: 13 died in the ICD group and 17 died in the control group. There was no difference in cumulative 2-, 4-, or 6-year survival between groups. Cumulative survival was 92%, 86%, and 73% at 2, 4, and 6 years in the ICD group vs 93%, 80%, and 68% in the control group (p=NS). The major predictor of total mortality was depressed LVEF.

Concl.   ICD therapy did not provide a survival benefit in patients with recent onset dilated cardiomyopathy.

CIDS

Canadian Implantable Defibrillator Study

Title	A randomized trial of the implantable cardioverter defibrillator against amiodarone.
Authors	Connolly SJ, Gent M, Roberts RS, et al.
Reference	Circulation 2000;101:1297-1302.
Disease	Ventricular fibrillation, ventricular tachycardia.
Purpose	To compare the efficacy of the implantable cardioverter defibrillator (ICD) to amiodarone for preventing death in patients with previous life threatening sustained ventricular arrhythmia.
Design	Randomized, multicenter.
Patients	659 patients with resuscitated ventricular fibrillation, ventricular tachycardia, or unmonitored syncope.
Follow-up	5 years.
Regimen	ICD vs amiodarone starting at ≥1200 mg/d for at least 1 week and then ≥300 mg/d. Could be lowered to 200 mg/d if side effects developed.
Add'l Tx	β-blocker, sotalol, digoxin, Class I antiarrhythmics. Note: There was imbalance in use of other antiarrhythmics between the 2 groups. Sotalol and other β-blockers more commonly used in the ICD group.
Results	Primary end point was all cause mortality. All cause mortality occurred in 10.2% per year of amiodarone patients vs 8.3% per year of ICD patients (19.7% relative risk reduction for ICD therapy; 95% CI=-7.7%-40.0%; p=0.142). Hence, this reduction in risk of all cause mortality with ICDs over amiodarone did not achieve statistical significance. Also there was a nonsignificant decrease in arrhythmic death from ICDs from 4.5% with amiodarone to 3.0% per year for ICDs (relative risk reduction =32.8%; 95% CI=-7.2%-57.8%; p=0.094). 1.9% per year of amiodarone patients experienced pulmonary infiltrate.

Concl.   There were nonsignificant trends toward reductions in all cause
           mortality and arrhythmic death in patients receiving ICDs vs
           amiodarone.

CTAF

Canadian Trial of Atrial Fibrillation

Title	Amiodarone to prevent recurrence of atrial fibrillation.
Authors	Roy D, Talajic M, Dorion P, et al.
Reference	N Engl J Med 2000;342:913-920.
Disease	Atrial fibrillation.
Purpose	To compare low dose amiodarone to sotalol or propafenone for the prevention of recurrence of atrial fibrillation.
Design	Prospective, nonblinded, randomized, multicenter.
Patients	403 patients who had at least 1 episode of symptomatic atrial fibrillation within the previous 6 months. 1 episode had to have lasted at least 10 minutes and be confirmed by ECG.
Follow-up	16 months.
Regimen	Amiodarone (10 mg/kg daily for 14 days; then 300 mg per day for 4 weeks; then 200 mg daily). Sotalol at doses varying by age, creatinine concentration, and weight; propafenone dose based on age and weight.
Add'l Tx	For atrial fibrillation lasting >48 hours, anticoagulant therapy. Electrical cardioversion if necessary (recommended if atrial fibrillation persisted after 14 days of loading doses of amiodarone and after 4 days of treatment with sotalol or propafenone).
Results	Primary end point was length of time to first ECG documented recurrence of atrial fibrillation. 71 (35%) of 201 patients assigned to amiodarone vs 127 (63%) of 202 patients assigned to sotalol or propafenone had recurrent atrial fibrillation (p<0.001). Median time for recurrence of atrial fibrillation in the sotalol or propafenone group was 98 days but was >468 days in the amiodarone group. The probability of staying in sinus rhythm for 1 year without recurrence of atrial fibrillation was 69% in amiodarone patients and 39% in the sotalol or propafenone group (39%; p<0.001). Drug therapy was discontinued due to adverse events in 18% of patients on amiodarone and 11% of those on sotalol or propafenone (p=0.06).

Concl.	Amiodarone was more effective than sotalol or propafenone for preventing recurrent episodes of atrial fibrillation.

CTOPP

Canadian Trial of Physiologic Pacing

Title	Effects of physiologic pacing vs ventricular pacing on the risk of stroke and death due to cardiovascular causes.
Authors	Connolly SJ, Kerr CR, Gent M, et al.
Reference	N Engl J Med 2000;342:1385-1391.
Disease	Randomized, multicenter.
Purpose	To determine whether there is a benefit of physiologic (dual chamber or atrial) pacing compared to single chamber (ventricular) pacing in patients with symptomatic bradycardia.
Design	Randomized, multicenter.
Patients	2568 patients scheduled for initial implantation of a pacemaker to correct symptomatic bradycardia and did not have chronic atrial fibrillation.
Follow-up	3 years.
Regimen	1474 patients were assigned to ventricular pacing and 1094 to physiologic pacing.
Add'l Tx	Anticoagulant, antiplatelet drugs; 11.5 and 12.6% on antiarrhythmic drugs in ventricular pacing and physiologic pacing groups, respectively.

Results   Primary outcome was occurrence of either stroke or death due to
             cardiovascular cause. Secondary outcome events were death from
             any cause, documented atrial fibrillation lasting more than 15
             minutes, and admission to the hospital for congestive heart fail-
             ure. Annual rate of stroke or death due to cardiovascular causes
             was 5.5% in the ventricular pacing group vs 4.9% in the physi-
             ologic pacing group (p=NS). Annual rate of atrial fibrillation was
             6.6% in the ventricular pacing group vs 5.3% in the physiologic
             pacing group (p=0.05). This benefit was not apparent until 2
             years after pacemaker implantation. Annual rate of death was
             6.6% for ventricular pacing and 6.3% for physiologic pacing
             (p=NS); rate for hospitalization for congestive heart failure was
             3.5% for ventricular pacing and 3.1% for physiologic pacing
             (p=NS). Annual rate of stroke was 1.1% in ventricular pacing
             and 1.0% in physiologic pacing group. Perioperative complica-
             tions were more common in the physiologic pacing (9.0%) vs
             ventricular pacing (3.8%) groups; p<0.001.

Concl.   Physiologic pacing was no better than ventricular pacing in pre-
             venting rate of stroke or death due to cardiovascular cause.

CTOPP

Canadian Trial of Physiological Pacing

Title	Canadian Trial of Physiological Pacing. Effects of physiological pacing during long-term follow-up.
Authors	Kerr CR, Connolly SJ, Abdollah H, et al.
Reference	Circulation 2004;109:357-362.
Disease	Arrhythmia.
Purpose	To assess a potential delayed benefit of physiological pacing over ventricular pacing.
Design	Randomized trial.
Patients	2568 patients requiring a pacemaker for symptomatic bradycardia.
Follow-up	6 years.
Regimen	Ventricular (n=1474) or physiological (n=1094) pacemakers.
Results	The original follow-up period was 3 years. At 3 years, the outcomes were similar, but atrial fibrillation (AF) was significantly less common with physiological pacemakers, so outcome was extended to 6 years to assess the possibility of a delayed benefit. At a mean follow-up of 6.4 years, there was no difference between the groups in the primary outcome of cardiovascular death or stroke, nor was there a significant difference in total mortality or stroke. There was a lower rate in the development of AF in the physiological pacing group (relative risk reduction 20.1%; 95% CI=5.4-32.5; p=0.009).
Concl.	The extended follow-up of 6 years did not reveal a difference in cardiovascular death or stroke or in total mortality or in stroke between patients receiving ventricular or physiological pacing. The reduced risk of AF with physiological pacing persisted; however, hard evidence in favor of physiological pacing remains unclear.

DAVID

Dual Chamber and VVI Implantable Defibrillator Trial

Title	Dual-chamber pacing or ventricular backup pacing in patients with an implantable defibrillator.
Authors	The DAVID Trial Investigators.
Reference	JAMA 2002;288:3115-3123.
Disease	Congestive heart failure; arrhythmias.
Purpose	To determine the effectiveness of dual-chamber pacing compared with backup ventricular pacing in patients who have an indication for implantable cardioverter-defibrillator (ICD) implantation but not indications for antibradycardia pacing.
Design	Randomized, single-blinded, parallel-arm, multicenter.
Patients	506 patients. All participants had a standard indication for ICD implantation because of ventricular tachyarrhythmia but not an indication for antibradycardia pacing. In addition to the arrhythmia, included patients also had to have a left ventricular ejection fraction ≤40%. Exclusion criteria were numerous and included: permanent pacemaker, pre-existing endocardial pacing leads, planned cardiac surgery or percutaneous intervention; symptomatic bradycardia or second- or third-degree AV block, disqualifying atrial fibrillation and atrial tachyarrhythmias, and others.
Follow-up	Median 8.4 months (range: 0-23.6 months).

Regimen	After implantation of the ICD, patients were randomized to have the pacing function of the device programmed to the VVI mode with a lower rate of 40/min (VVI-40) without supraventricular tachycardia detection enhancements or to the DDDR mode with a lower rate of 70/min (DDDR-70) and activation of supraventricular tachycardia detection enhancements. Medical therapy consisted of digoxin, diuretics, ACE inhibitors, and β-blockers. ACE inhibitors were used first, followed by β-blockers, and then diuretics were added as needed. Patients who had symptomatic CHF, New York Heart Association class II or III, received digoxin, 0.125 mg/d. Spironolactone was added at 12.5 mg/d to 25 mg/d if the patients continued to have functional class II or III CHF. Amiodarone for ventricular arrhythmia was given only in the event of sustained or symptomatic episodes, or to try and decrease the ICD shocks. Patients on antiarrhythmic medicines for supraventricular tachycardias or atrial fibrillation at randomization could stay on these medicines.
Results	The composite primary end point was the absence of death and absence of hospitalization from heart failure. The characteristics of the 2 groups were well matched at baseline. The average age was 65 years, the mean LVEF was 27%. Half of the patients were NYHA functional class I, and approximately 12% were functional class III-IV. Patients in the VVI-40 group had a reduced risk of the composite end point—death or hospitalization for new or worsening CHF (RR 1.61; 95% CI=1.06-2.44; p=0.03). Patients in the VVI-40 group also had trends toward reduced risk of first hospitalization for new or worsening CHF (RR 1.54; 95% CI=0.97-2.46; p=0.07), or all-cause death (RR 1.61; 95% CI=0.84-3.09; p=0.15).
Concl.	In patients who had a standard indication for ICD placement and a LVEF of 40% or less, dual-chamber pacing showed no clinical favorability over ventricular back-up pacing. Patients who received ventricular back-up pacing had a significant reduction in the composite end point of all-cause death and morbidity related to CHF compared to those who received dual-chamber pacing.

DEBUT

Defibrillator vs β-Blocker for Unexplained Death in Thailand

Title	Defibrillator vs β-blockers for unexplained death in Thailand, a randomized clinical trial.
Authors	Nademanee K, Veerakul G, Mower M, et al.
Reference	Circulation 2003;107:2221-2226.
Disease	Arrhythmias.
Purpose	To compare the annual death rates of patients with Sudden Unexplained Death Syndrome (SUDS) between those randomized to therapy with β-blockers and those who receive an implantable cardioverter defibrillator (ICD).
Design	Prospective, randomized, multicenter.
Patients	20 in the pilot study phase and 66 in the main trial. Patients were eligible if they had either survived SUDS or were likely to have SUDS. A survivor of SUDS was defined as someone without structural heart disease who survived unexpected ventricular fibrillation (VF) or cardiac arrest. A likely SUDS patients was someone without structural heart disease who had symptoms characteristic of SUDS, particularly during sleep, such as agonal respiration, transient episodes of stress, abnormal respiration combined with grasping and groaning, syncope, or seizure-like symptoms and right bundle-branch block with ST elevation in the right precordial leads and inducible ventricular tachycardia (VT)/VF in the electrophysiology lab.
Follow-up	3 years.
Regimen	Patients were randomized to receive either a transvenous ICD or β-blocker therapy. Patients in the β-blockade group received long-acting propanolol (40 mg/d-160 mg/d). Other β-blockers or amiodarone were allowed if side effects of propanolol were intolerable.

Add'l Tx	The primary study end point was all-cause death. The secondary end point was recurrent VT/VF or cardiac arrest. In the pilot study, 10 patients were randomized to ICD and 10 to β-block-ade. During the 2-year follow-up, there were 3 deaths in the β-blocker arm and no deaths in the ICD arm (p=0.07). In the main trial, 37 patients were randomized to ICD and 29 to β-blockade therapy. There were no differences in the baseline characteristics of the 2 groups. During the 3-year follow-up, there were 4 deaths, all in the β-blocker group (14% vs. 0%; p=0.02). The rate of death annually was approximately 10%. 7 patients in the ICD arm had recurrent VF, all of which were effectively treated by the ICD. The rate of events (sudden death or episodes of VF) in the pilot and main trials combined was 20% annually in the ICD group compared to 10% in the b-blocker group.
Results	The primary study end point was all-cause death. The secondary end point was recurrent VT/VF or cardiac arrest. In the pilot study, 10 patients were randomized to ICD and 10 to β-block-ade. During the 2-year follow-up, there were 3 deaths in the β-blocker arm and no deaths in the ICD arm (p=0.07). In the main trial, 37 patients were randomized to ICD and 29 to β-blockade therapy. There were no differences in the baseline characteristics of the 2 groups. During the 3-year follow-up, there were 4 deaths, all in the β-blocker group (14% vs. 0%; p=0.02). The rate of death annually was approximately 10%. 7 patients in the ICD arm had recurrent VF, all of which were effectively treated by the ICD. The rate of events (sudden death or episodes of VF) in the pilot and main trials combined was 20% annually in the ICD group compared to 10% in the β-blocker group.
Concl.	Use of ICD was associated with complete protection against sudden death arising from SUDS-related VF. ICD use was superior to β-blockade.

DIAMOND

Danish Investigations of Arrhythmia and Mortality on Dofetilide

Title	a. Dofetilide in patients with left ventricular dysfunction and either heart failure or acute myocardial infarction: rationale, design, and patient characteristics of the DIAMOND studies. b. Effect of dofetilide in patients with recent myocardial infarction and left ventricular dysfunction: a randomised trial.
Authors	a. The DIAMOND Study Group. b. Kober L, Bloch Thompsen PE, Moller M, et al.
Reference	a. Clin Cardiol 1997;20:704-710. b. Lancet 2000;356:2052-2058.
Disease	Arrhythmia, acute myocardial infarction, congestive heart failure.
Purpose	To evaluate the effects of long-term treatment with dofetilide, a new class III antiarrhythmic agent, on mortality and morbidity of patients with left ventricular dysfunction following acute myocardial infarction.
Design	Randomized, double-blind, placebo-controlled, multicenter.
Patients	1510 patients, ≥18 years old, within 7 days of acute myocardial infarction, left ventricular dysfunction (echocardiographic wall motion index of ≤1.2. Patients with heart rate <50 beats per minute, sinoatrial or atrioventricular block not treated with a pacemaker, history of drug-induced proarrhythmia, long QT, diastolic blood pressure <80 mm Hg, systolic blood pressure >115 mm Hg, hypokalemia, hyperkalemia, previous treatment with dofetilide or use of other antiarrhythmic agents, creatinine clearance <20 mL/min, significant hepatic dysfunction, aortic stenosis, recent cardiac surgery, presence of an automatic implantable cardioverter/defibrillator and planned revascularization were excluded.

Follow-up	>12 months.
Regimen	Randomization to placebo (n=761) or dofetilide (n=749) (for patients in sinus rhythm: 0.50 mg bid when creatinine clearance was ≥60 mL/min, 0.25 mg bid when creatinine clearance was 40-60 mL/min, and 0.25 mg once daily when creatinine clearance was <40 mL/min. For patients in atrial fibrillation: 0.25 mg bid when creatinine clearance was ≥40 mL/min, and 0.25 mg once daily when creatinine clearance was <40 mL/min).
Add'l Tx	If creatinine clearance fell <20 mL/min the treatment was discontinued. If creatinine clearance decreased (but was ≥20 mL/min) or if QTc interval increased >20% from baseline (or >550 ms), the dose was decreased.
Results	The median duration of therapy was 458 days in the placebo group and 454 days in the dofetilide group. All-cause mortality was 31% in the dofetilide group and 32% in the placebo group (p=0.61). Cardiac mortality was 26% and 28%, respectively (p=0.30). Arrhythmic death occurred in 17% and 18% of the patients, respectively (p=0.55). Dofetilide did not adversely affect mortality in any of the predefined subgroups. There was no significant reduction in the risk of cardiac death (p=0.101), total arrhythmic death (p=0.139), or worsening heart failure (p=0.513) with dofetilide. There were 75 reinfarctions in the dofetilide group vs 104 in the placebo group (p=0.086). Among the 8% of the patients with atrial fibrillation or flutter at entry, dofetilide was significantly more effective than placebo in restoring sinus rhythm (42.4% vs 12.5%; p=0.002). Among the patients with sinus rhythm at entry, atrial fibrillation or flutter developed in 5 patients in the dofetilide group vs 14 patients in the placebo group (p=0.09). During follow-up, arrhythmias requiring withdrawal of the study drug and specific treatment occurred in 8% of the patients in the dofetilide group and 9% in the placebo group (p=0.59). Torsade de pointes occurred in 7 patients in the dofetilide group vs zero in the placebo group.
Concl.	Long-term therapy with dofetilide in patients with left ventricular dysfunction after recent myocardial infarction did not affect all cause mortality, cardiac mortality, and arrhythmic mortality. Dofetilide was effective and relatively safe in treating atrial fibrillation and flutter in these patients.

DIAMOND (Substudy)

Danish Investigations of Arrhythmia and Mortality on Dofetilide

Title	Efficacy of dofetilide in the treatment of atrial fibrillation-flutter in patients with reduced left ventricular function.
Authors	Pedersen OD, Bagger H, Keller N, et al.
Reference	Circulation 2001;104:292-296.
Disease	Atrial fibrillation-flutter.
Purpose	To determine the ability of dofetilide to restore and maintain sinus rhythm in patients with atrial fibrillation-flutter and left ventricular (LV) dysfunction.
Design	Pooled data from the 2 DIAMOND studies; randomized, double-blind, placebo-controlled, parallel-group, multicenter studies.
Patients	506 patients in the DIAMOND CHF/MI studies with reduced LV function and atrial fibrillation-flutter. Patients had to have an echocardiographic wall motion index of ≤1.2 corresponding to an LV ejection fraction (EF) of ≤35%.
Follow-up	12 months.
Regimen	Patients were randomized to either oral dofetilide 250 mg bid (n=249) vs placebo (n=257). Dose was adjusted based on creatinine clearance.

9. Arrhythmia

Results   Sinus rhythm was restored pharmacologically in 31 (12%) of the dofetilide-treated patients vs 5 (2%) of the placebo-treated patients at 1 month (p<0.001). Over 12 months pharmacologic or spontaneous cardioversion occurred in 44% of dofetilide and 14% of placebo patients (p<0.001). Cardioversion (including electrical) occurred in 148 (5%) of dofetilide patients vs 86 (34%) of placebo patients over the course of the study. In the cardioverted patients, probability of maintaining sinus rhythm for 12 months was 79% vs 42% in the dofetilide vs placebo groups, respectively (p<0.001). Mortality was similar in patients treated with dofetilide vs placebo. However, restoration and maintenance of sinus rhythm was associated with a decrease in mortality (risk ratio [RR] 0.44; 95% CI=0.30-0.64; p<0.0001). All-cause hospitalization and hospitalization for worsening congestive heart failure were delayed by dofetilide. 73 of 249 dofetilide patients (24%) and 102 of 257 placebo patients (40%) required hospitalization for worsening heart failure. With adjustment for wall motion index the RR of CHF hospitalization for dofetilide vs placebo was 0.69; 95% CI=0.51-0.93 (p≤0.02). Torsade de pointes occurred in 4 dofetilide treated patients (1.6%) and treatment was stopped, in these patients.

Concl.   Dofetilide increased the probability of achieving and maintaining sinus rhythm in patients with LV dysfunction. Dofetilide reduced hospitalizations for CHF.

ERAFT

European Rythmol/Rytmonorm Atrial Fibrillation Trial

Title	Efficacy and safety of propafenone sustained release in the prophylaxis of symptomatic paroxysmal atrial fibrillation.
Authors	Meinertz T, Lip GY, Lombardi F, et al.
Reference	Am J Cardiol 2002;90:1300-1306.
Disease	Atrial fibrillation.
Purpose	To determine whether a sustained-release formulation of propafenone is better than placebo in preventing the recurrence of symptomatic paroxysmal atrial fibrillation (AF).
Design	Double-blind, placebo-controlled, multicenter.
Patients	293 patients, age ≥18 years, all with documented evidence of symptomatic paroxysmal AF, treated or untreated. Patients taking rate-limiting medications could be entered in the trial if they had symptomatic AF while taking these medications. Exclusion criteria were numerous and included: New York Heart Association class III and IV heart failure or left ventricular ejection fraction <35%, acute myocardial infarction, unstable angina, persistent severe bradycardia, hypotension, various electrophysiologic abnormalities including high-grade sinoatrial and atrioventricular blocks, and others. Patients who had previously received treatment with propafenone for supraventricular arrhythmias for more than 4 days were excluded, in order to prevent patient bias among known responders.
Follow-up	95 days.
Regimen	Class I and III antiarrhythmic drugs were required to be washed out before study entry, and were not allowed as medications during the study. Patients who had taken a cumulative dose of amiodarone greater than 15 g had a required wash-out period of 6 months; if less than 15 g, the wash-out period was 3 months. Patients were randomized to receive either propafenone SR 325 mg or 425 mg or matched placebo bid. Steady-state concentrations were expected to be achieved by day 5 or 6 after study start, and the period thereafter was the "efficacy period," which lasted 91 days or until the first relapse of symptomatic AF.

Results   The final analysis included 107 patients in the propafenone SR 325 mg group, 83 patients in the propafenone SR 425 mg group, and 88 patients in the placebo group. The primary efficacy end point was the arrhythmia-free period of time during the efficacy period, starting at day 5 after randomization until the first symptomatic recurrence of documented atrial arrhythmia. The secondary efficacy end point was the arrhythmia-free period of time starting at day 1 (randomization) until the first symptomatic recurrence of documented atrial arrhythmia. Other efficacy end points were: heart rate during the first symptomatic recurrence of arrhythmia, time beginning from the steady state to first documented symptomatic or nonsymptomatic atrial arrhythmia, and time from steady state to treatment failure (first symptomatic arrhythmia or trial withdrawal for any reason). Adverse events were classified as "serious" and "nonserious." The 3 treatment groups were well balanced for baseline and demographic characteristics. For the primary outcome, there was an increase in the number of days to symptomatic atrial arrhythmia in the propafenone groups vs placebo: median time to first recurrence was 9 days in the placebo group, and 35 days (hazard ratio [HR] 0.60; 95% CI=0.43-0.86; p=0.004) and 44 days (HR 0.55; 95% CI=0.36-0.82; p=0.003) in the propafenone SR 325 and 425 mg groups, respectively. The time-to-recurrence between the 2 propafenone groups was not significant (HR 0.84; 95% CI=0.57-1.25, p=0.40). In the secondary efficacy outcome, there was also a significantly increased time to first recurrence in the propafenone groups vs placebo: propafenone 325 mg, 23 days, HR 0.61, 95% CI=0.43-0.85, p=0.003; propafenone 425 mg, 28 days, HR 0.66, 95% CI=0.45-0.96, p=0.03, placebo=9 days. There was no difference between the propafenone groups (HR 0.99, 95% CI=0.69-1.43, p=0.96). There was a significant reduction in the average heart rate (approximately 10 bpm) during the first symptomatic recurrence in the 325 mg propafenone group vs the placebo group. The median time to atrial arrhythmia, symptomatic or asymptomatic, was 23, 29, and 8 days for the propafenone 325 mg, 425 mg, and placebo groups, respectively. The median time to treatment failure was 8 days in the placebo group, 19 days in the propafenone 325 mg group (p=0.002), and 24 days in the propafenone 425 mg group (p=0.006). The number of patients reporting an adverse event was greater in the propafenone groups vs placebo; (propafenone 325 mg, 53.2%: 425 mg, 51.7%; and placebo, 28.0%). The number of patients with at least 1 serious adverse event was higher in the propafenone groups vs placebo (propafenone 325 mg, 9.9%; 425 mg, 11.2%; and placebo, 1.1%). The most common adverse events in the propafenone groups were first-degree atrioventricular block and sinus bradycardia. There was a higher incidence of serious adverse cardiovascular events in the propafenone groups vs placebo; 1% in the placebo group vs 5% and 7% in the propafenone SR 325 mg and 425 mg groups, respectively. Events occurring most frequently were AF (5 patients) in the placebo group and atrial flutter (2 patients).

GEMICA

Grupo de Estudios Multricentricos en Argentina

Title	Morbidity and mortality following early administration of amiodarone in acute myocardial infarction.
Authors	Elizari MV, Martinez JM, Belziti C, et al.
Reference	Eur Heart J 2000;21:198-205.
Disease	Acute myocardial infarction.
Purpose	To evaluate the effects of amiodarone on mortality and morbidity in the first few hours after acute myocardial infarction.
Design	Randomized, double-blind, placebo-controlled, multicenter.
Patients	1073 patients within 24 hours of onset of an acute myocardial infarction. Patients with systolic BP <100 mm Hg, heart rate <60 bpm, atrioventricular block, intraventricular block, long QT, severe heart failure, ventricular or supraventricular arrhythmia, significant liver disease, or amiodarone treatment within the last 3 months were excluded.
Follow-up	180 days.
Regimen	Randomization to either placebo (n=531) or amiodarone (n=542). Study drug was initiated within the first 24 hours of onset of symptoms, and in those receiving thrombolytic therapy, amiodarone was administered immediately after the thrombolytic drug. Patients received amiodarone IV for 48 hours for a total dose of 2700 mg. Oral amiodarone 600 mg bid was initiated immediately and continued for 4 days. From day 5 to day 90 patients received placebo or amiodarone 400 mg/d, and then 200 mg/d for the next 90 days. After the first 516 patients were analyzed, the Safety and Monitoring Board suggested changing the IV amiodarone dose to 1200 mg over 48 hours and the oral amiodarone to 800 mg/d for 2 days, 400 mg/d from day 3 to day 90, and then 200 mg/d for the next 90 days.

Add'l Tx	Reperfusion therapy by either thrombolytic drugs or PCI was permitted. Aspirin, nitrates, β-blockers, digitalis, diuretics, calcium channel blockers, and ACE inhibitors were permitted.
Results	The study was terminated early by the Safety and Monitoring Board, because amiodarone did not have an effect on 30-day survival. A total of 270 patients received high dose amiodarone and 246 received placebo. Total mortality was 16.3% with amiodarone vs 10.2% with placebo (OR 1.72; 95% CI=0.99-3.01; p=0.04). Cardiac mortality was 9.6% vs 7.7%, respectively (OR 1.27; 95% CI=0.66-2.47; p=0.40), and noncardiac mortality was 6.7% vs 2.4% (OR 2.86; 95% CI=1.05-8.19; p=0.02). More patients in the amiodarone group were hospitalized (32.6% vs 23.2%; p=0.01). However, fewer patients in the amiodarone group had postinfarction angina (19.6% vs 30.9%; p=0.003). Amiodarone did not reduce the incidence of nonfatal arrhythmic events (9.6% vs 10.6%; p=0.70). Hypotension was detected more often in the amiodarone group (11.5% vs 4.9%). A total of 272 patients received the lower dose of amiodarone and 285 patients received the placebo. Total mortality was 6.6% in the amiodarone group vs 9.5% in the placebo group (p=0.20). Cardiac mortality was 3.3% vs 6.0% (p=0.10), and noncardiac mortality was 3.3% vs 3.5% (p=0.80). Fewer patients in the amiodarone group had postinfarction angina (19.1% vs 29.8%; OR 0.56; 95% CI=0.37-0.84; p=0.004). There was no difference in readmission rate (25.7% vs 27.4%; p=0.60). Hypotension occurred in 4.0% of the amiodarone vs 4.6% in the control group.
Concl.	Early administration of high dose amiodarone was associated with increased mortality, especially noncardiac mortality. Low dose amiodarone did not significantly affect mortality. Early administration of low dose amiodarone in acute MI may be used only to treat life threatening arrhythmia.

MADIT-II

Multicenter Automatic Defibrillator Implantation Trial-II

Title	Prophylactic implantation of a defibrillator in patients with myocardial infarction and reduced ejection fraction.
Authors	Moss AJ, Zareba W, Hall WJ, et al.
Reference	N Engl J Med 2002;346:877-883.
Disease	Myocardial infarction, left ventricular dysfunction, arrhythmia.
Purpose	To investigate the effects of prophylactic implantation of automatic defibrillator (AD) on survival of patients with left ventricular (LV) dysfunction (LV ejection fraction ≤30%) after myocardial infarction.
Design	Randomized, open-label, multicenter.
Patients	1232 patients, >21 years old, with a prior myocardial infarction (>1 month before enrollment), and LVEF ≤30%. Patients with FDA approved indication for AD implantation, New York Heart Association (NYHA) class IV, revascularization in the preceding 3 months, advanced cerebrovascular disease, serious non-cardiac disease, and myocardial infarction within the preceding month were excluded.
Follow-up	Average 20 months (range 6 days to 53 months).
Regimen	Randomization to AD implantation (Guidant, St. Paul, MN) or conventional medical therapy in a ratio of 3:2.
Results	54 crossovers occurred (4.5% of the patients in the conventional therapy received AD, 2.8% of the patients in the AD group did not undergo AD implantation, and in 1.5% the AD was removed during follow-up). Mortality was 14.2% in the AD group vs 19.8% in the conventional therapy group (hazard ratio 0.69; 95% CI=0.51-0.93; p=0.016). The survival curves began to separate at approximately 9 months after enrollment and continued to diverge. Mortality was reduced by 12% after 1 year, 28% after 2 years, and 28% after 3 years. Subgroup analysis according to age, gender, LVEF, NYHA class, or the QRS interval showed similar survival effect in all subgroups.

Concl.   Prophylactic implantation of an AD in patients with LVEF
           ≤30% after myocardial infarction resulted in improved sur-
           vival. AD implantation should be considered for patients with
           advanced LV dysfunction after myocardial infarction.

MOST

Mode Selection Trial in Sinus-Node Dysfunction

Title	Ventricular pacing or dual-chamber pacing for sinus-node dysfunction.
Authors	Lamas GA, Lee KL, Sweeney MO, et al.
Reference	N Engl J Med 2002;346:1854-1862.
Disease	Sinus node dysfunction.
Purpose	To determine whether dual-chamber (atrioventricular) pacing results in better outcome than single-chamber (ventricular) pacing in patients requiring pacing for bradycardia due to sinus-node dysfunction.
Design	Randomized, blinded, controlled, and multicenter.
Patients	2010 patients with sinus-node dysfunction requiring a pacemaker.
Follow-up	33.1 months.
Regimen	Following positioning of atrial and ventricular leads, pacemaker programmed to rate-modulated dual-chamber pacing (n=1014) or rate-modulated ventricular pacing (n=996) before implantation.
Results	Primary end point was death or nonfatal stroke. Primary end point occurred in 21.5% of patients with dual-chamber pacing vs 23.0% of patients with ventricular pacing (p=0.48). There was no difference in rate of hospitalization for heart failure, stroke, or death between groups. The risk of atrial fibrillation was lower in patients with dual-chamber pacing (hazard ratio [HR] 0.79; 95% CI=0.66-0.94; p=0.008). 10.3% of patients randomized to dual-chamber pacing were hospitalized for heart failure vs 12.3% of patients that received ventricular pacing (HR 0.82; 95% CI=0.63-1.06; p=0.13). There was a small increase in quality of life in the dual-chamber pacing groups.
Concl.	In patients with sinus-node dysfunction dual-chamber pacing did not reduce rate of death or nonfatal stroke but did reduce the risk of atrial fibrillation, reduced hospitalizations for heart failure, and improved quality of life.

MUSTT

Multicenter Unsustained Tachycardia Trial Investigation

Title	A randomized study of the prevention of sudden death in patients with coronary artery disease.
Authors	Buxton AE, Lee KL, Fisher JD, et al.
Reference	N Engl J Med 1999;341:1882-1890.
Disease	Sudden death, coronary artery disease.
Purpose	To determine whether electrophysiologically guided antiarrhythmic therapy would decrease sudden cardiac death in patients with coronary heart disease, LV ejection fraction of ≤40%, and asymptomatic, unsustained ventricular tachycardia (VT).
Design	Multicenter, randomized.
Patients	704 patients with coronary artery disease, LV ejection fraction of ≤40%, asymptomatic unsustained VT who had inducible sustained VT on electrophysiologic testing.
Follow-up	5 years.
Regimen	Antiarrhythmic therapy guided by results of electrophysiologic testing or no antiarrhythmic therapy. Drugs were assigned randomly with the exception of amiodarone (amiodarone could be given if 2 tests had failed). Implantable defibrillator could be given after 1 unsuccessful drug test.
Add'l Tx	ACE inhibitors, β-blockers in some patients.

Results	Of 704 patients who were randomized 351 were assigned to electrophysiologically guided therapy and 353 to no antiarrhythmic therapy. The primary end point of cardiac arrest or death from arrhythmia was reached in 25% of patients receiving electrophysiologically guided therapy vs 32% of patients assigned to no antiarrhythmic therapy (RR 0.73; 95% CI=0.53-0.99) representing a 27% reduction in risk (p=0.04). 5 year estimates of overall mortality were 42% and 48% in treated vs nontreated group (RR 0.80; 95% CI=0.64-1.01; p=0.06). Treatment with implantable defibrillators was associated with a lower risk of cardiac arrest or death from arrhythmias than patients discharged without defibrillators (RR 0.24; 95% CI=0.13-0.45; p<0.001). Rate of cardiac arrest or death from arrhythmia nor overall mortality rate was lower among patients assigned to electrophysiologically guided therapy and treated with antiarrhythmic drugs compared to patients in the untreated group that did not receive antiarrhythmic drugs.
Concl.	While electrophysiologically guided therapy with subsequent therapy with implantable defibrillators reduced the risk of cardiac arrest or death from arrhythmias in high risk patients, antiarrhythmic drugs alone were not successful.

MUSTT

Multicenter Unsustained Tachycardia Trial (Substudy)

Title	Effect of implantable defibrillators on arrhythmic events and mortality in the multicenter unsustained tachycardia trial.
Authors	Lee KL, Hafley G, Fisher JD, et al.
Reference	Circulation 2002;106:233-238.
Disease	Arrhythmias.
Purpose	To analyze the previously published Multicenter Unsustained Tachycardia Trial (MUSTT) and determine the contribution of defibrillators in reducing the risk of arrhythmic death or cardiac arrest in patients with inducible sustained ventricular tachycardia (VT) who were randomized to antiarrhythmic therapy.
Design	Retrospective analysis of a multicenter, randomized, prospective study.
Patients	704 patients with coronary artery disease, LV ejection fraction of ≤40%, and asymptomatic unsustained VT with inducible sustained VT electrophysiologic testing.
Follow-up	5 years.
Regimen	Per MUSTT.
Add'l Tx	Per MUSTT.

Results   704 patients were randomized: 353 to control and 351 to electro-physiologically (EP)-guided therapy. Patients in the EP-guided therapy group either received an implantable defibrillator (ICD) together with antiarrhythmic drug therapy (n=196) or antiarrhythmic drug therapy alone (n=155). Control patients received no antiarrhythmic treatment. The primary end point in the analyzed study was death due to arrhythmia or resuscitated cardiac arrest. Study results were reanalyzed to determine if there was a benefit from EP-guided therapy according to enrollment date, frequency of ICD use at site, and whether use of ICD was independently associated with a decreased risk of arrhythmic death or cardiac arrest. Patients enrolled before Jan 1, 1994 comprised 41% of the entire cohort. Patients in the EP-guided group were less likely to have received an ICD prior to this date (41% vs 66% ICD placement after Jan 1, 1994); this was due to post-1994 availability of non-thoracotomy ICD systems and a protocol change allowing defibrillator implantation after only 1 drug trial failure. No benefit in arrhythmic death or cardiac arrest was observed for EP-guided therapy vs no-anti-arrhythmic therapy group in the pre-1994 cohort (hazard ratio [HR] 1.03; 95% CI=0.68-1.57; p=0.874), but benefit was seen in the post-1994 cohort (HR 0.46; 95% CI=0.28-0.76; p=0.002) during which time use of ICD was markedly increased. Study sites varied in the percentage of patients who received ICDs; implantation rates ranged from 0-100%. Sites were grouped according to frequency of ICD usage and categorized as low (less than one third of patients on EP-guided therapy received ICDs), medium (one third to two thirds received ICDs) and high-use (more than two thirds received ICDs). The low-use group had an ICD implantation rate of 24% of patients in the EP-guided therapy group; medium, 52%, and high, 84%. There was no observable benefit of EP-guided therapy in the low-use group; rather, there was a higher risk of arrhythmic death or cardiac arrest in the therapy group vs control (HR 1.30; 95% CI=0.68-2.48; p=0.427). In sites with medium-level usage of ICDs, there was a trend favoring EP-guided therapy vs control (HR 0.75; 95% CI=0.49-1.15; p=0.182). Sites with high-level usage of ICD showed a significant benefit for EP-guided therapy (HR 0.36; CI=0.17-0.75; p=0.004). The risk of arrhythmic death or cardiac arrest in patients who received ICD was decreased by >70% (p<0.001) vs EP-guided patients who did not receive an ICD, or control. In addition, ICD placement decreased the risk of all-cause mortality by >50% (p<0.001). Patients in the EP-guided group who did not receive an ICD had a slightly worse outcome than control patients (HR for arrhythmic death or cardiac arrest 1.12 [0.79-1.59] and total mortality 1.08 [0.82-1.42]).

Concl.	Observed benefits in patients who underwent EP-guided therapy in the MUSTT trial were due to improved outcomes from ICD placement and not antiarrhythmic drug therapy.

ORCA

Optimized Response to Cardiac Arrest

Title	Multicenter, randomized, controlled trial of 150-J biphasic shocks compared with 200- to 360-J monophasic shocks in the resuscitation of out-of-hospital cardiac arrest victims. Optimized Response to Cardiac Arrest (ORCA) investigators.
Authors	Schneider T, Martens PR, Paschen H, et al.
Reference	Circulation 2000;102:1780-1787.
Disease	Ventricular fibrillation, cardiac arrest.
Purpose	To compare a 150-J impedance-compensating biphasic truncated exponential waveform automatic external defibrillator with traditional, energy escalating monophasic AEDs for victims of cardiac arrest in out-of-hospital situations.
Design	Prospective, randomized, multicenter.
Patients	115 patients with known or suspected cardiac arrest, who were attended by emergency medical services, and had presented with ventricular fibrillation.
Follow-up	Through hospital discharge.
Regimen	150-J impedance-compensating biphasic truncated exponential AEDs or 200- to 360-J monophasic AEDs. For the former, a sequence of 3 consecutive 150-J biphasic shocks delivered; for later 200, 200- to 360-J monophasic shocks delivered.
Add'l Tx	CPR, local protocols if above failed.

Results	Primary end point was percentage of patients with ventricular fibrillation who were defibrillated in the first series of ≤3 shocks. Secondary end points were defibrillation with ≤2 shocks, first-shock defibrillation, survival to hospital admission and discharge. The 150-J biphasic waveform defibrillated at higher rates, resulting in more patients who had a return of spontaneous circulation. For the primary end point of defibrillation with first 1-3 shocks, 53 of 54 (98%) were successful with 150-J biphasic shocks vs 42 of 61 (69%) with 200- to 360-J monophasic shocks (p<0.0001). 96% were defibrillated with the initial biphasic shock vs with the initial monophasic shock (59%; p<0.0001). After 150-J biphasic-waveform defibrillation, 76% of patients achieved return of spontaneous circulation vs 54% with high-energy monophasic-waveform defibrillation (54%; p=0.01). Survival rates to hospital admission and discharge did not differ between groups. Of patients surviving to hospital discharge, 87% resuscitated with 150-J biphasic shocks had good cerebral status vs 53% with high-energy monophasic shocks (p=0.04).
Concl.	Low-energy impedance-compensating biphasic waveform resulted in superior defibrillation vs escalating high-energy monophasic shocks in out-of-hospital cardiac arrest.

PIAF

Pharmacologic Intervention in Atrial Fibrillation

Title	Rhythm or rate control in atrial fibrillation-Pharmacologic Intervention in Atrial Fibrillation (PIAF): a randomised trial.
Authors	Hohnolser SH, Kuck K-H, Lilienthal J, for the PIAF Investigators.
Reference	Lancet 2000;356:1789-1794.
Disease	Atrial fibrillation.
Purpose	To compare 2 strategies in patients with atrial fibrillation: maintaining sinus rhythm with antiarrhythmic drugs or ventricular rate control without attempting to convert to sinus rhythm.
Design	Randomized, open-label, prospective, pilot study.
Patients	252 patients, 18-75 years old, with symptomatic persistent (7-360 days duration) atrial fibrillation. Patients with congestive heart failure, New York Heart Association class IV, unstable angina, recent (<30 days) myocardial infarction, slow (<50 BPM) ventricular response, known sick sinus syndrome, Wolf-Parkinson-White syndrome, recent (<3 months) cardiac surgery, intracardiac thrombus, embolisation within 3 months, hypertrophic cardiomyopathy, amiodarone therapy within the past 6 months, acute thyroid dysfunction, pacemaker, pregnancy and contraindications for anticoagulation therapy were excluded.
Follow-up	1 year.
Regimen	Patients were randomized to either ventricular rate control or cardioversion with an attempt to maintain sinus rhythm using antiarrhythmic drugs. In the rate control group patients received diltiazem (90 mg X2-3/d). If diltiazem was not sufficient to control ventricular rate, additional therapy was left to the discretion of the treating physician. In the rhythm control group patients underwent pharmacological cardioversion with amiodarone 600 mg/d for 3 weeks. If sinus rhythm had not been restored, patients underwent electrical cardioversion. Thereafter, patients received amiodarone 200 mg/d. In case of recurrence of atrial fibrillation, therapeutic decisions were left to the treating physicians.

Add'l Tx	All patients received anticoagulation therapy with a target international normalized ratio of 2.0-3.0 throughout the entire study period.
Results	There were 125 patients in the rate control group and 127 in the rhythm control group. Only 23% of the patients in the rhythm control group converted to sinus rhythm with amiodarone loading. The rest of the patients in this group underwent at least 1 electrical cardioversion. In the rate control group only 10% of the patients were in sinus rhythm after 1 year, compared with 56% of the patients in the rhythm control group (p<0.001). During follow-up, 2 patients in each group died. 4 patients crossed over from rate control to rhythm control strategy and 6 from rhythm control to rate control strategy. Symptomatic improvement occurred in a similar percentage of patients in both groups. At 1 year improvement was noted in 61% of the patients in the rate control group vs 55% in the rhythm control group; p=0.317). In contrast, 6-minute walk test was better in the rhythm control group than in the rate control group (p=0.008 at 1 year). More patients in the rhythm control group were hospitalized (69% vs 24%; p=0.001). The most frequent cause for admission in the rhythm control group was admission for electrical cardioversion (67% of all admissions) or for amiodarone-related adverse effects (27%). In the rate control group, most admissions were related to drug-related adverse effects (68% of all admissions).
Concl.	Both treatment strategies were comparable with respect to symptomatic improvement. However, exercise performance was better with the rhythm control strategy, although it resulted in more hospital admissions. The results of the PIAF study may have important implications for therapeutic decisions in patients with symptomatic persistent atrial fibrillation.

SAFIRE-D

Symptomatic Atrial Fibrillation Investigative Research on Dofetilide Study

Title	Efficacy and safety of oral dofetilide in converting to and maintaining sinus rhythm in patients with chronic atrial fibrillation or atrial flutter: The SAFIRE-D study.
Authors	Singh S, Zoble RG, Yellen L, et al.
Reference	Circulation 2000;102:2385-2390.
Disease	Atrial fibrillation/atrial flutter.
Purpose	To determine efficacy and safety of dofetilide in converting atrial fibrillation or atrial flutter to sinus rhythm and maintaining sinus rhythm for 1 year.
Design	Randomized, double-blind, placebo-controlled, dose-ranging, multicenter.
Patients	325 patients with atrial fibrillation or atrial flutter.
Follow-up	12-month.
Regimen	Randomized to 125, 250, or 500 μg dofetilide or placebo twice daily. Dosages adjusted for QTc response and creatinine clearance.
Add'l Tx	If after receiving a minimum of 5 doses of study drug without pharmacologic cardioversion, electrical cardioversion attempted. Anticoagulation before cardioversion and continued for 3-4 weeks after sinus rhythm re-established.

Results   277 patients (85%) had atrial fibrillation and 48 (15%) had atrial flutter. Pharmacologic cardioversion occurred at 6.1%, 9.8%, and 29.9% at the 125, 250, and 500 μg dose of dofetilide, respectively vs only 1.2% for placebo (p=0.015, 250 μg dose vs placebo; p<0.001 for 500 μg dose vs placebo). 70% of pharmacologic cardioversions occurred within 24 hours of dofetilide and 91% within 36 hours. Probability of remaining in sinus rhythm for those who cardioverted with dofetilide was 0.40, 0.37, and 0.58 at the 125, 250, and 500 μg dofetilide dose, respectively; vs 0.25 for placebo (p=0.001 for 500 μg dose vs placebo). Torsade de pointes occurred in 1 case on day 2 and 1 case on day 3 (0.8% of all patients on dofetilide); there was 1 case of sudden death thought to be pro-arrhythmic on day 8 (0.4% of all patients on active drug).

Concl.   The new class III antiarrhythmic drug, dofetilide, was moderately effective in cardioverting atrial fibrillation or flutter to sinus rhythm and effective in maintaining sinus rhythm for 1 year.

STAF

The Strategies of Treatment of Atrial Fibrillation

Title	Randomized trial of rate-control vs rhythm-control in persistent atrial fibrillation.
Authors	Carlsson J, Miketic S, Windeler J, et al.
Reference	J Am Coll Cardiol 2003;41:1690-1696.
Disease	Atrial fibrillation.
Purpose	To compare 2 treatment strategies: rhythm control vs rate control in patients with atrial fibrillation who were at high risk of arrhythmia recurrence.
Design	Open, randomized, controlled pilot trial, multicenter.
Patients	200 patients with persistent atrial fibrillation. Had to be ≥18 years and have 1 or more of the following criteria: atrial fibrillation for >4 weeks; left atrium greater than 45 minutes in diameter, CHF-NYHA class II or worse; LVEF <45%; or ≥1 prior cardioversion with recurrence of arrhythmia. Exclusion criteria included permanent atrial fibrillation for more than 2 years, a history of paroxysmal atrial fibrillation, left atrium >70 mm; LVEF <20%, Wolff-Parkinson-White syndrome, and others.
Follow-up	19.6±8.9 months.
Regimen	Patients randomized to rhythm-control to be cardioverted by external or internal cardioversion; Class I antiarrhythmic agents or sotalol if no CAD and if LV function normal. Patients with CAD or LV dysfunction to receive β-blocker and or amiodarone. Patients randomized to rate-control received β-blockers, digitalis, calcium channel blockers, or AV node ablation, modification with or without pacemaker.
Add'l Tx	Oral anticoagulants for both treatments given according to published guidelines.

Results	Primary end point was combination of death, stroke, transient ischemic attack, systemic embolism, and CPR. At 19.6 months primary end point was similar between rhythm-control (9/100; 5.54%/yr) vs rate-control (10/100; 6.09%/yr; p=0.99). Only 23% of patients in the rhythm control group were still in sinus rhythm after up to 4 cardioversions, at 36 months. Total mortality was 2.5% and 4.9%/yr in the rhythm-controlled vs the rate-control group, respectively. The rhythm-control group experienced 3.1%/yr cerebrovascular events vs 0.6% in the rate-control group. 18/19 primary end points occurred while patients were in atrial fibrillation; only 1 (stroke) occurred while a patient was in sinus rhythm. As expected, hospitalizations were more common in the rhythm control group (n=54) vs the rate control group (n=26).
Concl.	There was no difference in rhythm control (restoration and maintenance of sinus rhythm) vs rate control (pharmacologic or invasive rate control and anticoagulation) for the primary end points in patients with atrial fibrillation.

STAF

The Strategies of Treatment of Atrial Fibrillation

Title	Randomized trial of rate-control vs rhythm control in persistent atrial fibrillation.
Authors	Carlsson J, Miketic S, Windeler J, et al.
Reference	J Am Coll Cardiol 2003;41:1690-1696.
Disease	Atrial fibrillation.
Purpose	To compare a rhythm control strategy (restoration and maintenance of sinus rhythm) vs a rate-control strategy (pharmacologic or invasive rate control + anticoagulation) in patients with atrial fibrillation.
Design	Open, randomized, controlled, multicenter.
Patients	200 patients with persistent atrial fibrillation. Patients had to have 1 or more of the following: atrial fibrillation for more than 4 weeks; left atrial size >45 mm; congestive heart failure class II or greater; left ventricular ejection fraction <45%; or ≥1 prior cardioversion with arrhythmia recurrence. Patients were excluded if they had permanent atrial fibrillation >2 years, history of paroxysmal atrial fibrillation, left atrial size >70 mm, left ventricular ejection fraction <20%, Wolff-Parkinson White syndrome, contraindications to oral anticoagulation, and others.
Follow-up	Average follow-up 19.6 months. Up to 36 months.
Regimen	For patients randomized to rhythm control: cardioversion by external or internal cardioversion and prophylaxis of recurrent atrial fibrillation including class I antiarrhythmic drugs or sotalol in the absence of coronary artery disease and in patients with normal left ventricular function. Those with coronary artery disease or impaired left ventricular function were to receive a β-blocker and/or amiodarone. Repeated cardioversion could be performed. Patients randomized to rate control could receive β-blockers, digitalis, calcium blocker, or atrioventricularnode ablation modification with or without pacemaker. Oral anticoagulation therapy was given in both strategies according to guidelines of the American College of Chest Physicians.

Results   The primary end point was the combined end point of death, cardiopulmonary resuscitation, cerebrovascular event, and systemic embolism. There was no significant difference in the end point between the rhythm control (9/100; 5.54%/y) vs the rate-control (10/100; 6.09%/y; p=0.99) groups at 19.6 months. 18 primary end points occurred while patients were in atrial fibrillation vs only 1 while they were in sinus rhythm. At 36 months, the percent of patients in sinus rhythm in the rhythm-control group (after even multiple cardioversions) was only 23%. Total mortality was 2.5% with rhythm control and 4.9% with rate control. Cerebrovascular events occurred at a rate of 3.1%/y in the rhythm control group vs 0.6%/y in the rate-control group. Of 5 cerebrovascular events that occurred in the rhythm control group, 3 occurred under full anticoagulation (international normalized ratio [INR] >2); and 2 at an INR of <2. There was no difference in occurrence of syncope or bleeding complications between groups. 54 hospitalizations for cardiovascular disease were reported in the rhythm control group vs 26 in the rate-control group (p<0.001).

Concl.   There were no differences between rhythm or rate control for atrial fibrillation for the primary end points. Hospitalizations were more frequent in the rhythm control group.

SVA-3

Azimilide Supraventricular Arrhythmia Program-3

Title	Antiarrhythmic effects of azimilide in atrial fibrillation: efficacy and dose-response.
Authors	Pritchett ELC, Page RL, Connolly SJ, et al.
Reference	J Am Coll Cardiol 2000;36:794-802.
Disease	Atrial fibrillation.
Purpose	To assess effectiveness of azimilide in decreasing frequency of symptomatic arrhythmia in patients with atrial fibrillation and/or flutter.
Design	Randomized, placebo-controlled, multicenter.
Patients	384 patients with history of symptomatic atrial fibrillation, atrial flutter, or both and judged to be candidates for anti-arrhythmic therapy. Electrocardiograph showing atrial fibrillation or flutter within 24 hours of randomization; patients had to be in sinus rhythm at time of randomization.
Follow-up	180 day efficacy phase.
Regimen	Patients randomized to placebo (n=93) or azimilide 50 mg (n=101), 100 mg (n=97), or 125 mg (n=93). There was a 3 day loading period in which the drug was given twice a day and then reduced to once-a-day for 180 day efficacy period.

Results   Primary end point was time to first symptomatic arrhythmia
             recurrence documented by an ECG (transtelephonic ECG
             recording) showing atrial fibrillation, atrial flutter or paroxys-
             mal supraventricular arrhythmia in combined azimilide 100 mg
             and 125 mg dose vs placebo using log-rank test. Of initial 384
             randomized patients, 367 entered efficacy phase in sinus rhythm
             after loading dose phase. Time to first symptomatic arrhythmia
             recurrence was significantly prolonged in combined azimilide
             dose group vs placebo (chi-square 7.96; p=0.005; hazard ratio
             [HR] [placebo:azimilide] 1.58; 95% CI=1.15-2.16). Median
             time to event was 17 days in the placebo group vs 60 days in
             the combined azimilide group. During the loading dose period
             19.3% of placebo patients had an event vs 15.8% of combined
             azimilide patients. Efficacy improved at higher doses of azimil-
             ide. Median time to first symptomatic arrhythmia recurrence
             was 17 days in placebo vs 22, 41, and 130 in the azimilide 50
             mg once daily, 100 mg and 125 mg dose, respectively. HR
             (placebo:azimilide) for placebo vs 100 mg dose was 1.38 (95%
             CI=0.96-1.98; p=0.08) and for 125 mg dose was 1.83 (95%
             CI=1.24-2.70; p=0.002).

Concl.   Azimilide (100 mg-125 mg) lengthened the symptomatic arrhyth-
             mia-free interval in patients with fibrillation and/or atrial flutter.

TRACE (Atrial Fibrillation Substudy)

Trandolapril Cardiac Evaluation

Title	Trandolapril reduces the incidence of atrial fibrillation after acute myocardial infarction in patients with left ventricular dysfunction.
Authors	Pedersen OD, Bagger H, Kober L, et al.
Reference	Circulation 1999;100:376-380.
Disease	Atrial fibrillation.
Purpose	To determine whether the ACE inhibitor trandolapril could reduce the incidence of atrial fibrillation in patients with left ventricular dysfunction following acute myocardial infarction.
Design	Randomized, double-blind, placebo-controlled, multicenter study.
Patients	Of 1749 patients who had been entered into the original TRACE study, 1577 had sinus rhythm at randomization. Impaired LV function by echocardiography with randomization between 3-7 days after onset of acute myocardial infarction.
Follow-up	4 years.
Regimen	790 patients randomized to trandolapril; 787 to placebo. Trandolapril initially given as 1 mg/d, then increased to 2 mg/d before hospital discharge. At about 4 weeks after myocardial infarction dose was increased to 4 mg/d. Dose adjustment if necessary.
Add'l Tx	As per physician.
Results	During the follow-up period, 42 (5.3%) patients developed atrial fibrillation in the placebo group vs 22 (2.8%) in the trandolapril group (p<0.05). After adjusting for a number of baseline characteristics, trandolapril significantly decreased the risk of developing atrial fibrillation (risk reduction [RR]=0.45; 95% CI=0.26-0.76; p<0.01). Factors associated with development of atrial fibrillation included severe congestive heart failure at baseline, LV function, male sex, digitalis use at baseline, age, and systolic blood pressure. There was a nonsignificant trend toward higher mortality in patients that developed atrial fibrillation (RR 1.2; 95% CI=0.73-2.06; p=NS).

Concl.   Trandolapril decreased the incidence of atrial fibrillation in post MI patients with LV dysfunction.

UKPACE

United Kingdom Pacing and Cardiovascular Events Trial

Reference	Presented by Toff WD at the ACC 52nd Annual Scientific Session, Chicago, IL 2003.
Disease	High-degree AV block; arrhythmia.
Purpose	To compare the long-term costs and clinical outcomes of DDD vs VVI and VVIR (rate-adaptive single-chamber ventricular pacing) in patients ≥70 years old with high-degree AV block undergoing permanent pacemaker implantation for their first time.
Design	Randomized, open-label, multicenter.
Patients	2021 patients, ≥70 years old, with high-degree AV block undergoing permanent pacemaker implantation for their first time. Patients with chronic atrial fibrillation, advanced cancer, New York Heart Association class IV heart failure, total immobility, or advanced cognitive impairment were excluded.
Follow-up	Median 4.6 years.
Regimen	Randomization to single-chamber pacing (25% of the patients VVI, 25% of the patients VVI-R) or to DDD pacing (50% of the patients).
Results	There was no difference in all-cause mortality (hazard ratio [HR] for VVI + VVI-R vs DDD 0.96; 95% CI=0.83-1.11; p=0.56) between the groups. The primary end point (atrial fibrillation ≥15 minutes, heart failure, stroke, transient ischemic attack (TIA), thromboembolism, revision of pacing system, new-onset angina, new onset ischemic heart disease, and MI) occurred at a similar rate in all 3 groups. No significant difference in the rate of atrial fibrillation was seen between the groups over a median follow-up of 3 years. Stroke, transient ischemic attack (TIA), and thromboembolism occurred more frequently in the VVI group than in the DDD group (HR 1.58; 95% CI=1.03-2.42; p=0.035). There was no difference in the rate of this outcome between the VVI-R and the DDD group (p=0.93). There was no difference in the incidence of heart failure (p=0.41), new onset angina/ ischemic heart disease (p=0.22), MI (p=0.22), or revision of pacing system (p=0.83) between the VVI + VVI-R groups and the DDD group.

| Concl. | No significant differences were found between VVI or VVI-R pacing and DDD pacing, although VVI pacing was associated with an increased risk for stroke, TIA, and thromboembolism. |

VPS II

Second Vasovagal Pacemaker Study

Title	Pacemaker therapy for prevention of syncope in patients with recurrent severe vasovagal syncope.
Authors	Connolly SJ, Sheldon R, Thorpe KE, et al.
Reference	JAMA 2003;289:2224-2229.
Disease	Syncope, arrhythmia.
Purpose	To determine whether pacing decreases the risk of syncope in patients who have recurrent vasovagal syncope.
Design	Randomized, double-blind, multicenter.
Patients	100 patients, >19 years, with a characteristic history of recurrent vasovagal syncope, having at least 6 episodes in their lifetime, or at least 3 episodes in the 2 years before enrollment. Patients were also required to have a positive head-up tilt table test. Exclusion criteria included important valvular, coronary artery, or myocardial disease, an abnormality on electrocardiogram, or other major disease.
Follow-up	6 months.
Regimen	Patients were randomized to receive either dual-chamber pacing (DDD) or sensing without pacing (ODO). Patients in the DDD group also received rate drop response pacing, which instituted rapid DDD pacing if a rapid decrease in heart rate was detected. The initial rate drop was set to be a drop size of at least 20 beats, a drop rate of 70 bpm, and an intervention rate of 100/min for 2 minutes.

Results	The primary study end point was syncope, defined as a transient loss of consciousness followed by prompt spontaneous recovery. Patients had a median of 4 syncopal episodes in the year before the study. The 2 groups were generally well matched. 12% of patients in the ODO group and 19% in the DDD group received b-blockers to treat vasovagal syncope; 10% and 2% received fludrocortisone, respectively, and 12% and 13% received selective serotonin reuptake inhibitors. 22 of the 52 patients in the ODO group had syncope within 6 months, compared with 16 of 48 patients in the DDD group. The cumulative risk of syncope at 6 months was 40% (95% CI=25-52%) in the ODO group and 31% (95% CI=17-43%) in the DDD group. The relative risk reduction on DDD pacing was 30% (95% CI=-33% to 63%; p=0.14). Subgroup analyses by age, duration of tilt test before syncope, and minimum heart rate of less than 50/min during the tilt test did not clarify in which groups of patients pacing was beneficial. Patients who received isoproterenol during the tilt test were significantly more likely to see benefit from pacing vs those who did not receive isoproterenol.
Concl.	The use of pacing therapy was not associated with a reduced risk of recurrent syncope in patients with recurrent vasovagal syncope.

Title	A randomized comparison of atrial and dual-chamber pacing in 177 consecutive patients with sick sinus syndrome: echocardiographic and clinical outcome.
Authors	Nielsen JC, Kristensen L, Andersen HR, et al.
Reference	J Am Coll Cardiol 2003;42:614-623.
Disease	Arrhythmia.
Purpose	To compare single-chamber atrial and dual-chamber pacing in patients with sick sinus syndrome.
Design	Multicenter, randomized trial.
Patients	177 consecutive patients with sick sinus syndrome.
Follow-up	Mean 2.9±1.1 years.
Regimen	Treatment with 1 of 3 rate-adaptive pacemakers: single-chamber atrial rate adaptive (AAIR) (n=54), dual-chamber rate adaptive (DDDR) with a short atrioventricular delay (DDDR-s, n=60), or DDDR with a fixed long atrioventricular delay (DDDR-l, n=63).
Results	Patients in the AAIR group showed no significant changes in echocardiographically measured left atrial (LA) or LV diameters or LV fractional shortening (LVFS). LA diameter increased in both DDDR groups (p<0.05); in the DDDR-s group, LVFS decreased (p<0.01). Atrial fibrillation was less common with AAIR (7.4% vs 23.3% in the DDDR-s group and 17.5% in the DDDR-l group; p=0.03). Mortality, thromboembolism, and CHF rates did not differ significantly; the annual mortality rate was 5.4%, 8.4%, and 8%, respectively, in the AAIR, DDDR-S, and DDDR-l groups. During follow-up, 31% vs 30% vs 46% of patients improved at least 1 New York Heart Association functional class, respectively.

Concl.   This is the first randomized trial to compare AAIR and DDDR
          pacing in patients with sick sinus syndrome and normal atrio-
          ventricular conduction. DDDR pacing increased LA diam-
          eter and DDDR-s pacing also decreased LVFS. There were no
          changes in LA or LV diameters or LVFS with AAIR pacing.
          Atrial fibrillation is less common with AAIR pacing. AAIR pac-
          ing is the preferred pacing mode in this patient population.

ATTEST

Atrial Therapy Efficacy and Safety Trial

Title	The effect of atrial pacing therapies on atrial tachyarrhythmia burden and frequency: results of a randomized trial in patients with bradycardia and atrial tachyarrhythmias.
Authors	Lee MA, Weachter R, Pollak S, et al.
Reference	J Am Coll Cardiol 2003;41:1926-1932.
Disease	Arrhythmia.
Purpose	To evaluate the efficacy and safety of preventive pacing and anti-tachycardia pacing (ATP) in patients with symptomatic atrial fibrillation or atrial tachycardia.
Design	International, multicenter, prospective, randomized study.
Patients	368 patients with symptomatic atrial fibrillation or atrial tachycardia.
Follow-up	3 months.
Regimen	Implantation of a DDDRP (Medtronic, Inc., Minneapolis, MN) pacemaker with 3 atrial preventive pacing algorithms and 2 ATP algorithms; random assignment 1 month postimplantation to all prevention and ATP therapies ON or OFF.
Results	A total of 271 patients had 17,018 atrial fibrillation/atrial tachycardia (AT/AF) episodes with stored electrograms. Appropriate detection was confirmed in 17,004 (99.9%). Activation of the prevention algorithms increased the relative amount of atrial pacing from 75% to 98% (p<0.001). The median amount of ventricular pacing was 99% in the ON group and 98% in the OFF group (p=0.005). ATP terminated 8590 (54%) of 15,789 treated episodes. The median AT/AF burden over 3 months was 4.2 h/mo ON vs 1.1 OFF (p=0.2). The median AT/AF frequency was 1.3 episodes/mo ON vs 1.2 off. System-related, complication-free survival at 4 months was 90.2% (Kaplan-Meier estimate). There were no significant differences in burden, total frequency, or symptomatic frequency between the ON and OFF groups.

Concl. The DDDRP pacemaker is safe, accurately detects AT/AF, and provides ATP with 54% efficacy. Atrial prevention and termination therapies combined did not reduce AT/AF burden or frequency. The failure of the atrial therapies to reduce burden or frequency may have been partially due to suppression of bradycardia-induced AT/AF by DDDR pacing.

DEFINITE

Defibrillators in Nonischemic Cardiomyopathy Treatment Evaluation

Title	Prophylactic defibrillator implantation in patients with nonischemic dilated cardiomyopathy.
Authors	Kadish A, Dyer A, Daubert JP, et al.
Reference	N Eng J Med 2004;350:2151-2158.
Disease	Dilated cardiomyopathy.
Purpose	To determine whether an implantable cardioverter-defibrillator can reduce the risk of death in patients with nonischemic cardiomyopathy and moderate to severe left ventricular dysfunction.
Design	Prospective, randomized, investigator-initiated study based on observational data.
Patients	458 patients with nonischemic dilated cardiomyopathy, left ventricular ejection fraction <36%, and premature ventricular complexes or nonsustained ventricular tachycardia.
Follow-up	Mean 29±14.4 months.
Regimen	Standard medical therapy (n=229) (angiotensin-converting enzyme inhibitors or, if contraindicated, hydralazine or nitrate or angiotensin receptor blocker; β-blocker required if tolerated) or standard medical therapy plus a single-chamber implantable cardioverter-defibrillator (n=229).
Add'l Tx	Digoxin, diuretics, to manage clinical symptoms.

Results	Mean LVEF was 21%. 86% of patients were taking ACE inhibitors and 85% β-blockers. 68 patients died: 28 in the implantable cardioverter-defibrillator (ICD) group and 40 in the standard therapy group (hazard ratio [HR] 0.65; 95% CI=0.40-1.06; p=0.08). At 2 years, the mortality rate was 14.1% in the standard-therapy group (annual mortality rate 7%) and 7.9% in the ICD group. There were 17 sudden deaths from arrhythmia: 3 in the ICD group and 14 in the standard therapy group (HR 0.20; 95% CI=0.06-0.71; p=0.006). 11 patients in the standard-therapy group and 9 in the ICD group died from CHF. There were 3 complications (1.3%) during ICD implantation: 1 hemothorax, 2 pneumothorax, and 1 cardiac tamponade. No patient died from a procedure-related complication. There were 10 complications during follow-up (4.4%): 6 lead dislodgements or fractures, 3 cases of venous thrombosis, and 1 infection. 41 patients received 91 appropriate ICD shocks and 49 received inappropriate shocks, primarily for atrial fibrillation or sinus tachycardia.
Concl.	ICD implantation in these patients with severe nonischemic dilated cardiomyopathy reduced the risk of sudden death from arrhythmia and was associated with an NS in mortality risk. Other large-scale trials evaluating the effect of prophylactic ICD implantation for prevention of sudden death focused on patients with CAD. Routine implantation of a ICD cannot be recommended for all patients with nonischemic cardiomyopathy and severe LV dysfunction; ICDs should be considered on a case-by-case basis.

Vasopressin vs Epinephrine for Cardiopulmonary Resuscitation

Title	A comparison of vasopressin and epinephrine for outof-hospital cardiopulmonary resuscitation.
Authors	Wenzel V, Krismer AC, Arntz HR, et al.
Reference	N Engl J Med 2004;350:105-113.
Disease	Out-of-hospital cardiac arrest.
Purpose	To determine the effects of vasopressin vs epinephrine on survival among adults who have an out-of-hospital cardiac arrest.
Design	Double-blind, prospective, multicenter, randomized, controlled.
Patients	1186 patients with out-ofhospital cardiac arrest presenting with ventricular fibrillation, pulseless electrical activity, or asystole requiring cardiopulmonary resuscitation.
Follow-up	Through hospital discharge.
Regimen	Patients with pulseless electrical activity or asystole were randomized immediately while those with ventricular fibrillation had 3 attempts at defibrillation and then were randomized if defibrillation was not successful. Either 1 mg of epinephrine or 40 IU of vasopressin was injected IV followed by 20 mL of normal saline. If spontaneous circulation did not occur within 3 minutes of the first injection, the same drug at the same dose was administered a second time. If the second injection did not restore circulation the patient was given an additional injection of epinephrine at the discretion of the physician. 589 patients were randomized to vasopressin vs 597 to epinephrine.
Add'l Tx	Sodium bicarbonate, atropine, lidocaine, amiodarone, fibrinolysis given at the discretion of the physician.

Results   The primary end point was survival to hospital admission. Secondary end point was survival to hospital discharge. Patients in both groups had similar baseline characteristics. 36.3% of the vasopressin group vs 31.2% of the epinephrine group survived to hospital admission (p=0.06). 9.9% of both groups achieved hospital discharge. In patients who presented with asystole, vasopressin was associated with higher rates of hospital admission (29% vs 20% in the epinephrine group; p=0.02) and hospital discharge (4.7% vs 1.5%; p=0.04). Hospital admission rates between the 2 groups were similar in those patients who presented with ventricular fibrillation (46.2% in the vasopressin group vs 43.0% in the epinephrine group; p=0.48). Hospital admission rates between the 2 groups also were similar in those patients who presented with pulseless electrical activity (33.7% in the vasopressin group vs 30.5% in the epinephrine group; p=0.65). Spontaneous circulation was not restored with 2 injections in 732 patients. In this group of patients additional epinephrine improved rates of survival to hospital admission in the vasopressin group (25.7%) vs the epinephrine group (16.4%; p=0.002). The additional epinephrine also improved rates of hospital discharge in the vasopressin group (6.2% vs 1.7%; p=0.002). The degree of cerebral performance among patients who survived to discharge did not differ between the vasopressin or epinephrine group. Also of note, rate of survival to hospital admission was higher among patients with a witnessed cardiac arrest (38.3%) than those with an unwitnessed cardiac arrest (16.1%; p<0.001). The rate of hospital admission was higher in patients who received basic life support within 10 minutes than those who received it more than 10 minutes after cardiac arrest (43.8% vs 20.7%; p<0.001).

Concl.   Vasopressin was superior to epinephrine in treating patients with asystole but was similar to epinephrine for treating those patients with ventricular fibrillation and pulseless electrical activity presenting for out-of-hospital cardiopulmonary resuscitation.

RAFT

Rythmol Atrial Fibrillation

Title	Efficacy and safety of sustained-release propafenone (propafenone SR) for patients with atrial fibrillation.
Authors	Pritchett EL, Page RL, Carlson M, et al.
Reference	Am J Cardiol 2003;92:941-946.
Disease	Atrial fibrillation.
Purpose	To study the efficacy of sustained-release preparation of propafenone in patients with atrial fibrillation.
Design	Randomized, placebo-controlled, multicenter.
Patients	523 patients, ≥21 years old, with a history of documented symptomatic atrial fibrillation, an indication for antiarrhythmic medications and sinus rhythm at enrollment. Patients with prior treatment with propafenone were excluded. Patients who had taken a class I or class III antiarrhythmic drug were required to discontinue it for 5 half-lives before enrollment; patients who had taken amiodarone were required to discontinue it for 6 months. Patients with permanent atrial fibrillation; New York Heart Association class III or IV angina pectoris; heart failure; Wolff-Parkinson-White syndrome; second- or third-degree atrioventricular block; QRS duration in sinus rhythm of >160 ms; heart rate of <50 bpm; blood pressure <90/60 mm Hg; implantable cardioverter-defibrillator implanted; history of sustained ventricular tachycardia or ventricular fibrillation; and neurologic symptoms were not included. In addition, patients with cardiac or thoracic surgery or acute pericarditis in the preceding 6 months or acute myocardial infarction/acute coronary syndrome within the preceding 12 months were not included.

9

Follow-up	Up to 39 weeks. Recurrent symptomatic arrhythmias were documented by transtelephone electrocardiographic monitoring.
Regimen	Patients were randomized to receive placebo or propafenone SR 225, 325, or 425 mg bid.
Add'l Tx	Patients were allowed to continue taking β-blockers, digitalis, and verapamil or diltiazem if they were taking these before randomization.
Results	The median time to the occurrence of a primary outcome event (symptomatic atrial arrhythmia) was 41 days in the placebo group, 112 days in the propafenone 225 group (hazard ratio [HR] 0.672; 95% CI=0.488-0.927; p=0.014 vs placebo), 291 days in the propafenone 325 group (HR 0.434; 95% CI=0.309-0.609; p<0.001 vs placebo), and >300 days in the propafenone 425 group (HR 0.353; 95% CI=0.243-0.513; p<0.001 vs placebo). Adverse effects leading to withdrawal from the study occurred more frequently in the propafenone 425 group than in the other 4 groups (13.5% in the placebo and 12.7%, 14.1%, and 25% in the propafenone 225, 325, and 425 groups, respectively). Fatigue, dizziness, dyspnea, taste disturbance, and constipation were reported more frequently in the propafenone groups than in the placebo group. Propafenone SR increased the PR interval and QRS duration in a dose-dependent way, but did not alter the QTc interval. None of the patients died or experienced ventricular tachycardia during the study.
Concl.	Propafenone SR was safe and effective in preventing recurrence of symptomatic atrial arrhythmia in stable patients with atrial fibrillation.

SPPAF

The Pilot Study of Prevention of Postoperative Atrial Fibrillation

Title	A comparison between oral antiarrhythmic drugs in the prevention of atrial fibrillation after cardiac surgery: the pilot study of prevention of postoperative atrial fibrillation (SPPAF), a randomized, placebo-controlled trial.
Authors	Auer J, Weber T, Berent R, et al.
Reference	Am Heart J 2004;147:636-643.
Disease	Atrial fibrillation.
Purpose	To determine whether oral drug regimens (oral amiodarone + metoprolol, metoprolol alone, or sotalol) were superior to placebo for preventing postoperative atrial fibrillation in patients undergoing cardiac surgery.
Design	Randomized, double-blinded, placebo-controlled trial.
Patients	253 patients undergoing cardiac surgery without congestive heart failure or left ventricular dysfunction. Cardiac surgery included coronary artery bypass graft surgery, valve surgery, or both.
Follow-up	Entire hospital stay.
Regimen	Patients were randomly assigned to 1 of 4 therapies: 1) metoprolol (50 mg bid) + oral amiodarone (1200 mg qd for 2 days divided into 3 single doses; then amiodarone 800 mg qd for the next 2 days; then 400 mg qd for 5 days); 2) metoprolol 50 mg bid; 3) 240 mg sotalol (divided into three daily doses); 4) placebo therapy started 24-48 hours prior to surgery and was continued for up to 8 days following surgery.

Results | The primary end point was development of atrial fibrillation (AF) detected by ECG. 35 of 65 (53.8%) patients in the placebo group developed AF vs 25 of 62 (40.3%) in the metoprolol alone group (p=0.16 vs placebo) vs 20 of 63 (31.7%) in the sotalol group (p=0.013 vs placebo) vs 19 of 63 (30.2%) in the amiodarone + metoprolol group (p=0.008 vs placebo). Adverse events such as postoperative ventricular tachycardia, in-hospital death, and hypotension were similar among the groups. Dose reduction or drug withdrawal due to bradycardia was necessary in 3.1% of the placebo patients, 3.2% of the combined amiodarone and metoprolol patients, 12.7% of the sotalol patients (p<0.05 vs placebo); and 16.1% of the metoprolol alone patients (p<0.05 vs placebo). There was an NS trend for patients in the placebo group to have a longer hospital stay (13.1 days) compared to those receiving active therapy (11.3 days).

Concl. | Atrial fibrillation is a common postoperative complication of cardiac surgery. Prophylaxis with amiodarone + metoprolol or sotalol reduced the rate of postoperative atrial fibrillation. Metoprolol alone resulted in an NS trend toward lowering post-operative atrial fibrillation.

9.Arrhythmia

VEPARAF

Verapamil Plus Antiarrhythmic Drugs Reduce Atrial Fibrillation

Title	VErapamil Plus Antiarrhythmic drugs Reduce Atrial Fibrillation recurrences after an electrical cardioversion (VEPARAF Study).
Authors	De Simone A, De Pasquale M, De Matteis C, et al.
Reference	Eur Heart J 2003;24:1425-1429.
Disease	Atrial fibrillation.
Purpose	To evaluate the efficacy of verapamil added to class IC or III antiarrhythmic drugs in reducing recurrence of atrial fibrillation after electrical cardioversion.
Design	Randomized, open label, multicenter.
Patients	363 patients, 18-85 years old, with persistent atrial fibrillation. Patients with atrial fibrillation for ≤21 days or ≥18 months, sick-sinus syndrome or pause >2.5 seconds during 24-hour Holter monitoring, trifascicular block or atrioventricular block, major liver or renal disease, myocardial infarction or revascularization within the preceding 6 months, severe congestive heart failure or respiratory insufficiency, and left ventricular ejection factor <0.35 were not included. In addition, patients with implantable pacing device, previous history of ventricular arrhythmia, long QT syndrome, cardiac arrest, and evidence of left atrial thrombus were excluded.
Follow-up	3 months.

Regimen	Randomization to: 1) oral amiodarone started 4 weeks before cardioversion; 2) oral amiodarone started 4 weeks before cardioversion + oral verapamil 240 mg/d; 3) oral flecainide 200 mg/d started 3 days before cardioversion; and 4) oral flecainide 200 mg/d started 3 days before cardioversion + verapamil 240 mg/d.
Add'l Tx	β-blockers, calcium channel blockers, and all other antiarrhythmic agents were stopped for ≥5 half lives and amiodarone was stopped for ≥1 month before randomization. All patients received warfarin with target international normalized ratio 2-3.
Results	There were 23 patients who converted to sinus rhythm spontaneously before cardioversion, without difference among the 4 groups. 13 patients dropped out because of study drug adverse effects. The final study group included 324 patients. During the 3 month follow-up period, 89 patients (27.5%) had recurrence of atrial fibrillation. Verapamil significantly reduced the recurrence rate of atrial fibrillation in both the amiodarone- and flecainide-treated patients (from 35% to 20%; p=0.004). The effect was significant in the flecainide treated patients (from 38% to 21%; p=0.02), but not in the amiodarone groups (from 32% to 20%; p=0.08). Stepwise logistic regression analysis showed that age, duration of atrial fibrillation, and the use of verapamil, but not amiodarone vs flecainide, were significantly associated with the risk of recurrence. Each of the 89 patients who had recurrence of atrial fibrillation was switched to the alternative group (patients who were on verapamil stopped their verapamil and patients who were off verapamil started verapamil). An additional episode of atrial fibrillation was detected in 77% of the patients who were now on amiodarone + verapamil, in 57% of those who were on flecainide + verapamil, in 81% of those who were on amiodarone alone, and in 88% who were on flecainide. Hence, the addition of verapamil to those who had recurrence on amiodarone alone or flecainide alone significantly reduced the risk of another episode vs discontinuing verapamil in the 2 combination groups (p=0.03).
Concl.	Verapamil, added to amiodarone or flecainide, reduced the risk of recurrence of atrial fibrillation after electrical cardioversion.

10. Anticoagulation for Atrial Fibrillation

ACUTE

Assessment of Cardioversion Using Transesophageal Echocardiography

Title	Use of transesophageal echocardiography to guide cardioversion in patients with atrial fibrillation.
Authors	Klein AL, Grimm RA, Murray RD, et al.
Reference	N Engl J Med 2001;344:1411-1420.
Disease	Atrial fibrillation.
Purpose	To compare conventional anticoagulation strategy with transesophageal echocardiography-guided short-term anticoagulant therapy in patients with atrial fibrillation considered for electrical cardioversion.
Design	Controlled, randomized, multicenter.
Patients	1222 patients with atrial fibrillation for more than 2 days duration.
Follow-up	8 weeks.
Regimen	Patients randomized to treatment strategy based on transesophageal echocardiography with brief anticoagulation or conventional anticoagulation guidelines. In TEE-guided group, in-patients received IV unfractionated heparin with TEE and cardioversion within 24 hours. Out-patients received warfarin (international normalized ratio 2.0-3.0) and TEE and cardioversion scheduled for 5 days later. Patients assigned to conventional therapy received warfarin for 3 weeks before cardioversion. All groups received warfarin for 4 weeks after cardioversion. Patients with thrombus detected by TEE received warfarin for 3 weeks and repeat TEE. If no thrombus was observed then direct current cardioversion was done; if thrombus was observed at end of 3 weeks, they received an additional 4 weeks of warfarin.

Results	Primary end point was composite of cerebrovascular accident, transient ischemic attack, and peripheral embolism. Secondary end points were major and minor hemorrhage, death, cardiac death, return to and maintenance of sinus rhythm, functional status. Of 619 patients assigned to TEE 425 (68.7%) had early cardioversion at a mean of 3 days; in 344 patients (80.9%) cardioversion was successful. 124 patients had TEE but no early electrical cardioversion (20%) and cardioversion was postponed in 76 (61%) due to visualization of thrombi. Of 603 in the conventional treatment group 333 (55%) underwent electrical cardioversion at a mean of 30 days and in 266 (80%) cardioversion was successful. Of 270 who did not undergo electrical cardioversion, 127 had spontaneous or chemical cardioversion. Patients in TEE group had a greater overall rate of successful restoration of sinus rhythm (71%) vs patients in conventional group (65%; p=0.03). Rate of embolism was low and similar between groups: 5 of 619 (0.8%) patients in TEE group vs 3 of 603 (0.5%) in convention therapy group (p=0.50). Hemorrhagic events were lower in TEE group (2.9%) vs conventional therapy (5.5%; p=0.03). There were no differences among groups in rates of death, maintenance of sinus rhythm or functional status at 8 weeks.
Concl.	TEE guided management of anticoagulation/cardioversion for atrial fibrillation is a clinically effective alternative strategy to conventional longer-term anticoagulation.

AFASAK 2

Copenhagen Atrial Fibrillation, Aspirin, and Anticoagulation 2

Title	Bleeding during warfarin and aspirin therapy in patients with atrial fibrillation.
Authors	Gulløv AL, Koefold BG, Petersen P.
Reference	a. Arch Intern Med. 1999;159:1322-1328. b. Arch Intern Med. 1998;158:1513-1521.
Disease	Atrial fibrillation.
Purpose	To determine the rate of bleeding as part of the AFASAK 2 study. Both major and minor bleeding was assessed.
Design	As per AFASAK 2.
Patients	670 patients in AFASAK 2 study.
Follow-up	≈3.5 years.
Regimen	Patients were randomized to: 1) warfarin sodium 1.25 mg/d; 2) warfarin sodium, 1.25 mg/d plus aspirin, 300 mg/d; 3) aspirin 300 mg/d; or 4) adjusted dose warfarin therapy to obtain an INR of 2.0-3.0 U.

Results   Major bleeding was defined as fatal life threatening or potentially life threatening. Minor bleeding was nonthreatening including overt or occult gastrointestinal bleeding, hemoptysis, gross hematuria, nose bleeding, bruising, symptomatic anemia due to bleeding, chronic bleeding. Median age was 77 years—range of 67-89 years. 19.2% (130 of 677 randomized patients) experienced any bleeding. 13 major (1 woman and 12 men) and 139 minor bleeding events occurred. 4 patients had intracranial bleeds; 2 of these were fatal. The annual rate of major bleeding was 0.8% for mini dose warfarin, 0.3% for warfarin plus aspirin, 1.4% for aspirin, and 1.1% for adjusted dose warfarin (p=0.20). Following 3 years of therapy, cumulate rate of bleeding was 24.7% in patients on mini dose warfarin, 24.4% on warfarin plus aspirin, 30.0% on aspirin, and 41.1% on adjusted dose warfarin (p=0.003 for adjusted dose warfarin vs the other groups). Independent risk factors for bleeding included adjusted dose warfarin therapy and prior myocardial infarction. Risk for bleeding increased with higher INR values.

Concl.   Incidence of major bleeding was low in patients on adjusted dose warfarin. This finding plus a lack of influence of age on risk of bleeding suggests that even elderly patients with atrial fibrillation can tolerate adjusted dose warfarin to an INR of 2-3.

10

PATAF

Primary Prevention of Arterial Thromboembolism in Nonrheumatic Atrial Fibrillation

Title	Primary prevention of arterial thromboembolism in non-rheumatic atrial fibrillation in primary care: randomised controlled trial comparing two intensities of coumarin with aspirin.
Authors	Hellemons BSP, Langenberg M, Lodder J, et al.
Reference	BMJ 1999;319:958-964.
Disease	Atrial fibrillation.
Purpose	To compare the effect of very low intensity (target international normalized ratio 1.1-1.6) and standard intensity (target INR 2.5-3.5) anticoagulation and of aspirin in patients with non-rheumatic atrial fibrillation.
Design	Randomized, primary-care-based, single-blind trial.
Patients	729 patients, ≥60 years old, with chronic or paroxysmal atrial fibrillation. Patients with treatable causes of atrial fibrillation, previous stroke, rheumatic valvular disease, cardiovascular disease, myocardial infarction within a year of randomization, left ventricular ejection fraction <40%, congestive heart failure, cardiac aneurysm, history of systemic embolism, retinal infarction or anticoagulant use in the preceding 3 months before randomization were excluded. In addition, patients with contraindications to aspirin or coumarin, hemoglobin <7.0 mmol/L, coagulation disorder, and severe hepatic or renal disease, permanent pacemaker, and a life expectancy of <2 years were not included.
Follow-up	Up to 4 years. Mean follow-up 2.7 years.
Regimen	Randomization to aspirin 150 mg/d, low anticoagulation (target INR 1.1-1.6) or standard anticoagulation (target INR 2.5-3.5). Patients who had exclusion criteria for standard anticoagulation (age ≥78 years, retinopathy, peptic ulcer, history of gastrointestinal or genitourinary bleeding and blood pressure >185/105 mm Hg) were randomized to aspirin 150 mg/d or low anticoagulation. Patients were single-blinded for the 2 intensities of anticoagulation.

Results	Of the patients without contraindication to standard antico-agulation, 131 patients were randomized to standard antico-agulation, 122 to low anticoagulation and 141 to aspirin. 335 patients had contraindications to standard anticoagulation and were randomized to aspirin (n=178) or low anticoagulation (n=157). The mean INR was 3.1±1.2 for the standard antico-agulation group and 1.4±0.4 for the low anticoagulation group. 48% of the measurements in the standard anticoagulation group and 75% in the low anticoagulation group were within the target INR. There were 10 primary events (stroke, systemic arterial embolisation, major hemorrhage or vascular death) in the standard anticoagulation group, 8 in the low anticoagulation and 12 in the aspirin group. Among patients with contraindications to standard anticoagulation, there were 10 primary events in the low anticoagulation and 10 in the aspirin group. The hazard ratio (HR) for low anticoagulation compared with aspirin was 0.91 (95% CI=0.61 to 1.4), and for standard anticoagulation compared with aspirin it was 0.78 (95% CI=0.34-1.8). The hazard nonvascular mortality was lower in the low anticoagula-tion group than in the aspirin group (HR 0.41; 95% CI=0.20 to 0.82). The rate of bleedings was 3.9 per 100 patient-years in the low anticoagulation group, 4.0 per 100 patient-years in the standard anticoagulation group and 3.7 per 100 patient-years in the aspirin group. The HR of standard anticoagulation vs aspirin was 1.3 (95% CI=0.59-3.0) and for low anticoagulation vs aspirin 1.02 (95% CI=0.58-1.8).
Concl.	In patients with non-rheumatic atrial fibrillation, standard anti-coagulation and low anticoagulation were not better than aspirin in preventing stroke, systemic embolisation, major hemorrhage or vascular mortality. Aspirin may be the first choice in patients with non-rheumatic atrial fibrillation without clear indication for anticoagulation therapy.

SPORTIF II

Stroke Prevention by Oral Thrombin Inhibitors in Atrial Fibrillation

Title	Ximelagatran vs warfarin for stroke prevention in patients with nonvalvular atrial fibrillation. SPORTIF II. A dose-guiding, tolerability, and safety study.
Authors	Peterson P, Grind M, Adler J, et al.
Reference	J Am Coll Cardiol 2003;41:1445-1451.
Disease	Nonvalvular atrial fibrillation.
Purpose	To assess the tolerability and safety of 3 doses of ximelagatran (an oral direct thrombin inhibitor) vs warfarin in patients with nonvalvular atrial fibrillation.
Design	Randomized, parallel-group, dose-guiding study.
Patients	254 patients, ≥18 years with a history of chronic, paroxysmal, or persistent nonvalvular atrial fibrillation plus at least 1 predefined risk factor for stroke.
Follow-up	12 weeks.
Regimen	Patients received 20, 40, or 60 mg bid of oral ximelagatran in a double-blind fashion or dose-adjusted warfarin (goal was an INR of 2.0-3.0) in an open label fashion.
Add'l Tx	Aspirin was not recommended; however, low does (up to 160 mg/d) could be used at the discretion of the investigator.

Results	Primary end point was number of thromboembolic events and bleeding. 4 neurologic events occurred: 1 nonfatal ischemic stroke and 1 transient ischemic attack in ximelagatran group; 2 transient ischemic attacks in the warfarin group. There was 1 major bleed in the warfarin group but no major bleeds in the ximelagatran group. Minor bleeds occurred in 4, 5, and 7 taking 20, 40, and 60 of ximelagatran, respectively, vs 6 in the warfarin group. There was an increase in S-alanine aminotransferase in 8 patients (4.3%) on ximelagatran; this abnormality resolved with continued treatment or cessation of therapy.
Concl.	Fixed oral doses of ximelagatran were well tolerated without the need for either anticoagulation monitoring or for dose adjustment.

10

SPORTIF III

Stroke Prevention Using an Oral Thrombin Inhibitor in Atrial Fibrillation

Title	Stroke prevention with the oral direct thrombin inhibitor ximelagatran compared with warfarin in patients with non-valvular atrial fibrillation (SPORTIF III): randomized controlled trial.
Authors	Executive Steering Committee on behalf of the SPORTIF III Investigators.
Reference	Lancet 2003;362:1691-1698.
Disease	Stroke.
Purpose	To compare the safety and efficacy of ximelagatran with warfarin in patients with atrial fibrillation at risk for ischemic stroke.
Design	Randomized, multicenter, open-label, parallel-group trial.
Patients	3410 patients with atrial fibrillation and at least 1 stroke risk factor.
Follow-up	Mean±SD 17.4±4.1 months.
Regimen	Open-label warfarin (adjusted-dose, international normalized ratio 2.0-3.0) or ximelagatran (fixed-dose, 36 mg bid).

Results	Primary end point was stroke or systemic embolism. During 4941 years of patient exposure, 96 patients had primary events (56 receiving warfarin and 40 ximelagatran). The primary event rate by intention to treat was 2.3% per year with warfarin and 1.6% per year with ximelagatran, yielding an absolute risk reduction of 0.7% (p=0.10; 95% CI=-0.1 to 1.4) and a relative risk reduction of 29% (95% CI=-6.5 to 52). All-cause mortality was 3.2% per year in both treatment groups (79 patients receiving warfarin and 78 receiving ximelagatran). 33 patients died from vascular causes in the warfarin group and 40 in the ximelagatran group (p=0.478). There were 9 fatal strokes in the warfarin group and 10 in the ximelagatran group. Nonfatal disabling stroke occurred in 8 patients in the warfarin group and 5 in the ximelagatran group. There were 67 cases of ischemic stroke, transient ischemic stroke, or systemic embolism in the warfarin group (2.9% per year) and 48 in the ximelagatran group (2.1% per year), yielding an absolute risk reduction of 0.8% per year with ximelagatran (95% CI=-0.2 to 1.7, p=0.1086). International normalized ratios at the time of these events were below 2.0 in 17 (25%) warfarin-treated patients. There were no differences in the composite end point of death, stroke, systemic embolism, and definite MI. The rate of combined minor and major hemorrhages was lower with ximelagatran than with warfarin (25.8% vs 29.8% per year, p=0.0007, relative risk reduction 14% [95% CI=4-22]). Patients receiving ximelagatran more often had elevated alanine aminotransferase (ALT) levels (6% vs 1% with warfarin; p<0.0001). ALT elevations with ximelagatran typically took place between 2 and 6 months after initiation of therapy and returned toward baseline either spontaneously or after cessation of treatment.
Concl.	Fixed-dose oral ximelagatran was at least as effective as well-controlled warfarin for prevention stroke and systemic embolism. Although anticoagulation intensity was not monitored or regulated in patients receiving ximelagatran, these patients had less bleeding than those receiving warfarin.

ACE

Anticoagulation in Cardioversion Using Enoxaparin

Title	Safety and efficacy of enoxaparin compared with unfractionated heparin and oral anticoagulants for prevention of thromboembolic complications in cardioversion of nonvalvular atrial fibrillation: the Anticoagulation in Cardioversion using Enoxaparin (ACE) trial.
Authors	Stellbrink C, Nixdorff U, Hofmann T, et al.
Reference	Circulation 2004;109:997-1003.
Disease	Arrhythmia.
Purpose	To compare the safety and efficacy of SC enoxaparin with IV unfractionated heparin followed by the oral anticoagulant phenprocoumon in patients scheduled for cardioversion of atrial fibrillation.
Design	Multicenter, randomized, open-label, prospective trial.
Patients	496 patients scheduled for cardioversion of atrial fibrillation >48 hours and ≤1 year in duration.
Follow-up	Up to ≈49 days.
Regimen	Enoxaparin or unfractionated heparin + phenprocoumon.
Add'l Tx	Cardioversion without (stratum A) or with (stratum B) guidance by transesophageal electrocardiogram.
Results	The aim was to demonstrate noninferiority of enoxaparin with regard to the primary end point (a composite of embolic events, all-cause death, and major bleeding complications). Secondary end points were successful cardioversion, maintenance of sinus rhythm until study end, and minor bleeding. 428 of the 496 patients were analyzed per protocol. Enoxaparin was noninferior to unfractionated heparin (UFH) + phenprocoumon with regard to the incidence of the composite primary end point (per-protocol analysis, 7 of 216 vs 12 of 212 patients; p=0.016; intention-to-treat analysis, 7 of 248 vs 12 of 248 patients; p=0.013). The groups did not differ with regard to rate of reversion to sinus rhythm.

Concl.   This study showed enoxaparin to be noninferior to UFH + phenprocoumon for prevention of ischemic and embolic events, bleeding complications, and death in transesophageal echocardiography-guided cardioversion of atrial fibrillation. Because of the easier application and more stable anticoagulation afforded by enoxaparin, it may be the preferred drug for initiation of anticoagulation in this setting.

ATRIA Substudy

Anticoagulation and Risk Factors in Atrial Fibrillation

Title	Effect of intensity of oral anticoagulation on stroke severity and mortality in atrial fibrillation.
Authors	Hylek EM, Go AS, Chang Y, et al.
Reference	N Engl J Med 2003;349:1019-1026.
Disease	Atrial fibrillation.
Purpose	To assess the effect of the intensity of anticoagulation on the severity of ischemic stroke and on the 30-day mortality rate after stroke in patients with nonvalvular atrial fibrillation, and to determine the rates of ischemic stroke and intracranial hemorrhage according to the intensity of anticoagulation.
Design	Cohort study.
Patients	13,559 patients with nonvalvular atrial fibrillation.
Follow-up	30 days.
Regimen	Warfarin or aspirin.

Results   Patients who had suffered strokes were identified through hospital databases and medical records, which also provided information on anticoagulation and antiplatelet therapy. Severity of stroke was graded by a modified Rankin scale; 30-day mortality data were obtained from hospitalization and mortality files. 596 ischemic strokes were identified; 32% occurred during warfarin, 27% during aspirin, and 42% during neither therapy. Among the 188 patients who had a stroke while taking warfarin, 15% of those with an international normalized ratio (INR) level <2.0 on admission had a severe stroke or died in the hospital, compared with 5% who had an INR >2.0. Among patients who had been taking aspirin, 13% had a severe stroke or died in the hospital, and 22% taking neither warfarin nor aspirin had a severe stroke or died in hospital. The 30-day mortality rate was 6% among patients taking warfarin and who had an INR of ≥2, compared with 16% among those who were taking warfarin and had an INR <2, 15% among those taking aspirin, and 24% among those taking neither. There was no significant difference in mortality rates between patients taking warfarin who had an INR of 1.5-1.9 and those with an INR <1.5. The risk of intracranial hemorrhage did not increase until INR exceeded 3.9.

Concl.   In patients with nonvalvular atrial fibrillation (AF), anticoagulation that produces an INR of ≥2 reduces the frequency of ischemic stroke as well as its severity and the risk of death from ischemic stroke. Lower INR target levels cannot be recommended in patients with AF.

11. Deep Vein Thrombosis/Pulmonary Embolism

11. Deep Vein Thrombosis/ Pulmonary Embolism

Low-Molecular-Weight Heparin in the Treatment of Patients with Venous Thromboembolism

Title	Low-molecular-weight heparin in the treatment of patients with venous thromboembolism.
Authors	The Columbus Investigators.
Reference	N Engl J Med 1997;337:657-662.
Disease	Venous thromboembolism.
Purpose	To determine whether fixed dose, subcutaneous, low-molecular-weight heparin and adjusted dose, IV, unfractionated heparin infusion have equivalent efficacy in patients with symptomatic venous thromboembolism.
Design	Randomized, open-label, multicenter.
Patients	1021 patients with acute symptomatic deep vein thrombosis, pulmonary embolism, or both. Diagnosis had to be documented by ultrasonography or venography, lung scanning, or pulmonary angiography.
Follow-up	12 weeks.
Regimen	Reviparin sodium (low-molecular-weight heparin) given subcutaneously at various fixed doses by range of weight: 6300 u x2/d for patients > 60 kg; 4200 u x2/d for patients 46-60 kg; and 3500 u x2/d for patients 35-45 kg. Unfractionated heparin was given as IV bolus 5000 IU, followed by infusion of 1250 IU per hour and adjusted as needed. Study drug was continued for at least 5 days. Oral anticoagulant was started in the first or second day and continued for 12 weeks.
Results	510 patients assigned to low-molecular-weight heparin reviparin and 511 patients to unfractionated heparin. 5.3% of patients receiving reviparin had recurrent thromboembolic events vs 4.9% of patients receiving unfractionated heparin. Major bleeding occurred in 3.1% of reviparin and 2.3% of unfractionated heparin group. Mortality rates were similar in the 2 groups at 7.1 and 7.6%, respectively.

Concl.   Fixed dose, subcutaneous, low-molecular-weight heparin was as effective and safe as infusion of unfractionated heparin in patients with venous thromboembolism with or without pulmonary embolus.

Low-Molecular-Weight Heparin Prophylaxis vs Warfarin in Hip Arthroplasty

Title	Low-molecular-weight heparin prophylaxis using dalteparin in close proximity to surgery vs warfarin in hip arthroplasty patients. A double-blind, randomized comparison.
Authors	Hull RD, Pineo GF, Francis C et al for North American Fragmin(r) Trial Investigators.
Reference	Arch Intern Med 2000;160:2199-2207.
Disease	Deep vein thrombosis prophylaxis.
Purpose	To determine whether administration of low-molecular-weight heparin just prior to hip arthroplasty is more effective in preventing venous thrombosis than to warfarin.
Design	Randomized, double-blind, multicenter.
Patients	1472 patients undergoing elective hip replacement.
Follow-up	≈6 days.
Regimen	Patients randomized to preoperative dalteparin sodium received 2500 IU subcutaneously within 2 hours of surgery; they received a second dose 4 hours postoperatively. Patients randomized to postoperative dalteparin received placebo injection before surgery and dalteparin at least 4 hours postoperatively. On subsequent days patients in both of these groups received 5000 IU dalteparin subcutaneously q am. Patients randomized to warfarin received initial postoperative dose in the evening of the day of surgery. Initial dose was 10 mg (less in patients 70 or older or weighing less than 57 kg). Warfarin then adjusted to maintain international normalized ratio from 2.0-3.0. Placebo injections given to warfarin patients. Placebo capsules given to dalteparin patients.

Results	Primary end point was deep vein thrombosis detected with contrast venography performed on a mean of day 5.7. Deep vein thrombosis assessed by interpretable venograms was observed in 36/337 (10.7%) preoperative dalteparin patients; 44/336 (13.1%) postoperative dalteparin patients vs 81/338 (24.0%) warfarin patients (p<0.001 for both preoperative and postoperative dalteparin vs warfarin). Proximal deep vein thrombosis developed in 3/354 (0.8%) in preoperative dalteparin group, 3/358 (0.8%) in postoperative dalteparin group, and 11/363 (3.0%) of warfarin group (p=0.04 and p=0.03 for preoperative and postoperative dalteparin vs warfarin, respectively). Symptomatic venous thrombi were less frequent in preoperative dalteparin group (1.5%) vs warfarin group (4.4%; p=0.02). Major bleeding at surgical sites was more common in patients receiving preoperative dalteparin vs warfarin (2.2 vs 0.4% on days 2-8, =0.01).
Concl.	Dalteparin given in close proximity to surgery decreased the risk of deep vein thrombosis. Dalteparin initiated postoperatively was more effective than warfarin without increasing bleeding.

11

Title	Fondaparinux compared with enoxaparin for the prevention of venous thromboembolism after hip-fracture surgery.
Authors	Eriksson BI, Bauer KA, Lassen MR, et al.
Reference	N Engl J Med 2001;345:1298-1304.
Disease	Venous thromboembolism.
Purpose	To determine whether a new antithrombotic agent, a synthetic pentasaccharide, may reduce the risk of venous thromboembolism following surgery for hip fracture.
Design	Randomized, double-blind, multicenter.
Patients	1711 patients undergoing surgery for fracture of the upper third of the femur.
Follow-up	6 weeks.
Regimen	Patients were randomized to either 2.5 mg of fondaparinux subcutaneously once daily begun postoperatively or 40 mg of enoxaparin subcutaneously given preoperatively. Therapy continued for 5-9 days.
Results	Primary efficacy was rate of venous thromboembolism (deep vein thrombosis, pulmonary embolism, or both) up to day 11. Diagnosis of venous thromboembolism was defined as deep vein thrombosis diagnosed by mandatory bilateral venography or documented symptomatic pulmonary embolism (confirmed by lung scan, pulmonary angiography, helical computed tomography, or autopsy). By postoperative day 11, 8.3% (52 of 626 patients) in the fondaparinux group vs 19.1% (119 of 624 patients) in the enoxaparin group had venous thromboembolism (p<0.001). RR reduction with fondaparinux was 56.4% (95% CI=39.0%-70.3%; p<0.001). By postoperative day 49 incidence of symptomatic venous thromboembolism was similar in 2 groups at 2.0% and 1.5% in the fondaparinux and enoxaparin group respectively. Major bleeding occurred in 18 of 831 patients in the fondaparinux group and 19 of 842 in the enoxaparin group by day 11. Minor bleeding was more common with fondaparinux (4.1%) vs enoxaparin (2.1%; p=0.02). Death occurred in 4.6% of patients in the fondaparinux vs 5.0% of patients in the enoxaparin group.

Concl.   Fondaparinux was more effective than enoxaparin for preventing venous thromboembolism during the first 11 days after hip-fracture surgery.

Ximelagatran Prophylaxis Against Venous Thromboembolism

Title	Comparison of the oral direct thrombin inhibitor ximelagatran with enoxaparin as prophylaxis against venous thromboembolism after total knee replacement. A phase 2 dose-finding study.
Authors	Heit JA, Colwell CW, Francis CW, et al.
Reference	Arch Intern Med 2001;161:2215-2221.
Disease	Venous thromboembolism.
Purpose	To test the efficacy and safety of a novel direct inhibitor of free and clot-bound thrombin, ximelagatran, as prophylaxis against deep vein thrombosis (DVT).
Design	Randomized, blinded, parallel study design, multicenter, dose-finding.
Patients	600 adults undergoing elective total knee replacement.
Follow-up	4 weeks.
Regimen	Patients received either ximelagatran twice a day orally of 8, 12, 18, 24 mg vs open-label enoxaparin 30 mg, subcutaneously twice a day beginning 12-24 hours after surgery and continuing for 6-12 days. Patients underwent venography of the operative leg between 6-12 days after surgery.
Results	443 patients were evaluable for efficacy. Primary end point was 6-12 day cumulative incidence of symptomatic or venographic DVT or symptomatic pulmonary embolism. Bleeding rates also were assessed. Venous thromboembolism occurred in 27%, 19.8%, 28.7%, and 15.8% of patients on the 8, 12, 18, and 24 mg doses of ximelagatran, respectively. Rates with enoxaparin (22.7%) were similar. Rates of proximal DVT or pulmonary embolism were 7%, 2%, 6%, and 3% at 8, 12, 18, 24 mg ximelagatran vs 3% enoxaparin. Major bleeding occurred at 0%, 0%, 2%, and 0% of 8, 12, 18, and 24 mg ximelagatran, respectively vs 1% in the enoxaparin group.
Concl.	Oral ximelagatran, 24 mg twice a day, given after surgery for total knee replacement appeared as safe and effective as subcutaneous enoxaparin for prophylaxis against venous thromboembolism

Title	Fondaparinux compared with enoxaparin for the prevention of venous thromboembolism after elective major knee surgery.
Authors	Bauer KA, Eriksson BI, Lassen MR, et al.
Reference	N Engl J Med 2001;345:1305-1310.
Disease	Venous thromboembolism.
Purpose	To determine whether fondaparinux is more efficacious than enoxaparin in reducing the incidence of venous thromboembolism following major knee surgery.
Design	Double-blind, randomized, multicenter.
Patients	1049 patients undergoing elective major knee surgery.
Follow-up	Primary efficacy evaluated between postoperative days 5-9. Clinical follow-up to 49 days.
Regimen	Patients randomized to receive subcutaneous doses of either 2.5 mg fondaparinux once a day or 30 mg enoxaparin twice daily starting postoperatively.
Add'l Tx	Graduated-compression stockings and physiotherapy.
Results	Primary efficacy outcome was venous thromboembolism up to postoperative day 11. Venous thromboembolism was defined as deep vein thrombosis (DVT) assessed by mandatory venography, documented symptomatic DVT, or documented symptomatic pulmonary embolism. 724 patients were included in the primary efficacy analysis and 1034 were available for safety analysis in which the end point was major bleeding. By day 11, venous thromboembolism occurred in 27.8% (101 of 363 patients) in the enoxaparin group vs 12.5% (45 of 361 patients) in the fondaparinux group. The reduction in risk for fondaparinux was 55.2% (95% CI=36.2-70.2; $p<0.001$). Fondaparinux decreased the incidence of proximal DVT by 55% ($p=0.06$) compared to enoxaparin and decreased distal DVT by 55.9% ($p<0.001$). There were no cases of fatal bleeding or bleeding into a critical organ in either group. However, there were 11 major bleeding episodes with fondaparinux vs 1 in the enoxaparin group ($p=0.006$). Bleeding leading to reoperation occurred in 0.4% of fondaparinux patients vs 0.2% of enoxaparin patients.

Concl.   Fondaparinux was more effective than enoxaparin in preventing DVT following major knee surgery, but was associated with more bleeding.

Title	3 months vs one year of oral anticoagulant therapy for idiopathic deep venous thrombosis.
Authors	Agnelli G, Prandoni P, Santamaria G, et al.
Reference	N Engl J Med 2001;345:165-169.
Disease	Deep venous thrombosis.
Purpose	To determine if there was an added benefit of treating patients who had a first episode of idiopathic deep venous thrombosis and had completed 3 months of oral anticoagulation therapy with additional 9 months of therapy.
Design	Randomized, multicenter, open trial with independent, blinded assessment of outcome.
Patients	267 patients with a first episode of idiopathic proximal deep venous thrombosis who had completed 3 months of anticoagulation therapy.
Follow-up	≈37 months.
Regimen	Oral anticoagulation with an international normalized ratio (INR) between 2.0-3.0 during most of the study.
Add'l Tx	About 20% of patients received low-molecular-weight heparin as initial therapy.

Results	Primary intention-to-treat outcome was recurrence of symptomatic, objectively confirmed deep venous thromboembolism for at least 2 years. Objective measures were positive results on compression ultrasonography or venography. Objective evidence for pulmonary embolism was diagnostic angiogram, high probability ventilation-perfusion lung scan, or indeterminant lung scan with high degree of clinical suspicion and objective recurrence of deep venous thrombosis. Results of primary intention-to-treat analysis revealed that of 134 patients assigned to the additional 9 months of anticoagulation, 21 (15.7% over average follow-up of 37.8 months) had recurrent venous thromboembolism, whereas 21 of 133 (15.8%, average follow-up was 37.2 months) patients assigned to discontinue anticoagulation therapy after 3 months, had a recurrence of thromboembolism (p=NS). However, during the initial 9 months after randomization (that is during the active therapy in the 9-month treatment group), 1 patient had a recurrence of thromboembolism on anticoagulation therapy (0.7%) while 11 in the discontinuation group (8.3%; p=0.003) had recurrence. Nonfatal major bleeding occurred in 4 patients that received extended anticoagulation therapy.
Concl.	In patients with idiopathic deep venous thrombosis extension of anticoagulation therapy for an additional 9 months (after 3 months of therapy) was only beneficial during the therapy itself. Once anticoagulation therapy was stopped the benefit was not maintained long-term.

Prolonged Thromboprophylaxis with Oral Anticoagulants After Total Hip Arthroplasty

Title	Prolonged thromboprophylaxis with oral anticoagulants after total hip arthroplasty.
Authors	Prandoni P, Bruchi O, Sabbion P, et al.
Reference	Arch Int Med 2002;162:1966-1971.
Disease	Venous thromboembolism/pulmonary embolism.
Purpose	To determine the benefit of continuing oral anticoagulation after hospital discharge in patients who have undergone total hip arthroplasty.
Design	Randomized, controlled, prospective.
Patients	360 patients who received warfarin during their hospitalization after elective total hip arthroplasty. Patients who had previous hip surgery on the same side or history of thromboembolic disorders were excluded. Patients who developed venous thromboembolic complications or major bleeding or had ultrasound-demonstrated DVT (deep venous thrombosis) before hospital discharge and those in need of long-term anticoagulation were also excluded.
Follow-up	3 months.
Regimen	All study patients received 5 mg/d of warfarin starting on the 2nd preoperative day. After surgery, dosage was adjusted to a target INR of 2-3. At hospital discharge, eligible patients were randomized to discontinue oral anticoagulant therapy (n=176) or to continuation for 4 more weeks (n=184), with a target international normalized ratio between 2.0 and 3.0.

Results	The primary outcome of the study was a composite of symptomatic venous thromboembolic events and asymptomatic proximal DVT during the first 4 weeks after hospital discharge. The secondary study outcome was the number of such events in the entire follow-up period. Also, the association between selected clinical parameters (ie, age, sex, obesity, prolonged immobilization, length of hospital stay, quality of in-hospital anticoagulation, and presence of varicose veins, cancer, heart/lung failure, and estrogen therapy) with development of postoperative thromboembolism was investigated. During the first 4 weeks of follow-up, the primary outcome occurred in 9/176 (5.1%) of the control patients and 1/184 (0.5%) of the treated patients. The relative risk (RR) of developing venous thromboembolism in control patients was 9.4 (95% CI=1.2-73.5). Of the 9 events in the control group, 4 were symptomatic (3 proximal DVT and 1 pulmonary embolism) and 5 asymptomatic. During the entire 3-month follow-up a total of 12 thromboembolic events were recorded, 9 in the control group and 3 in the treated group. The RR for developing venous thromboembolism in the control group vs the treated group was 3.1 (95% CI=0.9-11.4), which was not statistically significant. Among the investigated parameters, only old age (OR 9.35; 95% CI=1.14-76.4) and presence of varicose veins (OR 12.6; 95% CI=2.9-54.2) were associated with development of post-operative thromboembolism. 1 patient in the extended prophylaxis group experienced major (retroperitoneal) bleeding, and there was no major bleeding in the control group.
Concl.	Continuing oral anticoagulation therapy a few weeks beyond hospital discharge is potentially beneficial in reducing venous thromboembolic complications in patients who have undergone total hip arthroplasty.

Heparin Plus Alteplase Compared with Heparin Alone in Patients with Submassive Pulmonary Embolism

Title	Heparin plus alteplase compared with heparin alone in patients with submassive pulmonary embolism.
Authors	Konstantinides S, Geibel A, Heusel G, et al.
Reference	N Engl J Med 2002;347:1143-1150.
Disease	Pulmonary embolism (PE).
Purpose	To determine whether alteplase together with heparin is superior to heparin alone in determining the clinical course of hemodynamically stable patients with submassive PE.
Design	Randomized, prospective, double-blind, placebo-controlled, multicenter.

Patients	256 patients were randomized: 118 to the heparin plus alteplase group, 138 to the heparin-placebo group. Eligible patients had acute PE with at least 1 of the following: right ventricular dysfunction detected on echocardiography, defined as right ventricular enlargement combined with loss of inspiratory collapse of the inferior vena cava, with no left ventricular or mitral valve disease; echocardiographically detected pulmonary artery hypertension, followed by confirmation of pulmonary embolism (by ventilation-perfusion scanning, computed tomography, or pulmonary angiography); precapillary pulmonary hypertension based on catheterization of the right side of the heart, defined as a mean pulmonary artery pressure >20 mm Hg, and a pulmonary-capillary wedge pressure <18 mm Hg, followed by confirmation of pulmonary embolism; or new signs of right ventricular strain on electrocardiography, followed by confirmation of pulmonary embolism. Exclusion criteria included 1 or more of the following: age >80 years; hemodynamic instability; onset of symptoms more than 96 hours prior to diagnosis; thrombolytic treatment, major surgery, or biopsy within the prior 7 days; major trauma within the preceding 10 days; stroke, transient ischemic attack, craniocerebral trauma, or neurologic surgery within the past 6 months; gastrointestinal bleeding within the previous 3 months; uncontrolled hypertension; bleeding disorder; intolerance to alteplase; diabetic retinopathy; current oral anticoagulant use; current pregnancy or lactation; life expectancy of less than 6 months due to underlying disease; or planned use of thrombolytic agents for extensive deep-vein thrombosis.
Follow-up	30 days.
Regimen	All patients received a 5000 U bolus of unfractionated heparin intravenously. Patients were then randomized (1:1) to receive 100 mg of alteplase in a 10 mg bolus, followed by 90 mg intravenously over the next 2 hours, or matching placebo.
Add'l Tx	All patients received unfractionated heparin as an IV infusion, starting at 1000 U per hour, and thereafter adjusted to maintain the activated partial-thromboplastin time at 2.0-2.5 times the upper limit of normal. Oral anticoagulant therapy was overlapped on the third day after randomization, with the dosage adjusted to maintain an international normalized ratio of 2.5-3.5.

Results	The primary end point was in-hospital death or clinical deterioration that necessitated an escalation of treatment. Escalation of treatment was defined as any of the following: catecholamine infusion because of persistent arterial hypotension or shock (except for dopamine infusion at a rate ≤5 mg/kg body weight/min); secondary thrombolysis (for any of the following indications: worsening clinical symptoms [i.e., dyspnea], or worsening respiratory failure due to PE; arterial hypotension or shock; and persistent or worsening pulmonary hypertension or right ventricular dysfunction detected by echocardiography or right heart catheterization); endotracheal intubation; CPR; and emergency surgical embolectomy or thrombus fragmentation by catheter. Secondary study end points included recurrent PE, major bleeding, and ischemic stroke. At study entry, there were no significant differences in clinical characteristics such as systolic or diastolic BP, heart rate, dyspnea severity, or arterial hypoxemia between the 2 patient groups. Pulmonary artery pressures as determined by right heart catheterization were similar between patients in the 2 groups. The primary end point occurred in 13/118 (11.0%) of patients in the heparin-alteplase group, and 34/138 (24.6%) in the heparin-placebo group (relative risk 2.63; 95% CI=1.32-5.26; p=0.006). The difference was primarily accounted for by the increased number of treatment escalations in the placebo group (34/138 vs. 12/118 in the alteplase group; p=0.004). There were 4/118 deaths in the alteplase group and 3/138 in the placebo group. There were no significant differences in the occurrences of the secondary end points between the groups. The likelihood of 30-day event-free survival was higher in the heparin-alteplase group vs heparin-placebo group (p=0.005). Certain baseline patient characteristics predicted an increased risk of in-hospital death or escalation of treatment; these were: age >70 years, female sex, and presence of arterial hypoxemia. Bleeding complications were uncommon in both groups, and there was no significant difference in the incidence of bleeding between the heparin-alteplase and heparin-placebo groups.
Concl.	The addition of alteplase to heparin improves the clinical course of hemodynamically stable patients with acute submassive PE compared to heparin alone. There was no increased risk of bleeding associated with alteplase.

DOTAVK

Duree Optimale du Traitement Antivitamines K

Title	Comparison of 3 and 6 months of oral anticoagulant therapy after a first episode of proximal deep vein thrombosis or pulmonary embolism and comparison of 6 and 12 weeks of therapy after isolated calf deep vein thrombosis.
Authors	Pinede L, Ninet J, Duhaut P, et al.
Reference	Circulation 2001;103:2453-2460.
Disease	Venous thromboembolism.
Purpose	To determine optimal duration of oral anticoagulation following a first episode of venous thromboembolism—for proximal deep vein thrombosis and/or pulmonary embolism or isolated calf deep vein thrombosis.
Design	Open-label, randomized, controlled trial, parallel-group, multicenter.
Patients	736 patients—with symptomatic calf deep vein thrombosis, proximal deep vein thrombosis, or pulmonary embolism. Confirmation by positive Doppler ultrasonography, venography, perfusion—ventilation lung scanning, pulmonary angiography.
Follow-up	Mean follow-up was 12 months.

Regimen	At the end of heparin therapy (≈5 days) all patients received oral anticoagulation with fluindione (a vitamin K antagonist). Oral anticoagulation was targeted to an international normalized ratio of 2.0-3.0. Dose of fluindione was then adjusted based upon INR. Patients were stratified to C-DVT (isolated calf deep vein thrombosis) or P-DVT (proximal deep vein thrombosis) and/or pulmonary embolism (PE). In P-DVT-PE patients 3 months vs 6 months of anticoagulation was compared. In patients with C-DVT 6 weeks vs 12 weeks of therapy were compared.
Results	Primary end point was recurrent venous thromboembolism; and major, minor, and fatal bleeding complications. There were 23 recurrences of venous thromboembolism in patients on short treatment regimen (6.4%) vs 26 (7.4%) in the longer treatment regimens group (p=NS). In C-DVT group 2.0% of short-term and 3.0% of long-term treatment had recurrence of venous thromboembolism; in P-DVT and/or PE group 8.1% of short-term and 8.7% of long-term treatment had recurrence. Hemorrhage (all) occurred in 15.5% vs 18.4% (p=NS) of short- and long-term treatment, respectively. Also, there were no significant differences between major or minor bleeds between the short- or long-term treatment regimens. Overall recurrence rates of venous thromboembolism were lower for patients with C-DVT (2.6%) vs P-DVT or PE (8.4%).
Concl.	Following isolated C-DVT, 6 weeks of oral anticoagulation is appropriate. 3 and 6 months of oral anticoagulation resulted in equivalent outcomes in patients with P-DVT or PE.

ENOXACAN II

Enoxaparin and Cancer

Title	Duration of prophylaxis against venous thromboembolism with enoxaparin after surgery for cancer.
Authors	Bergqvist D, Agnelli G, Cohen A, et al.
Reference	N Engl J Med 2002;346:975-980.
Disease	Postoperative thromboembolism associated with open surgery for abdominal or pelvic cancer.
Purpose	To compare 4 week and 1 week enoxaparin (low-molecular-weight heparin) therapy in patients undergoing surgery for abdominal or pelvic cancer.
Design	Prospective, placebo-controlled, double-blind, multicenter.
Patients	322 patients undergoing open, elective, curative surgery for malignant tumor of the abdomen or pelvis. Patients had to be 40 years or older with a life expectancy of at least 6 months.
Follow-up	3 months.
Regimen	40 mg subcutaneous enoxaparin daily for 6-10 days after surgery. Following this open treatment phase, patients randomized to 40 mg subcutaneous enoxaparin (n=165) vs placebo (n=167) for 19-21 days.

Results   Primary end point was deep vein thrombosis documented by venograms, symptomatic pulmonary embolism documented by ventilation-perfusion lung scanning and/or pulmonary angiography. Venograms were performed in a routine manner between days 25-31 or sooner if patients had symptoms of venous thromboembolism. Venous thromboembolism occurred in 12% of placebo patients vs 4.8% of the enoxaparin group (p=0.02). At 3 months this difference persisted at 13.8% in the placebo patients vs 5.5% in the enoxaparin patients (p=0.01). At 3 months proximal deep vein thrombosis had occurred in 2.4% of placebo and 1.2% of enoxaparin patients; distal deep vein thrombosis in 10.2% of placebo and 4.2% of enoxaparin patients; and pulmonary embolism in 1.2% of placebo and 0% of enoxaparin patients. Cumulative incidence of hemorrhage at 3 months was 4.4% in placebo vs 7.1% in enoxaparin groups (p=0.20).

Concl.   Prophylaxis with enoxaparin for 4 weeks after abdominal or pelvic surgery for cancer reduced incidence of venographically demonstrated thrombosis vs enoxaparin therapy for only 1 week.

EPHESUS

European Pentasaccharide Hip Elective Surgery Study

Title	Postoperative fondaparinux vs preoperative enoxaparin for prevention of venous thromboembolism in elective hip-replacement surgery: a randomized double-blind comparison.
Authors	Lassen MR, Bauer KA, Eriksson BI.
Reference	Lancet 2002;359:1715-1720.
Disease	Venous thromboembolism.
Purpose	To compare the efficacy and safety of a once-daily subcutaneous fondaparinux (a specific factor Xa inhibitor), started postoperatively, and twice daily subcutaneous enoxaparin, started preoperatively, for prevention of venous thromboembolism in patients undergoing elective hip-replacement surgery.
Design	Randomized, double-blind, multicenter.
Patients	2309 patients, ≥18 years old, scheduled for elective total hip-replacement surgery or a revision of ≥1 component of a previously implanted hip prosthesis. Patients undergoing bilateral hip replacement; patients with active bleeding; acute bacterial endocarditis; bleeding disorder; hemorrhagic stroke; recent spinal, brain, or eye surgery; hypersensitivity to heparin; hypersensitivity to iodinated contrast media; serum creatinine ≥180 mmol/L; and platelet count <100×109/L were excluded. Patients who had received anticoagulant, antiplatelet or fibrinolytic treatment, including dextran within 2 days prior to surgery, or who had an indication for anticoagulation therapy were not included. Use of aspirin before enrollment was not considered as exclusion criterion.
Follow-up	49 days.
Regimen	Randomization to fondaparinux (2.5 mg/d subcutaneous) or enoxaparin (40 mg/d subcutaneous). Therapy with fondaparinux was started a mean of 6±2 hours after surgery and enoxaparin was started 12 hours before surgery. Therapy was continued for 5-9 days.

11. Deep Vein Thrombosis/Pulmonary Embolism

Add'l Tx	Intermittent pneumatic compression, dextran, thrombolytic treatment, and any anticoagulant or antiplatelet agents were prohibited. The use of aspirin and nonsteroidal anti-inflammatory drugs was discouraged.
Results	Of the 2309 patients randomized, 1827 patients (79%) were assessed for primary efficacy outcomes (908 in the fondaparinux and 919 in the enoxaparin group). By day 11, fewer patients in the fondaparinux (4%) than the enoxaparin (9%) group had venous thromboembolism (relative risk reduction 55.9%; 95% CI=72.8-33.1; $p<0.0001$). Deep vein thrombosis was detected in 4% and 9%, respectively (RR reduction 56.1%; 95% CI=73.2-32.9; $p<0.0001$). Proximal deep vein thrombosis was detected in 1% and 2%, respectively ($p=0.0021$). Nonfatal pulmonary embolism was detected in 0.2% of the patients in each group and fatal pulmonary embolism in none of the patients. 4% of the patients in the fondaparinux group vs 9% in the enoxaparin group were treated for venous thromboembolism by day 11 on the basis of local-site assessment ($p<0.0001$). Between day 1 and day 49, 1% of the patients in each group had symptomatic venous thromboembolism. 1 patient in the fondaparinux group and zero in the enoxaparin group had a fatal pulmonary embolism. 3 patients in each group had a nonfatal pulmonary embolism. Major bleeding occurred in 4% of the patients in the fondaparinux group and in 3% in the enoxaparin group. 63% vs 61% of the patients in the fondaparinux and enoxaparin groups, respectively, needed transfusion. Mortality was 0.2% and 0.5%, respectively ($p=0.45$).
Concl.	Fondaparinux, started after surgery, was more effective than once-daily enoxaparin started before surgery, in preventing venous thromboembolism after elective hip-replacement surgery.

MEDENOX

Prophylaxis in Medical Patients with Enoxaparin Study

Title	A comparison of enoxaparin with placebo for the prevention of venous thromboembolism in acutely ill medical patients.
Authors	Samama MM, Cohen AT, Darmon J-Y, et al.
Reference	N Engl J Med 1999;341:793-800.
Disease	Patients at risk for venous thromboembolism.
Purpose	To determine the frequency of deep vein thrombosis and pulmonary embolism in hospitalized medical patients and to determine safety and efficacy of regimens of low molecular weight heparin for their prevention.
Design	Randomized, multicenter.
Patients	1102 hospitalized patients over 40 years of age not immobilized for more than 3 days with risk factors for venous thromboembolism—congestive heart failure, acute respiratory failure, infection, acute rheumatic disorder, acute arthritis, acute inflammatory bowel disease, as well as other risk factors.
Follow-up	83-110 days.
Regimen	Placebo, 20 mg of enoxaparin, or 40 mg of enoxaparin subcutaneously once-a-day for 6-14 days.
Add'l Tx	Other standard therapy—elastic bandages, support stockings, physiotherapy as per usual practice.

Results   The primary outcome was venous thromboembolism (defined as deep vein thrombosis, pulmonary embolism, or both) between days 1-14. Secondary outcome was venous thromboembolism between days 1-10. Diagnosis was made by venography, venous ultrasonography, high probability lung scanning, pulmonary angiography, helical computed tomography, or at autopsy. Primary outcome could be determined in 866 patients. Incidence of venous thromboembolism was lower in the 40 mg enoxaparin group (5.5%; 16 of 291 patients) vs placebo group (14.9%; 43 of 288 patients; RR 0.37; 97.6% CI=0.22-0.63; p<0.001). The 20 mg enoxaprin had a rate of 15.0% that was not statistically different than the placebo group. The benefit observed in the 40 mg group persisted at 3 months. There was no difference in mortality among groups. Adverse events did not differ among groups.

Concl.   Prophylaxis with 40 mg of enoxaparin subcutaneously per day reduces risk of thromboembolism in patients hospitalized with acute medical illness.

METHRO II

Melagatran for Thrombin Inhibition in Orthopaedic Surgery

Title	Ximelagatran and melagatran compared with dalteparin for prevention of venous thromboembolism after total hip or knee replacement: the METHRO II randomised trial.
Authors	Eriksson BI, Bergqvist D, Kälebo P, et al.
Reference	Lancet 2002; 360:1441-1447.
Disease	Deep vein thrombosis/pulmonary embolism.
Purpose	To determine the safety and efficacy of sequential subcutaneous melagatran (MG) (a direct thrombin inhibitor, given subcutaneously) and oral ximelagatran (XM) (a direct thrombin inhibitor, given orally) in preventing deep venous thrombosis, and to compare these with dalteparin.
Design	Randomised, double-blind, multicenter.
Patients	1876 patients, aged 18-85 years, who weighed 50-100 kg, and who underwent primary elective total hip or total knee replacement. Exclusion criteria included: history of deep-vein thrombosis or pulmonary embolism, increased risk of bleeding due to medical condition, history of intracranial bleeding, ischemic stroke, intraocular or gastrointestinal bleeding, or objectively confirmed ulcer disease in the past 12 months, recent major surgery, malignancy, and others.
Follow-up	4-6 weeks.
Regimen	Randomization to either 5000 IU SC dalteparin qd or: 1) 1.00 mg SC MG followed by 8 mg oral XM; 2) 1.50 mg SC MG followed by 12 mg oral XM; 3) 2.25 mg SC MG followed by 18 mg oral XM; 4) 3.00 mg SC melagatran followed by 24 mg oral XM (all doses bid). The first dose of MG was given after regional anesthesia but before surgery start. The second dose was given 7-11 hours after surgery. Bid injections continued until oral XM was started, usually 1-3 days after surgery. Dalteparin was started the night before surgery and continued until the night before venography. All patients had bilateral venograms 7-10 days after surgery.

Add'l Tx	Heparins, oral anticoagulants, thrombolytics, dipyridamole, ticlopidine, non-steroidal anti-inflammatory drugs with half-life >20 hours, aspirin >500 mg daily, dextran 40, and dextran 70 were not allowed during the 7 days prior to surgery and during the study protocol period. Pneumatic compression devices were not allowed, but elastic compression stockings were permitted.

Results	The primary efficacy end point was the overall frequency of confirmed thromboembolic events (either deep venous thrombosis [DVT] or pulmonary embolism [PE]). DVT was confirmed with bilateral venography, and PE was verified with pulmonary perfusion and ventilation scintigraphy and chest radiography. DVT symptoms after the treatment period and during the follow-up were confirmed by either compression sonogram or venography. The safety end points included number of patients with severe bleeding, defined as intracranial, intraocular, intraspinal, or retroperitoneal, location of bleed, volume of blood loss, and transfused volume of red blood cells. 1495 patients were randomized to the XM and MG group and 381 to the dalteparin group. Two thirds of patients underwent total hip replacement and one third underwent total knee replacement. A total of 1477 patients were included in the primary efficacy analysis. In the population of patients randomized to XM, the percentage of patients with DVT or PE (the primary outcome) was 37.8%, 24.1%, 23.7%, 15.1% in the 1.0/8 mg XM, 1.5/12 mg XM, 2.25/18 mg XM, and 3/24 mg XM groups, respectively. The percentage of patients with DVT or PE in the dalteparin group was 28.2%. The dose-dependent decrease in the primary outcome was significant in both the hip replacement (p<0.0001) and knee replacement groups (p=0.0014). A decrease in the incidence of DVT, PE, or both with relation to dose was also significant (p=0.0002). The incidence of venous thromboembolism was significantly lower in the highest-dose XM group vs the dalteparin group (15.1% vs 28.2%, OR 0.45; 95% CI=0.30-0.68; p<0.0001). Differences between the other XM groups and the dalteparin group

were not significant. The incidence of VTE in the hip replacement group was significantly lower for the highest-dose XM group vs dalteparin (11.9% vs 25.5%, OR 0.39; 95% CI=0.23-0.67; p=0.0005). The incidence of VTE in the knee replacement group was lower in the highest-dose XM group vs dalteparin but did not reach significance (22.0% vs 33.7%, OR 0.56; CI=0.29-1.05; p=0.08). Blood transfusions were given to over 70% of patients in both XM and dalteparin groups. There was an increasing amount of blood volume transfused after total hip replacement with increasing doses of XM (p=0.0013). Volume of transfused blood after total knee replacement was similar in all XM groups and similar to dalteparin. The number of patients with excessive bleeding ranged from 1.1% to 5.0% in the XM group and 2.4% in the dalteparin group. The dose-response relation within the XM groups was significant (p=0.002), but the difference between the highest-dose XM and dalteparin was not significant. The frequency of adverse events was similar between the groups. There were small and temporary increases in the levels of alanine and aspartate transaminases; no patients had any symptoms of adversely affected liver function.

| Concl. | XM sequential therapy is as safe and effective as dalteparin for the prophylaxis of VTE in orthopaedic patients undergoing hip and knee replacement. |

NAFT

Low-Molecular-Weight Heparin Prophylaxis vs Warfarin in Hip Arthroplasty

Title	Low-molecular-weight heparin prophylaxis using dalteparin in close proximity to surgery vs warfarin in hip arthroplasty patients.
Authors	Hull RD, Pineo GF, Francis C, et al.
Reference	Arch Intern Med 2000;160:2199-2207.
Disease	Deep vein thrombosis prophylaxis.
Purpose	To determine whether administration of low-molecular-weight heparin just prior to hip arthroplasty is more effective in preventing venous thrombosis than to warfarin.
Design	Randomized, double-blind, multicenter.
Patients	1472 patients undergoing elective hip replacement.
Follow-up	≈6 days.
Regimen	Patients randomized to preoperative dalteparin sodium received 2500 IU subcutaneously within 2 hours of surgery; they received a second dose 4 hours postoperatively. Patients randomized to postoperative dalteparin received placebo injection before surgery and dalteparin at least 4 hours postoperatively. On subsequent days patients in both of these groups received 5000 IU dalteparin subcutaneously q am. Patients randomized to warfarin received initial postoperative dose in the evening of the day of surgery. Initial dose was 10 mg (less in patients 70 or older or weighing less than 57 kg). Warfarin then adjusted to maintain international normalized ratio from 2.0-3.0. Placebo injections given to warfarin patients. Placebo capsules given to dalteparin patients.

Results	Primary end point was deep vein thrombosis detected with contrast venography performed on a mean of day 5.7. Deep vein thrombosis assessed by interpretable venograms was observed in 36/337 (10.7%) preoperative dalteparin patients; 44/336 (13.1%) postoperative dalteparin patients vs 81/338 (24.0%) warfarin patients (p<0.001 for both preoperative and postoperative dalteparin vs warfarin). Proximal deep vein thrombosis developed in 3/354 (0.8%) in preoperative dalteparin group, 3/358 (0.8%) in postoperative dalteparin group, and 11/363 (3.0%) of warfarin group (p=0.04 and p=0.03 for preoperative and postoperative dalteparin vs warfarin, respectively). Symptomatic venous thrombi were less frequent in preoperative dalteparin group (1.5%) vs warfarin group (4.4%; p=0.02). Major bleeding at surgical sites was more common in patients receiving preoperative dalteparin vs warfarin (2.2 vs 0.4% on days 2-8, =0.01).
Concl.	Dalteparin given in close proximity to surgery decreased the risk of deep vein thrombosis. Dalteparin initiated postoperatively was more effective than warfarin without increasing bleeding.

11. Deep Vein Thrombosis/Pulmonary Embolism

NAFT

Dalteparin Extended Out-of-Hospital vs In-Hospital Warfarin/Out-of-Hospital Placebo, in Hip Arthroplasty

Title	Low-molecular-weight heparin prophylaxis using dalteparin extended out-of-hospital vs in-hospital warfarin/out-of-hospital placebo in hip arthroplasty patients. A double-blind, randomized comparison.
Authors	Hull RD, Pineo GF, Francis C, et al., for North American Fragmin(r) Trial Investigators.
Reference	Arch Intern Med 2000;160:2208-2215.
Disease	Deep vein thrombosis, prophylaxis.
Purpose	To determine the efficacy of extended out-of-hospital prophylaxis using dalteparin sodium vs placebo in patients undergoing elective hip surgery to prevent proximal vein thrombosis.
Design	Randomized, double-blind, multicenter.
Patients	569 patients undergoing hip arthroplasty.
Follow-up	≈35 days.
Regimen	Preoperative, postoperative dalteparin groups as described under "Low-Molecular-Weight Heparin Prophylaxis vs Warfarin in Hip Arthroplasty" Study. (Arch Intern Med 2000;160:2199-2207). In-hospital warfarin group: During extended out-of-hospital prophylaxis patients randomized to placebo discontinued warfarin and received placebo injection until day 35. Dalteparin patients received 5000 IU qd; subcutaneously until day 35.

Results   Venography performed on day 6 or at hospital discharge and
           at the end of the extended prophylaxis period (≈day 35). New
           out-of-hospital proximal vein thrombosis assessed by interpre-
           table venograms were observed in 1.3% of preoperative dalte-
           parin group; 0.7% of postoperative dalteparin group (p=0.04),
           and 1.0% (p=0.02) of combined dalteparin groups; vs 4.8% of
           the in-hospital warfarin/out-of-hospital placebo groups. Overall
           cumulative frequencies of all deep thrombosis (including in
           and out-of-hospital) were 17.2% (p<0.001), 22.2% (p=0.003)
           and 19.7% (p<0.001) in the preoperative, postoperative, com-
           bined dalteparin groups vs 36.7% for in-hospital warfarin/out-
           of-hospital placebo groups. Benefits of dalteparin were also seen
           for reducing proximal deep vein thrombosis. Major bleeding
           did not occur during the extended prophylaxis period.

Concl.   Extended dalteparin prophylaxis resulted in lower frequencies of
           proximal vein thrombosis vs in hospital warfarin.

PENTATHLON 2000

Fondaparinux vs Enoxaparin for Prevention of Venous Thromboembolism After Hip-Replacement Surgery

Title	Postoperative fondaparinux vs postoperative enoxaparin for prevention of venous thromboembolism after elective hip-replacement surgery: a randomized double-blind trial.
Authors	Turpie AGG, Bauer KA, Eriksson BI, et al.
Reference	Lancet 2002;359:1721-1726.
Disease	Venous thromboembolism.
Purpose	To compare the efficacy and safety of a once-daily subcutaneous fondaparinux (a specific factor Xa inhibitor) and twice daily subcutaneous enoxaparin for prevention of venous thromboembolism in patients undergoing elective hip-replacement surgery.
Design	Randomized, double-blind, multicenter.
Patients	1584 patients, ≥18 years old, undergoing a first elective total hip-replacement surgery or a revision of ≥1 component of a previously implanted hip prosthesis. Patients undergoing bilateral hip replacement; women of childbearing potential; patients with active bleeding; acute bacterial endocarditis; bleeding disorder; hemorrhagic stroke; recent spinal, brain, or eye surgery; hypersensitivity to heparin; hypersensitivity to iodinated contrast media; serum creatinine ≥180 mmol/L, and platelet count <100×109/L were excluded. Patients who had received anticoagulant, antiplatelet, or fibrinolytic treatment, including dextran within 1-week prior to surgery, or who had an indication for anticoagulation therapy were not included. Use of aspirin before enrollment was not considered as exclusion criterion.
Follow-up	49 days.
Regimen	Randomization to fondaparinux (2.5 mg/d subcutaneous) or enoxaparin (30 mg bid subcutaneous). Therapy with fondaparinux was started 4-8 hours after surgery and enoxaparin was started 12-24 hours after surgery. Therapy was continued for 5-9 days.

Results   Of the 2275 patients randomized, 1584 patients (70%) received the study medications and were available for follow-up (787 patients in the fondaparinux group and 797 patients in the enoxaparin group). By day 11, venous thromboembolism was detected in 6% of the patients receiving fondaparinux and in 8% of the patients receiving enoxaparin (relative risk reduction was 26.3%; 95% CI=-10.8 to 52.8; p=0.099). Any deep vein thrombosis occurred in 6% and 8% of the patients, respectively (RR reduction 31.3% (95% CI=-4.8 to 56.8; p=0.047). Between day 1 and day 49, more patients in the fondaparinux had symptomatic venous thromboembolism (3% vs 1%; p=0.013). 1% of the patients in the fondaparinux group vs 0.2% in the enoxaparin group had nonfatal pulmonary embolism. 49-day mortality was 0.5% with fondaparinux and 0.3% with enoxaparin. Bleeding leading to reoperation occurred in 0.2% of the patients in each group, and major bleeding in 2% of the patients in the fondaparinux group vs 0.7% in the enoxaparin group. 53% and 49% of the patients, respectively, needed postoperative transfusions. Thrombocytopenia <100×109/L was detected in 2% and 3%, respectively. Fondaparinux was safe and was not associated with adverse effects.

Concl.   2.5 mg fondaparinux administered subcutaneously once daily was comparable to enoxaparin in preventing venous thromboembolism after elective hip-replacement surgery.

PREVENT

Prevention of Recurrent Venous Thromboembolism

Title	Long-term, low-intensity warfarin therapy for the prevention of recurrent venous thromboembolism.
Authors	Ridker PM, Goldhaber SZ, Danielson E, et al.
Reference	N Engl J Med 2003;348:1425-143.
Disease	Deep vein thrombosis/pulmonary embolism.
Purpose	To determine if long-term, low-intensity warfarin therapy (target INR=1.5-2.0) is safe and effective in reducing the risk of venous thromboembolism in patients who have had an episode of idiopathic venous thromboembolism.
Design	Randomized, double-blind, placebo-controlled.
Patients	508 patients who were men and women at least 30 years of age, with idiopathic venous thromboembolism who had completed at least 3 continuous months of full-dose warfarin. Thromboembolic events were classified as idiopathic if they did not occur within 90 days of surgery or trauma. Exclusion criteria were history of metastatic cancer; major gastrointestinal bleeding; hemorrhagic stroke; life expectancy less than 3 years; treatment with dipyridamole, ticlopidine, clopidogrel, heparin, or >325 mg aspirin; known lupus anticoagulant disease, or antiphospholipid antibody syndrome.
Follow-up	Up to 4.3 years; mean was 2.1 years. Trial terminated early.
Regimen	Patients were randomized to low-intensity warfarin or placebo. The target INR in the warfarin group was 1.5-2.0, and the dose of warfarin was adjusted every 2 months based on the INR. Blood samples were obtained and evaluated for factor V Leiden and the G20210A prothrombin polymorphism.

Results	The primary end point was the composite of recurrent venous thromboembolism, major hemorrhage, and all-cause death. 253 patients were assigned to placebo and 255 assigned to warfarin. The median duration of the full-dose warfarin therapy before study start was 6.5 months. The median INR in the placebo group was 1.0, and the median INR in the warfarin group was 1.7. The median warfarin dose was 4.0 mg. The composite primary end point was reached in 8.0/100 person-years in the placebo group and 4.1/100 person-years in the warfarin group, (hazard ratio [HR] 0.52; 95% CI=0.31-0.87; p=0.01). 37/253 patients in the placebo group had a recurrent venous thromboembolism vs 14/255 in the low-intensity warfarin group; this was a risk reduction of 64% (HR 0.36; 95% CI=0.19-0.67; p<0.001). The warfarin had a similar effect in patients with and without either factor V Leiden or the prothrombin mutation; patients who had a thrombophilia and were in the warfarin group had a 75% RR vs those in the placebo group; patients without a thrombophilia who were in the warfarin group had a 58% RR, and the difference between these was not significant (for interaction, p=0.51). There were 2 episodes of bleeding requiring hospitalization in the placebo group vs 5 in the warfarin group, (HR 2.53; 95% CI=0.49-13.03; p=0.25). There were 34 incidences of minor bleeding in the placebo group vs 60 in the warfarin group, (HR 1.92; 95% CI=1.26-2.93; p=0.002). There were no significant differences between the groups in death, cancer, or MI.
Concl.	Long-term, low-intensity treatment with warfarin is an effective and safe method for preventing recurrent venous thromboembolism.

SACRE

Study Comparing Oral Anticoagulants with Reviparin

Title	Extended venous thromboembolism prophylaxis after total hip replacement.
Authors	Samama CM, Vray M, Barre J, et al.
Reference	Arch Intern Med 2002;162:2191-2196.
Disease	Deep vein thrombosis/pulmonary embolism.
Purpose	To compare the efficacy and safety of low-molecular-weight heparin with acenocoumarol in the prevention of symptomatic venous thromboembolism.
Design	Multi-center, randomized.
Patients	1279 patients, randomized to reviparin (n=643) or oral aceno-coumarol (n=636). Eligible patients were >18 years who were to undergo elective unilateral primary total hip replacement. Exclusion criteria included: current active bleeding, history of deep vein thrombosis or pulmonary embolism, heparin-induced thrombocytopenia, disorders in which anticoagulation therapy was contraindicated, and others.
Follow-up	Approximately 52 days.
Regimen	All patients received reviparin sodium (4200 IU, 1 SC injection) 12 hours before the surgery. Post-operatively, patients continued to receive the same amount of reviparin qd for 3±1 days. If there were no symptoms or signs of deep vein thrombosis, pulmonary embolism, or major bleeding, patients were then randomized to continue receiving reviparin or switched to acenocoumarol for 6 weeks postoperatively. Acenocoumarol was dosed to a target international normalized ratio (INR) of 2.0-3.0 for 2 consecutive days, after which reviparin was discontinued.

Results	The primary end point of the study was the composite outcome of a confirmed symptomatic thromboembolic event, major bleeding, and death. Patients were asked to report bleeding and thromboembolic episodes. Major bleeding was defined as clinically overt and meeting any of the following criteria: 1) associated with a decrease in the hemoglobin level of >20 g/L vs baseline; 2) required transfusion of 2 U or more of packed red blood cells during the study period; 3) digestive, intracranial, retroperitoneal, or intraocular in location; 4) bleeding at the surgical site that required reoperation; 5) bleeding leading to termination of study treatment. Minor bleeding was defined as clinically overt but without meeting the above major criteria. The primary end point occurred in 24 of 643 patients (3.7%) in the reviparin group vs 53 of 636 patients (8.3%) in the acenocoumarol group, an absolute difference of 4.6% and relative risk reduction of 55% (c2 p=0.001). In the reviparin group, 15/643 (2.3%) developed at least 1 thromboembolic event vs 21/636 (3.3%) in the acenocoumarol group; this was an absolute difference of 1.0% (95% CI=-0.8% to 2.8%, c2 p=0.30). 9 patients (1.4%) in the reviparin group had at least 1 major bleeding event vs 35 patients (5.5%) in the acenocoumarol group, which was an absolute difference of 4.1% (c2 p=0.001). 13 patients (2.0%) in the reviparin group had a minor bleeding episode vs 17 patients (2.7%) in the acenocoumarol group, a nonsignificant difference (c2 p=0.44).
Concl.	Reviparin was as effective as acenocoumarol but was associated with significantly fewer major bleeding episodes.

CLOT

Randomized Comparison of Low-Molecular-Weight Heparin vs Oral Anticoagulant Therapy for the Prevention of Recurrent Venous Thromboembolism in Patients with Cancer

Title	Low-molecular-weight heparin vs a coumarin for the prevention of recurrent venous thromboembolism in patients with cancer.
Authors	Lee AYY, Levine MN, Baker RI, et al.
Reference	N Engl J Med 2003;349:146-153.
Disease	Deep vein thrombosis/pulmonary embolism.
Purpose	To compare the efficacy of a low-molecular-weight heparin with that of an oral anticoagulant agent in preventing recurrent thrombosis in patients with cancer.
Design	Multicenter, randomized, open-label clinical trial.
Patients	672 patients with cancer who had acute, symptomatic proximal deep-vein thrombosis, pulmonary embolism, or both.
Follow-up	6 months.
Regimen	Low-molecular-weight heparin (dalteparin), 200 IU/kg body weight SC qd for 5-7 days and a coumarin derivative for 6 months (target international normalized ratio 2.5); or dalteparin alone for 6 months (200 IU/kg qd for 1 month, then 150 IU/kg/d for 5 months).
Results	During follow-up, 27 of 336 patients receiving dalteparin only and 53 of 336 receiving oral anticoagulant had recurrent venous thromboembolism (hazard ratio [HR] 0.48; p=0.002). The probability of recurrent thromboembolism at 6 months was 17% among patients receiving oral anticoagulant and 9% among those receiving dalteparin only. Rates of major bleeding were not significantly different between the groups, 4% with oral anticoagulant vs 6% with dalteparin only, nor were rates of any bleeding, 19% and 14%, respectively. The 6-month mortality rate was 39% in the dalteparin group and 41% in the oral anticoagulant group. 90% of the deaths in each group were due to progressive cancer.

Concl.   Dalteparin was more effective than an oral anticoagulant in reducing the risk of recurrent thromboembolism. Dalteparin did not increase the risk of bleeding. Long-term self-injection of this low-molecular-weight heparin was acceptable to the patients.

ELATE

Extended Low-Intensity Anticoagulation for Thromboembolism

Title	Comparison of low-intensity warfarin therapy with conventional-intensity warfarin therapy for long-term prevention of recurrent venous thromboembolism.
Authors	Kearon C, Ginsberg JS, Kovacs MJ, et al.
Reference	N Engl J Med 2003;349:631-639.
Disease	Venous thromboembolism.
Purpose	To compare low-intensity warfarin therapy with conventional-intensity warfarin therapy for long-term prevention of recurrent venous thromboembolism.
Design	Multicenter, randomized, double-blind study.
Patients	738 patients who had completed ≥3 months of warfarin therapy for unprovoked venous thromboembolism.
Follow-up	Average 2.4 years.
Regimen	Warfarin with a target international normalized ratio of 2-3 (conventional intensity, n=369) or a target international normalized ratio of 1.5-1.9 (low intensity, n=369).
Results	Mean international normalized ratio was 1.8 among patients receiving low-intensity therapy and 2.4 among those receiving conventional-intensity therapy. There were 16 episodes of recurrent venous thromboembolism among those receiving low-intensity therapy (1.9 per 100 person-years) vs 6 among those receiving conventional-intensity therapy (0.7 per 100 person-years) (hazard ratio [HR] 2.8; 95% CI=1.1-7). Major bleeding episodes occurred in 9 patients receiving low-intensity therapy (1.1 events per 100 person-years) and in 8 receiving conventional-intensity therapy (0.9 events per 100 person-years) (HR 1.2; 95% CI=0.4-3). Major bleeding was more common among patients ≥65 years (HR 2.6; 95% CI=1-6.9). The frequency of overall bleeding did not differ significantly between the groups. The length of warfarin therapy (>4 months vs 3-4 months) did not affect the risk of major bleeding.

Concl.   Conventional-intensity warfarin therapy is more effective than low-intensity therapy for long-term prevention of venous thromboembolism. Low-intensity therapy does not reduce the risk of clinically important bleeding.

EXULT A

Exanta Used to Lessen Thrombosis A

Title	Comparison of ximelagatran with warfarin for the prevention of venous thromboembolism after total knee replacement.
Authors	Francis CS, Berkowitz SD, Comp PC, et al.
Reference	N Engl J Med 2003;349:1703-1712.
Disease	Deep vein thrombosis.
Purpose	To determine whether ximelagatran 36 mg bid is superior to warfarin for prevention of deep vein thrombosis after total knee replacement.
Design	Randomized, double-blind trial.
Patients	1851 patients who had undergone total knee replacement (efficacy analysis).
Follow-up	6 weeks.
Regimen	Oral ximelagatran 24 or 36 mg bid for 7-12 days starting the morning after surgery or warfarin starting the evening of the day of surgery. The warfarin dose was adjusted to achieve an international normalized ratio of 2.5.
Results	Ximelagatran 36 mg bid was better than warfarin with respect to the primary composite end point of venous thromboembolism and death from all causes, 20.3% vs 27.6% (p=0.003). The incidence of the composite primary end point in the group receiving 24 mg of ximelagatran was 24.9% (p=0.28 for the comparison with warfarin). The incidence of major bleeding was similar (0.8% with ximelagatran 36 mg and 0.7% with warfarin), as were perioperative indicators of bleeding, wound characteristics and the composite secondary end point of proximal deep-vein thrombosis, pulmonary embolism, and death (2.7% vs 4.1%).

Concl.   Warfarin is the most widely used form of deep vein thrombosis prophylaxis after total knee replacement. It has a long safety record, it can be administered orally, and the rate of early bleeding is lower than with other agents; however, warfarin has a delayed onset of action, requires monitoring of coagulation and dose adjustment, and has the potential for interaction with food and other drugs. Fixed-dose ximelagatran, administered without coagulation monitoring, was significantly more effective than warfarin, with similar safety.

Matisse

Fondaparinux vs Heparin for Pulmonary Embolism

Title	Subcutaneous fondaparinux vs intravenous unfractionated heparin in the initial treatment of pulmonary embolism.
Authors	Matisse Investigators.
Reference	N Engl J Med 2003;349:1695-1702.
Disease	Pulmonary embolism.
Purpose	To determine whether fixed-dose, qd, subcutaneous administration of fondaparinux is as effective as unfractionated heparin for the initial treatment of symptomatic pulmonary embolism.
Design	Randomized, open-label trial.
Patients	2213 patients with acute symptomatic pulmonary embolism.
Follow-up	3 months.
Regimen	Fondaparinux (5, 7.5, or 10 mg in patients weighing <50, 50-100, or >100 kg, respectively) SC qd (n=1103) or continuous IV infusion of unfractionated heparin (ratio of activated partial thromboplastin time) to a control value, 1.5-2.5) (n=1110), both given for ≥5 days and until use of vitamin K antagonists resulted in an international normalized ratio >2.0.
Results	The primary efficacy outcome was 3-month incidence of the composite end point of symptomatic, recurrent pulmonary embolism (fatal or nonfatal) and new or recurrent deep-vein thrombosis. The rate of recurrent thromboembolic events among patients receiving fondaparinux was 3.8% vs 5% among those receiving unfractionated heparin (UFH) (95% CI=-3 to 0.5). Major bleeding occurred in 1.3% of fondaparinux-treated patients and 1.1% of UFH-treated patients. The 3-month mortality rate was 5.2% with fondaparinux and 4.4% with UFH, an NS difference. In the fondaparinux group, 14.5% of patients received the drug in part as outpatients.

| Concl. | Once-daily, SC fondaparinux was at least as safe as UFH for initial treatment of hemodynamically stable pulmonary embolism. Rates of adverse events were similar. Fondaparinux has the advantage of not requiring anticoagulation monitoring; further, it can be administered outside of the hospital. |

PENTHIFRA Plus

Pentasaccharide in Hip-Fracture Surgery Plus

Title	Duration of prophylaxis against venous thromboembolism with fondaparinux after hip fracture surgery: a multicenter, randomized, placebo-controlled, double-blind study.
Authors	Eriksson BI, Lassen MR, for the PENTasaccharide in Hip-FRActure Surgery Plus (PENTHIFRA Plus) Investigators.
Reference	Arch Intern Med 2003;163:1337-1342.
Disease	Deep vein thrombosis.
Purpose	To evaluate the benefit-to-risk ratio of fondaparinux sodium compared with placebo for prevention of venous thromboembolism in patients undergoing surgery for hip fracture.
Design	Multicenter, randomized, double-blind trial.
Patients	656 patients undergoing hip fracture surgery.
Follow-up	3 weeks.
Regimen	Once-daily subcutaneous injection of either fondaparinux sodium 2.5 mg or placebo for 19-23 days.
Results	The primary efficacy outcome, venous thromboembolism (VTE) occurring during the double-blind period, was assessed in 428 patients. The incidence of VTE (detected by bilateral venography) was significantly lower in patients receiving fondaparinux (3/208; 1.4%) compared with placebo (77/220; 35%), yielding a relative risk reduction of 95.9% (95% CI=87.2%-99.7%; p<0.001). The incidence of symptomatic VTE was also lower with fondaparinux (1/326; 0.3%) than with placebo (9/330; 2.7%) (relative risk reduction 88.8%, p=0.02). An additional 3 weeks of fondaparinux prophylaxis reduced the incidence of proximal deep vein thrombosis by 94%. There was a trend toward more major bleeding in the fondaparinux group (p=0.06), but the incidence of clinically relevant bleeding (leading to death, reoperation, or critical organ bleeding) did not differ. There were no differences between the 2 groups in the overall incidence of adverse events and overall mortality.

Concl.   Prophylaxis with fondaparinux for 3 weeks after hip fracture surgery produced a 96% reduction in risk of VTE and was well tolerated; it did not increase the rate of clinically relevant bleeding in this population of generally old and frail patients. The dramatic reduction in venographically detected VTE was associated with an 89% reduction in symptomatic events, suggesting that asymptomatic thrombosis detected by screening venography is a valid surrogate end point for symptomatic events.

THRIVE III

Thrombin Inhibitor in Venous Thromboembolism III

Title	Secondary prevention of venous thromboembolism with oral direct thrombin inhibitor ximelagatran.
Authors	Schulman S, Wåhlander K, Lundström T, et al.
Reference	N Engl J Med 2003;349:1713-1721.
Disease	Venous thromboembolism.
Purpose	To determine the long-term efficacy and safety of fixed-dose ximelagatran, a novel oral direct thrombin inhibitor, started after 6 months standard anticoagulation therapy for venous thromboembolism.
Design	Double-blind, randomized, placebo-controlled, multicenter.
Patients	1233 patients with venous thromboembolism (symptomatic, objectively confirmed deep venous thrombosis of the leg or pulmonary embolism) who had been treated for 6 months with standard anticoagulation therapy without recurrence.
Follow-up	18 months.
Regimen	After these patients had undergone 6 months of standard anticoagulation therapy, they were randomized for extended secondary prevention to either oral ximelagatran (n=612; 24 mg) or placebo (n=611) given bid without monitoring for anticoagulation for 18 months. Bilateral ultrasonography of the legs and perfusion lung scanning were performed at baseline.

11

Results	Primary outcome was time-to-confirmed new venous thromboembolic event. Secondary objective was to estimate overall mortality and other measures of safety such as bleeding. Symptomatic recurrent venous thromboembolism occurred in 12 patients in the ximelagatran group vs 71 patients in the placebo group (hazard ratio=0.16; 95% CI=0.09-0.30; p<0.001). Estimated cumulative risk of an event was 2.8% in the ximelagatran group vs 12.6% in the placebo group (p<0.001). Death occurred in 1.1% of the ximelagatran group vs 1.4% of the placebo group (p=NS). Bleeding occurred in 23.9% of the ximelagatran group vs 21.0% of the placebo group (p=0.17). Major bleeding occurred 6 times in the ximelagatran group vs 5 events in the placebo group; none of these were fatal. Cumulative risk of transient increase in the alanine aminotransferase liver enzymes >3× upper limit of normal was greater in the ximelagatran group (6.4%) vs the placebo group (1.2%; p<0.001).
Concl.	After 6 months of standard anticoagulant therapy for venous thromboembolism, an additional 18 months of treatment with the oral direct thrombin inhibitor ximelagatran extended prevention of venous thromboembolism. While it did not increase the frequency of bleeding, it did increase the number of patients that had transient increases in alanine aminotransferase levels.

12. Coronary Artery Disease, Atherosclerosis, Prevention of Progression

Ramipril in Patients with Coronary Disease

Title	Randomized, placebo-controlled trial of the angiotensin-converting enzyme inhibitor, ramipril, in patients with coronary or other occlusive arterial disease.
Authors	MacMahon S, Sharpe N, Gamble G, et al, for the PART-2 Collaborative Research.
Reference	J Am Coll Cardiol 2000;36:438-443.
Disease	Coronary, cerebrovascular, peripheral vascular disease.
Purpose	To determine the effects of the ACE inhibitor, ramipril, on carotid atherosclerosis in patients with atheroclerosis.
Design	2-Week tolerability phase followed by randomization to placebo vs ramipril; double-blind, parallel-group design, multicenter.
Patients	617 patients aged 75 years or less who had a diagnosis within 5 years of enrollment of acute MI, angina with CAD confirmed by angiography or exercise ECG, transient ischemic attack or intermittent claudication.
Follow-up	4 years.
Regimen	During 2 week tolerability phase ramipril 5 mg daily for the first week; then 10 mg daily for the second week. Then, depending on initial tolerability 5 mg or 10 mg ramipril once daily (n=308) vs placebo (n=309).
Results	Main outcomes were based on results of B mode ultrasound of the carotid arteries and LV mass assessed by M-mode echocardiography. Ramipril caused a 6 mm Hg reduction in systolic blood pressure and a 4 mm Hg reduction in diastolic blood pressure vs the placebo group (p<0.0001). There was no difference between groups in changes in common carotid artery wall thickness from baseline or in change in carotid plaque score. There was a 3.8 gm/m² decrease in LV mass index in the ramipril group vs placebo group (p=0.04). 16 patients in the ramipril group and 25 in the placebo group died (p=0.17); there was no difference in hospitalization rate.

Concl. The results did not support the hypothesis that ramipril reduced atherosclerosis as a mechanism for its benefit in such studies as HOPE. Benefits may have been due to its BP lowering effect or a reduction in LV mass or endothelial dysfunction.

United Kingdom Small Aneurysm Trial Participants

Title	Long-term outcomes of immediate repair compared with surveillance of small abdominal aortic aneurysms.
Authors	The United Kingdom Small Aneurysm Participants.
Reference	N Engl J Med 2002;346:1445-1452.
Disease	Small abdominal aortic aneurysm.
Purpose	To report the long-term survival analysis of surveillance by ultrasonography vs early elective surgery for patients with small abdominal aortic aneurysms in the United Kingdom Small Aneurysm Trial.
Design	Randomized, multicenter.
Patients	1090 patients 60-76 years old with asymptomatic small abdominal aortic aneurysms defined as a diameter of 4.0-5.5 cm.
Follow-up	8 years.
Regimen	Patients were randomized to surveillance with ultrasonography and offered surgery when the diameter of the aneurysm exceeded 5.5 cm, if the aneurysm expanded more than 1 cm per year, if patients developed symptoms or tenderness, or if repair of a proximal or iliac aneurysm was scheduled (n=527); or randomized to elective surgery (n=563).

Results   At 8 years (range 6-10 years) follow-up 254 died in the surveil-
           lance group vs 242 in the early surgery group. Mean duration
           of survival was 6.5 years in the surveillance group vs 6.7 in the
           early surgery group (p=0.29). As of August, 2001, the adjusted
           hazard ratio for death in the early surgery group was 0.83 (95%
           CI=0.69-1.00; p=0.05). Survival was initially worse in the early-
           surgery group (30-day mortality of 5.5%) whereas at 3 years
           the survival curves crossed and at 8 years, mortality in the early
           surgery group was 7.2% lower than in the surveillance group
           (p=0.03). Death due to ruptured abdominal aortic aneurysm
           occurred in 21 (8%) of patients in the surveillance group vs 10
           (4%) in the early surgery group. Death rates were associated with
           older age, larger diameter of aneurysm, worse lung function,
           current smoking. Death rates were lower among patients who
           stopped smoking. Death due to ruptured aneurysm was more
           common in women (14%) than men (5%) who died.

Concl.   There was no long-term difference in mean survival between
           early surgery and surveillance groups. Early mortality was high-
           er in the early surgery group but after 3 years survival curves
           crossed and at 8 years mortality in the early-surgery group was
           lower than the surveillance group.

Lyon Diet Heart Study

Title	Mediterranean diet, traditional risk factors, and the rate of cardiovascular complications after myocardial infarction. Final report of the Lyon Diet Heart Study.
Authors	DeLorgeril M, Salen P, Martin J-L, et al.
Reference	Circulation 1999; 99:779-785.
Disease	Coronary artery disease.
Purpose	To determine whether a Mediterranean diet vs a prudent Western diet decreases the recurrence of cardiac events after a first acute myocardial infarction.
Design	Randomized, single blind.
Patients	Consecutive patients who survived a first acute myocardial infarction, <70 years of age, were randomized between March 1988 and March 1992. 1383 and 1467 person-year follow-up mortality in control vs experimental groups.
Follow-up	Average 46 months per patient.
Regimen	Mediterranean diet vs prudent western diet. (Mediterranean diet is high in a-linolenic acid-rich foods, high intake of fresh fruits, vegetables, legumes, cereals, and B vitamins).
Results	Patients on the Mediterranean diet had a reduction in the composite end point of cardiac death and nonfatal myocardial infarction at 14 events vs 44 in the prudent Western diet (p=0.0001). They also had a reduction in the first composite end point plus unstable angina, stroke, heart failure, pulmonary or peripheral embolism (27 vs 90; p=0.0001); they also had a reduction in the 2 composite end points above plus minor events requiring hospitalization (95 vs 180; p=0.0002). Total cholesterol, systolic blood pressure, and leukocyte count were associated with increased cardiac risk; female sex and aspirin were associated with reduced risk.
Concl.	The Mediterranean diet was protective after a first myocardial infarction.

Estrogen Replacement and Atherosclerosis Trial

Title	Effects of estrogen replacement on the progression of coronary artery atherosclerosis.
Authors	Herrington DM, Reboussin DM, Brosnihan B, et al.
Reference	N Engl J Med 2000;343:522-529.
Disease	Coronary artery disease.
Purpose	To determine the effects of hormone replacement therapy on the progression of coronary atherosclerosis in women.
Design	Randomized, double-blind, placebo-controlled, multicenter.
Patients	309 women with angiographic evidence of coronary artery disease.
Follow-up	Mean of 3.2 years.
Regimen	Randomized to 0.625 mg of conjugated estrogen per day, 0.625 mg of conjugated estrogen plus 2.5 mg of medroxyprogesterone acetate per day, or placebo.
Results	Coronary angiography at baseline and at follow-up of about 3 years. Primary end point was mean minimal coronary artery diameter within each subject at follow-up. Mean minimal coronary artery diameters at follow-up were 1.87±0.02 mm in estrogen group, 1.84±0.02 mm in estrogen plus medroxyprogesterone acetate group, and 1.87±0.02 mm in placebo group, respectively (p=NS). Analyses of secondary angiographic outcomes showed similar results. Thus, neither treatment altered the progression of atherosclerosis. Patients assigned to estrogen had a decrease in plasma LDL cholesterol of 9.4±20.9% and patients assigned to estrogen plus medroxyprogesterone had reductions of LDL of 16.5±21.8% vs 1.3±21.5% in placebo (p=0.02 for comparison of estrogen vs placebo; and p<0.001 for estrogen plus progesterone vs placebo). Women in both treatment groups had significant increases in HDL cholesterol (18.8±20.8% and 14.2±17.1%) compared to women on placebo (6.8±15.6%; p<0.01).

12

Concl.   Neither unopposed estrogen nor estrogen plus medroxyproges-
          terone acetate altered the progression of coronary atherosclerosis
          in women with known CAD.

Women's Health Initiative Observational Study

Title	Inflammatory biomarkers, hormone replacement therapy, and incident coronary heart disease—prospective analysis from the Women's Health Initiative observational study.
Authors	Pradhan AD, Manson JE, Rossouw JE, et al.
Reference	JAMA 2002;288:980-987.
Disease	Development of coronary heart disease in postmenopausal women.
Purpose	To determine the association between baseline levels of C-reactive protein (CRP) and interleukin-6 (IL-6) and incidence of coronary heart disease (CHD), and determine the interactions between hormone replacement therapy (HRT), CRP, and IL-6 with regards to heart disease risk.
Design	Prospective, case-control.
Patients	304 case patients and 304 control patients. Case patients were free of cardiovascular disease and cancer at enrollment and developed a first myocardial infarction during follow-up. Controls were patients without cardiovascular disease or cancer at baseline who did not develop an MI during follow-up. Control and cases were matched 1:1 according to age (±2 years), smoking status, ethnicity, and length of follow-up (±6 months). Patients were excluded if they had a history of any of the following at baseline: angina, congestive heart failure, MI, coronary revascularization, stroke, or cancer.
Follow-up	Median 2.9 years.

Regimen	Hormone replacement therapy was classified as never, past, or current. This included unopposed estrogen or estrogen plus progestin. 82% of current estrogen users were taking oral conjugated equine estrogens; 74% were on 6.25 mg/d.
Results	Case patients had an increased prevalence of cardiovascular risk factors than control patients. Overall, 36.5% of patients were currently using HRT; duration of treatment or unopposed estrogen vs estrogen plus progestin use were not significantly different between cases and controls. Usage rates of aspirin, statin, or other lipid-lowering treatment at baseline were not significantly different. Levels of CRP and IL-6 at baseline were higher in the case group than control (CRP: 0.33 vs 0.25 mg/dL; p<0.001; IL-6: 1.81 vs 1.47 pg/mL; p<0.001). Case patients were also more likely to have had higher levels of total cholesterol, LDL-C, triglycerides, higher total cholesterol to HDL-C ratio, and lower HDL-C at baseline. Increased levels of CRP and IL-6 were both associated with increased risk of CHD. For CRP, the events OR for women with CRP levels in the highest quartile vs the lowest quartile was 2.3 (95% CI=1.4-3.7 p=0.002); for IL-6, it was 3.3 (95% CI=2.0-5.5; p<0.001). Adjustment of the ratios for levels of total and HDL cholesterol and baseline aspirin and statin use did not change the results. Full adjustment including adjustment for other cardiovascular risk factors yielded ORs between the highest and lowest quartile levels of 2.1 [1.1-4.2; p=0.03] and 2.0 [1.0-4.0; p=0.03] for CRP and IL-6, respectively. Higher baseline levels of CRP and IL-6 were associated with incremental increases in odds of CHD across all BMI categories. No relationship was observed between IL-6 levels and HRT use. CRP levels were 55% higher in current users vs nonusers of HRT in case patients (p=0.001), and 70% higher in current users vs nonusers in control patients (p<0.001). Increases in CRP were independently correlated with future CHD events regardless of HRT use at baseline.
Concl.	Increased levels of CRP and IL-6 were independently associated with increased risk of CHD events in healthy postmenopausal women. Hormone replacement therapy was associated with higher levels of CRP. Baseline levels of CRP or IL-6 were more important than HRT use status in predicting CHD events.

Indo-Mediterranean Diet Heart Study

Title	Effect of an Indo-Mediterranean diet on progression of coronary artery disease in high-risk patients (Indo-Mediterranean Diet Heart Study): a randomised single-blind trial.
Authors	Singh RB, Dubnov G, Niaz MA, et al.
Reference	Lancet 2002;360:1455-1461.
Disease	Coronary artery disease.
Purpose	To assess the effects of Indo-Mediterranean diet consisting of whole grains including fruits, vegetables, nuts, legumes and mustard or soybean oil in patients with established coronary artery disease or at high-risk for coronary artery disease.
Design	Randomized, single-blind, multicenter.
Patients	1000 patients, >25 years old, with hypercholesterolemia, hypertension, diabetes mellitus, or coronary artery disease. 418 patients had ≥1 risk factors, 105 patients had angina pectoris and 478 patients had previous myocardial infarction. Patients without major risk factors, cancer, chronic diarrhea, BUN >6.6 mmol/L, arthritis, refusal of laboratory testing, dislike of the intervention diet, and death before randomization were not included.
Follow-up	2 years.
Regimen	Randomization to a diet rich in whole grains, fruits, vegetables, walnuts, and almonds (n=499) or a local diet similar to the Step 1 NCEP diet.
Add'l Tx	Patients from both groups were advised to walk 3-4 km or jog for 10-15 minutes every day. Yoga meditation and breathing exercises were encouraged in both groups. There were no restrictions concerning drug therapy. Smoking and alcohol intake were discouraged.

Results	Non-fatal MI occurred in 4.2% of the patients in the intervention diet vs 8.6% in the control diet (adjusted risk ratio [RR] 0.47; 95% CI=0.28-0.79). Fatal MI occurred in 2.4% and 3.4%, respectively (adjusted RR 0.67; 95% CI=0.31-1.42). Sudden cardiac death occurred in 1.2% vs 3.2%, respectively (adjusted RR 0.33; 95% CI=0.13-0.86). Total cardiac end points (MI or sudden cardiac death) occurred in 7.8% in the intervention diet vs 15.2% in the control diet (adjusted RR 0.48; 95% CI=0.33-0.71; p<0.001). Angina pectoris (7% vs 11%; p=0.013), positive exercise test (16% vs 36%; p<0.0001), LV hypertrophy (5% vs 11%; p=0.0004), heart failure (2.2% vs 7.0%; p=0.0003), coronary revascularization (1.2% vs 3.2%; p=0.0304), and all-cause mortality (5% vs 8%; p=0.064) were lower in the intervention group. There was no difference in the incidence of cancer or accidents between the groups. Pre-existing CAD at enrollment, and presence of hypertension or hypercholesterolemia at baseline did not alter the effect of the intervention diet.
Concl.	An Indo-Mediterranean diet that is rich in a-linolenic acid is more effective that standard Step 1 NCEP prudent diet for primary and secondary prevention of coronary artery events.

ACADEMIC

Azithromycin in Coronary Artery Disease: Elimination of Myocardial Infection with Chlamydia Study

Title	Randomized secondary prevention trial of azithromycin in patients with coronary artery disease. Primary clinical results of the ACADEMIC study.
Authors	Muhlestein JB, Anderson JL, Carlquist JF, et al.
Reference	Circulation 2000;102:1755-1760.
Disease	Coronary artery disease.
Purpose	To determine the effect of azithromycin, an antibiotic effective against C. pneumoniae, in seropositive CAD patients, on clinical outcomes.
Design	Prospective, randomized, double-blind, secondary prevention trial.
Patients	302 patients with CAD and seropositive to C. pneumoniae (IgG titers ≥1:16). CAD documented by previous MI, bypass surgery, angiographic evidence.
Follow-up	2 years.
Regimen	Placebo vs azithromycin 500 mg/d for 3 days and then 500 mg/week for 3 months.
Results	Primary end point was cardiovascular events at 2 years: cardiovascular death, resuscitated cardiac arrest, nonfatal MI, stroke, unstable angina requiring hospitalization, or unplanned coronary intervention. At 2 years there were 22 events in the azithromycin arm and 25 in the placebo group. There was no statistically significant difference in combined primary end point between groups ($p=0.74$). Cardiovascular death occurred in 5 azithromycin and 4 placebo patients ($p=0.35$). Nonfatal MI occurred in 4 vs 6 and unstable angina in 8 vs 7, azithromycin vs placebo patients, respectively. There was a nonsignificant trend toward fewer unplanned revascularization procedures in the azithromycin group (n=9) vs the placebo group (n=15; $p=0.20$).
Concl.	Azithromycin did not reduce ischemic events over a course of 2 years. The authors note that a larger and longer trial may be needed.

ADAM

Aneurysm Detection and Management Veterans Affairs Cooperative Study

Title	Immediate repair compared with surveillance of small abdominal aortic aneurysms.
Authors	Lederle FA, Wilson SE, Johnson GR, et al.
Reference	N Engl J Med 2002;346:1437-1444.
Disease	Abdominal aortic aneurysms.
Purpose	To determine whether immediate open surgical repair or surveillance with ultrasound or computed tomography with repair for aneurysms that enlarge or become symptomatic is the better strategy for small abdominal aortic aneurysms.
Design	Randomized, multicenter.
Patients	569 patients ages 50-79 years with abdominal aortic aneurysm of 4.0-5.4 cm in diameter by computed tomography without high surgical risk.
Follow-up	Mean 4.9 years; range 3.5-8.0 years.
Regimen	Patients randomized to immediate repair group (n=569) had standard open repair with a synthetic graft. Patients randomized to the surveillance group (n=567) were followed without repair until aneurysm reached at least 5.5 cm in diameter or enlarged by at least 0.7 cm in 6 months or at least 1.0 cm in 1 year or until patients became symptomatic. At that point open repair was carried out. Surveillance patients had ultrasonography or computed tomography to follow aneurysm size.

Results	Primary outcome was rate of death. This was reached in 25.1% of the immediate repair group and 21.5% of the surveillance group (relative risk [RR] 1.21; 95% CI=0.95-1.54). At the end of the study 92.6% of patients in the immediate repair group actually underwent aneurysm repair and 61.6% of patients in the surveillance group underwent repair. There was a low operative mortality of 2.7% in the immediate-repair group. Analysis of data by prespecified subgroups by age, or diameter of aneurysm at entry did not favor immediate repair. Rate of death related to abdominal aortic aneurysm was 3.0% in the immediate repair group vs 2.6% in the surveillance group. 11 patients in the surveillance group ruptured their aneurysm (resulting in 7 deaths) vs 2 in the immediate repair group. 255 patients had other aneurysm-related hospitalizations in the immediate repair group vs 129 in the surveillance group.
Concl.	Elective repair of abdominal aortic aneurysms smaller than 5.5 cm did not improve survival compared to a surveillance approach.

APRES

ACE Inhibition Post-Revascularization Study

Title	The angiotensin-converting enzyme inhibition post revascularization study (APRES).
Authors	Kjøller-Hansen L, Steffensen R, Grande P.
Reference	J Am Coll Cardiol 2000;35:881-888.
Disease	Angina pectoris, coronary artery disease.
Purpose	To determine whether the ACE inhibitor ramipril could reduce the incidence of cardiac events following invasive revascularization in patients with asymptomatic LV dysfunction.
Design	Randomized, double-blind, placebo-controlled, single-center study.
Patients	159 patients with chronic stable angina, LVEF of 0.30-0.50, and no clinical congestive heart failure referred for invasive revascularization with CABG or PTCA.
Follow-up	Median of 33 months.
Regimen	If patients tolerated a test dose of 2.5 mg ramipril they were randomized to 5 mg ramipril daily vs placebo.
Add'l Tx	As per physician.
Results	The composite end point of cardiac death, acute myocardial infarction, or clinical heart failure occurred in 18 of 79 placebo patients and 8 of 80 ramipril patients (risk reduction [RR]=58%; 95% CI=7%-80%; p=0.031). The composite end point of cardiac death, acute myocardial infarction, clinical heart failure, or recurrent angina pectoris occurred in 41 of 79 placebo patients and 36 of 80 ramipril patients (p=NS). 2 patients (2.5%) died in the ramipril group and 8 patients (10%) died in the placebo group (p=0.053). Findings were consistent across various subgroups with regard to LVEF above or below 0.40 and whether CABG or PTCA was performed. Ramipril was well tolerated.

12. CAD Atherosclerosis Prevention of Progression

Concl. Long-term ramipril therapy reduced the composite end point of cardiac death, acute myocardial infarction, or clinical heart failure in patients with angina and asymptomatic moderate LV dysfunction who underwent revascularization.

AVERT

Atorvastatin vs Revascularization Treatment

Title	Aggressive lipid lowering therapy compared with angioplasty in stable coronary artery disease.
Authors	Pitt B, Waters D, Brown WV, et al.
Reference	N Engl J Med 1999;341:70-76.
Disease	Coronary artery disease, hyperlipidemia.
Purpose	To determine the effect of aggressive lipid lowering vs percutaneous coronary revascularization for decreasing the incidence of ischemic events in patients with coronary artery disease and stable angina.
Design	Open-label, randomized, multicenter study.
Patients	341 patients with stable coronary artery disease with stenosis of ≥50% of at least 1 coronary artery who had been recommended for treatment for angioplasty. Low density lipoprotein (LDL) cholesterol of at least 115 mg/dL, serum triglyceride of no more than 500 mg/dL. Patients either were asymptomatic or had mild to moderate angina and relatively normal LV function.
Follow-up	18 months.
Regimen	Atorvastatin 80 mg once daily (n=164) or percutaneous revascularization procedure (angioplasty) plus usual care which could induce lipid lowering as per the physician (n=177).
Add'l Tx	Atorvastatin group could not be on other lipid lowering drugs. Patients randomized to angioplasty could receive lipid lowering drugs as per usual care.

Results	The end point of ischemic events was defined as at least 1 of the following: death from cardiac disease, resuscitation after cardiac arrest, nonfatal myocardial infarction, cerebrovascular accident, coronary bypass surgery, angioplasty, and worsening angina with hospitalization. 22 (13%) of patients on high dose atorvastatin, vs 37 (21%) of patients who received angioplasty plus usual care developed ischemic events. This 36% lower incidence of ischemic events achieved a p value of 0.048 (this was not statistically significant following adjustment for interim analysis). Serum LDL was reduced by 46% to 77 mg/dL in the atorvastatin group vs the angioplasty plus usual care group that had a serum LDL reduced by 18% to a mean of 119 mg/dL (p<0.05). The decrease in ischemic events in the atorvastatin group was primarily secondary to a smaller number of revascularization procedures in that group (12%) compared to the angioplasty group (16%), a decrease in worsening angina with objective evidence of myocardial ischemia resulting in hospitalizations (6.7% vs 14.1% in atorvastatin vs angioplasty groups, respectively). Atorvastatin treatment was associated with a longer time to first ischemic event compared to the angioplasty (p=0.03). The incidence of adverse events was similar in the 2 groups.
Concl.	In patients with stable coronary artery disease, aggressive lipid lowering was associated with a trend toward reduced need for further revascularization procedures compared to patients treated with angioplasty and usual care.

BCAPS

β-Blocker Cholesterol-Lowering Asymptomatic Plaque Study

Title	Low-dose metoprolol CR/XL and fluvastatin slow progression of carotid intima-media thickness. Main results from the β-Blocker Cholesterol-Lowering Asymptomatic Plaque Study (BCAPS).
Authors	Hedblad B, Wikstrand J, Janzon L, et al.
Reference	Circulation 2001;103:1721-1726.
Disease	Atherosclerosis.
Purpose	To determine the effect of low-dose metoprolol CR/XL and fluvastatin on progression of carotid intima-media thickness (IMT), incidence of myocardial infarction and stroke in asymptomic patients with carotid plaques.
Design	Randomized, double-blind, placebo-controlled, single-center trial.
Patients	793 patients with carotid plaque but no symptoms of carotid artery disease.
Follow-up	36 months.
Regimen	Patients randomized to 1 of 4 groups: placebo/placebo; metoprolol CR/XL (25 mg once daily)/placebo; fluvastatin (40 mg once/daily)/placebo; metoprolol/fluvastatin once daily.

Results	Primary outcomes were change in mean IMT in the common carotid artery and carotid bulb. Clinical events also were monitored. In placebo patients the annual rate of IMT (mean) progression was 0.013 mm/year at the common carotid artery and 0.89 mm/year at the carotid bifurcation. Metoprolol CR/XL decreased progression of IMT (mean) in carotid bulb at both 18 and 36 months (-0.058 mm/year [p=0.004] and -0.023 mm/year [p=0.014], respectively). Incidence of adverse cardiovascular clinical events (including mortality, incidence of MI and stroke) tended to be lower in metoprolol (n=5) vs patients not treated with metoprolol (n=13; p=0.055). Rate of IMT (mean) progression in common carotid artery was reduced at 36 months by fluvastatin (-0.009 mm/year; p=0.002). 7 patients on fluvastatin and 11 not on fluvastatin had a cardiovascular event (p=0.350). Combined end point of all cause mortality and time to first cardiovascular event were lower in patients on metoprolol CR/XL (n=8) vs those not on metoprolol CR/XL (n=19; p=0.031). Women had an increased frequency of transiently high liver enzymes on fluvastatin.
Concl.	The β-blocker metoprolol CR/XL had a favorable effect in that it reduced the rate of progression of carotid IMT in asymptomatic subjects. Fluvastatin also reduced rate of IMT progression.

CAPRIE

Clopidogrel vs Aspirin in Patients at Risk of Ischemic Events (Substudy)

Title	Effectiveness of clopidogrel versus aspirin in preventing acute myocardial infarction in patients with symptomatic atherothrombosis (CAPRIE trial).
Authors	Cannon CP, on behalf of the CAPRIE Investigators.
Reference	Am J Cardiol 2002;90:760-762.
Disease	Acute myocardial infarction, coronary artery disease.
Purpose	To determine whether risk of acute myocardial infarction (AMI) could be predicted with baseline characteristics and if clopidogrel has a greater relative benefit than aspirin in high-risk patients.
Design	Retrospective analysis of a randomized, blind, multicenter study.
Patients	19,185 patients with recent ischemic stroke (>1 week, ≤6 months), recent myocardial infarction (≤35 days), or symptomatic atherosclerotic peripheral arterial disease. Exclusion criteria included age <21 years, carotid endarterectomy after stroke, uncontrolled hypertension, contraindications to study drug, and others (from Lancet 1996;348:1329-1339).
Follow-up	Average follow-up of 1.9 years (1-3 years).
Regimen	Clopidogrel 75 mg qd (n=9577), or aspirin 325 mg qd (n=9566).

Results	Patients who developed acute MI (AMI) were found to be older, more often men, and had a higher rate of previous cardiac surgery and CHF. Independent predictors of AMI were found to be: age ≥65 years (OR 1.229; 95% CI=1.040-1.452; p=0.0154), history of diabetes (OR 1.273; 95% CI=1.051-1.540; p=0.0134), previous AMI (OR 1.721; 95% CI=1.321-2.242; p<0.0001), peripheral arterial disease (OR 1.800; 95% CI=1.342-2.415; p<0.0001), previous angina (OR 1.874; 95% CI=1.581-2.221; p<0.0001), previous ischemic stroke (OR 1.448; 95% CI=1.000-2.095; p=0.0497), or baseline creatinine >1.3 mg/dL (OR 1.415; 95% CI=1.192-1.680; p<0.0001). Treatment with clopidogrel was protective against future MI (OR 0.801; 95% CI=0.683-0.941; p=0.0067). The risk of future AMI was also grouped according to the number of risk factors (1 through 5) patients had. Patients who received clopidogrel had a lower risk of AMI vs aspirin in all risk factor subgroups. Relative risk reductions with clopidogrel were 30%, 27%, 12%, 1%, and 30% in patients with 1, 2, 3, 4, and 5 risk factors, respectively.
Concl.	Certain baseline characteristics were predictive of the risk of acute MI, and clopidogrel was more effective than aspirin in preventing future AMI in patients across all risk categories.

CLARIFY

Clarithromycin Acute Coronary Syndrome Patients in Finland

Title	Effect of 3 months of antimicrobial treatment with clarithromycin in acute non-Q-wave coronary syndrome.
Authors	Sinisalo J, Mattila K, Valtoren V, et al.
Reference	Circulation 2002;105:1555-1560.
Disease	Acute non-Q-wave coronary syndrome; unstable angina.
Purpose	To determine whether the antibiotic clarithromycin reduces morbidity and mortality in patients with acute non-Q-wave myocardial infarction (MI) or unstable angina.
Design	Randomized, placebo-controlled, double-blind, multicenter.
Patients	148 patients with acute non-Q-wave MI or unstable angina.
Follow-up	552-557 days.
Regimen	Patients randomized in hospital to placebo (n=74) vs clarithromycin (n=74; 500 mg) daily for 85 days.
Add'l Tx	Usual other antianginal medicines. Decision to perform coronary angiography and revascularization (percutaneous transluminal coronary angioplasty, stenting, coronary artery bypass graft surgery) left up to discretion of physicians.

Results	Primary end point was composite of death, MI, unstable angina within the 3-month period of treatment. Occurrence of any cardiovascular event (defined as death, MI, unstable angina, ischemic stroke, critical peripheral ischemia requiring surgery) during average follow-up period of 555 days was the secondary end point. There was a nonsignificant trend toward fewer patients reaching the primary end point in the clarithromycin group (11) vs the placebo group (19); risk ratio [RR] 0.54; 95% CI=0.25-1.14; p=0.10). At the end of the follow-up period the secondary end point of any cardiovascular event was reached in 16 patients in the clarithromycin vs 27 patients in the placebo group (RR 0.49; 95% CI=0.26-0.92; p=0.03). At the end of follow-up there were 4 deaths in the clarithromycin group from ischemic heart disease and 1 death in the placebo group from cancer. 5 patients in the clarithromycin group vs 14 in the placebo group had MIs (p=0.01).
Concl.	Clarithromycin reduces risk of overall cardiovascular events in patients with acute non-Q-wave MI or unstable angina. It did not reduce mortality.

12

CUDAS

Perth Carotid Ultrasound Disease Assessment Study

Title	Antioxidant vitamins and the risk of carotid atherosclerosis. The Perth Carotid Ultrasound Disease Assessment Study (CUDAS).
Authors	McQuillan BM, Hung J, Beilby JP, et al.
Reference	J Am Coll Cardiol 2001;38:1788-1794.
Disease	Atherosclerosis.
Purpose	To assess the relationship between dietary intake or plasma levels of antioxidant vitamins and common carotid artery intima-media wall thickness (IMT) or focal plaque.
Design	Survey.
Patients	1024 asymptomatic subjects from Perth, Western Australia, 27-77 years old.
Regimen	Dietary vitamin intake was assessed and fasting plasma levels of vitamin A, C, and E, lycopene and a- and β-carotene. All patients underwent bilateral carotid artery B-mode ultrasound imaging.
Results	After adjusting for age and conventional risk factors, an inverse relation was found between dietary intake of vitamin E and mean IMT in men (p=0.02). In women there was a similar trend, but without statistical significance (p=0.10). However, dietary vitamin E intake accounted only for 1% of the variance in measured IMT in men. There was an inverse relation between plasma lycopene and mean IMT in women (p=0.047), but not in men. There were no other associations between either dietary intake or plasma levels of other vitamins and IMT or focal carotid artery plaque.
Concl.	There is only a weak correlation between dietary intake of vitamin E and IMT in men. There was an inverse relation between plasma lycopene and mean IMT in women. No other association was found between either intake or plasma levels of antioxidant vitamins and carotid artery atherosclerotic disease. There is no evidence that supplemental antioxidant vitamin use affect carotid atherosclerosis.

DAIS

Diabetes Atherosclerosis Intervention Study

Title	Effect of fenofibrate on progression of coronary artery disease in type 2 diabetes: the Diabetes Atherosclerosis Intervention Study; a randomized study.
Authors	Diabetes Atherosclerosis Intervention Study Investigators.
Reference	Lancet 2001;357:905-910.
Disease	Coronary artery disease; diabetes mellitus.
Purpose	To evaluate whether fenofibrate therapy will affect coronary atherosclerosis in patients with type 2 diabetes mellitus.
Design	Randomized, double-blind, placebo-controlled, multicenter.
Patients	418 patients with type 2 diabetes mellitus, 40-65 years old, with or without previous coronary intervention, and total cholesterol/high-density lipoprotein cholesterol ratio ≥4, and either a low-density lipoprotein cholesterol 3.5-4.5 mmol/L and triglyceride ≤5.2 mmol/L, or a triglyceride 1.7-5.2 mmol/L and LDL cholesterol ≤4.5 mmol/L. All patients underwent coronary angiography before randomization and there had to be ≥1 visible coronary lesion to be included. Patients with a recent (≤6 months) coronary intervention were excluded.
Follow-up	≥3 years with clinical and angiographic follow-up (39.8 months for the fenofibrate and 39.4 months for the placebo group).
Regimen	Randomization to fenofibrate or placebo.
Add'l Tx	The treating physician was allowed to adjust the glucose-lowering drug-therapy to optimize glycemic control.

12

Results   Of the 731 patients screened, 418 met the entry criteria. Compliance with fenofibrate was 95% and with placebo 97%. Total plasma cholesterol, LDL cholesterol and triglycerides decreased and HDL cholesterol increased with fenofibrate ($p<0.001$ vs placebo). The percentage of diameter stenosis increased on the average by $2.11\pm0.594\%$ in the fenofibrate vs $3.65\pm0.608\%$ in the placebo group ($p=0.02$). The minimum lumen diameter decreased by 0.06 ± 0.016 mm in the fenofibrate vs 0.10 ± 0.016 mm in the placebo group ($p=0.029$). Mean segment diameter was reduced by 0.06 ± 0.017 mm in the fenofibrate vs 0.08 ± 0.018 mm in the placebo group ($p=0.171$). 45 patients in the placebo group vs 46 patients in the fenofibrate group underwent coronary artery bypass surgery at least 6 months before randomization. There was no significant differences in the angiographic findings in the saphenous vein grafts or internal thoracic artery grafts between the fenofibrate and placebo groups. There were 38 cardiovascular events (death, myocardial infarction, admission for angina, or revascularization) in the fenofibrate group vs 50 in the placebo group.

Concl.   Fenofibrate reduced the angiographic progression of coronary atherosclerosis in patients with type 2 diabetes mellitus. The study was underpowered to test for clinical end points.

ELSA

European Lacidipine Study on Atherosclerosis

Title	Calcium antagonist lacidipine slows down progression of asymptomatic carotid atherosclerosis. Principal results of the European Lacidipine Study on Atherosclerosis (elsa), a randomized, double-blind, long-term trial.
Authors	Zanchetti A, Bond MG, Hennig M, et al.
Reference	Circulation 2002;106:2422-2427.
Disease	Hypertension, progression of atherosclerosis.
Purpose	To determine the effects of treatment with either lacidipine or atenolol on the mean of the maximum intima-media thicknesses (IMT) in the walls of the common carotid arteries and bifurcations.
Design	Multi-center, randomized, double-blind.
Patients	2334 patients, aged 45-75 years, with hypertension defined as sitting systolic blood pressure between 150-210 mm Hg, and diastolic blood pressure 95-115 mm Hg.
Follow-up	4 years.
Regimen	50 mg qd. After 1 month, if diastolic BP was not less than 95 mm Hg with a decrease of at least 5 mm Hg, the lacidipine could be increased to 6 mg and atenolol increased to 100 mg. After 3 months, open-label hydrochlorothiazide 12.5 mg daily could be added and at 6 months, 25 mg daily.

Results   The primary end point of the study was the change in mean maximum intima media thickness in the 4 far walls in the distal common carotid arteries and carotid bifurcations bilaterally (mean thickness=CBMmax) after 4 years. Secondary outcomes were the number of patients with an increase or decrease in number of plaques (defined as a focal IMT ≥1.3 mm) at the end of the study, incidences of fatal and nonfatal cardiovascular events, and total death. The 2 groups were well matched at baseline. In the intent-to-treat population, 49.7% and 46.6% of patients randomized to atenolol and lacidipine, respectively, stayed at the lowest dose. 12.2% and 11%, respectively, received the higher dose, and 35.9% and 31.8% received hydrochlorothiazide. The primary outcome variable, CBMmax, was changed significantly less in the lacidipine group vs the atenolol group. The estimated effect of treatment (lacidipine minus atenolol) was -0.0227 mm in the intent-to-treat group and -0.0281 mm in the completing group. This effect was significant in subgroups based on treatment, time points, and baseline CBMmax ($p<0.0001$). The progression of CBMmax was much slower in the lacidipine groups vs the atenolol group; the rate was 15% (intent-to-treat population) and 40% (completers) lower in the lacidipine group vs atenolol. In the intent-to-treat population, 25.9% of patients in the lacidipine group vs 29.0% in the atenolol group had plaque progression by follow-up, and 19.8% (lacidipine) vs 15.7% (atenolol) had plaque regression (chi-square test, $p=0.0404$). In the completer population, 25.3% of patients in the lacidipine group vs 31.3% in the atenolol group had plaque progression by follow-up, and 20.4% (lacidipine) vs 14.8% (atenolol) had plaque regression (chi-square test, $p=0.0036$). Systolic and diastolic BPs as measured in clinic decreased similarly in both groups (atenolol -21.6/-15.6 mm Hg), (lacidipine -21.8/-15.5 mm Hg). 24-hour ambulatory BPs were reduced significantly more ($p<0.0001$) in the atenolol group (-10.3/-8.7 mm Hg) vs the lacidipine group (-6.8/-4.9 mm Hg). There were no significant difference in the risk of stroke, major cardiovascular events, and cardiovascular or all death, but there was a trend in favor of lacidipine.

Concl.   Lacidipine had a greater positive effect on the progression of carotid intima media thickness progression vs atenolol. Atenolol reduced ambulatory BP significantly more than lacidipine.

ENCORE I

Evaluation of Nifedipine and Cerivastatin on Recovery of Coronary Endothelial Function

Title	Effect of nifedipine and cerivastatin on coronary endothelial function in patients with coronary artery disease. The ENCORE I study.
Authors	The ENCORE Investigators.
Reference	Circulation 2003;107:422-428.
Disease	Coronary artery disease.
Purpose	To evaluate the effects of a statin with and without a calcium channel blocker on coronary endothelial function.
Design	Randomized, double-blind, placebo-controlled, prospective.
Patients	Patients were >18 years of age, had LDL cholesterol <180 mg/dL, and a left coronary artery segment with ≤40% stenosis. Patients had to have at least 1 coronary artery segment that did not vasodilate in response to acetylcholine (a sign of endothelial dysfunction). There were numerous exclusion criteria, including: Q-wave myocardial infarction in the 2 weeks before study entry, stroke, major surgery in the 3 weeks before study entry, unstable angina, unstable diabetes, uncontrolled or symptomatic hypertension, left ventricular ejection fraction <40%, and others.
Follow-up	6 months.
Regimen	Patients underwent percutaneous coronary intervention, and were infused with acetylcholine at 2 mL/min for 3 minutes in the order: acetylcholine 0.36, 3.6, and 18 mg/mL; saline; adenosine 1.2 mg/mL; and 250 mg of nitroglycerin. Changes in coronary diameter were measured by angiography. Patients were then randomized to receive placebo, cerivastatin 0.4 mg/d, nifedipine 30 to 60 mg/d, or a combination of cerivastatin and nifedipine. Patients then underwent repeat acetylcholine infusion and angiography at 6 months.

Results   343 were randomized, and 334 patients received treatment. 243
           patients were evaluable for the intention-to-treat analysis. Of the
           patients treated with nifedipine, 84%-90% were taking 60 mg/d.
           217 of 243 patients were taking aspirin. 217 patients were taking
           ticlopidine and 62 were taking clopidogrel. 41% of patients had
           a history of hypertension. The primary end point was the effects
           of cerivastatin, nifedipine, or both vs placebo on the coronary
           vascular response induced by acetylcholine at the highest dose of
           acetylcholine applied at baseline and at follow-up. At baseline,
           all 3 doses of acetylcholine were infused in 92.8% of patients;
           in 4.8% of patients, there was marked vasoconstriction after 2
           doses; and in 1.8% of patients, there was severe vasoconstriction
           after 1 dose. At 6 months, the acetylcholine test was repeated in
           250 patients. In 96% of patients, all 3 doses were infused. Severe
           vasoconstriction was noted after the 2nd and 1st dose in 2% of
           patients each. The change in the mean luminal diameter from
           baseline to follow-up was 10.0%±3.0% in the placebo group,
           18.8%±3.0% in the nifedipine group (p=0.04), 11.1%±3.0%
           in the cerivastatin group (p=NS), and 12.9%±3.3% in the com-
           bination group (p=NS). Thus, nifedipine significantly reduced
           vasoconstriction to acetylcholine. Analyses of all coronary seg-
           ments (approximately 3 segments/patient) showed changes in
           luminal diameter from baseline to follow-up of 5.8%±1.6%,
           9.6%±1.8% (p=NS), 9.1%±1.8% (p=NS), and 10.4%±1.8%
           (p<0.05) with placebo, nifedipine, cerivastatin, and combina-
           tion, respectively.

Concl.   The combination of nifedipine and cervastatin had a trend
           toward improving endothelial function, but this was only sig-
           nificant when all coronary segments were analyzed.

ETICA

Exercise Training Intervention After Coronary Angioplasty

Title	Exercise training intervention after coronary angioplasty: the ETICA Trial.
Authors	Belardinelli R, Paolini I, Cianci G, et al.
Reference	J Am Coll Cardiol 2001;37:1891-1900.
Disease	Coronary artery disease.
Purpose	To determine effects of exercise training on functional capacity, quality of life, restenosis rates, and cardiac event rates in patients who received percutaneous coronary intervention: either percutaneous transluminal coronary angioplasty or stenting.
Design	Randomized, consecutive patients.
Patients	118 patients with CAD who underwent PTCA or stenting in 1 or 2 native coronaries.
Follow-up	6 months (angiographic); 33 months (clinical).
Regimen	Randomized to exercise group vs control (sedentary) group. Exercise consisted of 3 sessions per week at an intensity of 60% peak oxygen uptake (cycle ergometer at target work rate for 30 minutes). There was a warm-up and cool-down phase.
Add'l Tx	As needed.

12

Results	Clinical adverse outcome defined as mortality, from any cause, any cardiovascular morbidity. Exercise-trained patients only demonstrated significant improvements in peak VO2 (26%; $p<0.001$) and quality of life (26.8%; $p=0.001$ vs control group). Exercise did not affect the restenosis rates assessed by 6 month coronary angiograms (29% in the exercise group vs 33% in the control; p=NS). Residual diameter stenosis was 34% in the exercise group vs 49% in the control group ($p<0.001$) in patients that underwent PTCA, and 45% in the exercise group vs 58% in the control group ($p=0.005$) in patients who underwent stenting. Overall residual stenosis was lower in trained patients (-29.7%; $p=0.045$). Thallium uptake improved in the treated group (19%; $p<0.001$), but not control group, in patients with angiographic restenosis. Clinical adverse event rate at a mean of 33 months follow-up was lower in exercise patients (11.9%) vs controls (32.2%; RR 0.71; 95% CI=0.60-0.91; $p=0.008$). Hospital re-admission rates also were lower in exercise-treated patients (18.6% vs 46%; RR 0.69; 95% CI=0.55-0.93; $p<0.001$).
Concl.	Moderate exercise training improved functional capacity and quality of life in coronary artery patients who underwent either PTCA or stenting. Exercise trained patients developed fewer adverse cardiac events and had lower in-hospital re-admission rates but no change in restenosis rates.

12. CAD Atherosclerosis Prevention of Progression

HERS II

Heart and Estrogen/Progestin Replacement Substudy

Title	Statin therapy, cardiovascular events, and total mortality in the Heart and Estrogen/Progestin Replacement Study (HERS).
Authors	Herrington DM, Vittinghoff E, Lin F, et al.
Reference	Circulation 2002;105:2962-2967.
Disease	Coronary artery disease.
Purpose	To determine the effect of statins on cardiovascular disease prevention and total mortality in women, and the influence of statin use on the cardiovascular effects of hormone replacement therapy.
Design	Retrospective analysis of a randomized, placebo-controlled trial.
Patients	2763 postmenopausal women younger than 80 years, (mean age 66.7 years), with CAD and without a hysterectomy. Postmenopausal was defined by age ≥55 years and absence of natural menses for at least 5 years, or absence of menses for 1 year and follicle-stimulating hormone level >40 IU/L, or confirmed bilateral oophorectomy, or reported bilateral oophorectomy and follicle-stimulating hormone level >40 IU/L and estradiol less than 25 pg/mL. Confirmed CAD was established by at least 1 of the following: myocardial infarction, CABG surgery, percutaneous coronary revascularization, or greater than 50% occlusion of 1 or more major coronary arteries on angiography. There were numerous exclusion criteria (refer to JAMA 1998;280:606).
Follow-up	Mean 5.7 years.
Regimen	Patients were randomized to either 0.625 mg conjugated equine estrogens plus 2.5 mg medroxyprogesterone acetate together in 1 pill (n=1380), or placebo (n=1383). 1004 women (36.3%) were using statins at baseline and 426 (11.3%) were using other types of lipid-lowering medications. 708 women started statin therapy during the trial; 497 of these women were not using other lipid-lowering therapy at baseline.

12

Results	The primary outcome was death from coronary heart disease (CHD) or nonfatal MI. Secondary outcomes were unstable angina, coronary revascularization, stroke, transient ischemic events, venous thromboembolic events, and death from all causes. Women who were on statins at baseline or started during the trial had a significantly lower risk of having a primary CHD event (MI or cardiac death). The risk hazard for women who were on statin therapy for greater than 3 years was 0.74 (95% CI=0.57-0.96; p=0.02); the risk hazard for women who had used statins <3 years was 0.89 (95% CI=0.64-1.23; p=0.48). There were fewer primary CHD events among patients who were using statins at baseline vs those who were not (107/1004 vs. 209/1467; relative hazard [RH] 0.78; 95% CI=0.61-0.99; p=0.044), and fewer primary CHD events for patients who had any statin use vs those who had none (144/1270 vs 172/1467; RH 0.79; 95% CI=0.63-0.99; p=0.037). Nonfatal MI was also significantly reduced in the patients who had baseline use of statin (p=0.044). Statin use at baseline or at anytime also significantly reduced the incidence of venous thromboembolism (p=0.033 and 0.020, respectively). All-cause mortality was also significantly reduced with baseline statin use (75 deaths/1004 vs 159 deaths/1467; RH 0.74; 95% CI=0.56-0.99; p=0.040) and any statin use (100 deaths/1270 vs 134 deaths/1467; RH 0.67; 95% CI=0.51-0.87; p=0.003).
Concl.	In the HERS study, use of statins significantly reduced the risk of cardiovascular events, venous thromboembolism, and all-cause mortality.

HERS II

Heart and Estrogen/Progestin Replacement Study Follow-Up

Title	Cardiovascular disease outcomes during 6.8 years of hormone therapy.
Authors	Grady D, Herrington D, Bittner V, et al.
Reference	JAMA 2002;288:49-57.
Disease	Coronary artery disease.
Purpose	To determine if the reduced risk of coronary heart disease (CHD) events observed in the later years of HERS was maintained and resulted in a reduced overall risk of CHD events when including the additional years of follow-up.
Design	Randomized, blind, placebo-controlled, multicenter.
Patients	2763 in HERS; 2321 followed-up in HERS-II. Study participants were women younger than 80 years without previous hysterectomy and a history of at least 1 of the following: myocardial infarction, CABG surgery, percutaneous angioplasty, or greater than 50% angiographic narrowing of a coronary artery.
Follow-up	6.8 years.
Regimen	Patients were randomized to receive 0.625 mg/d of conjugated estrogens and 2.5 mg/d of medroxyprogesterone acetate (n=1380), or placebo (n=1383) during HERS. During HERS-II, open-label hormone therapy was given at the discretion of personal physicians.

12

Results	The primary end point was nonfatal MI and coronary heart disease (CHD) death. The secondary end points were coronary revascularization, hospitalization for unstable angina or CHF, nonfatal ventricular arrhythmia, sudden death, stroke or transient ischemic attack, and peripheral arterial disease. The rate of CHD events in the 2 groups was similar during HERS, HERS-II, and overall: (HERS: relative hazard [RH] 0.99; 95% CI=0.81-1.22; HERS-II: RH 1.00; 95% CI=0.77-1.29; overall: RH 0.99; 95% CI=0.84-1.17; all p values nonsignificant). During the entire follow-up, there were 132 CHD deaths in the hormone group and 122 in the placebo group. The rates of CHD death were also similar between the 2 groups during HERS, HERS-II and overall: (HERS: RH 1.20; 95% CI=0.85-1.69; HERS-II: RH 0.99; 95% CI=0.70-1.41; overall: RH 1.09; 95% CI=0.85-1.39; all p values non-significant). The rates of nonfatal MI were similar between the 2 groups during HERS, HERS-II and overall: (HERS: RH 0.92; 95% CI=0.72-1.17; HERS-II: RH 0.98; 95% CI=0.69-1.40; overall: RH 0.94; 95% CI=0.77-1.15; all p values nonsignificant). There were also no significant differences between the groups during HERS, HERS-II, and overall for any of the secondary outcomes except nonfatal ventricular arrhythmia. Women assigned to hormone treatment had a higher risk: in HERS-II, RH 3.30; 95% CI=1.08-10.1; p=0.04; overall, RH 1.97; 95% CI=1.10-3.53; p=0.02). The analyses were adjusted for differential statin use between the 2 groups and was also limited to those who were more than 80% adherent to their assigned regimen. Results from these analyses were very similar to the unadjusted intention-to-treat analyses for the risk of CHD events.
Concl.	After 6.8 years of follow-up, hormone replacement therapy did not reduce the risk of coronary heart disease death or events in women with existing coronary heart disease.

HOPE

Heart Outcomes Prevention Evaluation (Substudy)

Title	Effect of long-term therapy with ramipril in high-risk women.
Authors	Lonn E, Roccaforte R, Yi Q, et al.
Reference	J Am Coll Cardiol 2002;40:693-702.
Disease	Coronary artery disease, atherosclerosis.
Purpose	To determine the effect of angiotensin-converting enzyme inhibitor therapy on cardiovascular outcomes in women at high-risk for ischemic cardiovascular disease.
Design	Randomized, prospective, placebo-controlled, multicenter.
Patients	As per HOPE. In this analysis only women were included.
Follow-up	Mean 4.5 years.
Regimen	Patients were randomized to receive either ramipril 2.5 mg a day for 1 week, 5 mg for the next 3 weeks and 10 mg thereafter, or matching placebo. There was also a vitamin E vs placebo study reported elsewhere in this book. (from N Engl J Med 2000;342:146).

Results	The primary outcome of the study was a composite of MI, stroke, or cardiovascular death. Secondary outcomes were all-cause death, revascularization procedures, hospital admissions for unstable angina or heart failure, and complications related to diabetes. Other studied outcomes were: all heart failure, cardiac arrest, worsening angina, unstable angina with ECG changes, new onset diabetes, and diabetic complications. 2480 women were included in the analysis. The primary outcome occurred less frequently in patients in the ramipril group vs placebo: 11.3% vs 14.9%, (relative risk [RR] 0.77; 95% CI=0.62-0.96; p=0.019). Compared to the placebo group, women in the ramipril group experienced fewer strokes (3.1% vs 4.8%, RR 0.64; 95% CI=0.43-0.96; p=0.029) and less CV death (4.2% vs 6.9%, RR 0.62; 95% CI=0.44-0.88; p=0.0068). Women in the ramipril group also had a lower incidence of MI but this did not reach statistical significance (RR 0.89; 95% CI=0.69-1.17; p=0.43). There was a trend toward benefit for all secondary outcomes in the ramipril group, but none of these was statistically significant. There was also a trend toward benefit in the other studied outcomes, except for unstable angina with ECG changes, which favored placebo (RR 1.30; 95% CI=0.86-1.97; p=NS). Worsening angina was the only subcategory that resulted in benefit in favor of ramipril that was statistically significant (RR 0.88; 95% CI=0.74-0.94; p<0.05). Permanent discontinuation of a study drug occurred at a similar frequency between the 2 groups (placebo group, 31.7%, ramipril group, 29.8%). However, discontinuation due to cough and angioedema occurred more often in the ramipril group (cough: 11.3% vs 2.2%; p<0.0001; angioedema: 0.7% vs 0.1%; p<0.05).
Concl.	Ramipril is beneficial in reducing the risk of stroke and CV death in high-risk women with CAD, preserved LV function, and without heart failure.

HOPE

Heart Outcomes Prevention Evaluation Study (Substudy)

Title	Prevention of heart failure in patients in the heart outcomes prevention evaluation study.
Authors	Arnold JMO, Yusuf S, Young J, et al.
Reference	Circulation 2003;107:1284-1290.
Disease	Heart failure.
Purpose	To determine the effect of the angiotensin-converting enzyme inhibitor ramipril on preventing the development of heart failure in patients without known heart failure or low ejection fraction.
Design	Randomized, double-blind, placebo-controlled, multicenter.
Patients	4.5 years.
Follow-up	4.5 years.
Regimen	Patients were randomized to ramipril 10 mg od or matched placebo.

Results	The substudy end point was all heart failure that was defined as heart failure leading to death, heart failure that required hospitalization, heart failure requiring open-label ACE inhibitors, or development of signs and symptoms of heart failure. The mean age of the participants was 66 years, 73% male, 53% with previous MI, 47% with hypertension, and 38% with diabetes mellitus. Any sort of heart failure occurred in 951 patients (10.2% of all randomized) during the follow-up period. Developing heart failure increased the risk of death 4.01 times (95% CI=3.42-4.71; $p<0.0001$), and increased the risk of cardiovascular death 4.35 times (95% CI=3.56-5.31; $p<0.0001$). Patients who developed heart failure were more likely to be older, have a higher BMI, higher systolic pressure, pulse pressure, and heart rate. The incidence of heart failure in the placebo group was 11.5% compared to 9.0% in the ramipril group (relative risk [RR] 0.77; 95% CI=0.68-0.87; $p<0.0001$). The incidence of cardiovascular death and all heart failure was 17.4% in the placebo group and 13.4% in the ramipril group (RR 0.76; 95% CI=0.69-0.84; $p<0.0001$). Ramipril reduced the risk of all heart failure by 9% (RR 0.91; 95% CI=0.75-1.10) in those with baseline systolic pressure less than the median (139 mm Hg), but 33% (RR 0.67; 95% CI=0.57-0.80) in those with baseline systolic pressure equal to or greater than the median. Ramipril reduced the risk of heart failure after MI by 13% (RR 0.87; 95% CI=0.66-1.15; $p=0.32$). In patients who did not have a MI during follow-up, ramipril reduced the risk of heart failure by 22% (RR 0.78; 95% CI=0.62-0.97; $p=0.023$).
Concl.	Ramipril significantly reduced the risk of developing heart failure in those at high cardiovascular risk.

HOPE (Ramipril Study)

Heart Outcomes Prevention Evaluation

Title	Effects of an angiotensin-converting enzyme inhibitor, ramipril, on cardiovascular events in high risk patients.
Authors	The Heart Outcomes Prevention Evaluation Study Investigators.
Reference	N Engl J Med 2000;342:145-153.
Disease	Patients at high risk for cardiovascular events; coronary artery disease.
Purpose	To determine whether ramipril could reduce the incidence of myocardial infarction, stroke, or death from cardiovascular causes in patients at high risk for cardiovascular events without heart failure or LV dysfunction.
Design	Double-blind, multicenter, 2 x 2 factorial design evaluating ramipril and vitamin E (vitamin E results given elsewhere).
Patients	9297 high risk patients, men and women at least 55 years old with "history of coronary artery disease, stroke, peripheral vascular disease, or diabetes plus at least 1 other cardiovascular risk factor." Patients could not have heart failure or LV ejection fraction <40%.
Follow-up	5 years.
Regimen	Ramipril 10 mg once-a-day orally vs matched placebo.
Add'l Tx	There was also a randomization to 400 IU of vitamin E vs placebo.

Results	The primary outcome was the composite of myocardial infarction, stroke, or death from cardiovascular causes. 826 (17.8%) patients in the placebo group achieved the primary end point vs 651 (14.0%) in the ramipril group. (relative risk [RR]=0.78; 95% CI=0.70-0.86; p<0.001). Ramipril significantly reduced death from cardiovascular causes, myocardial infarction, stroke, and death from any cause (10.4% vs 12.2%; RR 0.84; p=0.005). Ramipril decreased the need for revascularization procedures (16.0% vs 18.3%; RR 0.85; p=0.002), cardiac arrest, heart failure and complications of diabetes. Blood pressure at the start of the study was 139/79 mm Hg in both groups. At the end of the study, blood pressure was 136/76 mm Hg in the ramipril group and 139/77 mm Hg in the placebo group. Ramipril did not alter the hospitalizations for unstable angina. The benefit of ramipril on the composite end point was observed within 1 year after randomization.
Concl.	Ramipril reduced death, myocardial infarction, and stroke in high risk patients without heart failure or LV dysfunction.

HOPE (Substudy)

Heart Outcomes Prevention Evaluation

Title	Comparative effects of ramipril on ambulatory and office blood pressure. A HOPE Substudy.
Authors	Svensson P, de Faire U, Sleigut P, et al.
Reference	Hypertension 2001;38:e28-e32.
Disease	Coronary artery disease (CAD); risk factors for CAD.
Purpose	To determine the effect of ramipril on 24-hour blood pressure (BP) monitoring in a subgroup of patients with peripheral arterial disease. The concern was that ramipril reduced office BP by only 3/2 mm Hg, in the HOPE trial. Since measurement of office BP took place ≈10-18 hours after drug, could reduction in BP by ramipril have been underestimated?
Design	Substudy of HOPE.
Patients	38 patients in HOPE trial with peripheral arterial disease who had 24-hour ambulatory BP monitoring before randomization and at 1 year.
Follow-up	1 year.
Regimen	As per HOPE. In this cohort, 20 patients received ramipril and 18 received placebo.
Add'l Tx	As per HOPE.
Results	At baseline, office-based BP was 152±21/83±7 mm Hg in the ramipril group and 149±19/79±12 mm Hg in the placebo group (p=NS); 24-hour ambulatory BP was 148±19/78±9 and 153±18/80±8 mm Hg, respectively (p=NS). While ramipril did not significantly reduce office BP (-8/-2 mm Hg; p=NS) or daytime ambulatory BP (-6/-2 mm Hg; p=NS) after 1 year, it did significantly reduce 24 hour ambulatory BP (-10/-4 mm Hg; p=0.03) primarily because of a greater fall in nighttime BP (-17/-8 mm Hg; p<0.001). At 1 year, the night/d ratio of mean arterial pressure was reduced by ramipril (0.82±0.06) vs placebo (0.89±0.07; p<0.01).

Concl.   The effects of ramipril on cardiovascular morbidity and mortality in HOPE might have been related to effects of the BP pattern over the 24-hour period, rather than just the small changes observed with office BP.

HOPE (Substudy)

Heart Outcomes Prevention Evaluation

Title	Ramipril and the development of diabetes.
Authors	Yusuf S, Gerstein H, Hoogwerf B, et al.
Reference	JAMA 2001;286:1882-1885.
Disease	Diabetes.
Purpose	To determine the effectiveness of ramipril, an angiotensin-converting enzyme inhibitor, on preventing the development of diabetes in high-risk patients.
Design	As per HOPE.
Patients	5720 patients >55 years, with no evidence of left ventricular dysfunction or heart failure, who had evidence of vascular disease and, in this substudy, no diabetes at baseline.
Follow-up	4.5 years.
Regimen	Patients were randomized to receive up to 10 mg ramipril (n=2837) per day vs placebo (n=2883).
Results	Primary outcome was new diagnosis of diabetes. Hemoglobin A1C and medications used among those diagnosed with diabetes were also assessed. Diabetes developed in 102 (3.6%) patients in the ramipril group vs 155 (5.4%) in the placebo group (relative risk [RR] 0.66; 95% CI=0.51-0.85; p<0.001). The RR for diagnosis of diabetes and hemoglobin A1c >110% was 0.60 (95% CI=0.43-0.85) with ramipril. Ramipril use was associated with a lower RR for initiation of glucose lowering therapy (0.56 [95% CI=0.41-0.77]). In the vitamin E limb of the HOPE trial there was no evidence that vitamin E reduced the development of diabetes. Ramipril was effective in preventing diabetes in a number of subgroups: those with a waist-hip ratio >0.93, body mass index >27.7 kg/m^2, patients with hypertension, microalbuminuria, patients on β-blockers, and patients on diuretics.
Concl.	Ramipril was associated with lower rates of newly diagnosed diabetes.

HOPE (Vitamin E Study)

Heart Outcomes Prevention Evaluation

Title	Vitamin E supplementation and cardiovascular events in high risk patients.
Authors	The Heart Outcomes Prevention Evaluation Study Investigators.
Reference	N Engl J Med 2000;342:154-160.
Disease	Patients at high risk for cardiovascular events; coronary artery disease.
Purpose	To determine whether a high dose of vitamin E (400 IU per day) reduced the composite of myocardial infarction, stroke, and death from cardiovascular causes.
Design	Double-blind, multicenter, randomized trial within a 2 x 2 factorial design evaluating ramipril and vitamin E (ramipril data presented elsewhere).
Patients	9541 patients ≥55 years at high risk of cardiovascular events as they had known cardiovascular disease or diabetes plus at least 1 other risk factor (see ramipril limb of study for more details).
Follow-up	4.5 years.
Regimen	Patients were randomly assigned to placebo (n=4780) or 400 IU of vitamin E (n=4761) from natural sources.
Add'l Tx	Also randomized to ramipril vs placebo (see ramipril study).
Results	The primary outcome measure was the composite end point of myocardial infarction, stroke, and death from cardiovascular causes. Primary outcome was reached in 15.5% of patients on placebo and 16.2% on vitamin E (p=NS). There were no significant differences in numbers of death due to cardiovascular cause, myocardial infarction, or stroke. There were no significant differences between groups in the secondary outcomes of unstable angina, congestive heart failure, new onset angina, worsening angina, claudication, hospitalization for heart failure, or complications of diabetes.

Concl.	Vitamin E did not affect cardiovascular outcomes in patients at high risk of cardiovascular events.

MICRO-HOPE

Microalbuminuria, Cardiovascular and Renal Outcomes—Heart Outcomes Prevention Evaluation

Title	Effect of ramipril on cardiovascular and microvascular outcomes in people with diabetes mellitus: Results of the HOPE study and MICRO-HOPE substudy.
Authors	Heart Outcomes Prevention Evaluation (HOPE) Study Investigators.
Reference	Lancet 2000;355:253-259.
Disease	Cardiovascular disease, atherosclerosis, diabetes mellitus.
Purpose	To assess the effects of ramipril, an ACE inhibitor on the risk of overt nephropathy in patients with diabetes mellitus.
Design	Randomized, 2 x 2 factorial, placebo-controlled, multicenter.
Patients	3577 patients, ≥55 years old, with diabetes mellitus and a history of cardiovascular disease or at least 1 other cardiovascular risk factor (hypercholesterolemia, low HDL, hypertension, known microalbuminuria, or current smoking). Patients with overt proteinuria, diabetic nephropathy, other severe renal disease, hyperkalemia, congestive heart failure, LVEF <40%, uncontrolled hypertension, recent myocardial infarction or stroke, or use of or hypersensitivity to ACE inhibitors or vitamin E were excluded.
Follow-up	4.5 years.
Regimen	All patients completed a run-in phase, during which they received ramipril 2.5 mg/d for 7-10 days, followed by matching placebo for 10-14 days. Patients were randomized to ramipril 10 mg X1/d or matching placebo and to vitamin E 400 IU/d or matching placebo.

Results	The HOPE study was stopped prematurely after 4.5 years by the data safety and monitoring board because of consistent benefit of ramipril. At the end of the study, 65% of the surviving participants assigned to ramipril and 66% of those assigned to placebo were taking their study medications, whereas 12% and 15%, respectively, were taking open-label ACE inhibitors. The primary end point of cardiovascular death, myocardial infarction, or stroke occurred in 15.3% of the ramipril group vs 19.8% of the placebo group (relative risk reduction [RRR] 25%; 95% CI=12%-36%; p=0.0004). Cardiovascular mortality was 6.2% in the ramipril group vs 9.7% in the placebo group (RRR 37%; 95% CI=21%-51%; p=0.0001). Myocardial infarction occurred in 10.2% and 12.9% of the ramipril vs placebo groups, respectively (RRR 22%; 95% CI=6%-36%; p=0.01), whereas stroke occurred in 4.2% vs 6.1% (RRR 33%; 95% CI=10%-50%; p=0.0074). Total mortality was lower in the ramipril group (10.8% vs 14.0%; RRR 24%; 95% CI=8%-37%; p=0.004). Less patients in the ramipril group developed overt nephropathy (6.5% vs 8.4%; RRR 24%; 95% CI=3%-40%; p=0.027). Ramipril reduced the rate of heart failure (11.0% vs 13.3%; p=0.019), transient ischemic attack (4.4% vs 5.9%; p=0.04), worsening angina (20.1% vs 22.4%; p=0.057), and the combined end point of over nephropathy, need for laser therapy or dialysis (15.1% vs 17.6%; p=0.036). Ramipril benefit was noted in the subset of patients with and without a history of cardiovascular events, those with and without hypertension, and those with or without microalbuminuria. Ramipril was effective both in patients with type 1 and type 2 diabetes and irrespective of the current medications for diabetes. After adjustment for the changes in systolic (2.4 mm Hg) and diastolic (1.0 mm Hg) blood pressure between the groups, ramipril was still associated with lower risk of the combined primary end point by 25% (95% CI=12%-36%; p=0.0004).
Concl.	Ramipril was effective in reducing the risk of cardiovascular events, overt nephropathy, and death in patients with diabetes mellitus and an additional ≥ cardiovascular risk factor or cardiovascular disease. The effect on cardiovascular mortality and morbidity was greater than that can be ascribed to the mild reduction in systolic and diastolic blood pressure by ramipril.

MORE

Multiple Outcomes of Raloxifene Evaluation (Secondary Analysis)

Title	Raloxifene and cardiovascular events in osteoporotic postmenopausal women. Four-year results from the MORE Randomized Trial.
Authors	Barrett-Connor E, Grady D, Sashegyi A, et al.
Reference	JAMA 2002;287:847-857.
Disease	Coronary artery disease.
Purpose	To determine the effects of raloxifene (a selective estrogen receptor modulator) on cardiovascular events of osteoporotic postmenopausal women.
Design	Secondary analysis of a randomized, double-blind, placebo-controlled, multicenter study.
Patients	7705 osteoporotic, postmenopausal women, mean age of 67 years.
Follow-up	4 years.
Regimen	Patients randomized to raloxifene 60 mg/d (n=2557), 120 mg/d (n=2572), vs placebo (n=2576) for 4 years.
Add'l Tx	500 mg of calcium per day. 400-600 IU of cholecalciferol per day.

Results	For this substudy main outcome was cardiovascular events (including MI, unstable angina, myocardial ischemia) and cerebrovascular events (stroke, transient ischemic attack) collected as safety end points. Cardiovascular risk at study entry was also determined. There were no significant differences in combined coronary and cerebrovascular events among the groups (3.7% with placebo, 3.2% with the 60 mg/d raloxifene, and 3.7% with 120 mg/d of raloxifene). Any coronary event occurred in 2.1%, 1.8%, and 2.2% of the placebo, 60 mg, and 120 mg dose, respectively (p=NS). Any cerebrovascular event occurred in 1.6%, 1.4%, and 1.5% (p=NS) of the 3 groups respectively. In a subset of 1035 women who were identified at baseline to have a higher cardiovascular risk, patients receiving raloxifene had a lower risk of cardiovascular events (7.8% in the 2 raloxifene groups vs 12.9% in the placebo group; p=0.03; relative risk [RR] 0.60; 95% CI=0.38-0.95). During the first year, the number of cardiovascular events did not differ among the groups, either for the total cohort, or those identified at increased cardiovascular risk.
Concl.	Raloxifene therapy did not reduce the risk of cardiovascular or cerebrovascular events in an overall cohort of postmenopausal, osteoporotic women. It did reduce the risk of cardiovascular events in a subset of women identified with increased cardiovascular risk.

PACIFIC

Prevention with a Combined Inhibitor and Folic Acid in Coronary Heart Disease

Title	Dose-dependent effects of folic acid on plasma homocysteine in a randomized trial conducted among 723 individuals with coronary heart disease.
Authors	PACIFIC Study Group.
Reference	Eur Heart J 2002;23:1509-1515.
Disease	Coronary artery disease.
Purpose	To evaluate the effects of 2 doses of folic acid on homocysteine levels in patients with coronary artery disease.
Design	Randomized, double-blind, placebo-controlled, 3 x 3 factorial, multicenter.
Patients	723 patients with a history of myocardial infarction or unstable angina, LVEF ≥40%, and a high risk for recurrent myocardial infarction or coronary heart disease death (age ≥65 years, current smokers, diabetic, history of recurrent myocardial infarction, or Canadian Cardiovascular Society angina grade ≥2). Patients with a definite indication or contraindication to angiotensin-converting enzyme inhibitors or folic acid were excluded.
Follow-up	7 months.
Regimen	Patients were randomized in a 3 x 3 factorial design to 1 of 3 folic acid treatment groups (placebo, 0.2 mg/d, or 2.0 mg/d), and 1-3 omapatrilat treatment groups (placebo, 20 mg/d, or 40 mg/d).

Results	This paper reports the results of the folic acid treatment. After 6 months of therapy, serum folate increased by 11.2 nmol/L in the folate 0.2 mg/d group and by 22.2 nmol/L in the folate 2.0 mg/d group compared to placebo. Red blood cell folate levels increased by 283 nmol/L and 759 nmol/L, respectively. The effect of the folate 2.0 mg/d was significantly greater than the effect of the folate 0.2 mg/d treatment ($p < 0.001$ for both serum folate and red blood cell folate levels). Blood homocysteine was reduced by 1.2 µmol/L (95% CI=0.8-1.7; $p < 0.001$) in the folate 0.2 mg/d group compared with the placebo group, and by 1.8 µmol/L (95% CI=1.3-2.3; $p < 0.001$) in the folate 2.0 mg/d group compared with the placebo group. Folate 2.0 mg/d was more effective than 0.2 mg/d in reducing homocysteine levels ($p=0.01$). There was no significant interaction of the methylene tetrahydrofolate reductase polymorphism with the effect of the folate treatment ($p=0.7$). Omapatrilat therapy was associated with an increase in homocysteine levels (20 mg vs placebo 0.7 µmol/L increase; $p=0.006$); (40 mg vs placebo 0.8 µmol/L increase; $p < 0.001$).
Concl.	Both doses of folic acid reduced homocysteine levels. The effect of the 2.0 mg/d was greater than that of 0.2 mg/d.

12

PART-2

Prevention of Atherosclerosis with Ramipril Trial-2

Title	Randomized, placebo-controlled trial of the angiotensin-converting enzyme inhibitor, ramipril, in patients with coronary or other occlusive arterial disease.
Authors	MacMahon S, Sharpe N, Gamble G, et al.
Reference	J Am Coll Cardiol 2000;36:438-443.
Disease	Atherosclerosis.
Purpose	To evaluate the effects of ramipril, an angiotensin-converting-enzyme inhibitor, on carotid atherosclerosis and left ventricular hypertrophy in patients with coronary, cerebrovascular or peripheral arterial atherosclerotic disease.
Design	Randomized, double-blind, placebo-controlled, multicenter.
Patients	617 patients, ≤75 years old, with a previous myocardial infarction, angina with documented coronary artery disease, transient ischemic attack or intermittent claudication. Patients with congestive heart failure, a definite indication or a contraindication for ACE inhibitor, serious nonvascular disease, blood pressure above 160/100 mm Hg, hypotension <100 mm Hg systolic blood pressure and women of childbearing potential were excluded.
Follow-up	4 years. B-mode ultrasound of the carotid arteries and M-mode echocardiogram at baseline, 2 and 4 years.
Regimen	All patients underwent a tolerability open-label phase of ramipril 5 mg/d for 1 week and 10 mg/d for an additional week. Only those tolerant to the drug were randomized to ramipril 5 or 10 mg/d (n=308) or to placebo (n=309).

Results	83% of the patients randomized to ramipril received 10 mg/d and 17% received 5 mg/d. At 4 years follow-up 72% of the ramipril group and 75% of the placebo group were still taking study drugs. On average, systolic blood pressure decreased by 6 mm Hg and diastolic blood pressure by 4 mm Hg in the ramipril group compared with the placebo group (p<0.0001). There was no significant difference in the change in common carotid far wall thickness between the ramipril (0.80, 0.82, and 0.83 mm at baseline, 2, and 4 years, respectively) and the placebo group (0.79, 0.81, and 0.81 mm Hg, respectively) (p=0.58). Carotid plaque score was 9.2, 11.1, and 12.0 mm at baseline, 2, and 4 years, respectively, in the ramipril group and 9.8, 11.7, and 13.0 mm, respectively, in the placebo group (p=0.93). After 4 years there was a significant decrease in LV mass index in the ramipril group (from 96.9 g/m^2 to 89.3 g/m^2) compared with the placebo group (from 98.3 g/m^2 to 94.6 g/m^2; p=0.04). In addition, there was a small increase in LV end diastolic diameter in the placebo group (from 52.6 mm to 54.0 mm), compared to the ramipril group (from 53.4 mm to 53.9 mm) (p=0.004). There was no difference in mortality between the ramipril group (n=16) and the placebo group (n=25) (RR 0.64; 95% CI=0.34-1.20; p=0.17); neither was there a difference in the number of patients hospitalized (279 vs 289; p=0.18). Death from cardiovascular disease or hospital admission for major cardiovascular event occurred in 73 patients in the ramipril group vs 77 in the placebo group (RR 0.95; 95% CI=0.69-1.31). There were nonsignificant trends toward lower cardiovascular mortality (8 vs 18; RR 0.45; 95% CI=0.19-1.03) and fewer major coronary events (22 vs 33; RR 0.66; 95% CI=0.39-1.14) in the ramipril group.
Concl.	Ramipril does not reduce carotid atherosclerosis in patients with coronary or other occlusive arterial disease. In contrast, ramipril lowered blood pressure and reduced left ventricular mass.

PPP

Primary Prevention Project

Title	Low-dose aspirin and vitamin E in people at cardiovascular risk: a randomised trial in general practice.
Authors	Collaborative Group of the Primary Prevention Project (PPP).
Reference	Lancet 2001; 357: 89-95.
Disease	Atherosclerosis.
Purpose	To assess the efficacy of aspirin and vitamin E in primary prevention of cardiovascular events in patients with ≥1 major risk factors.
Design	Randomized, open-label, multicenter.
Patients	4495 patients, ≥50 years old, with ≥1 major cardiovascular risk factors (age ≥65 years; systolic blood pressure ≥160 mm Hg; diastolic blood pressure ≥95 mm Hg; total blood cholesterol ≥6.4 mmol/L; diabetes mellitus; obesity; and a family history of myocardial infarction before the age of 55 years). Patients with antiplatelet treatment; chronic use of anti-inflammatory agents or anticoagulants, contraindications to aspirin; and severe illness with predictable poor short-term prognosis were excluded.
Follow-up	The mean follow-up was 3.6±1.0 years (median 4.0 years).
Regimen	Randomized to aspirin 100 mg/d or no aspirin, and to vitamin E 300 mg/d or no vitamin E.
Add'l Tx	66% of the patients received antihypertensive drugs, 12% received antidiabetic drugs, and 16% received lipid-lowering drugs.

Results	Mean age was 64.4±7.6 years, 57.7% of the patients were women. At the end of the study, in 99.3% of the patients there was information concerning vital status. At the end of the study, 19.3% of the patients assigned to aspirin and 13.6% of those assigned to vitamin E had stopped the study medications. At the end of the study, 7.2% of the patients not assigned to aspirin were taking aspirin and 0.2% of those not assigned to vitamin E were taking vitamin E. The combined end point of cardiovascular death, nonfatal myocardial infarction, and nonfatal stroke occurred in 2.0% of the aspirin group vs 2.8% of the no-aspirin group (relative risk [RR] 0.71; 95% CI=0.48-1.04). Total mortality was 2.8% vs 3.4%, respectively (RR 0.81; 95% CI=0.58-1.13), and cardiovascular mortality was 0.8% vs 1.4% (RR 0.56; 95% CI=0.31-0.99; p=0.049). Myocardial infarction occurred in 0.8% and 1.2% of the aspirin and no-aspirin groups (RR 0.69; 95% CI=0.38-1.23), and strokes in 0.7% and 1.1%, respectively (RR 0.67; 95% CI=0.36-1.27). The combined end point of cardiovascular death, nonfatal myocardial infarction, and nonfatal stroke occurred in 2.5% of the vitamin E group vs 2.3% of the no-vitamin E group (RR 1.07; 95% CI=0.74-1.56). Total mortality was 3.2% vs 3.0%, respectively (RR 1.07; 95% CI=0.77-1.49), and cardiovascular mortality was 1.0% vs 1.1% (RR 0.86; 95% CI=0.49-1.52). Vitamin E had no effect on the risk of myocardial infarction or stroke. However, the incidence of peripheral artery disease was lower in the vitamin E group (0.7%) than in the no-vitamin E group (1.3%) (RR 0.54; 95% CI=0.30-0.99; p=0.043). Neither aspirin nor vitamin E were associated with an increased risk for cancer. Bleeding complications occurred more often in the aspirin group (1.1% vs 0.3%; p=0.0008).
Concl.	In patients ≥50 years old with ≥1 cardiovascular risk factors, low-dose aspirin was effective in reducing cardiovascular events. In contrast, vitamin E was not effective in reducing the incidence of cardiovascular events, except for a reduced risk for peripheral artery disease.

PREVENT

Prospective Randomized Evaluation of the Vascular Effects of Norvasc Trial

Title	Effect of amlodipine on the progression of atherosclerosis and the occurrence of clinical events.
Authors	Pitt B, Byington RP, Furberg CD, et al.
Reference	Circulation 2000;102:1503-1510.
Disease	Coronary artery disease.
Purpose	To determine whether amlodipine could slow the progression of early coronary atherosclerosis and slow the progression of intimal-medial thickness in the carotid arteries.
Design	Randomized, placebo-controlled, double-masked, multicenter.
Patients	825 patients with angiographic evidence of coronary artery disease.
Follow-up	36 months.
Regimen	Placebo vs amlodipine (initiated at 5 mg once daily and increased to 10 mg once daily after 2 weeks, if tolerated).

Results	Primary outcome was effect of amlodipine on progression of early atherosclerotic segments in the coronaries assessed by quantitative coronary angiography. A secondary hypothesis was to test effect of amlodipine on progression of atherosclerosis in carotid arteries by measuring IMT with B-mode ultrasound. Prespecified clinical events were all cause mortality and major fatal/nonfatal vascular events or procedures. Average reductions in minimal coronary diameters were similar in placebo (0.084 mm) vs amlodipine group (0.095mm; p=0.38). IMT of the carotids increased by 0.033 mm in placebo patients while it decreased by 0.013 mm in the amlodipine group (p=0.007). Estimated 3-year change in common carotid artery segment was +0.011 mm progression in the placebo group vs -0.046 mm regression in the amlodipine group (95% CI on difference=-0.090 to -0.024 mm). Amlodipine had no effect on all cause mortality. Amlodipine decreased the combination of hospitalized nonfatal CHF and unstable angina (61 amlodipine; 88 placebo; hazard ratio [HR] 0.65 [0.47 to 0.91]), a difference mainly secondary to a decreased rate of unstable angina (60 vs 85; HR=0.67 [0.48 to 0.93]). Amlodipine decreased the rate of coronary revascularizations (53 vs 86; HR=0.57 [0.41 to 0.81]). This benefit was independent of use of lipid-lowering agents, β-blockers, nitrates. 23 amlodipine and 28 placebo patients had fatal and nonfatal coronary and cerebrovascular events, combined (HR=0.82 [95% CI=0.47 to 1.42]). Combining major and other events and procedures, there were fewer events with amlodipine (86 vs 116; HR=0.69 [0.52-0.92]) mainly secondary to reduced unstable angina and revascularization.
Concl.	Amlodipine did not alter atherosclerotic progression of coronary arteries determined by angiography, but reduces carotid IMT by ultrasound. Amlodipine use reduces hospitalization for unstable angina and revascularization procedures.

PREVENT (Post Hoc Analysis)

Prospective Randomized Evaluation of the Vascular Effects of Norvasc Trial

Title	Post hoc analysis of coronary findings from the Prospective Randomized Evaluation of the Vascular Effects of the Norvasc Trial (PREVENT).
Authors	Mancini GBJ, Miller ME, Evans GW, et al.
Reference	Am J Cardiol 2002;89:1414-1416.
Disease	Coronary artery disease.
Purpose	To re-evaluate whether amlodipine has an effect on progression and/or regression of coronary artery lesions as assessed by angiography.
Design	Retrospective post hoc analysis of a prospective study.
Patients	696 patients with angiographic evidence of coronary artery disease at baseline (≥1 focal lesion with ≥30% diameter stenosis (nonintervened and noninfarcted) and ≥ lesion with 5%-20% diameter stenosis in a vessel without ≥60% diameter stenotic lesion) who underwent follow-up angiogram. In the present post hoc analysis, vessels that had been previously intervened upon at the time of randomization were excluded. However, the preprocedural angiograms of vessels not intervened upon at the time of randomization and requiring intervention during follow-up were included in an augmented data set.
Follow-up	36 months.
Regimen	Placebo or amlodipine.

Results	86% of the amlodipine group and 83% of the placebo group had follow-up angiograms. Multivariate analysis of covariance showed a significant interaction between categorized baseline percent diameter stenosis and the effect of amlodipine on lesion progression ($p=0.013$ for the original data set; $p=0.0031$ for the augmented data set). Lesion progression was also dependent on the coronary segment and baseline minimum luminal diameter. Smaller baseline minimum diameter (more severe lesions) had regression. In contrast, lesions with a larger minimum diameter showed progression. Lesions with >70% diameter stenosis at baseline showed more regression with amlodipine than with placebo ($p<0.0001$).
Concl.	Post hoc analysis of the angiographic data from the PREVENT trial suggests that amlodipine has a favorable effect on regression of coronary lesions with >70% diameter stenosis at baseline.

QUIET

Quinapril Ischemic Event Trial

Title	The Quinapril ischemic event trial (QUIET): evaluation of chronic ACE inhibitor therapy in patients with ischemic disease and preserved left ventricular function.
Authors	Pitt B, O'Neill B, Feldman R, et al.
Reference	Am J Cardiol 2001;87:1058-1063.
Disease	Coronary artery disease.
Purpose	To determine whether the angiotensin-converting enzyme inhibitor quinapril would reduce ischemic events and progression of CAD in patients without systolic left ventricular dysfunction.
Design	Double-blind, placebo-controlled, randomized, multicenter.
Patients	1750 patients with CAD who had undergone successful coronary angioplasty or atherectomy at baseline, and had at least 1 coronary artery not receiving revascularization. Patients had to have normal left ventricular function.
Follow-up	Mean of 27 months.
Regimen	Quinapril 20 mg per day (n=878) vs placebo (n=872).
Add'l Tx	Patients on lipid lowering medicines, ACE inhibitors or calcium blockers were excluded.

Results   Angiographic data reported elsewhere. Primary clinical outcome was time to first cardiac event of the following: cardiac death; resuscitated cardiac arrest, nonfatal MI, CABG, PTCA, hospitalization for angina. Frequency of primary event was 38% in both groups (RR 1.04; 95% CI=0.89-1.22; p=0.6). Cardiac death occurred in 1.5% of placebo and 1.4% of quinapril patients. Nonfatal MI occurred in 4.6% vs 4.1%; resuscitated cardiac arrest in 0.5% vs 0%; CABG in 11.9% vs 13.2%; PTCA 26.7% vs 25.4%; hospitalization for unstable angina in 5.6% vs 5.9%, in placebo vs quinapril, respectively (all p=NS). There was no significant difference in incidence of patients with angiographic evidence of progression or coronary atherosclerosis. Also rate of development of new lesions was similar between groups. Incidence of angioplasty for new (originally nonintervened) vessels was lower in the quinapril group (79) vs the placebo group (114; p=0.018).

Concl.   Quinapril did not affect overall frequency of primary clinical end point or progression of coronary atherosclerosis. It did lower incidence of angioplasty for new coronary lesions.

QUIET (Angiographic Study)

Quinapril Ischemic Event Trial

Title	Angiotensin-converting enzyme inhibition as antiatherosclerotic therapy: no answer yet.
Authors	Cashin-Hemphill L, Holmvang G, Chan RC, et al.
Reference	Am J Cardiol 1999;83:43-47.
Disease	Coronary artery disease.
Purpose	To determine the effect of long-term treatment with quinapril in coronary artery disease patients who had normal LV function and normal blood pressure, and normal cholesterol, on cardiac events and the progression of coronary atherosclerosis.
Design	Double-blind, placebo-controlled, randomized, multicenter.
Patients	1750 patients with normal LV function undergoing successful coronary angioplasty or atherectomy. Exclusion criteria included LDL cholesterol >165 mg/d, systolic BP >160 mm Hg, diastolic BP >100 mm Hg, LVEF <40%, and others. Quantitative coronary angiographic analysis reported in 477 patients.
Follow-up	3 years.
Regimen	Quinapril (20 mg) or placebo once daily for 3 years.
Results	Quantitative coronary angiography showed similar findings at baseline. At 3 years 111 of 234 (47%) of quinapril patients and 119 of 243 (49%) of placebo patients had progression of atherosclerosis (p=NS). Mean change in minimum lumen diameter index was -0.18±0.03 mm in quinapril patients and -0.21±0.03 mm in placebo patients (p=NS). 50 (22%) patients in the quinapril group developed new stenoses vs 44(19%) in the placebo group. Percent diameter stenosis index was +3.5±1.0 with quinapril and +5.1±1.0 with placebo (p=NS). Quinapril apparently did not reduce clinical end points (time to first cardiac event defined as cardiac death, resuscitated cardiac arrest, nonfatal MI, revascularization, hospitalization for angina pectoris). Discussion reviews some of the limitations of this study including dose and an increase in LDL cholesterol in both groups.

| Concl. | Quinapril had a neutral effect on quantitative coronary angiographic parameters of progression and nonprogression. |

SCAT

Simvastatin/Enalapril Coronary Atherosclerosis Trial

Title	Long term effects of cholesterol lowering and angiotensin-converting enzyme inhibition on coronary atherosclerosis: The SCAT trial.
Authors	Teo KK, Burton JR, Buller CE, et al.
Reference	Circulation 2000;102:1748-1754.
Disease	Coronary artery disease.
Purpose	To determine the effect of cholesterol lowering with simvastatin and ACE inhibition with enalapril alone or together on CAD progression and regression in normo-cholesterolemic patients.
Design	Randomized, double-blind, placebo-controlled, multicenter, 2 x 2 factorial study.
Patients	460 patients with total serum cholesterol between 4.1 and 6.2 mmol/L, high-density lipoprotein cholesterol <2.2 mmol/L, angiographically detectable coronary disease in ≥3 major coronary segments, left ventricular ejection fraction >35%.
Follow-up	Average follow-up 47.8 months.
Regimen	Starting doses were simvastatin/placebo 10 mg daily and enalapril/placebo 2.5 mg twice daily. Upward dose titration during first 3 months to simvastatin 40 mg daily and enalapril 10 mg twice daily. Of 460 patients; 230 received simvastatin and 230 received a simvastatin placebo; 229 received enalapril and 231 an enalapril placebo. Some patients received both drugs and some received double placebo. National Cholesterol Education Program diet was encouraged in all patients.

Results	Primary end points were quantitative coronary angiographic measures and clinical events (death, myocardial infarction, stroke, hospitalization for angina, revascularization, cancer). During therapy average per-patient mean absolute coronary diameter decreased by 0.07±0.20 mm with simvastatin vs 0.4±0.25 mm with placebo (p=0.004). Average decreases in minimal absolute diameters were 0.09±0.17 and 0.16±0.20 in simvastatin vs placebo patients (p=0.0001). Increase in percent diameter stenosis was 1.67±5.01% in simvastatin vs 3.83±6.58% in placebo patients (p=0.0003). There was no benefit of enalapril on quantitative coronary angiography. There was no additive benefit of both groups together on quantitative coronary angiography. Fewer simvastatin patients required PTCA (8 vs 21 events; p=0.020). Fewer enalapril patients had combined end point of death, MI, stroke (16 vs 30; p=0.043) vs placebo. There was no difference in all cause mortality among groups.
Concl.	Lipid lowering therapy had beneficial effects on coronary angiography. Enalapril did not alter the degree of atherosclerotic narrowing; however, it did reduce events.

SECURE

Study to Evaluate Carotid Ultrasound Changes in Patients Treated with Ramipril and Vitamin E

Title	Effects of ramipril and vitamin E on atherosclerosis. The study to evaluate carotid ultrasound changes in patients treated with ramipril and vitamin E (SECURE).
Authors	Lonn EM, Yusuf S, Dzavik V, et al.
Reference	Circulation 2001;103:919-925.
Disease	Atherosclerosis.
Purpose	To assess the effects of ramipril and vitamin E on the progression of carotid atherosclerosis.
Design	Randomized, double-blind, placebo-controlled, multicenter (a substudy of the HOPE trial).
Patients	732 patients, ≥55 years old, with vascular disease or diabetes mellitus and ≥1 additional cardiovascular risk factors and adequate B-mode carotid ultrasound image. Patients with heart failure, left ventricular ejection fraction <40%, myocardial infarction, unstable angina or stroke in the month preceding randomization, current use of ACE inhibitors or vitamin E, uncontrolled hypertension, or nephropathy were excluded.
Follow-up	4-5 years (mean 4.5 years).
Regimen	After a single-blind, run-in phase of 7-10 days with ramipril 2.5 mg/d, patients were randomized to placebo, ramipril 10 mg/d or 2.5 mg/d, and to vitamin E 400 IU/d or placebo.

Results	Ramipril 2.5 mg/d and 10 mg/d reduced systolic and diastolic blood pressure vs placebo, without a significant difference between the 2 ramipril groups. Vitamin E had no effect on blood pressure. The progression slope of the mean maximum carotid intimal-medial thickness was 0.0217 mm/year in the placebo group, 0.0180 mm/year in the ramipril 2.5-mg/d group, and 0.0137 mm/year in the ramipril 10-mg/d group (p=0.033). Vitamin E did not have an effect on the rate of progression of the carotid intimal-medial thickness. The primary clinical end point of the HOPE study (cardiovascular death, myocardial infarction or stroke) occurred in 16.8% of the placebo group, 13.9% in the ramipril 2.5-mg/d group, and in 12.7% in the ramipril 10-mg/d group (p=NS). The primary clinical end point occurred in 15.1% and 13.9% of the patients receiving placebo or vitamin E (p=NS).
Concl.	Long-term administration of ramipril reduced the rate of progression of carotid intimal-medial thickness. In contrast, vitamin E had no effect on the progression of carotid atherosclerosis.

SUAVIS-Arterial Arm

Sulodexide Arterial Venous Italian Study—Arterial Arm

Title	Sulodexide in the treatment of intermittent claudication. Results of a randomized, double-blind, multicentre, placebo-controlled study.
Authors	Coccher S, Scondotto G, Agnelli G, et al.
Reference	Eur Heart J 2002;23:1057-1065.
Disease	Peripheral artery disease.
Purpose	To assess the effects of sulodexide, a standardized extractive glycosaminoglycan containing 80% "fast moving" heparin and 20% dermatan-sulfate, in patients with peripheral arterial disease and intermittent claudication.
Design	Randomized, double-blind, placebo-controlled, multicenter.
Patients	286 patients, 45-75 years old, with chronic obliterative peripheral artery disease and intermittent claudication for ≥6 months, without deterioration in the preceding 3 months, maximum walking distance of 100-300 m. Patients with osteoarthritis, arthritis, low back pain, cardiopulmonary insufficiency, ischemic heart disease, arrhythmias, polyneuropathy, or other conditions preventing the performance of treadmill test were not included. In addition, patients with abdominal aortic aneurysm (>3 cm), severe hemodynamic stenosis of the pelvic arteries, prior surgical revascularization on the affected limb, prior gangliotomy of the affected limb, type 1 diabetes, severe liver or kidney disease, malignant hypertension, cancer, vasculitis, and hypersensitivity to extractive mucopolysaccharides were excluded. Patients who needed treatment with oral anticoagulants, ticlopidine, or NSAIDs were not included.

Follow-up	Clinical follow-up and repeat treadmill tests for 6 months.
Regimen	Randomization to sulodexide (60 mg/d by intramuscular injection for the first 20 days, and then 50 mg bid orally for 6 months) (n=143) or placebo (n=143). Total treatment duration was 27 weeks.
Results	17 patients in the sulodexide and 34 in the placebo group did not complete the treatment phase (p=0.013). Doubling of pain-free walking distance was achieved by 23.8% of the patients in the sulodexide and by 9.1% in the placebo group (p=0.001). Doubling the maximum walking distance was achieved by 25.9% and 6.3% of the patients, respectively (p<0.001). The pain-free walking distance increased by 83.2±8.6 m in the sulodexide group and by 36.7±6.2 m in the placebo group (p=0.001). The maximum walking distance increased by 142.3±15.8 m and 54.5±8.4 m, respectively (p=0.001). Non-fatal acute MI occurred in 2 patients in the placebo group and in 0 of the patients in the sulodexide group. Fatal acute MI occurred in 3 and 1 patient(s), respectively. 1 patient in the sulodexide and 4 in the placebo group died. At the end of the study plasma fibrinogen levels decreased by 31.9±8.8 mg/dL in the sulodexide group and increased by 30.2±10.0 mg/dL in the placebo group (p=0.001). The effect of sulodexide was comparable for nondiabetic patients and for patients with type 2 diabetes.
Concl.	Sulodexide improved the walking ability and decreased plasma fibrinogen levels in patients with peripheral artery disease and intermittent claudication. The treatment was safe and well tolerated.

12

TPT (Angina)

Thrombosis Prevention Trial

Title	Antithrombotic treatment and the incidence of angina pectoris.
Authors	Knottenbelt C, Brennan PJ, Meade TW, et al.
Reference	Arch Intern Med 2002;162:881-886.
Disease	Angina pectoris; coronary artery disease.
Purpose	To determine the effects of antithrombotic treatment on the incidence of angina pectoris.
Design	Double-blind, placebo-controlled, randomized.
Patients	5499 men aged 45-69 years at increased risk of coronary heart disease.
Follow-up	6.8 years.
Regimen	Factorial design with patients randomized to active warfarin and active aspirin; active warfarin and placebo aspirin; placebo warfarin and active aspirin; placebo warfarin and placebo aspirin. Warfarin started at 2.5 mg/d and adjusted by increments or decrements of 0.5 mg/d or 1.0 mg/d at monthly intervals to an international normalized ratio (INR) of about 1.5. Aspirin was given as 75 mg/d in a controlled-release form.
Results	There was a trend (although not statistically significant) for warfarin to decrease the incidence of stable angina by 16% (95% CI=-14 to 38); while aspirin increased the incidence by 39% (95% CI=0-91; p=0.05). Stable angina was 37% less in patients on warfarin vs those on aspirin (p=0.05). Total coronary heart disease was defined as a combination of coronary deaths, nonfatal MI, and incident angina. Warfarin decreased total coronary heart disease by 18% (95% CI=4-30; p=0.01); aspirin reduced total coronary heart disease by 8% (95% CI=-10 to 22; p=0.36).
Concl.	The results suggest (although not definitively) that warfarin has a durable effect on chronic pathologic conditions underlying angina; further research in this field is needed.

VEAPS

The Vitamin E Atherosclerosis Prevention Study

Title	Alpha-tocopherol supplementation in healthy individuals reduces low-density lipoprotein oxidation but not atherosclerosis.
Authors	Hodis HN, Mack WJ, LaBree L, et al.
Reference	Circulation 2002;106:1453-1459.
Disease	Coronary artery disease; atherosclerosis hyperlipidemia.
Purpose	To determine whether vitamin E supplementation reduces the progression of atherosclerosis.
Design	Prospective, randomized, placebo-controlled.
Patients	353 patients, who were ≥40 years old with LDL ≥3.37 mmol/L (130 mg/dL), without any clinical signs or symptoms of cardiovascular disease. Patients were excluded if their fasting triglycerides were >5.64 mmol/L (500 mg/dL), had diabetes or fasting glucose ≥3.62 mmol/L (140 mg/dL), usual vitamin E supplement intake for more than 1 year, lipid standardized plasma vitamin E >35 mmol/L, diastolic blood pressure ≥100 mm Hg, untreated disease of the thyroid, serum creatinine >2.5 mg/dL, serious disease with life expectancy <5 years, and alcohol ingestion greater than 5 drinks/d.
Follow-up	Average 3 years.
Regimen	Patients were assigned to placebo (n=176) and vitamin E (n=177). Vitamin E was given as DL-a-tocopherol 400 IU/d. Patients were instructed to take the study medication with the highest-fat meal of the day.

12

Results   The primary study end point was the rate of change of the intima media thickness (IMT) in the right distal common carotid artery as assessed by computer image-processed B-mode ultrasonograms. Of the 353 originally randomized study participants, 258 completed the entire follow-up period through the end of the study. The placebo and vitamin E groups were similar at baseline. Baseline measurements of IMT were similar between the placebo and vitamin E groups (placebo=0.760±0.131 vs vitamin E=0.746±0.132 mm; p=0.35). The rate of IMT progression in the placebo group overall was 0.0023±0.0007 mm/yr and in the vitamin E group, 0.0040±0.0007; p=0.08. Adjustment for baseline LDL cholesterol yielded a p-value of 0.13. There were no differences in IMT progression between the groups according to gender, baseline vitamin E level, baseline vitamin C level, or levels of LDL cholesterol, HDL, or triglycerides during the trial. Levels of vitamin E rose in the vitamin E group from baseline (22.1±6.3-53.3±12.7 mmol/L; p<0.0001). Differences in plasma vitamin E levels between the 2 groups were significant at follow-up (p<0.0001). There were 14 cardiovascular events (fatal or nonfatal MI, non-Q-wave MI, CABG surgery, percutaneous transluminal coronary angioplasty, unstable angina, transient ischemic attack, and cerebrovascular accident) in the placebo group and 11 events in the vitamin E group (p=0.81).

Concl.   Supplementation with vitamin E does not reduce the progression of atherosclerosis in healthy men and women.

WAVE

Women's Angiographic Vitamin and Estrogen Trial

Title	Effects of hormone replacement therapy and antioxidant vitamin supplements on coronary atherosclerosis in postmenopausal women: a randomized controlled trial.
Authors	Waters DD, Alderman EL, Hsia J, et al.
Reference	JAMA 2002;288:2432-2440.
Disease	Coronary artery disease.
Purpose	To determine if hormone replacement therapy (HRT) or antioxidant vitamin supplements, singly or together, can alter the progression of coronary artery disease.
Design	Randomized, double-blind, placebo-controlled, multicenter.
Patients	423 postmenopausal women, who had a coronary angiogram performed in the 4 months prior to enrollment which showed at least 1 15%-75% coronary stenosis in an artery that was not treated with intervention. If the angiography was performed within 2 weeks of a myocardial infarction, the infarct should not have been related to the stenosis that qualified the patient for the study. Exclusion criteria included: current use of greater than 60 mg/d of vitamin C or 30 IU of vitamin E and no intention of discontinuing use, suspected breast, uterine, or cervical cancer, uncontrolled diabetes or hypertension, MI in the previous 4 weeks, past or planned CABG surgery, and others.
Follow-up	Mean 2.8 years.
Regimen	Patients were randomized into 4 different groups. Patients received 400 IU of vitamin E and 500 mg of vitamin C, or a placebo bid. Also, women received either HRT or no HRT; women with a past hysterectomy took 0.625 mg of conjugated equine estrogens (Premarin) daily or placebo, and women without a hysterectomy received either 1 tablet of conjugated equine estrogens and medroxyprogesterone acetate (0.625/2.5 mg of Prempro) daily, or placebo.

12

Results	The main outcome measure was the change in the minimum lumen diameter of the original lesion of interest. There were greater decreases in minimum lumen diameter (MLD) and average lumen diameter in each of the 3 groups that contained an active-treatment vs the placebo-only group, but these differences were not significant. There was no statistically significant interaction between any of the treatments and any angiographic outcomes (p=0.31 for interaction for MLD). The groups were combined according to specific treatments (HRT groups, vitamin groups) and then analyzed; the MLD showed a greater decrease in the HRT groups vs placebo (-0.047 mm/yr vs 0.024 mm/yr), but this was not significant (p=0.17). Patients who were treated with vitamins showed a greater decrease in MLD vs placebo; this decrease was not significant (-0.044 mm/yr vs -0.028 mm/yr; p=0.32). The rate of death was lowest in the placebo-only group (1.9%), highest in the treatment groups (9.4% for HRT and vitamins), and between these values in the other groups (3.9% for HRT/placebo and 5.7% for placebo/vitamins); this trend was not significant (p=0.08). A composite of death, nonfatal MI, or stroke was more frequent in women in the HRT groups compared with placebo (26/210 vs 15/213, hazard ratio [HR] 1.9; 95% CI=0.97-3.6; p=0.07). Women assigned to the vitamin group had a significantly higher rate of all-cause death vs placebo patients (16/212 vs 6/211, HR 2.8; 95% CI=1.1-7.2; p=0.047). There was a similar trend for death or nonfatal MI (20/212 vs 10/211, HR 2.1; 95% CI=0.99-4.5; p=0.09).
Concl.	In this trial consisting of postmenopausal women, neither HRT nor vitamin C and E use was associated with any cardiovascular benefit. There was a trend towards harm with each treatment.

WHI

Women's Health Initiative

Title	Risks and benefits of estrogen plus progestin in healthy postmenopausal women—principal results from the Women's Health Initiative randomized controlled trial.
Authors	Writing Group for the Women's Health Initiative Investigators.
Reference	JAMA 2002;288:321-333.
Disease	Healthy postmenopausal women; development of coronary heart disease (CHD).
Purpose	To determine the chief health benefits and risks associated with combination hormone replacement therapy (HRT) in healthy postmenopausal women.
Design	Randomized, controlled, multicenter, blinded.
Patients	16,608 patients, 8506 randomized to estrogen plus progestin, 8102 to placebo. Patients were women age 50-79, postmenopausal, and likely to remain at the same residence for 3 years. Exclusion criteria included any medical condition with an expected survival of <3 years, prior breast cancer or other cancer, and conditions (alcoholism, dementia) that would interfere with compliance and retention.
Follow-up	Mean 5.2 years.
Regimen	Patients randomized to receive active medication received 1 daily tablet that contained conjugated equine estrogen 0.625 mg and medroxyprogesterone acetate 2.5 mg (Prempro). A matching placebo was given to the control group.

12

Results	The primary end point was CHD which was defined as acute MI requiring overnight hospitalization, silent MI, or CHD death. Invasive breast cancer was the primary adverse outcome. The trial was terminated early due to study results that showed evidence of harm from breast cancer as well as some increase in stroke, CHD, and pulmonary embolism. This harm was deemed to outweigh the small benefits of HRT for fractures and colon cancer that were seen in the trial. Baseline characteristics between the 2 groups were similar. The levels of cardiovascular risk factors were similar to those expected in a generally healthy population of postmenopausal women. The rate of cardiovascular events was increased by 29% in the combination treatment group compared to placebo (37 vs 30 per 10,000 person-years, hazard ratio [HR] 1.29; adjusted 95% CI=0.85-1.97), which was nominally significant. Most of the excess risk was accounted for by nonfatal MI. No differences were noted in numbers of CHD deaths or revascularization procedures. Rate of stroke was also higher in the treatment group (29 vs 21 per 10,000 person-years, HR 1.41; adjusted 95% CI=0.86-2.31). Rate of venous thromboembolism (VTE) was 2 times higher in the treatment group (151/8506 vs 67/8102, HR 2.11; 95% CI=1.58-2.82). A small subgroup of women (n=400) had preexisting cardiovascular disease (ie, previous MI or revascularization). These women were also at increased risk of future coronary events, (HR 1.28; 95% CI=0.64-2.56). Women who did not have preexisting disease had the same increased risk (HR 1.28; 95% CI=1.00-1.65). Women with a past history of VTE seemed to be an increased risk of VTE with HRT use (HR 4.90; 95% CI=0.58-41.06) vs those without such a history (HR 2.06; 95% CI=1.54-2.76), but only a few women had a previous VTE. Prior history of stroke did not increase the future risk while on HRT.
Concl.	Estrogen plus progestin therapy in healthy postmenopausal women appeared to be associated with an increased risk of adverse coronary events compared to placebo.

WHI

Women's Health Initiative

Title	Estrogen plus progestin and the risk of coronary heart disease.
Authors	Manson JE, Hsia J, Johnson KC, et al.
Reference	N Engl J Med 2003;349:523-534.
Disease	Prevention of coronary heart disease.
Purpose	To determine whether estrogen + progestin would reduce the incidence of nonfatal myocardial infarction or death due to coronary heart disease in postmenopausal women as primary prevention.
Design	Randomized, primary prevention study, placebo-controlled, blinded, multicenter.
Patients	Postmenopausal women ages 50-79 (N=16,608).
Follow-up	Mean follow-up of 5.2 years (initial planned duration of the study was 8.5 years).
Regimen	Patients were randomized to receive conjugated estrogens (0.625 mg/d) + medroxyprogesterone acetate (2.5 mg/d) or placebo.
Results	Primary efficacy end point was nonfatal MI or death due to coronary heart disease. The data and safety monitoring board recommended terminating the trial as the risks exceeded the benefits. Hormone therapy was associated with an increased hazard ratio for the primary end point of 1.24 (95% CI=1.00-1.60). For nonfatal MI, the hazard ratio was 1.28 and for death due to coronary heart disease it was 1.10. This elevated risk was most apparent at 1 year, at which time the hazard ratio for the primary outcome was increased at 1.81 (95% CI=1.09-3.01). Estrogen + progestin was associated with a 5.4% decrease in total cholesterol, a 12.7% decrease in LDL cholesterol, and a 7.3% increase in HDL cholesterol. Systolic BP was 1 mm Hg higher among women receiving hormones than among those receiving placebo. Higher baseline LDL was associated with increased risk of coronary heart disease among women on hormone therapy. However, higher baseline levels of C-reactive protein did not modify treatment related risk of coronary heart disease.

Concl.   Estrogen + progestin did not protect healthy postmenopausal women from the development of coronary heart disease and, in fact, appeared to increase the risk, especially during the first year of therapy.

WHI

Women's Health Initiative

Title	Effects of conjugated equine estrogen in postmenopausal women with hysterectomy: the Women's Health Initiative randomized controlled trial.
Authors	Women's Health Initiative Steering Committee.
Reference	JAMA 2004;291:1701-1712.
Disease	Prevention of disease with hormone therapy.
Purpose	To assess the effects on major disease incidence of conjugated equine estrogen, the most commonly used postmenopausal hormone therapy in the United States.
Design	Multicenter, randomized, double-blind, placebo-controlled, disease-prevention trial.
Patients	10,739 ethnically/racially diverse, postmenopausal women, aged 50-79 years, with prior hysterectomy.
Follow-up	7 years.
Regimen	Conjugated equine estrogen (CEE) 0.625 mg/d or placebo.
Results	The primary outcome was coronary artery disease (CAD) incidence (nonfatal MI or CAD death). Invasive breast cancer incidence was the primary safety outcome. In February 2004, the National Institutes of Health terminated the intervention phase of the trial early. Estimated hazard ratios (95% CI) for conjugated equine estrogen (CEE) vs placebo for some of the major clinical outcomes (average follow-up 6.8 years) were: CAD, 0.91 (0.75-1.12) with 376 cases; breast cancer, 0.77 (0.59-1.01) with 218 cases; stroke, 1.39 (1.10-1.77) with 276 cases; and pulmonary embolism, 1.34 (0.87-2.06) with 85 cases. The composite outcome was, for total coronary vascular disease (CVD), 1.12 (1.01-1.24).

Concl.   Use of CEE does not affect CAD incidence in postmenopausal
          women with prior hysterectomy over an average of 6.8 years.
          The burden of incident disease events was equivalent in the
          treatment and placebo groups, indicating no overall benefit.
          CEE should not be routinely recommended for chronic disease
          CVD prevention in postmenopausal women.

Recombinant ApoA 1 Milano

Title	Effect of recombinant ApoA 1 Milano on coronary atherosclerosis in patients with acute coronary syndromes: a randomized controlled trial.
Authors	Nissen SE, Tsunoda T, Tuzcu EM, et al.
Reference	JAMA 2003;290:2292-2300.
Disease	Acute coronary syndromes, coronary artery disease, unstable angina, non-ST elevation myocardial infarction or ST elevation myocardial infarction.
Purpose	In a small village in Northern Italy live about 40 carriers with a naturally occurring mutant of apolipoprotein A 1 which is associated with longevity and less atherosclerosis than expected in those patients who have very low high-density lipoprotein cholesterol levels (10-30 mg/dL). Recombinant ApoA 1 Milano formulated with phospholipid complexes (ETC-216) was administered IV to patients with acute coronary syndromes to determine whether it could lower the atheroma burden.
Design	Double-blind, randomized, placebo-controlled, multicenter, intravascular ultrasound study.
Patients	123 patients consented; 47 completed the protocol. Patients had to be 30-75 years and required diagnostic coronary angiography within 14 days of an acute coronary syndrome (unstable angina, non-ST elevation myocardial infarction, or ST-elevation myocardial infarction). They had to have an obstructive lesion in a major epicardial coronary vessel with at least a 20% luminal diameter narrowing. Target vessel for baseline intravascular ultrasound interrogation could have no more than 50% luminal narrowing.
Follow-up	About 7 weeks.
Regimen	Patients randomized to 3 treatment groups in 1:2:2 ratio. Therapies were placebo (n=11), low-dose (15 mg/kg, n=21), or high-dose (45 mg/kg; n=15) ETC-216. Study drug was given IV once a week for 5 doses. Patients had repeat intravascular ultrasound within 2 weeks of final dose.

Results	Primary outcome was change (%) in atheroma volume (follow-up minus baseline) assessed by intravascular ultrasound. Secondary outcomes included average change in total atheroma volume, change in average maximal atheroma thickness, and change in atheroma volume in most and least severely diseased segments. In the combined treatment group (patients receiving either low- or high-dose ETC-216), the change in mean percent atheroma volume was -1.06% ±3.17% (mean ± SD). Median was -0.81% (95% CI=-1.53% to -0.34%; p=0.02 vs baseline). In the placebo group, the mean change was 0.14%±3.09%; median was 0.03% (95% CI=-1.11% to 1.43%; p=0.97 vs baseline). The mean change in the total atheroma volume in the combined treatment group was -14.1 mm^3±39.5 mm^3; median was -13.3 mm^3; 95% CI=-20.7 to -7.2; p<0.001). In the placebo group, this mean change was -2.9 mm^3±23.3 mm^3 and the median change was -0.2 mm^3 (95% CI=-8.6 to 8.2; p=0.97). Mean change in maximum atheroma thickness for combined treatment was -0.042 mm±0.08 mm; median was -0.035 mm (95% CI=-0.058 to -0.020; p<0.001), while for the placebo group the mean change from baseline in maximum atheroma thickness was -0.008 mm±0.061 mm; and the median was -0.009 (95% CI=-0.035 to 0.026; p=0.83). The effect of ETC-216 was mainly due to regression of disease in the most severely diseased subsegments.
Concl.	Recombinant ApoA 1 Milano/phospholipid complex (ETC-216) given IV for 5 doses at weekly intervals produced significant regression of coronary atherosclerosis measured by intravascular ultrasound.

BRAVO

Blockade of the Glycoprotein IIb/IIIa Receptor to Avoid Vascular Occlusion

Title	Randomized, double-blind, placebo-controlled, international trial of the oral IIb/IIIa antagonist lotrafiban in coronary and cerebrovascular disease.
Authors	Topol EJ, Easton D, Harrington RA, et al.
Reference	Circulation 2003;108:399-406.
Disease	Coronary artery disease, atherosclerosis.
Purpose	To report preliminary results of the BRAVO trial, which was stopped prematurely because of excess mortality in the lotrafiban group.
Design	International, randomized, double-blind, placebo-controlled trial.
Patients	9190 patients from 23 countries and 690 hospitals. 41% had cerebrovascular disease and 59% coronary artery disease at the time of entry.
Follow-up	Planned for 2 years.
Regimen	Lotrafiban 30 or 50 mg bid (on the basis of age and predicted creatinine clearance) or placebo.
Add'l Tx	Aspirin 75-325 mg/d.
Results	Trial enrollment was completed on June 26, 2000. The trial was terminated early, on December 12, 2000, because of a significant excess of mortality with lotrafiban, 3% vs 2.3% with placebo (hazard ratio [HR] 1.33; 95% CI=1.03-1.72; p=0.026). The cause of excess death was vascular related. The primary end point (composite of all-cause mortality, MI, stroke, recurrent ischemia requiring hospitalization, urgent revascularization) did not differ significantly between groups (17.5% placebo vs 16.4% lotrafiban). Serious bleeding was more common with lotrafiban (8% vs 2.8% with placebo; p<0.001); it was also more common in patients receiving larger doses of aspirin (>162 mg/d), with or without lotrafiban.

Concl.   The BRAVO trial confirms the increased risk of death and serious bleeding for oral glycoprotein IIb/IIIa inhibitors shown in other trials. It also demonstrates, for the first time, that the increased mortality risk is extended to patients with cerebrovascular disease. Finally, although higher aspirin doses resulted in an increased risk of the primary composite end point, serious bleeding, and transfusion, it decreased mortality risk.

DCCT/EDIC

The Diabetes Control and Complications Trial/Epidemiology of Diabetes Interventions and Complications Study

Title	Intensive diabetes therapy and carotid intima-media thickness in type 1 diabetes mellitus.
Authors	Diabetes Control and Complications Trial (DCCT)/Epidemiology of Diabetes Interventions and Complications (EDIC) Research Group.
Reference	N Engl J Med 2003;348:2294-2303.
Disease	Atherosclerosis.
Purpose	To examine the progression of carotid intima-media thickness, a measure of atherosclerosis, in a population with type 1 diabetes.
Design	Long-term follow-up epidemiologic study.
Patients	1229 patients with type 1 diabetes (participants in the DCCT) who underwent B-mode ultrasonography of the internal and common carotid arteries in 1994-1996 and again in 1998-2000.
Follow-up	6 years.
Regimen	Random assignment in the DCCT to receive conventional diabetes treatment (n=611, mean hemoglobin A1c of 9%) or intensive diabetes treatment (n=618, mean hemoglobin 7.2%).

Results	At 1 year of the EDIC study, the carotid intima-media thickness in the study population was similar to that in an age- and sex-matched control population. After 6 years, the intima-media thickness was significantly greater in the diabetic patients than in the controls. Among patients in the DCCT, progression of intima-media thickness was significantly less among those receiving intensive than among those receiving conventional therapy (progression of 0.032 vs 0.046 mm; p=0.01; progression of the combined intima-media thickness of the common and internal carotid arteries, -0.155 vs 0.007; p=0.02) after adjusting for other risk factors. Progression was associated with age, EDIC baseline BP, smoking, ratio of LDL to HDL cholesterol, and urinary albumin excretion rate, and with the mean hemoglobin A1c value during the DCCT (mean duration 6.5 years).
Concl.	Patients with type 1 diabetes are at high risk of cardiovascular disease, but the specific risk factors and whether chronic hyperglycemia has a role are unknown. Carotid intima-media thickness is a measure of atherosclerosis. Intensive therapy during the DCCT resulted in decreased progression of intima-media thickness 6 years after the end of the trial.

EUROPA

European Trial on Reduction of Cardiac Events with Perindopril in Stable Coronary Artery Disease

Title	Efficacy of perindopril in reduction of cardiovascular events among patients with stable coronary artery disease: randomised, double-blind, placebo-controlled, multicenter trial (The EUROPA Study).
Authors	The EUROPA Investigators.
Reference	Lancet 2003;362:782-788.
Disease	Coronary artery disease.
Purpose	To determine whether the angiotensin-converting enzyme inhibitor perindopril decreases cardiac event rate in patients with low-risk, stable coronary artery disease and no apparent clinical heart failure.
Design	Randomized, double-blind, placebo-controlled, multicenter.
Patients	12,218 patients randomized. Patients ≥18 years of age with no clinical evidence of congestive heart failure, but with evidence of coronary artery disease as documented by previous myocardial infarction (>3 months prior to screening), percutaneous coronary intervention or coronary artery bypass graft (>6 months prior to screening), or angiographic evidence of at least 70% narrowing of one or more major coronary arteries, or men with chest pain and a positive stress test.
Follow-up	Mean follow-up was 4.2 years.

12

Regimen	There was an initial run-in period of 4 weeks in which all of the patients received perindopril. Then the patients were randomized to perindopril 8 mg qd (n=6110) or placebo (n=6108).
Add'l Tx	92% were taking antiplatelet agents; 62% were on β blockers, and 58% on lipid-lowering agents.
Results	The primary end point was a composite of cardiovascular death, nonfatal MI, and cardiac arrest with successful resuscitation. 488 (8%) perindopril patients vs 603 (10%) placebo patients developed the primary end point. Thus, the relative risk reduction was 20% (95% CI=9-29; p=0.0003). Mean age of patients was 60 years. 85% of the patients were men. During the run-in phase, when all patients took perindopril, BP fell from 137/83 mm Hg at baseline to 128/78 mm Hg. Average BP in the placebo group during double-blind treatment phase was 5/2 mm Hg higher than in the perindopril group. Cardiovascular mortality was 3.5% in the perindopril group vs 4.1% in the placebo group (p=0.11). Nonfatal MI was 4.8% in the perindopril group vs 6.2% in the placebo group (p=0.001). Cardiac arrest occurred in 0.1% of perindopril vs 0.2% of placebo patients (p=0.22). Perindopril was associated with a 14% reduction in total mortality, nonfatal MI, unstable angina, and cardiac arrest (95% CI=6-21, p=0.0009). Perindopril was associated with a 39% reduction in heart failure admissions. The benefit of perindopril was observed across a wide array of subgroups, including patients on lipid-lowering drugs or β blockers. The drug was well tolerated.
Concl.	Perindopril improved cardiac outcome in patients with stable coronary heart disease without heart failure.

GOES

Secondary CAD Prevention with Folic Acid

Title	Secondary prevention with folic acid: effects on clinical outcomes.
Authors	Liem A, Reynierse-Buitenwerf GH, Zwinderman AH, et al.
Reference	J Am Coll Cardiol 2003;41:2105-2113.
Disease	Coronary artery disease.
Purpose	To assess the effect of folic acid in secondary prevention of stable coronary artery disease.
Design	Randomized, open-label.
Patients	593 patients with stable coronary artery disease.
Follow-up	Mean 24 months.
Regimen	Folic acid 0.5 mg/d (n=300) or standard care (n=293, control group).
Add'l Tx	Statin treatment.
Results	In patients receiving folic acid, plasma homocysteine levels decreased by 18%, from 12±4.8 to 9.4±3.5 μmol/L; homocysteine did not change in the control group (p<0.001 between groups). The primary end point was all-cause mortality and a composite of vascular events (sudden death, fatal recurrent MI, fatal stroke, and other cardiovascular deaths). A primary end point occurred in 31 (10.3%) patients receiving folic acid and in 28 (9.6%) in the control group, a nonsignificant difference (relative risk 1.05; 95% CI=0.63-1.75). In a multifactorial survival model with adjustments for clinical factors, the most predictive laboratory variables were creatinine clearance, plasma fibrinogen, and homocysteine. On-treatment lipid values, including apolipoprotein A and apolipoprotein B, were not predictive.
Concl.	Low-dose folic acid supplementation for 2 years does not appear to reduce clinical end points in patients with stable CAD. The study does not support routine folic acid supplementation.

HPS

Heart Protection Study (Antioxidant Vitamins)

Title	MRC/BHF Heart Protection Study of antioxidant vitamin supplement in 20,536 high-risk individuals: a randomised placebo-controlled trial.
Authors	Heart Protection Study Collaborative Group.
Reference	Lancet 2002;360:23-33.
Disease	Atherosclerosis.
Purpose	To assess the effects of antioxidant vitamins on vascular and non-vascular morbidity and mortality in a large cohort of patients at high risk.
Design	Randomized, double-blind, 2 × 2 factorial, placebo-controlled, multicenter.
Patients	20,536 patients, 40-80 years old, with a history of coronary artery disease, peripheral vascular disease, stroke, diabetes, or hypertension and low-to-average total or low-density lipoprotein cholesterol (≥3.5 mmol/L [135 mg/dL]). Patients in whom statin therapy was considered indicated by their physicians were not included. Patients with chronic liver disease, creatinine >200 μmol/L, severe renal disease; inflammatory muscle disease, creatine kinase >750 IU/L, cyclosporine, fibrates, on niacin therapy, women with child-bearing potential, severe heart failure, severe chronic lung disease, or other life-threatening disease were excluded.
Follow-up	5 years.

Regimen	After 2-month run-in period of active vitamins, patients were randomized to vitamins (vitamin E 600 mg, vitamin C 250 mg, and β-carotene 20 mg) (n=10,269) or placebo (n=10,267) and to either simvastatin (40 mg/d) or placebo.
Results	83% of the patients in each group were compliant with the study medication. All-cause mortality was 14.1% in the vitamin group and 13.5% in the placebo group (rate ratio 1.04; 95% CI=0.97-1.12; p=0.3). Coronary mortality was 6.5% and 6.1%, respectively, and vascular mortality was 8.6% in the vitamin group and 8.2% in the placebo group (rate ratio 1.05; 95% CI=0.95-1.15; p=0.3). Nonvascular mortality was 5.5% and 5.3%, respectively (rate ratio 1.04; 95% CI=0.92-1.17; p=0.5). Major coronary events occurred in 10.4% of the patients in the vitamin group vs 10.2% in the placebo group (p=0.7). Stroke occurred in 5.0% of the patients in each group (p=0.8). Vitamins did not reduce the rate of coronary (6.1% vs 6.0%) or noncoronary (4.6% vs 5.0%) revascularization. Major vascular events occurred in 22.5% of the patients in each group (p>0.9). Subgroup analysis did not identify treatment benefit in any of the different prior-disease categories. Vitamins had no effect on incidence of cancer or on hospitalization for any other nonvascular cause.
Concl.	Among high-risk patients, 5-year treatment with antioxidant vitamins did not reduce morbidity and mortality.

WELL-HART

Women's Estrogen-Progestin Lipid-Lowering Hormone Atherosclerosis Regression Trial

Title	Hormone therapy and the progression of coronary artery atherosclerosis in postmenopausal women.
Authors	Hodis HN, Mack WJ, Azen SP, et al.
Reference	N Engl J Med. 2003;349:535-545.
Disease	Coronary artery disease.
Purpose	To compare the effects of oral micronized 17β-estradiol with or without sequentially administered medroxyprogesterone acetate on the progression of atherosclerosis in postmenopausal women with angiographic coronary artery disease.
Design	Randomized, double-blind, placebo-controlled trial.
Patients	226 postmenopausal women, mean age 63.5 years, with at least 1 coronary artery lesion.
Follow-up	Median 3.3 years.
Regimen	Usual care (control group, n=76), estrogen with micronized 17β-estradiol alone (estrogen group, n=76), or 17β-estradiol + sequentially administered medroxyprogesterone acetate (estrogen-progestin group, n=74).
Add'l Tx	Lipid-lowering therapy (dietary intervention and, if needed, lipid-lowering agent, usually statins) to reduced low-density lipoprotein cholesterol to <130 mg/dL.

Results	The mean (±SE) change in percent stenosis from baseline in the 169 participants who had a pair of matched angiograms was 1.89±0.78 percentage points in the control group, 2.18±0.76 in the estrogen group, and 1.24±0.80 in the estrogen-progestin group, yielding no significant difference (p=0.66) among the 3 groups. The mean difference in percent stenosis between the estrogen group and the control group was 0.29 percentage point (95% CI=-1.88 to 2.46) and the mean difference between the estrogen-progestin group and the control group was -0.65 percentage point (95% CI=-2.87 to 1.57). There were no significant differences among the groups in the number of cardiovascular events occurring during the first year of study treatment. Breast cancer was diagnosed in 1 patient in the control group and uterine cancer was not diagnosed in any participant.
Concl.	Neither estrogen nor estrogen-progestin therapy had a significant effect on progression of atherosclerosis in these postmenopausal women with established CAD. These results are similar to those of previous randomized, controlled trials in elderly women with CAD.

STOP-NIDDM

STOP-Non-Insulin-Dependent Diabetes Mellitus Trial

Title	Acarbose treatment and the risk of cardiovascular disease and hypertension in patients with impaired glucose tolerance: the STOP-NIDDM Trial.
Authors	Chiasson JL, Josse RG, Gomis R, et al., for the STOP-NIDDM Trial Research Group.
Reference	JAMA 2003;290:486-494.
Disease	Coronary artery disease, hypertension.
Purpose	To evaluate the effect of decreasing postprandial hyperglycemia with acarbose, an α-glucosidase inhibitor, on the risk of cardiovascular disease and hypertension in patients with impaired glucose tolerance.
Design	International, multicenter, double-blind, placebo-controlled, randomized trial.
Patients	1429 patients with impaired glucose tolerance.
Follow-up	Mean 3.3±1.2 years.
Regimen	Acarbose 100 mg tid (n=714) or placebo (n=715).

Results	The primary end point was development of major cardiovascular events (CAD, cardiovascular death, CHF, cerebrovascular event, peripheral vascular disease) and hypertension (≥140/90 mm Hg). About one fourth of patients (n=341; 211 receiving acarbose, 130 placebo) discontinued participation prematurely; these patients were followed for outcome parameters. The decrease in postprandial hyperglycemia associated with acarbose yielded a 49% relative risk (RR) reduction in the development of cardiovascular events (hazard ratio [HR] 0.51; 95% CI=0.28-0.95; p=0.03) and a 2.5% absolute risk reduction. For major cardiovascular events, the major reduction in risk with acarbose was for MI (HR 0.09; 95% CI=0.01-0.72; p=0.02). Acarbose was also associated with a 34% RR reduction in the incidence of new cases of hypertension (HR 0.66; 95% CI=0.49-0.89; p=0.006) and a 5.3% absolute risk reduction. After adjusting for major risk factors, the reduction in risk of cardiovascular events (HR 0.47; 95% CI=0.24-0.90; p=0.02) and hypertension (HR 0.62; 95% CI=0.45-0.86; p=0.004) associated with acarbose treatment remained significant.
Concl.	In patients with impaired glucose tolerance, treatment with acarbose produces a significant reduction in the risk of cardiovascular disease and hypertension. This is the first prospective intervention study to test the "postprandial hyperglycemia hypothesis," ie, that postprandial hyperglycemia is a risk factor for cardiovascular disease.

12. CAD Atherosclerosis Prevention of Progression

13. Valvular Heart Disease

Low-Molecular-Weight Heparin After Mechanical Heart Valve Replacement

Title	Low-molecular-weight heparin after mechanical heart valve replacement.
Authors	Montalescot G, Polle V, Collet JP, et al.
Reference	Circulation 2000;101:1083-1086.
Disease	Valvular heart disease. Mechanical heart valve replacement.
Purpose	To compare consecutive patients with mechanical heart valve replacement who received low-molecular-weight heparin (LMWH) to a similar series who received unfractionated heparin.
Design	Comparative, nonrandomized.
Patients	208 consecutive patients undergoing single or double heart valve replacement with mechanical valves.
Follow-up	In-hospital.
Regimen	Subcutaneous unfractionated heparin (3 injections per day at 500 IU/kg/d adjusting activated partial thromboplastin time (APTT) to 1.5-2.5 times control. LMWH -72% received enoxaparin at 100 anti-Xa IU/kg (1 mg/kg) subcutaneously every 12 hours. Other patients received nadroparin at 87 anti-Xa IU/kg at 12 hour intervals. Over first part of study 106 patients received unfractionated heparin (UH); over the second phase similar patients received LMWH. Oral anticoagulation was also begun at the same time. The heparins were given until oral anticoagulation was effective.

Results	End points included effectiveness of anticoagulation and in-hospital events. Mean duration of therapy with UH was 13.6 days and with LMWH was 14.1 days (p=NS). On day 2 of treatment anti-Xa activity had reached the range of efficacy (0.5-1 IU/mL) in 87% of LMWH patients. Only 9% of UH patients attained a therapeutic APTT level (1.5-2.5 times control) by this time (p<0.0001). On the final day of treatment, all LMWH patients had achieved anti-Xa activity >0.5 IU/mL; 19% were above 1 IU/mL level. At this time 27% of patients in the UH group reached an APPT >1.5 times control; however, 62% were over-anticoagulated (level of APPT >2.5 times control). 1 patient in the UH group had 2 successive transient ischemic strokes after aortic valve replacement. 2 episodes of major bleeding occurred in each group.
Concl.	Anticoagulation with LMWH appeared feasible and effective compared with UH anticoagulation following mechanical heart valve replacement. Randomized studies are warranted.

Early and Long-Term (1 Year) Effects of the Association of
Aspirin and Oral Anticoagulant on Thrombi and Morbidity
After Replacement of the Mitral Valve with the St. Jude
Medical Prosthesis

Title	Early and long-term (one year) effects of the association of aspirin and oral anticoagulant on thrombi and morbidity after replacement of the mitral valve with the St. Jude medical prosthesis. A clinical and transesophageal echocardiographic study.
Authors	Laffort P, Roudaut R, Roques X, et al.
Reference	J Am Coll Cardiol 2000;35:739-746.
Disease	Mitral valve disease; mitral valve replacement.
Purpose	To assess low dose aspirin therapy with standard oral anticoagulants vs standard oral anticoagulation alone in decreasing strands, thrombi (assessed by transesophageal echocardiography) and thromboembolic events after mechanical mitral valve replacement.
Design	Randomized, controlled.
Patients	229 patients with mechanical mitral valve replacement.
Follow-up	1 year.
Regimen	Patients were randomized to oral anticoagulation alone to maintain international normalized ratio (INR) between 2.5-3.5 (n=120) or oral anticoagulation plus 200 mg or aspirin per day (aspirin group; n=109).

Add'l Tx	Anti-ulcer treatment. Mechanical mitral valve replacement was the St. Jude medical prosthesis.
Results	Primary composite was death, major thromboembolic event, or major hemorrhage at 1 year. On day 9 postop on trans-esophageal echocardiography there was a decreased incidence of thrombi in the aspirin group (4.8%) vs the oral anticoagulation alone group (13.1%; p=0.03), but the incidence of strands was similar between the 2 groups. At 5 months strands were present in 58.6% in the aspirin group and 63.6% in the oral anticoagulation group alone. Thrombi were less frequent than in the early postoperative phase. There was a trend toward a lower incidence of thrombi in the aspirin group (4.5%) vs the oral anticoagulation alone group (8%; p=NS). At 1 year mortality was 9% in the aspirin group and 4% in the oral anticoagulation alone group. Total thromboembolic events occurred in 9% of the aspirin group and 25% of the oral anticoagulation alone group (p=0.004). Gastrointestional bleeding was more common in the aspirin group (7%) vs the oral anticoagulation alone group (0%). The composite primary end point was 29% in the aspirin and 16% in the oral anticoagulation alone group (p=NS). Valve related events occurred in 36% of both groups. Thromboembolic events occurred in 30% of patients with early thrombus on echo vs 13.6% of patients without early thrombus (1.3%; p=NS; p=0.0003).
Concl.	In patients with mitral valve replacement with the St. Jude mechanical prosthesis combining aspirin with oral anticoagulation decreased thrombi and thromboembolic events but not overall morbidity due to an increase in hemorrhagic complications.

Mechanical vs Bioprosthetic Valves

Title	Outcome 15 years after valve replacement with a mechanical vs a bioprosthetic valve: final report of the Veterans Affairs randomized trial.
Authors	Hammermeister K, Sethi GK, Henderson WG, et al.
Reference	J Am Coll Cardiol 2000;36:1152-1158.
Disease	Mitral, aortic valve disease.
Purpose	To compare long-term survival and valve related complications between bioprosthetic vs mechanical heart valves in aortic and mitral positions.
Design	Randomized, multicenter, Dept. of Veterans Affairs trial.
Patients	394 men undergoing aortic value replacement; 181 men undergoing mitral valve replacement.
Follow-up	15 years.
Regimen	Patients randomized to Bjork-Shiley spherical disc mechanical prosthesis or Hancock porcine bioprosthetic valve.
Add'l Tx	Anticoagulation where indicated.

Results	Primary study end points were time to death from any cause and time to first occurrence of the following complications: "systemic embolism, clinically important bleeding, prosthetic valve endocarditis, valve thrombosis, nonthrombotic valve obstruction, prosthetic valve regurgitation, reoperation." Operative mortality was 7.7% with no difference between mechanical or bioprosthetic valve. All-cause mortality was lower in patients undergoing AVR with a mechanical valve (66±3%) vs those with a bioprosthetic valve (79±3%; p=0.02). There was no significant difference in long-term mortality in patients receiving a mechanical vs bioprosthetic valve in the mitral position (15 year mortality both >70%). In patients receiving AVR, valve-related death accounted for 37% of all deaths with mechanical and 41% with bioprosthetic valves. For patients receiving MVR, valve related deaths accounted for 44% in mechanical group and 57% in bioprosthetic group. Primary valve failure occurred primarily in patients <65 years old (bioprosthetic 26% vs mechanical 0%; p<0.001 for AVR and 44% vs 4%; p=0.0001 for MVR). In patients 65 or older 9±6% and 0% had primary valve failure of bioprosthetic vs mechanical valve (p=0.16) in the aortic valve position. Bioprosthetic valves required reoperation more frequently than mechanical valves. Bleeding was more common for the mechanical valve group than bioprosthetic group for both AVR (51 vs 30%; p=0.0001) and for MVR (53 vs 31%; p=0.01) patients. There were no significant differences between groups in other complications such as thromboembolism.

Concl.	At 15 years patients undergoing AVR had better survival with mechanical vs bioprosthetic valve mainly due to absence of valve failure with mechanical values. Primary valve failure was more common with bioprothesis for AVR and MVR and occurred more frequently in patients less than 65 years old. Reoperation was more common with bioprosthetic valves; bleeding more common with mechanical valves.

13

Clinical and Echocardiographic Follow-Up of Patients Previously Treated with Dexfenfluramine or Phentermine/Fenfluramine

Title	Clinical and echocardiographic follow-up of patients previously treated with dexfenfluramine or phentermine/fenfluramine.
Authors	Gardin JM, Weissman NJ, Leung C, et al.
Reference	JAMA 2001;286:2011-2014.
Disease	Valvular heart disease.
Purpose	To determine changes in valve morphology and regurgitation, and clinical parameters 1 year after initial echocardiograms (ECHOs) in patients treated with dexfenfluramine or phentermine/fenfluramine vs untreated controls.
Design	Reader-blinded, echocardiographic and clinical follow-up study; multicenter.
Patients	1142 obese patients who had follow-up ECHOs. Follow-up time from discontinuation of drug to follow-up ECHO was 17.5-18.7 months.
Follow-up	As above.
Regimen	Assessment of ECHOs 13-26 months after discontinuation of diet drugs.
Results	Primary outcome was echocardiographic change in valvular regurgitation, valve morphology, and mobility. 8 controls had changes in aortic regurgitation (1.7% had decreases; 0.2% had an increase); 29 dexfenfluramine patients had changes in aortic regurgitation (6.4% had decreases; 1.7% had increases; p<0.001 vs controls); and 15 phentermine/fenfluramine had changes in aortic regurgitation (4.5%—all decreases; p=0.03 vs controls). There were no other significant differences between control patients or those having received drugs for mitral regurgitation, aortic or mitral leaflet mobility or thickness, pulmonary artery systolic pressure or ejection fraction. There were no differences in cardiovascular events, changes in medical histories or physical findings among groups.

Concl.   Progression of valvular abnormalities is unlikely 13-16 months after discontinuation of dexfenfluramine and phentermine/fenfluramine.

SCT

Smoking Cessation Therapy (Fenfluramine Analysis)

Title	Echocardiographic examination of women previously treated with fenfluramine. Long-term follow-up of randomized, double-blind, placebo-controlled trial.
Authors	Davidoff R, McTiernan A, Constantine G, et al.
Reference	Arch Intern Med 2001;161:1429-1436.
Disease	Valvular heart disease.
Purpose	To evaluate the presence of valvular abnormalities by echo in subjects randomly assigned to fenfluramine hydrochloride.
Design	Randomized, double-blind, placebo-controlled, single-center study to evaluate role of fenfluramine in women attempting to stop smoking.
Patients	619 female smokers. Data from 530 were available (276 in fenfluramine group; 254 in placebo group).
Follow-up	Up to 4.9 years.
Regimen	Fenfluramine hydrochloride (60 mg daily) vs matched placebo for up to 3 months.
Results	No significant differences were observed in prevalence of aortic or mitral regurgitation by echo between fenfluramine and placebo groups. Aortic regurgitation (mild or greater) was observed in 6.2% of treated and 4.3% of control groups (RR vs control 1.42; 95% CI=0.68-2.98; p=0.44); and mitral regurgitation in 5.1% of treated vs 4.7% of control; RR 1.07; 95% CI=0.51-2.28; p>0.99. There also was no difference in aortic or mitral valve leaflet mobility or thickening, pulmonary artery pressures or left ventricular ejection fraction by echo analysis between groups. There also were no significant differences in cardiovascular status by physical examination or development of serious cardiac events between groups.
Concl.	There was no evidence of significant valvular heart disease during a 4.9-year period among women on fenfluramine (60 mg/d) for 3 months as part of a smoking cessation program.

Multicenter Aspirin Study in Infective Endocarditis

Title	A randomized trial of aspirin on the risk of embolic events in patients with infective endocarditis.
Authors	Kwan-Leung C, Dumesnil JG, Cujec B, et al.
Reference	J Am Coll Cardiol 2003;42:775-780.
Disease	Infective endocarditis (valvular heart disease).
Purpose	To determine the effect of aspirin on the development of embolic events in the setting of infective endocarditis.
Design	Randomized, double-blind, placebo-controlled, multicenter.
Patients	115 patients with endocarditis defined by the presence of 2 of the 3 criteria: 1) multiple positive blood cultures with no known extracardiac source, 2) echocardiographic evidence of vegetation, 3) at least 2 of the following clinical presentations: fever, new or changing heart murmur, preexisting heart disease, and microvascular phenomena. Patients with perivalvular abscess were excluded.
Follow-up	≈4-6 weeks.
Regimen	Patients were randomized to receive either aspirin 325 mg/d or placebo for 4 weeks. Patients encouraged to have baseline cerebral computed tomography and follow-up study after antibiotic therapy at 4-6 weeks. Transthoracic echocardiograms obtained at baseline and after completion of antibiotic therapy.
Add'l Tx	In patients with mechanical prosthetic heart valves, anticoagulation was continued.

13

Results   Primary outcome was clinical embolic event involving brain
           or other organs. Cutaneous micro-infarcts were not included.
           Secondary outcomes included subclinical stroke assessed by
           computed tomography, death, major or minor bleeding, valve
           surgery, and increased valvular involvement assessed by echo-
           cardiography. The primary outcome occurred in 17 patients
           (28.3%) of the patients on aspirin vs 11 patients (20.0%) of the
           patients on placebo (OR=1.62; 95% CI=0.68-3.86; p=0.29).
           Embolization occurred to the central nervous system in 8
           patients on aspirin vs 3 on placebo. Major or minor bleeding
           episodes occurred in 17 (28.8%) of the patients on aspirin vs 8
           (14.5%) on placebo (OR=1.92; 95% CI=0.76-4.86). There was
           no difference between the groups in the need for valvular sur-
           gery. There were no differences between groups in intracerebral
           abnormalities detected by computed tomography. By echocar-
           diography, the vegetations decreased in size over the course of
           the study in both groups to a similar degree; aspirin also had no
           effect on echo-assessed valvular dysfunction.

Concl.   The addition of aspirin to endocarditis patients receiving antibi-
           otic therapy did not confer any benefit. Aspirin did not reduce
           the risk of embolic events and increased the risk of bleeding.

13. Valvular Heart Disease

14. Preliminary Reports

In recent years numerous studies have been conducted on various cardiovascular subjects. In the previous chapters we describe some of the major studies that have already been completed and published in the medical literature. Nevertheless, preliminary results have been published as abstracts or presented at major medical meetings; some of these trials are ongoing.

In this chapter we review some of these preliminary reports.

a. Acute Myocardial Infarction

AMIHOT

Acute Myocardial Infarction with Hyperoxemic Therapy

Title	Acute Myocardial Infarction with Hyperoxemic Therapy (AMIHOT): A Prospective, Randomized Multicenter Trial.
Authors	O'Neill WW, et al.
Reference	Presented at the American College of Cardiology 2004 meeting.
Disease	Acute myocardial infarction.
Purpose	To assess the effects of hyperoxemic therapy during primary stenting in patients with ST elevation acute myocardial infarction. This presentation concentrated on ST resolution.
Design	A phase I trial.
Patients	250 patients with ST elevation acute myocardial infarction eligible for primary angioplasty.
Follow-up	3 months.
Regimen	Randomization to primary angioplasty with stenting alone or angioplasty + stenting with hyperoxemic therapy (mixing 3 mL of aqueous oxygen with 70 mL/min of the patient's blood which was then infused through a catheter in the infarct artery in the region of stent implantation).
Results	Overall, there was no significant difference between the 2 groups in terms of ST-segment resolution. Among patients with anterior acute MI there was a trend toward better ST-segment resolution with hyperoxemic therapy compared with angioplasty alone (p=0.09). A subgroup of 68 patients having 3-month postintervention follow-up show approximately a 60% improvement in regional wall motion.
Concl.	Hyperoxemic therapy during primary angioplasty may improve outcome of patients with ST elevation acute MI.

CASTEMI

Caldaret in ST Elevation Myocardial Infarction

Title	Reduction of infarct size and improved left ventricular function with IV caldaret [MCC-135] in patients with ST elevation myocardial infarction undergoing primary PCI.
Authors	Tzivoni D, et al.
Reference	Presented at the American College of Cardiology 2004 meeting.
Disease	Acute myocardial infarction.
Purpose	To evaluate whether IV caldaret (an inhibitor of calcium overload through sodium calcium exchange inhibition and enhancement of uptake of calcium by the sarcoplasmic reticulum) can further reduce infarct size and improve left ventricular function in patients with ST-elevation myocardial infarction who undergo primary percutaneous coronary intervention.
Design	Randomized, double-blind, placebo-controlled, multicenter.
Patients	387 patients with ST-elevation acute myocardial infarction suitable for primary angioplasty.
Follow-up	Single-photon emission computed tomography (SPECT) at 7 days, clinical follow-up for 30 days.
Regimen	Randomization to: 1) placebo; 2) low-dose IV caldaret (57.5 mg); or 3) high-dose IV caldaret (172.5 mg) infusions initiated during coronary intervention and continued for 48 hours.

14a

Results	SPECT imaging at day 7 did not show a difference in infarct size among the 3 groups. Total mortality in the study was low (2.3%) and without differences among the 3 groups. Among patients with anterior MI and TIMI 0 or 1 flow, high-dose caldaret was associated with significant reductions in LV end-systolic volume and LV end-diastolic volume at day 7 and 30 vs placebo. Global LVEF was significantly greater at day 7 with high-dose caldaret vs placebo; however, the difference by day 30 was no longer statistically significant. High-dose caldaret was also associated with a significant reduction in all cardiac markers vs placebo. Caldaret was not associated with any hemodynamic, biochemical, or ECG abnormalities.
Concl.	IV caldaret is safe and may improve LV function in patients with anterior ST-elevation acute MI undergoing primary percutaneous interventions.

EMERALD

Enhanced Myocardial Efficacy and Removal by Aspiration of Liberated Debris

Title	Primary Angioplasty in Acute Myocardial Infarction With Distal Protection of the Microcirculation: Principal Results From the Prospective, Randomized EMERALD Trial.
Reference	Presented by Stone GW at the American College of Cardiology 2004 meeting.
Disease	Acute myocardial infarction.
Purpose	To compare outcome of primary coronary intervention with and without the use of distal protection device. The primary end points were ST segment resolution 30 minutes after the procedure measured with 24-hour continuous electrocardiogram monitoring, and infarct size assessed by technetium-99m-sestamibi single-photon emission computed tomography imaging at days 5-14.
Design	Randomized, open-label.
Patients	501 patients within 6 hours of onset of ST ($\geq$2 mm in $\geq$2 adjacent leads) elevation acute myocardial infarction.
Follow-up	ST resolution at 30 minutes. Sestamibi single-photon emission computed tomography at day 5 to 14. 30 days clinical follow-up.
Regimen	All patients underwent primary percutaneous coronary interventions. Patients were randomized to intervention with or without the use of GuardWire Plus distal protection device (Medtronic, Inc, Minneapolis, MN).

14a

Results	There was no difference in the percentage of patients achieving complete ST resolution between the distal protection group (60.6%) and the control group (62.2%). Infarct size (by sestamibi) was 17.1% in the distal protection group and 14.3% in the control group (p=0.09). Post-procedure TIMI 3 flow was achieved by 91.8% of the patients in the distal protection group vs 89.3% in the control group (p=0.36). The mean TIMI frame count postprocedure was 22.1 and 23.0, respectively (p=0.48). Postprocedure grade 3 myocardial blush was achieved in 60.1% of distal protection group vs in 52.7% of the control group (p=0.13). The percentages of patients achieving grade 1 or 2 myocardial blush were comparable between the groups. The GuardWire Plus system was successful in removing clot and atheromatous debris from 70% of arteries and the procedure was safe. MACE within the first 30 days occurred at a similar rate in both groups. 30-day mortality was 2.1% and 2.9%, respectively (p=0.77). Heart failure occurred in 2.1% and 0.4%, respectively (p=0.12), hypotension in 11.1% of the patients in each group, and readmission for heart failure in 0.8% and 0 of the patients, respectively (p=0.25).
Concl.	The use of GuardWire Plus distal protection device did not reduce infarct size or improve ST resolution in patients treated with primary percutaneous intervention for ST elevation acute MI.

EXPEDITION

The Sodium-Proton Exchange Inhibition to Prevent Coronary Events in Acute Cardiac Conditions

Title	Effects of Na^+/H^+ exchange inhibition by cariporide on death and nonfatal myocardial infarction in patients undergoing coronary artery bypass graft surgery: The EXPEDITION study.
Authors	Presented by Mentzer RM at the American Heart Association 2003 meeting.
Disease	Coronary artery disease, coronary artery bypass graft.
Purpose	To study the safety and efficacy of cariporide (a Na^+/H^+ exchange inhibitor) on mortality and infarction in patients undergoing coronary artery bypass graft.
Design	Randomized, double-blind, placebo-controlled, multicenter.
Patients	5770 patients scheduled for coronary artery bypass graft.
Follow-up	6 months.
Regimen	Randomization to placebo or cariporide (IV 180 mg/kg preoperatively, followed by 40 mg/h for 24 hours and then, 20 mg/h for an additional 24 hours.
Results	At day 5, death or MI occurred in 20.3% of the patients in the placebo group and in 16.6% in the cariporide group (relative risk reduction [RRR] 18.28%; p=0.00020). After 6 months, death or MI occurred in 23.9% in the placebo and in 20.2% of the patients in the cariporide group (RRR 15.72%; p=0.0005). However, 5-day mortality was higher in the cariporide group (2.2% vs 1.5%; RRR -53.50%; p=0.028). 6-month mortality was also higher in the cariporide group (6.4% vs 5.4%; RRR -18.17%; p=0.11). On the other hand, cariporide reduced the MI rate at both day 5 (14.4% vs 18.9%; RRR 23.81%; p=0.000005), and at 6 months (13.8% vs 18.5%; RRR 25.58%; p=0.0000001). Overall, cerebrovascular events occurred in 4.8% in the cariporide group and in 2.7% in the placebo group (p<0.001).
Concl.	Cariporide administered for 48 hours, starting before CABG reduced the rate of MI, but was associated with increased mortality and cerebrovascular events.

14. Preliminary Reports
b. Unstable Angina/ Non-Q-Wave Infarction/ Non-ST-Elevated Myocardial Infarction or Acute Coronary Syndrome

14. Preliminary Reports — b. Unstable Angina/Non-Q-Wave Infarction/
Non-ST-Elevated Myocardial Infarction or Acute Coronary Syndrome

1331

SYNERGY

Superior Yield of the New Strategy of Enoxaparin, Revascularization, and Glycoprotein IIb/IIIa Inhibitors

Title	The SYNERGY trial: study design and rationale.
Authors	Presented by Mahaffwy KW, Califf RM, and Ferguson JJ at the American College of Cardiology 2004 meeting.
Reference	Am Heart J 2002;143:952-960.
Disease	Coronary artery disease, percutaneous coronary intervention.
Purpose	To compare the safety and efficacy of enoxaparin and unfractionated heparin (UHF) in patients with non-ST-elevation acute coronary syndromes treated with an early invasive strategy.
Design	Randomized, open-label, multicenter.
Patients	10,027 patients ≥60 years, with non-ST-elevation acute coronary syndrome, with either electrocardiogram changes or abnormal cardiac markers were included. Pregnant patients and patients with allergy to pork or pork products, contraindications to heparin, recent or planned epidural anesthesia, percutaneous coronary intervention within the preceding 24 hours, thrombolytic therapy within the preceding 24 hours, ischemic stroke within the preceding year, history of hemorrhagic stroke, tumor or intracranial aneurysm, recent trauma or major surgery, and active bleeding were excluded. In addition, patients with international normalized ratio >1.5, bleeding disorder, thrombocytopenia, history of glycoprotein IIb/IIIa inhibitor-induced or heparin-induced thrombocytopenia, secondary angina, blood pressure >180 mm Hg despite therapy, anemia, valvular disease, congenital heart disease, hypertrophic restrictive or constrictive cardiomyopathy, and thyrotoxicosis were not included. Also, patients with severe liver disease, renal insufficiency, and contraindications to coronary angiography or percutaneous coronary intervention were not included.
Follow-up	30 days.

Regimen	Patients were randomized to IV infusion of UFH (60 U/kg bolus followed by 12 U/kg/h infusion) or to enoxaparin (1 mg/kg subcutaneous bid). Treatment was continued at least through angiography and percutaneous coronary intervention, or until the patient required no further anticoagulation therapy.
Add'l Tx	In the enoxaparin group, catheterization was performed at any time after the last dose. No additional enoxaparin was given if percutaneous coronary intervention was performed ≤8 hours since the last dose. An IV dose of 0.3 mg/kg was given when percutaneous coronary intervention was performed 8-12 hours after the last dose. Enoxaparin was discontinued 8 hours prior to elective coronary artery bypass graft and was stopped immediately before urgent coronary artery bypass graft. In the UFH group, UFH was continued during catheterization but UFH infusion was stopped prior to percutaneous coronary intervention and IV boluses were used instead to achieve an ACT of 250 seconds. UFH was discontinued at least 6 hours prior to elective coronary artery bypass graft and stopped immediately in cases of urgent coronary artery bypass graft. All patients received aspirin 162-325 mg/d. In case of allergy or contraindications to aspirin, clopidogrel was given. Glycoprotein IIb/IIIa inhibitors were encouraged for high-risk patients and during percutaneous coronary intervention. All other medications were permitted.
Results	After 30 days of follow-up, MI occurred in 12.7% of the UFH treated patients and in 11.7% of the enoxaparin group. 30-day mortality was 3.1% in the UFH group and 3.2% in the enoxaparin group. The combined end point of 30-day mortality or MI occurred in 14.5% and 14.0% of the patients, respectively. In-hospital cardiac events were similar in both treatment groups. Bleeding events were uncommon, but occurred more frequently in the enoxaparin patients. Thrombotic complications following PCIs occurred at comparable rates between the treatment groups.
Concl.	SC enoxaparin is a safe and effective alternative to UFH for the early invasive management of high-risk acute coronary syndrome patients. However, enoxaparin was not superior to UHF.

14b

14. Preliminary Reports — b. Unstable Angina/Non-Q-Wave Infarction/
Non-ST-Elevated Myocardial Infarction or Acute Coronary Syndrome

14. Preliminary Reports
c.   Interventional Cardiology

CREST

Cilostazol for Restenosis

Title	CREST (cilostazol for restenosis trial).
Authors	Presented by Douglas J, et al., at the American Heart Association 2003 meeting.
Reference	Clin Cardiol 2003;26:451-454.
Disease	Restenosis, coronary stenting.
Purpose	To assess the effect of cilostazol, a phosphodiesterase III inhibitor, to prevent restenosis following coronary stent implantation for de novo coronary artery lesions.
Design	Randomized, double-blind, placebo-controlled, multicenter.
Patients	705 patients, mean age 60 years, after successful stent implantation in native coronary artery lesions (50%-100% diameter stenosis, with stented segments <40 mm). Patients with acute myocardial infarction, bifurcation lesions, thrombus, and liver or renal insufficiency were excluded.
Follow-up	Repeat coronary angiography at 6 months. Clinical follow-up for 6 months.
Regimen	Randomization to cilostazol (100 mg bid, n=354) or placebo (n=351).
Add'l Tx	All patients received aspirin and clopidogrel.

Results	507 patients underwent follow-up angiography at 6 months. At 6-months, in-segment minimal lumen diameter (MLD) was 1.61 mm in the placebo group and 1.77 mm in the cilostazol group (p=0.006). Late loss (0.52 mm vs 0.70 mm; p=0.0035), in-stent MLD, in-stent late loss, and >50% diameter restenosis (20.9% vs 34.6%; p=0.0006) rates were significantly better in the cilostazol group. In-stent restenosis occurred in 20.1% of the patients in the cilostazol vs 31.4% in the control group (p=0.0038). Subgroup analysis revealed that cilostazol was effective in reducing the rate of restenosis in diabetic patients (16.9% vs 37.0%; p=0.0108), and in vessels <3 mm in diameter (21.9% vs 34.4%; p=0.0071). There was no difference in the rate of major adverse cardiac events (death, MI, target vessel revascularization, and stroke) between the groups. The rates of bleeding and readmission were comparable.
Concl.	Oral cilostazol decreased the rate of in-stent restenosis; however, it was not associated with better clinical outcomes.

14c

14. Preliminary Reports
d. Hypertension

AVALON

Atorvastatin Plus Amlodipine When Compared with Either Therapy Alone in the Treatment of Patients with Concomitant Dyslipidemia and Hypertension

Title	Atorvastatin plus amlodipine when compared with either therapy alone in the treatment of patients with concomitant dyslipidemia and hypertension.
Authors	Flack JM, Houston M, Neutel J, et al.
Reference	a. Flack JM, Houston M, Neutel J, et al. Rationale and design of the AVALON study (Atorvastatin plus amlodipine when compared with either therapy alone in the treatment of patients with concomitant dyslipidemia and hypertension) [poster]. Presented at: The 13th International Symposium on Atherosclerosis 2003; September 28 October 2; Kyoto, Japan.
	b. Flack J, Houston M, Neutel J, et al. Rationale and design of the AVALON study (Atorvastatin plus amlodipine when compared with either therapy alone in the treatment of patients with concomitant dyslipidemia and hypertension) [abstract]. Presented at: The 13th International Symposium on Atherosclerosis 2003; September 28 October 2; Kyoto, Japan.c. Flack J, Houston M, Neutel J, et al. Efficacy and safety of atorvastatin plus amlodipine versus either agent alone in patients with concomitant dyslipidemia and hypertension: The AVALON study [abstract]. Presented at: The 20th Scientific Meeting of the International Society of Hypertension 2004; February 15 19,2004; Sao Paulo SP, Brazil.
Disease	Hypertension, dyslipidemia.
Purpose	Avalon was designed to evaluate the efficacy and safety of amlodipine 5 mg and atorvastatin 10 mg administered together vs placebo or either agent alone in the treatment of coexisting hypertension and dyslipidemia in patients with varying degrees of risk for coronary heart disease.
Design	North American, multicenter, randomized, double-blind, placebo-controlled, 2 × 2 factorial design study.

Patients	Men and women 18-75 years of age were eligible to participate in the study if they were diagnosed with concurrent hypertension and dyslipidemia.
Follow-up	8-week double-blind treatment phase.
Regimen	Patients received qd doses of atorvastatin 10 mg with placebo, amlodipine 5 mg with placebo, atorvastatin 10 mg with amlodipine 5 mg, or placebo with placebo.
Results	The percentage of combination-treated patients who reached their National Cholesterol Education Program Adult Treatment Panel III LDL cholesterol goal at week 8 was significantly greater than that in the amlodipine-alone group. Similarly, significantly more combination- than atorvastatin-treated patients reached their Joint National Committee on Prevention, Detection, Evaluation, and Treatment of High Blood Pressure (JNC) VI BP goal. Almost half (45.5%) of patients receiving atorvastatin 10 mg + amlodipine 5 mg reached both their LDL cholesterol and BP goals. The number of patients in the active treatment arms reporting 1 or more adverse events was comparable to placebo (combination 50.2%, atorvastatin 52.0%, amlodipine 50.7%, placebo 52.3%). The percentage of patients discontinuing was slightly higher in the placebo group (9.6%) than the active treatment groups (combination 7.7%, atorvastatin 7.5%, and amlodipine 7.0%).
Concl.	These data demonstrate that atorvastatin 10 mg and amlodipine 5 mg administered in combination is an effective and well-tolerated treatment for coexisting hypertension and dyslipidemia, which helps patients achieve their goals for both conditions, compared with placebo.

14d

GEMINI

Glycemic Effects in Diabetes Mellitus: Metroprolol Comparison in Hypertension

Title	Amlodipine/atorvastatin single pill dual therapy improves goal attainment in the treatment of concomitant hypertension and dyslipidemia: the Gemini study.
Authors	Blank R, LaSalle J, Reeves R, et al.
Reference	a. Blank R, LaSalle J, Reeves R, et al. Amlodipine/atorvastatin single pill dual therapy improves goal attainment in the treatment of concomitant hypertension and dyslipidemia: The Gemini Study [poster]. Presented at: the American College of Cardiology Scientific Sessions 2004; March 7, 2004; New Orleans, LA. b. Blank R, LaSalle J, Reeves R, et al. Amlodipine/atorvastatin single pill dual therapy improves goal attainment in the treatment of concomitant hypertension and dyslipidemia: The Gemini Study [abstract]. J Am Coll Cardiol 2004;43(suppl A):447A.
Disease	Hypertension, dyslipidemia.
Purpose	To evaluate the efficacy, safety, and clinical utility of single-pill amlodipine/atorvastatin therapy, administered as initial, add-on (to existing non-calcium channel blocker antihypertensive), substitution (for amlodipine or atorvastatin), or switch (from other calcium channel blocker and/or lipid-lowering therapies) therapy in the treatment of concomitant hypertension and dyslipidemia.
Design	14-week, open label, non-comparative, multicenter trial.

Patients	Men and women 18-80 years of age were eligible to participate in the study if they were diagnosed with concurrent hypertension and dyslipidemia. The patient's blood pressure had to be uncontrolled (with or without treatment) based on Joint National Committee on Prevention, Detection, Evaluation, and Treatment of High Blood Pressure (JNC VI) guidelines and low-density lipoprotein cholesterol could be controlled (with medication) or uncontrolled (with or without medication) based on National Cholesterol Education Program Adult Treatment Panel (NCEP ATP) III guidelines. Eligible participants were assigned to 1 of 3 cardiovascular risk categories (Group I: hypertension and dyslipidemia with no additional cardiovascular risk factors; Group II: hypertension and dyslipidemia with >1 additional cardiovascular risk factor; Group III: hypertension and dyslipidemia with coronary heart disease or coronary heart disease risk equivalent), based on criteria outlined in the JNC VI and the NCEP ATP III guidelines.
Follow-up	14 weeks.
Regimen	8 dosage strengths of single-pill amlodipine/atorvastatin therapy (5/10 mg, 10/10 mg, 5/20 mg, 10/20 mg, 5/40 mg, 10/40 mg, 5/80 mg, and 10/80 mg) were used in addition to lifestyle modification. The initial amlodipine/atorvastatin dosage was based on each patient's current level of blood pressure and low-density lipoprotein control and their use of blood pressure and/or lipid-lowering medications at screening. Dose adjustment was determined by the individual physician to titrate their patients to blood pressure and lipid goals based on published JNC VI and NCEP ATP III guidelines. The amlodipine component Caduet (Pfizer, New York, NY) was either initial antihypertensive therapy, substitution therapy for patients already receiving amlodipine, switch therapy for patients on other calcium channel blockers, or add-on therapy to other non-calcium channel blocker antihypertensive regimens. Similarly, the atorvastatin component of the combination tablet was either initial therapy for dyslipidemia, substitution therapy for patients already receiving atorvastatin, or switch therapy for patients on lipid lowering agents, including statins; however, the atorvastatin component was not add-on therapy or used with other lipid lowering agents.

14d

Add'l Tx	There was no wash-out of existing antihypertensive and lipid-lowering medications. For patients receiving antihypertensive and/or lipid-lowering therapy, doses of medication must have been stable for at least 6 weeks.
Results	In total, 1220 patients received treatment and 1095 (89.8%) patients completed the study. The age of participants was 60.9±10.9 years. At baseline, mean (± SD) SBP/DBP was 146.6±11.0/87.9±8.6 mm Hg and mean LDL cholesterol concentration was 152.9±33.4 mg/dL. The mean dose of Caduet administered at the end of the study period was 7.08/26.18 mg. At end point, 57.7% of patients reached both their BP and LDL cholesterol therapeutic goals. In the ITT study population, similar percentages of patients in CV risk Groups I and II attained both their BP and LDL-C goals (77.2% and 76.1%, respectively). A smaller percentage of patients in Group III (37.2%) reached both of their targets compared with Groups I and II.
Concl.	Treating hypertension and dyslipidemia with a single pill that combines amlodipine and atorvastatin offers an effective and well-tolerated approach to get patients to their BP and LDL cholesterol goals.

Respond

Title	The efficacy and safety of fixed-dose combinations of amlodipine and atorvastatin in the treatment of patients with concomitant hypertension and dyslipidemia.
Authors	Preston RA, Harvey P, Herfert O, et al.
Reference	a. Presented at the American Society of Hypertension Meeting, May 18-22, 2004, New York, NY. b. Am J Heart 2004;17:185A.
Disease	Hypertension, dyslipidemia.
Purpose	To compare the safety and efficacy of fixed doses of amlodipine + atorvastatin to amlodipine monotherapy, atorvastatin monotherapy, and placebo in 1660 patients with concurrent hypertension and dyslipidemia.
Design	Prospective, randomized, double-blind, double-dummy, placebo-controlled, multicenter, 3×5 factorial study.
Patients	1660 patients aged 18-75 years. Patients had both hypertension and dyslipidemia.
Follow-up	8-week double-blind treatment phase.
Regimen	Patients were treated for 8 weeks with amlodipine (5 or 10 mg), atorvastatin (10, 20, 40, or 80 mg), 8 combinations of these amlodipine/atorvastatin doses, or placebo.

14d

Results	Baseline LDL cholesterol was 182 mg/dL and mean SBP was 148 mm Hg. The 8 amlodipine/atorvastatin dose combinations decreased LDL cholesterol by 37%-49% greater than placebo (p<0.001). Of interest, amlodipine 5 mg/atorvastatin 10 mg decreased LDL cholesterol significantly more than 10 mg of atorvastatin alone (39% vs 34%; p<0.01). However, neither the 5 nor 10 mg dose of amlodipine affected LDL cholesterol when given in combination with other doses of atorvastatin. All 8 amlodipine/atorvastatin combinations decreased SBP (13-18 mm Hg) more than placebo (p<0.001). Atorvastatin added to amlodipine did not affect amlodipine's BP-lowering efficacy. A total of 83 (5.0%) patients discontinued drug due to adverse events. The majority of adverse events were mild to moderate and not associated with discontinuation. Peripheral edema (7.3%), headache (6.2%), and increased γ-glutamyl transferase (1.6%) were the most common treatment-emergent events. Myalgia occurred in only 1.6% of patients.
Concl.	Coadministration of amlodipine and atorvastatin is efficacious at reducing SBP and LDL cholesterol levels and safe when administered to patients with concomitant hypertension and dyslipidemia. Specifically, all 8 amlodipine + atorvastatin treatment groups demonstrated significant, dose-related reductions in LDL cholesterol, SBP, and DBP compared to placebo (all p<0.001), with no modification of effect of either component on LDL cholesterol, SBP, and DBP. Patients treated with amlodipine + atorvastatin did not experience any increase in adverse events compared with either amlodipine or atorvastatin monotherapy.

14. Preliminary Reports
e. Congestive Heart Failure

SCD-HeFT

Sudden Cardiac Death in Heart Failure Trial

Title	Sudden Cardiac Death in Heart Failure Trial (SCD-HeFT)
Authors	Brady G, et al.
Reference	Presented at the American College of Cardiology 2004 meeting.
Disease	Congestive heart failure, arrhythmia.
Purpose	To assess the effects of amiodarone and programmed shock-only implantable cardioverter-defibrillator on mortality in patients with left ventricular ejection fraction ≤35% and congestive heart failure (New York Heart Association Class II-III).
Design	Randomized, open-label, multicenter.
Patients	2521 patients with left ventricular ejection fraction ≤35% and congestive heart failure (New York Heart Association class II-III). Median age was 60.1 years. The etiology of congestive heart failure was ischemic in 48% of the patients and nonischemic in 52% of the patients.
Follow-up	A median follow-up of 45.5 months.
Regimen	Randomization to: 1) implantable cardioverter-defibrillator implantation; 2) amiodarone (800 mg/d for 1 week, followed by up to 400 mg/d for 2-4 weeks, and then a weight-adjusted dose); or 3) placebo.
Add'l Tx	All patients were receiving optimal heart failure medical therapy. The use of angiotensin-converting enzyme inhibitors and/or angiotensin receptor blockers and β-blockers was encouraged.

Results	The mortality rate in the placebo group was 36.1% (7.2% per year). The mortality rate in the implantable-cardioverter defibrillator group was 28.9% (hazard ratio [HR] vs placebo 0.77; 97.5% CI=0.60-0.96; p=0.007). The mortality in the amiodarone group was comparable to the placebo group (HR vs placebo 1.06; 97.5% CI=0.86-1.30; p=0.529). However, among patients with NYHA class III there was a 44% increase in mortality with amiodarone as compared with placebo (HR 1.44; 97.5% CI=1.05-1.97).
Concl.	Routine implantable-cardioverter defibrillator implantation in patients with CHF (NYHA class II-III) and LVEF ≤35% reduced mortality risk, whereas amiodarone treatment was associated with increased risk of death, especially in patients with more severe (NYHA class III) CHF.

14e

WATCH

Warfarin and Antiplatelet Therapy in Heart Failure Trial

Title	Final Results of the Warfarin and Antiplatelet Trial in Chronic Heart Failure (WATCH): A Randomized Comparison of Warfarin, Aspirin, and Clopidogrel.
Authors	Presented by Massie BM at the American College of Cardiology 2004 meeting.
Reference	J Card Fail 2004 10:101-112.
Disease	Congestive heart failure.
Purpose	To compare outcome of patients with congestive heart failure and sinus rhythm treated with aspirin, clopidogrel and warfarin.
Design	Randomized, multicenter.
Patients	Symptomatic heart failure patients in sinus rhythm with ejection fractions ≤35%, treated with angiotensin-converting enzyme inhibitors, if tolerated, and diuretics. The trial was designed to enroll 4500 patients; it was terminated 18 months prematurely in June 2003 by the VA Cooperative Study Program because of poor enrollment. A total of 1587 patients were enrolled.
Follow-up	2-5 years.
Regimen	Randomization to: 1) open-label warfarin (target international normalized ratio 2.5-3.0); 2) double-blind antiplatelet therapy with aspirin 162 mg/d; or 3) double-blind antiplatelet with clopidogrel 75 mg/d.

Results	The primary combined end point of death, nonfatal MI, or stroke occurred at similar rates in the 3 treatment groups. The OR for warfarin vs aspirin was 0.99 and that for clopidogrel vs aspirin was 1.10. The combined end point of death, nonfatal MI, stroke, hospitalization for CHF, embolism, and unstable angina occurred less frequently with warfarin than with aspirin (OR 0.94). The OR for clopidogrel vs aspirin was 1.03. In the warfarin group there was a 27% reduction in the end point of hospitalization for worsening CHF compared to the aspirin group (p=0.01). There was no significant difference between the clopidogrel and aspirin groups in hospitalization for worsening CHF. The reduction in CHF hospitalization seen with warfarin treatment represents a 31% reduction compared to the aspirin use per 100 patient-years. In the clopidogrel group there was a trend toward less CHF hospitalizations; however, the difference did not reach statistical significance.
Concl.	There were no significant differences in mortality or MI and stroke rates between warfarin, aspirin, and clopidogrel in patients with chronic heart failure with sinus rhythm; however, warfarin was associated with reduced rate of hospitalization for heart failure exacerbation compared to aspirin and to clopidogrel.

14e

14. Preliminary Reports
f. Lipid-Lowering Studies

ALLIANCE

Aggressive Lipid-Lowering Initiation Abates New Cardiac Events

Title	Comparison of clinical outcomes in managed care patients with coronary heart disease treated in aggressive lipid lowering programs using atorvastatin vs usual care.
Authors	Koren M, Hunninghake D, on behalf of the ALLIANCE investigators.
Reference	Program and abstracts from the American College of Cardiology, 53rd Annual Scientific Session, March 7-10, 2004, New Orleans. Late Breaking Clinical Trials I.
Disease	Coronary artery disease.
Purpose	To test the hypothesis that aggressive treatment of low-density lipoprotein cholesterol to levels beyond currently recommended ones can provide incremental benefit in terms of reducing the incidence of major coronary events in patients with coronary artery disease.
Design	Ongoing 4-year, population-based, randomized, open-label study.
Patients	2441 adults, aged 18-75 years, with coronary artery disease. Low-density lipoprotein cholesterol had to be ≥130 but ≤250 mg/dL without lipid-lowering medication or ≥110 but ≤200 mg/dL with medication.
Follow-up	Mean 52 months.
Regimen	Atorvastatin (mean 40.5 mg/d) or usual care as prescribed by primary care physician.

Results	LDL cholesterol fell from a mean of 147 mg/dL in both groups to 95 mg/dL in the atorvastatin group (p<0.0001) and 111 mg/dL in the usual-care group. 72% of the atorvastatin group achieved their LDL cholesterol goal (<100 mg/dL). Total and HDL cholesterol and triglyceride levels improved significantly more with atorvastatin vs usual care. The primary end point (cardiac death, nonfatal MI, resuscitated cardiac arrest, revascularization, or unstable angina requiring hospitalization) was 17% lower in the atorvastatin group compared with the usual care group (p=0.026). Patients receiving atorvastatin also had 47% fewer nonfatal MIs than usual care (p<0.0002). NS reductions were also seen in the atorvastatin group for the other individual variables of the primary composite end point: cardiac death, cardiac revascularization, unstable angina requiring hospitalization, and resuscitated cardiac arrest. The rate of serious adverse events was similar in the atorvastatin and usual-care groups (40% vs 42%). Among the atorvastatin patients, aspartate aminotransferase and alanine aminotransferase levels >3× upper level of normal occurred in 8 (0.7%) and 16 (1.3%) patients, respectively. No cases of rhabdomyolysis or myopathy were recorded.
Concl.	Aggressive lipid-lowering to levels below those recommended by the National Cholesterol Education Program provide additional benefits over usual care.

14f

CARDS

The Collaborative Atorvastatin Diabetes Study

Title	The Collaborative Atorvastatin Diabetes Study.
Authors	CARDS Investigators.
Reference	Preliminary Results Presented in June 2004, American Diabetes Association Meeting, Orlando, FL.
Disease	Diabetes, hypercholesterolemia.
Purpose	To determine whether 10 mg atorvastatin vs placebo decreases incidence of major coronary events or revascularization in patients with type 2 diabetes without known coronary artery disease (Primary Prevention Trial).
Design	Multicenter, randomized, double-blind, placebo-controlled trial.
Patients	2838 patients with type 2 diabetes and no previous history of myocardial infarct or known coronary heart disease. Men and women ages 40-75 years were eligible. Patients had to have at least 1 other coronary heart disease risk factor (smoking, hypertension, retinopathy, microalbuminuria or macroalbuminuria) plus LDL-C ≤160 mg/dL and triglycerides ≤600 mg/dL.
Follow-up	Initially planned for 4 years, but study stopped early due to significant benefit in atorvastatin group.
Regimen	After 6-week placebo baseline period, patients randomized to placebo vs atorvastatin 10 mg qd.

Results	Primary end point is time from randomization to occurrence of a major cardiovascular event (ie, cardiovascular-related death, nonfatal MI, stroke, resuscitated cardiac arrest, coronary revascularization procedure). Randomization was completed in 2001 and study was stopped in May 2003. Atorvastatin reduced major cardiovascular events by 37% (p=0.001) and decreased strokes by 48%. Atorvastatin reduced acute coronary events by 36% and coronary revascularization by 31%. There was a trend for atorvastatin to reduce all-cause mortality by 27% (p=0.059). Benefits of atorvastatin occurred regardless of baseline lipids, gender, or age. Of note, baseline LDL in this study was only 118-119 mg/dL. Atorvastatin reduced LDL cholesterol by 40%.
Concl.	Atorvastatin 10 mg prevented cardiac events in type 2 diabetes patients who previously did not have a history of CAD.

EASE

Ezetimibe Add-on to Statin for Effectiveness

Title	Ezetimibe Added to Statin Therapy Reduces LDL-C and Improves Goal Attainment in Patients with Hypercholesterolemia
Authors	Pearson TA, et al.
Reference	Presented at the American College of Cardiology 2004 meeting.
Disease	Hyperlipidemia.
Purpose	To assess the safety and efficacy of ezetimibe 10 mg/d, compared with placebo, added to standard statin therapy in patients who were not at their National Cholesterol Education Program Adult Treatment Panel III low-density lipoprotein cholesterol goal despite statin monotherapy.
Design	Randomized, double-blind, placebo-controlled, multicenter.
Patients	3030 patients with hypercholesterolemia who did not reach their National Cholesterol Education Program Adult Treatment Panel III low-density lipoprotein cholesterol goal with a stable dose of any statin.
Follow-up	6 weeks.
Regimen	Randomization in a 2:1 ratio to either ongoing statin + ezetimibe 10 mg/d (n=2020) or ongoing statin + placebo (n=1010).

Results	Overall, LDL cholesterol was reduced by 25.8% in the ezetimibe group, compared to only 2.7% in the placebo group (p<0.001). The difference between the ezetimibe and placebo treatment groups was consistent and significant in all National Cholesterol Education Program (NCEP) coronary heart disease (CHD) risk categories. In the overall study population and in each NCEP Adult Treatment Panel (ATP) III risk category, the percentage of patients who reached their LDL cholesterol goal was significantly greater in the ezetimibe group than in the placebo group (71.0% vs 20.6%; p<0.001). 69.5% of patients with CHD or CHD risk equivalents who were assigned ezetimibe achieved their LDL cholesterol goal compared with only 17.3% of placebo group (p<0.001). Among patients with multiple risk factors, 75.1% vs 32.2% in the ezetimibe and placebo group, respectively, achieved their LDL cholesterol goal (p<0.001), and among those with <2 risk factors, 90.7% vs 52.4%, respectively, reached their LDL cholesterol goal. Ezetimibe was more effective than placebo in increasing HDL cholesterol (+1.3% vs -0.8%, respectively; p<0.0001) and reducing triglycerides (12.8% vs 1.6%; p<0.001), non-HDL cholesterol, and apolipoprotein B (p<0.001 for all between-treatment differences). Subgroup analyses showed that ezetimibe was effective across all ages, in both men and women, and in all ethnicities. Ezetimibe was effective in patients with and without diabetes mellitus and in patients with and without metabolic syndrome. Ezetimibe was effective in reducing LDL cholesterol when added to all brands of statins and at all doses used. Elevations in liver enzyme (aspartate aminotransferase or alanine aminotransferase) >3 × the upper limit of normal occurred in 0.1% to 0.4% of the patients and without a difference between the groups. No patient in either group had an elevation in creatine kinase >10 × the upper limit of normal, with or without muscle symptoms.
Concl.	Ezetimibe added to a stable dose of statin significantly reduced LDL cholesterol from baseline, significantly improved NCEP ATP III LDL cholesterol goal achieved, significantly improved triglycerides, HDL cholesterol, non-HDL cholesterol, apolipoprotein B levels, and showed consistent efficacy across subgroups defined by age, sex, race, NCEP ATP III risk category, diabetes, metabolic syndrome, and brands of statin and dose.

14f

TNT

The Treating to New Targets Study

Title	Treating to New Targets (TNT) study: does lowering low-density lipoprotein cholesterol levels below currently recommended guidelines yield incremental clinical benefit?
Authors	Waters DD, Guyton JR, Herrington DM, et al.
Reference	Am J Cardiol 2004;93:154-158.
Disease	Hypercholesterolemia, coronary artery disease.
Purpose	To determine whether reducing low-density lipoprotein cholesterol aggressively to about 75 mg/dL will provide a greater reduction in coronary heart disease events than lowering low-density lipoprotein cholesterol more moderately to 100 mg/dL in patients with known coronary artery disease (a secondary prevention study).
Design	Multicenter, randomized, double-blind, parallel-group trial.
Patients	10,000 patients with known coronary heart disease. Includes men and women aged 35-75 years with low-density lipoprotein cholesterol of 130-250 mg following drug wash-out/ dietary therapy.
Follow-up	≈5 years.
Regimen	All patients begin with open label atorvastatin 10 mg/d. Patients who achieved a low-density lipoprotein cholesterol <130 mg/dL are randomized (≈10,000 patients) to 5 years of atorvastatin 10 mg/d with estimated mean low-density lipoprotein cholesterol target of 100 mg/dL vs atorvastatin 80 mg/d with estimated mean low-density lipoprotein cholesterol of 75 mg/dL.

Results	Primary end point is occurrence of a major coronary event (ie, coronary heart disease death or nonfatal MI, resuscitated cardiac arrest, fatal or nonfatal stroke). Secondary end points are the occurrence of other cardiovascular/coronary events, cerebro-vascular events, peripheral arterial disease, hospitalization with the primary diagnosis of CHF, and all-cause mortality. Results should be available in 2004 or 2005.
Concl.	When finalized, this important lipid-lowering trial should answer the question of how low-LDL cholesterol should be reduced in patients with CAD.

14f

14. Preliminary Reports
g. Arrhythmia

DINAMIT

Defibrillator in Acute Myocardial Infarction Trial

Title	Randomized trial of prophylactic implantable defibrillator therapy vs optimal medical treatment early after myocardial infarction: defibrillator in acute myocardial infarction trial (DINAMIT).
Authors	Presented by Hohnloser S at the American College of Cardiology 2004 meeting.
Reference	Card Electrophysiol Rev 2003;7:447-451.
Disease	Acute myocardial infarction, arrhythmia.
Purpose	To evaluate the impact of an implantable cardioverter-defibrillator early therapy after acute myocardial infarction.
Design	Randomized, open label, multicenter.
Patients	674 patients with recent (6-40 days before enrollment) myocardial infarction, a left ventricular ejection fraction ≤35%, and a depressed heart rate variability (in 24-hour Holter monitoring). Patients who had undergone extensive coronary revascularization (coronary artery bypass graft surgery or three-vessel percutaneous coronary intervention) were excluded from the study.
Follow-up	Mean 2.5 years (range: 15-48 months).
Regimen	Randomization to implantable cardioverter-defibrillator (n=332) or control (n=342).
Add'l Tx	The use of angiotensin-converting enzyme inhibitors, β-blockers and statins was encouraged in both groups.

Results	The cumulative risk of all-cause mortality was comparable between the implantable cardio-defibrillator (ICD) (7.5%) and the control group (6.9%; hazard ratio [HR] 1.08; p=0.66). The cumulative risk of arrhythmic death was reduced significantly by 58% in the ICD recipients (1.5% vs 3.5%; HR 0.42; p=0.009). However, there was a 75% greater risk of nonarrhythmic death in the ICD group (6.1% vs 3.5%; HR 1.75; p=0.016). Death due to cardiovascular disease accounted for the majority of nonarrhythmic deaths.
Concl.	ICD therapy did not reduce all-cause mortality in patients with depressed LV systolic function combined with autonomic dysfunction early after MI. The reduction in arrhythmic death with an ICD in these patients was offset by an increase in nonarrhythmic death.

14g

PAD

Public Access Defibrillation

Title	The Public Access Defibrillation (PAD) Trial.
Authors	Ornato JP.
Reference	Presented at the American Heart Association 2003 meeting, Orlando, FL.
Disease	Arrhythmia, cardiac arrest.
Purpose	To study whether the use of automated external defibrillators by laypersons trained to perform cardiopulmonary resuscitation could increase survival after out of hospital cardiac arrest, as compared to cardiopulmonary resuscitation without automated external defibrillators.
Design	Randomized, open-label, community-based, multicenter.
Patients	Patients, ≥8 years old, with confirmed, treatable out of hospital cardiac arrest.
Follow-up	Survival to hospital discharge.
Regimen	993 community units were randomized to training volunteer laypersons to perform cardiopulmonary resuscitation alone (497 sites) or cardiopulmonary resuscitation with defibrillation using automated external defibrillators (496 sites). The course lasted 2-4 hours.

Results	A total of 19,762 volunteers underwent training. In cardio-pulmonary resuscitation (CPR)-only units there were 1593 reported events. In the CPR + automated external defibrillator (AED) units there were 1819 events. In the CPR-only units 15 patients survived to hospital discharge (0.94%). In the CPR + AED units there were 29 patients who were discharged alive from the hospital (1.59%; p=0.042). Adverse events occurred at similar rates in the CPR alone (0.2%) and CPR + AED (0.3%) groups. There were no inappropriate delivered shocks in the CPR + AED group. The success rate of resuscitation in residential units was very low in both the CPR alone (1 patient) and CPR + AED (1 patient) groups. However, in public units there was a significant higher rate of survival with CPR + AED than with CPR alone. Overall, there were more survivors with CPR + AED than with CPR alone (29 vs 15; p=0.042).
Concl.	Adding AED to CPR performed by trained volunteers doubled the survival rates of patients with cardiac arrest in public locations. In contrast, the survival rate of patients with out-of-hospital cardiac arrest at residential locations is low and adding AED to CPR did not improve survival. Trained laypersons can safely use AEDs to provide early defibrillation for out of hospital cardiac arrest.

PAPABEAR

Prophylactic Amiodarone for the Prevention of Arrhythmias That Begin Early After Revascularization, Valvular Repair, or Replacement

Title	Prophylactic amiodarone for the prevention of arrhythmias that begin early after revascularization, valvular repair, or replacement (PAPABEAR): Preliminary results.
Authors	Mitchell LB, Exner DV, Wyse DG, et al.
Reference	Presented at the American Heart Association 2003 meeting, Orlando, FL.
Disease	Arrhythmia, cardiac surgery.
Purpose	To assess the safety and efficacy of amiodarone for prevention of atrial fibrillation after cardiac surgery.
Design	Randomized, placebo-controlled, multicenter.
Patients	601 patients scheduled to undergo cardiac surgery.
Follow-up	6 days after surgery.
Regimen	Randomization to oral placebo or amiodarone (10 mg/kg/d) for 6 days prior to surgery, the day of surgery and for 6 days following surgery.

Results	The primary outcome of atrial fibrillation for >5 minutes that prompted therapy in the postoperative period occurred less frequently in the amiodarone group (16.1%) than in the placebo group (29.6%; hazard ratio (HR) 0.48; 95% CI=0.34-0.69; p<0.001). Amiodarone reduced the rate of the primary end point in patients younger than 65 years (11.2% vs 21.2%; p=0.02), older than 65 years (21.7% vs 41.2%; p=0.001), undergoing CABG alone (10.9% vs 23.3%; p=0.002), undergoing valvular surgery and CABG (24.5% vs 41.7%; p=0.0060, those who received β-blockers (15.3% vs 25.1%; p=0.03), and those who did not receive β-blockers (16.3% vs 35.8%; p=0.001). During atrial fibrillation episodes, the ventricular rate was slower in the amiodarone group (105±24 vs 131±25 bpm; p<0.001). Withdrawal from the study drug due to adverse effects occurred in 11.4% of the patients in the amiodarone group vs only 5.3% in the placebo group (p=0.02). Postoperative complications occurred in 9.4% of the patients in the amiodarone group vs 11.3% in the placebo group (p=NS). In-hospital mortality was comparable (2.3% vs 3.3%, respectively; p=NS). Postsurgical hospital stay tended to be shorter in the amiodarone group (8.2±7.4 vs 8.9±8.1 days; p=0.11).
Concl.	Amiodarone, started 6 days prior to surgery, was safe and reduced the rate of atrial fibrillation postoperatively in a wide range of patients undergoing elective cardiac surgery.

14g

14. Preliminary Reports
h. Coronary Artery Disease, Atherosclerosis, Prevention of Progression

CAMELOT

Comparison of Amlodipine vs Enalapril to Limit Occurrences of Thrombosis

NORMALISE

Norvasc for Regression of Manifest Atherosclerotic Lesions by Intravascular Sonographic Evaluation

Disease	Coronary artery disease.
Purpose	To evaluate the effectiveness of amlodipine vs. enalapril or placebo in preventing clinical events in a population of patients with known coronary artery disease. To determine the correlation between blood pressure and the incidence of clinical events in a population of patients with known coronary artery disease.
Design	Multicenter, randomized, double-blind, placebo-controlled trial. This includes a substudy entitled Norvasc for Regression of Manifest Atherosclerotic Lesions by Intravascular Sonographic Evaluation (NORMALISE).
Patients	3000 patients. 2,250 randomized patients without intravascular ultrasound; 750 randomized patients with intravascular ultrasound. Patients will be male or female, 30-75 years, in whom coronary angiography is clinically indicated. There must be at least one segment of a native coronary artery that has >20% decrease in lumen diameter by angiography. Patients must have stable coronary artery disease.
Follow-up	24 months.

Regimen	Patients will be randomized to amlodipine 5-10 mg, enalapril 10-20 mg, or placebo daily. Patients will be followed over 24 months for the occurrence of cardiovascular events. Primary end points will be the combined incidence of major adverse cardiovascular events that occur in patients treated with amlodipine vs enalapril vs placebo. The major adverse cardiovascular events include: cardiovascular death, nonfatal MI, resuscitated cardiac arrest, need for coronary revascularization, hospitalization for angina pectoris, hospitalization for CHF, stroke or transient ischemic attacks, new diagnosis of peripheral vascular disease or admission for a procedure to treat peripheral vascular disease. Secondary end points: death from any cause, the influence of amlodipine on requirements for revascularization in vessels that have undergone stent placement. The primary end point for the NORMALISE substudy is the percent change (end of treatment minus baseline) in total plaque area for all slices of anatomically comparable segments of the target coronary artery.
Results	The study is ongoing at this point; results not yet available.

PERSUADE

Perindopril Substudy in Coronary Artery Disease and Diabetes

Title	Cardiovascular morbidity and mortality in patients with diabetes in the EUROPA study: results from the PERSUADE substudy.
Authors	Fox KM.
Reference	Presented at the American College of Cardiology 2004 meeting.
Disease	Coronary artery disease, diabetes mellitus.
Purpose	A substudy of EUROPA that assessed the effect of perindopril 8 mg/d, added to standard therapy on cardiovascular morbidity and mortality in patients with coronary artery disease and diabetes mellitus and without heart failure.
Design	Randomized, double-blind, placebo-control, multicenter.
Patients	1502 patients with coronary artery disease and diabetes mellitus and without heart failure. Mean age was 62.9 years.
Follow-up	Mean 4 years.
Regimen	Randomization to placebo or perindopril 8 mg/d.
Results	Perindopril reduced the primary end point (cardiovascular mortality, nonfatal MI, and cardiac arrest) (relative risk reduction of 19%). Perindopril was associated with relative risk reduction of 23% in fatal and nonfatal MI, and a relative risk reduction of 46% in developing heart failure. These reductions in risk with perindopril were similar to those observed in the overall EUROPA study population. The beneficial effect of perindopril on clinical outcomes was apparent irrespective of baseline BP or the degree of reduction in BP. The number needed to treat to prevent one cardiovascular death or MI in the PERSUADE population is 27 patients over 4 years.
Concl.	Perindopril reduced cardiovascular morbidity and mortality when given to diabetic patients with established CAD.

PREVEND IT

Prevention of Renal and Vascular Endstage Disease Intervention Trial

Title	Effects of fosinopril and pravastatin on cardiovascular events in microalbuminuric subjects without hypertension and hypercholesterolemia: a single-center, double blind, randomized, placebo-controlled trial with 2 × 2 factorial design (PREVEND IT).
Authors	Presented by Asselbergs FW, et al., at the American Heart Association 2003 meeting.
Reference	Diercks GFH, Janseen WMT, van Boven AJ, et al. Rationale, design, and baseline characteristics of a trial of prevention of cardiovascular and renal disease with fosinopril and pravastatin in nonhypertensive, nonhypercholesterolemic subjects with microalbumunuria (the Prevention of REnal and Vascular ENdstage Disease Intervention Trial (PREVEND IT). Am J Cardiol 2000;86:635-638.
Disease	Microalbuminuria, cardiovascular disease.
Purpose	To assess whether fosinopril, an angiotensin-converting enzyme inhibitor, and pravastatin will reduce cardiovascular and renal morbidity in patients with microalbuminuria and without hypercholesterolemia or hypertension.
Design	A substudy of the PREVEND study. Randomized, single-center, placebo controlled, 2 × 2 factorial.
Patients	864 patients, 28-75 years old, with persistent microalbuminuria, and without hypertension (<160/100 mm Hg) and hypercholesterolemia (total cholesterol <8.0 mmol/L or <5.0 mmol/L in case of previous myocardial infarction). Patients receiving antihypertensive or lipid-lowering medications were excluded. Patients with creatinine clearance <60% of normal age-adjusted values, hyperkalemia, chronic liver disease, elevated liver enzymes, use of angiotensin-converting enzyme inhibitors or angiotensin receptor blockers, use of insulin, intolerance to the study drugs, and pregnant or lactating women were not included.
Follow-up	Mean 46 months.

Regimen	Randomized to fosinopril 20 mg/d or placebo and to pravastatin 40 mg/d or placebo.
Results	854 patients were eligible for analysis. Urinary albumin excretion was reduced by 23% with fosinopril (p<0.001). Pravastatin did not affect urinary albumin excretion. Fosinopril reduced the incidence of the primary end point (cardiovascular mortality, admission for cardiovascular morbidity, and end stage renal disease) by 44% (hazard ratio [HR] 0.56; 95% CI=0.30-1.04; p=0.07; covariate adjusted HR 0.53; 95% CI=0.28-0.995; p=0.048). Pravastatin reduced the incidence of the primary end point by 25% (HR 0.75; 95% CI=0.41-1.38; p=0.35).
Concl.	Fosinopril decreased urinary albumin secretion in patients with microalbuminuria without hypertension or hypercholesterolemia. Fosinopril was associated with a trend toward reduced rates of cardiovascular events, however, the effect of pravastatin did not reach statistical significance.

Trials Index

Trials are listed alphabetically by recognized acronym followed by those trials not having recognized acronyms.

IDX

B

C

D

IDX

E

IDX

Index   1385

F

G

H

IDX

I

J

K

L

M

IDX

N

IDX

Q

IDX

R

S

IDX

T

IDX

U

V

W

X

IDX

About the Editors

ROBERT A. KLONER, MD, PhD

Robert A. Kloner, MD, PhD, is a professor of medicine in the Cardiovascular Division, Keck School of Medicine, University of Southern California, Los Angeles, CA. He is also director of research at the Heart Institute of Good Samaritan Hospital in Los Angeles, CA, and an attending cardiologist at Los Angeles County/University of Southern California Medical Center.

Dr. Kloner received his MD and PhD degrees from Northwestern University, Chicago, IL, and is a member of Alpha Omega Alpha honor society. He completed internship and residency in internal medicine at Peter Bent Brigham Hospital in Boston, MA. Additional training included clinical and research fellowships in medicine and cardiology at Harvard Medical School, Boston, MA, and at Brigham and Women's Hospital, Boston, MA. He served as assistant and then associate professor of medicine at Harvard Medical School and as an attending cardiologist at Brigham and Women's Hospital. There he received an Established Investigator Award from the American Heart Association. Dr. Kloner is a fellow of the American College of Cardiology, an Inaugural Fellow of the Council on Basic Cardiovascular Sciences of the American Heart Association, and was elected to the American Society of Clinical Investigation.

Among Dr. Kloner's major research interests are cardiac cell transplantation, protection of ischemic myocardium, cardiac function following coronary artery occlusion, the effect of toxins on the heart, preventative cardiology, hypertension, and PDE5 inhibition. He is currently participating in studies funded by the National Institutes of Health (NIH) on cardiac cell transplantation, doxorubicin cardiomyopathy, functional analysis of cardiac grafts, and stem cells. He has served on the NIH Cardiovascular Study Section A and has participated in a number of NIH Workshops.

A frequent contributor to the medical and scientific literature, Dr. Kloner has contributed 463 original papers, 183 chapters or monographs, and 389 abstracts. Dr. Kloner is the author or editor of 17 medical texts, including: *Cardiovascular Trials Reviews, The Guide to Cardiology, Stunned Myocardium, Ischemic Preconditioning, VIAGRA, Heart Disease and Erectile Dysfunction,* and three novels: *The Beta Virus, Mind Cure,* and *The Deity Genes.*

Among his editorial responsibilities, Dr. Kloner serves as associate editor of the *Journal of Cardiovascular Pharmacology and Therapeutics* and is on the editorial boards of *Journal of the American College of Cardiology, Circulation, American Journal of Cardiology, American Journal of Geriatric Cardiology, Journal of Molecular and Cellular Cardiology, Heart, Heart Disease,* and *Basic Research in Cardiology.* Among his many career distinctions, Dr. Kloner has been listed in *Who's Who in America* and *The Best Doctors in America* and was recently identified by the Institute for Scientific Information on ISIHighlycited.com as one of the world's most frequently cited authors.

YOCHAI BIRNBAUM, MD

Yochai Birnbaum, MD, is a professor of medicine in the Cardiology Division at the University of Texas Medical Branch (UTMB), Galveston, TX. He is also the director of the Cardiac Intensive Care Unit and the Heart Station at UTMB Hospital.

Dr. Birnbaum received his MD degree from the Hadassah School of Medicine, the Hebrew University, Jerusalem, Israel. He completed internship in Hadassah Medical Center, Jerusalem, and residency in internal medicine at Kaplan Hospital in Rehovot, Israel. Additional training included clinical fellowship in cardiology at Rabin Medical Center, Petah-Tiqva, Israel, and research fellowships at the Heart Institute, Good Samaritan Hospital, and at Cedars Sinai Medical Center, Los Angeles, CA. He served as assistant and then associate professor of medicine at Sackler School of Medicine, Tel Aviv University, Israel, and as an attending cardiologist and director of the Cardiac Intensive Care Unit, Rabin Medical Center, Petah-Tiqva, Israel. In August 2001 he assumed the position of medical director of the Cardiac Intensive Care Unit in the Division of Cardiology at UTMB as an associate professor of medicine. In August 2002, Dr. Birnbaum assumed the position of medical director of the Heart Station. In September 2002 he was appointed professor of medicine. In 2004 Dr. Birnbaum was named the recipient of the Edward D. & Sally M. Futch Professorship in Cardiology at the University of Texas, Galveston. Dr. Birnbaum is a fellow of the American College of Cardiology.

Dr. Birnbaum's research interests are in both clinical and basic cardiology. His clinical studies are mainly related to electrocardiography in acute ischemia and echocardiography. His basic research interests include modulation of ischemia-reperfusion injury and ultrasound-assisted thrombolysis.

A frequent contributor to the medical and scientific press, Dr. Birnbaum has contributed over 150 original papers, seven chapters or monographs, and 82 abstracts.

Praise for the Eighth Edition

"As the number of cardiovascular clinical trials grows, so does the value of *Cardiovascular Trials Review*. Drs. Kloner and Birnbaum deserve the thanks of the entire cardiovascular community for this fine review. This new edition is remarkably up-to-date and includes important trials that have been presented but not yet published."
  Eugene Braunwald, MD
  Harvard Medical School, Boston, MA

"Once again, a Herculean effort has been completed that chronicles and organizes a dizzying number of cardiovascular clinical trials. The ease of navigation and the succinct summaries make this truly one of the most resourceful guides for the busy clinician's bookshelf. Kudos to Dr. Kloner!"
  Clyde W. Yancy, MD
  University of Texas Southwestern Medical Center, Dallas, TX

"In my presidential address at the 2003 ACC Annual Scientific sessions, I used data from each edition of *Cardiovascular Trials Review* published from 1996–2002 to demonstrate the phenomenal growth of clinical trials in recent years. It is a challenge to remember the key findings of a small fraction of the nearly 200 new trials reported every year. This is where *Clinical Trials Review* can help busy clinicians and academics who need concise and up-to-date summaries of clinical trials that are helping us provide better care to patients with cardiovascular disease."
  W. Bruce Fye, M.D
  Mayo Clinic College of Medicine, Rochester, MN

"Well-organized, concise, timely resource for the clinician and the clinical investigator."
  Nanette K. Wenger, MD
  Emory University School of Medicine, Grady Memorial Hospital, Atlanta, GA

"I am impressed with the timeliness of the many trials. The editors have done a superb job of putting this into such an easy format… I find the descriptions to be accurate, compact, and right to the point."
  Gary S. Francis, MD
  The Ohio State University, Cleveland Clinic Foundation Medical Center, Cleveland, OH